ACUTE CARE
ONCOLOGY
NURSING

Second Edition

ACUTE CARE ONCOLOGY NURSING

Cynthia C. Chernecky, PhD, RN, CNS, AOCN®, FAAN
Professor
Department of Physiological & Technological
Nursing
Medical College of Georgia
School of Nursing
Augusta, Georgia

Kathleen Murphy-Ende, RN, PhD, AOCNP®
Palliative Care and Pain Nurse Practitioner
Clinical Assistant Professor
University of Wisconsin Hospital and Clinics
University of Wisconsin
School of Nursing
Madison, Wisconsin

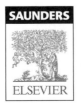

SAUNDERS

ELSEVIER

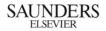

SAUNDERS
ELSEVIER

11830 Westline Industrial Drive
St. Louis, Missouri 63146

Notice

Knowledge and best practice in this field are constantly changing. As new research and experience broaden our knowledge, changes in practice, treatment, and drug therapy may become necessary or appropriate. Readers are advised to check the most current information provided (i) on procedures featured or (ii) by the manufacturer of each product to be administered, to verify the recommended dose or formula, the method and duration of administration, and contraindications. It is the responsibility of practitioners, relying on their own experience and knowledge of the patient, to make diagnoses, to determine dosages and the best treatment for each individual patient, and to take all appropriate safety precautions. To the fullest extent of the law, neither the Publisher nor the Authors assumes any liability for any injury and/or damage to persons or property arising out of or related to any use of the material contained in this book.

The Publisher

Previous edition copyrighted 1998
International Standard Book Number 978-1-4160-3734-7

Senior Acquisitions Editor: Sandra E. Clark
Senior Developmental Editor: Cindi Anderson
Publishing Services Manager: John Rogers
Project Manager: Helen Hudlin
Design Direction: Julia Dummitt

Working together to grow libraries in developing countries

www.elsevier.com | www.bookaid.org | www.sabre.org

ELSEVIER   BOOK AID International   Sabre Foundation

Printed in the United States of America

Last digit is the print number: 9   8   7   6   5   4   3   2   1

Michael I. Agugo, BSc, BSN
Registered Nurse
The Sydney Kimmel Comprehensive
    Cancer Center
Johns Hopkins Hospital
Baltimore, Maryland
Chapter 30. Hypomagnesemia

Lyle Stuart Baker, Jr., BSN, RN
Nurse Clinician III
The Sidney Kimmel Comprehensive
    Cancer Center
Johns Hopkins Hospital
Baltimore, Maryland
Chapter 30. Hypomagnesemia

Cynthia Brown, MS, AOCNP®,
    ACHPN, APRN-BC
Hospice Nurse Practitioner
Life Path Hospital and Palliative Care
Tampa, Florida
Chapter 13. End-of-Life Care

Lori Ann Brown, RN, BSN, CCRN
Critical Care Nurse
University Hospital
Augusta, Georgia
Chapter 14. Esophageal Varices

Patricia C. Buchsel, RN, MSN, FAAN
Clinical Instructor
Seattle University College of Nursing
Seattle, Washington
Chapter 42. Sinusoid Occlusive Syndrome

Jill K. Burleson, MSN, ANP-C
Adult Nurse Practitioner
Duke University Hospitals
Durham, North Carolina
Chapter 18. Graft Versus Host Disease

Nancy Jo Bush, RN, MN, MA, AOCN®
Oncology Nurse Practitioner
Premiere Oncology
Santa Monica, California
Assistant Clinical Professor
University of California Los Angeles
    School of Nursing
Los Angeles, California
Chapter 7. Cognitive Dysfunction,
Chapter 8. Depression and Anxiety

Kristin Casey, RN, MS, CPNP, CPON
Pediatric Nurse Practitioner
University of Wisconsin Children's
    Hospital
Madison, Wisconsin
Chapter 25. Hyperleukocytosis in
Childhood Leukemia

Cynthia C. Chernecky, PhD, RN, CNS,
    AOCN®, FAAN
Professor
Department of Physiological &
    Technological Nursing
Medical College of Georgia
School of Nursing
Augusta, Georgia
Chapter 12. Dyspnea and Airway
Obstruction, Chapter 20. Hemorrhage
Secondary to Cervical Cancer, Chapter 31.
Hyponatremia, Chapter 37. Pathologic
Fractures, Chapter 39. Pulmonary Fibrosis

Brenda K. Cobb, PhD, RN
Adjunct Associate Professor
Department of Health Environments
    and System
Medical College of Georgia
School of Nursing
Augusta, Georgia
*Chapter 20. Hemorrhage Secondary to
Cervical Cancer*

Diane G. Cope, PhD, ARNP, BC,A
Nurse Practitioner
Florida Cancer Specialists
Fort Meyers, Florida
Chapter 38. Pleural Effusions: Malignant

Angela L. Daniel, MSN, MBA, RN
Medical College of Georgia
Augusta, Georgia
*Chapter 16. Fever, Chapter 31.
Hyponatremia*

Jean Ellsworth-Wolk, RN, MS, AOCN®
Oncology Clinical Nurse Specialist
Cancer Wellness Program Coordinator
The Cleveland Clinic Cancer Center at
    Fairview Hospital
Cleveland, Ohio
Chapter 1. Acute Pancreatitis

Cathy Fortenbaugh, RN, MSN, AOCN®
Clinical Nurse Specialist
AIM Higher Program Coordinator
Pennsylvania Oncology Hematology
    Associates
Philadelphia, Pennsylvania
Chapter 21. Hemorrhagic Cystitis

Jacqueline R. Gannuscio, MSN, ACNP
Nurse Practitioner
Heart Failure Program
Veterans Administration Medical Center
Washington, District of Columbia
Chapter 19. Heart Failure

Carol D. Gaskamp, PhD, RN, CNE
Assistant Professor of Clinical Nursing
School of Nursing
University of Texas at Austin
Austin, Texas
*Chapter 44. Spiritual Distress in People
with Cancer*

Marcia Grant, RN, DNSc, FAAN
Director and Professor
Nursing Research and Education
City of Hope Cancer Center
Duarte, California
Chapter 35. Malnutrition and Cachexia

**Jeanne Held-Warmkessel, MSN, RN,
    AOCN®, APRN, BC**
Clinical Nurse Specialist
Fox Chase Cancer Center
Philadelphia, Pennsylvania
*Chapter 47. Syndrome of Inappropriate
Antidiuretic Hormone*

Demica N. Jackson, MSN, RN
Medical College of Georgia
Augusta, Georgia
Chapter 31. Hyponatremia

Nancy Kelly, RN, MSN, CNS, AOCNS®
Clinical Nurse Specialist
Hillcrest Hospital: A Cleveland Clinic
    Hospital
Mayfield Heights, Ohio
Chapter 46. Superior Vena Cava Syndrome

Kathy G. Kravits, RN, MA
Senior Research Specialist
City of Hope Cancer Center
Duarte, California
Chapter 35. Malnutrition and Cachexia

Teresa Kuntzsch, RN, BSN
Chemotherapy Services Manager
University of Wisconsin Hospitals and
 Clinics
Madison, Wisconsin
Chapter 27. Hypersensitivity Reactions to
Chemotherapy

Molly Loney, RN, MSN, CNS, AOCNS®
Oncology Clinical Nurse Specialist
Hillcrest Hospital: A Cleveland Clinic
 Hospital
Mayfield Heights, Ohio
Chapter 46. Superior Vena Cava Syndrome

Mary P. Lovely, PhD, RN
Assistant Adjunct Professor
University of California San Francisco;
Consultant
National Brain Tumor Foundation
San Francisco, California
Chapter 40. Seizures

Mary Pat Lynch, MSN, CRNP, AOCN®
Cancer Center Administrator
Joan Karnell Cancer Center at
 Pennsylvania Hospital
University of Pennsylvania Health
 System
Philadelphia, Pennsylvania
Chapter 24. Hyperkalemia, Chapter 29.
Hypokalemia

Yvonne D. Martin, MSN, RN, OCN®
Nurse Retention and Community
 Outreach Coordinator
Medical University of South Carolina
Charleston, South Carolina
Chapter 4. Bronchiolitis Obliterans

Martha Meraviglia, RN, CNS, PhD
Assistant Professor of Clinical Nursing
School of Nursing
The University of Texas at Austin
Austin, Texas
Chapter 44. Spiritual Distress in People
with Cancer

Christine Miaskowski, RN, PhD, FAAN
Professor
Department of Physiological Nursing
University of California San Francisco
San Francisco, California
Chapter 36. Pain Management:
Nociceptive and Neuropathic; Chapter 43.
Spinal Cord Compression

Laura Milligan, RN, MSN, FNP,BC,
 AOCN®
Nurse Practitioner
Medical University of South Carolina
Charleston, South Carolina
Chapter 4. Bronchiolitis Obliterans

Libby Montoya, MSN, APRN,BC
Clinical Nurse Specialist
Leukemia, Lymphoma, Hematology
 Services
St. Jude Children's Research Hospital
Memphis, Tennessee
Chapter 12. Dyspnea and Airway
Obstruction, Chapter 28. Hyperuricemia

Deborah Murphy, MSN, RN, CCRN,
 CMSRC, CLNC
Clinical Nurse Educator
Paoli Hospital
Paoli, Pennsylvania
Chapter 3. Malignant Ascites

Kathleen Murphy-Ende, RN, PhD, AOCN®
Palliative Care and Pain Nurse Practitioner
Clinical Assistant Professor
University of Wisconsin Hospital and Clinics
University of Wisconsin School of Nursing
Madison, Wisconsin
Chapter 13. End-of-Life Care; Chapter 17. Gastrointestinal Obstruction: Biliary, Gastric, and Bowel Obstructions; Chapter 22. Hepatic Encephalopathy; Chapter 45. Suicidal Ideation

Kaci L. Osenga, MD
University of Wisconsin Children's Hospital
Madison Wisconsin
Chapter 49. Typhlitis in Pediatrics

Kathryn E. Pearson, RN, CNS, AOCN®
Oncology Clinical Nurse Specialist
St. Jude Medical Center
Virginia K. Crosson Cancer Center
Fullerton, California
Chapter 23. Tumor-Induced Hypercalcemia

Kara L. Penne, RN, MSN, ANP, AOCNP®
Adult Nurse Practitioner
Hematology-Oncology
Duke University Medical Center
Durham, North Carolina
Chapter 32. Increased Intracranial Pressure

Marlene M. Rosenkoetter, PhD, RN, FAAN
Professor
Medical College of Georgia
Augusta, Georgia
Chapter 15. Ethics in Adult Oncology and Critical Care Nursing

Catherine Sargent, MS, RN,C, AOCN®
Oncology Clinical Nurse Specialist/ Educator
Bryn Mawr Hospital
Bryn Mawr, Pennsylvania
Chapter 6. Carotid Artery Rupture; Chapter 33. Lactic Acidosis, Type B

Dionne T. Savage, RN, BSN
Oncology Nursing Coordinator
The Sidney Kimmel Comprehensive Cancer Center
Johns Hopkins Hospital
Baltimore, Maryland
Chapter 34. Lambert-Eaton Myasthenic Syndrome

Kathy A. Shane, RN, BSN
Oncology Shift Coordinator
Johns Hopkins Hospital
Baltimore, Maryland
Chapter 41. Sepsis and Septic Shock

Brenda K. Shelton, MSN, RN, CCRN, AOCN®
Clinical Nurse Specialist
The Sidney Kimmel Comprehensive Cancer Center
Johns Hopkins Hospital
Baltimore, Maryland
Chapter 5. Cardiac Tamponade and Pericardial Effusions, Chapter 11. Disseminated Intravascular Coagulation (DIC), Chapter 30. Hypomagnesemia, Chapter 48. Tumor Lysis Syndrome

Mady Stovall, RN, MSN, NP
Neuro-Oncology Nurse Practitioner
University of California Los Angeles
Los Angeles, California
Chapter 26. Hypernatremia

Rebecca R. Sutter, RN, MN, DDiv(h)
Assistant Professor of Clinical Nursing
    (Retired)
School of Nursing
University of Texas at Austin
Austin, Texas
*Chapter 44. Spiritual Distress in People
with Cancer*

**Jennifer U. Varma, MSN, APRN-BC,
    NP-C**
Nurse Practitioner
Division of Neurosurgery
University of California Los Angeles
David Geffen School of Medicine
Los Angeles, California
Chapter 9. Diabetes Insipidus

Cassie A. Voge, RN, MS, AOCN®
Clinical Assistant Professor
University of Wisconsin—Madison
    School of Nursing
Madison, Wisconsin
*Chapter 27. Hypersensitivity Reactions to
Chemotherapy*

Kathleen R. Wren, CRNA, PhD
Acting Associate Dean
Louisiana State University Health
    Sciences Center
New Orleans, Louisiana
Chapter 10. Diabetes Mellitus

Timothy L. Wren, RN, DNP
Assistant Professor of Adult Nursing
Louisiana State University Health
    Sciences Center
New Orleans, Louisiana
Chapter 10. Diabetes Mellitus

Mercedes K. Young, MSN, NP
Nurse Practitioner
Division of Hematology
Keck School of Medicine
University of Southern California
Los Angeles, California
*Chapter 2. Acute Respiratory Distress
Syndrome*

Carolyn Becker, MSN, APN, AOCN®
Advanced Practice Nurse
The Rocky Mountain Blood and
    Marrow Transplant Program
Rocky Mountain Cancer Center
Denver, Colorado

Audrey G. Gift, PhD, RN, FAAN
Professor
College of Nursing
Michigan State University
East Lansing, Michigan

Daniel Mulkerin, MD
Assistant Professor
Department of Medicine
University of Wisconsin
Madison, Wisconsin

Bari K. Platter, MS, RN, CS
Clnical Nurse Specialist/Educator
Department of Psychiatric Services
University of Colorado Hospital
Denver, Colorado

Lisa N. Sherven, RN, BSN, CHPN
Manager of Admissions and Clinical
    Outreach
HospiceCare, Inc.
Madison, Wisconsin

**Janet H. Van Cleave, MSN, AOCNP,
    ACNP-CS**
Acute Care Nurse Practitioner
Division of Medical Oncology
The Mt. Sinai Medical Center of New
    York City
New York, New York

The specialty of oncology, within the acute or critical care setting, is a reality in the practice of cancer nurses. The vast amount of knowledge required to give compassionate and effective care can be overwhelming. This book is an attempt to provide clinical expertise condensed into a useful format for professional nurses. The content includes the physiological, psychological, spiritual, social, and ethical realms of care. Each chapter includes pathophysiology, risk profile, diagnoses, treatment approaches, patient/family education, anticipatory guidance for home care, and research findings applicable to clinical practice. This book is a resource to guide nurses in implementing care in an efficient manner for the goal of cure, comfort, palliation, and the best possible quality of life. An understanding of complex problems is necessary in order for nurses to provide detailed patient care. Professional nurses are expected to apply knowledge to practice and are accountable for proper assessment, treatment, and evaluation of care. This book is our combined effort to contribute to nursing because we care about patients, family, significant others, society, and humanity, as well as the future of nursing practice. The result is a reference that provides needed information to work collaboratively with health care providers, patients, family members and significant others.

Cynthia C. Chernecky
Kathleen Murphy-Ende

The following is a list of body systems and the primary oncologic complications that affect each. Each primary oncologic complication listed corresponds to a chapter title, where the reader can find necessary information helpful in caring for a client experiencing the complication or body system alteration. The reader is advised that four chapters, "Depression and Anxiety," "End-of-Life Care," "Ethics in Adult Oncology and Critical Care Nursing," and "Spiritual Distress in People with Cancer" provide valuable assistance when working with clients experiencing any type or location of cancer throughout the continuum of care.

CARDIOVASCULAR
Cardiac tamponade and pericardial effusions
Cognitive dysfunction
Carotid artery rupture
Disseminated intravascular coagulation
Heart failure
Hemorrhage secondary to cervical cancer
Hypercalcemia, tumor induced
Hyperkalemia
Hypernatremia
Hypersensitivity reactions to chemotherapy
Hypokalemia
Malignant ascites
Pulmonary fibrosis
Sepsis and septic shock
Spinal cord compression
Superior vena cava syndrome
Syndrome of inappropriate antidiuretic hormone secretion
Tumor lysis syndrome

ENDOCRINE
Acute pancreatitis
Diabetes insipidus
Diabetes mellitus
Fever
Syndrome of inappropriate antidiuretic hormone secretion

FLUID AND ELECTROLYTE BALANCE/ HEMODYNAMICS
Acute respiratory distress syndrome
Bronchiolitis obliterans

Cardiac tamponade and pericardial effusions
Carotid artery rupture
Cognitive dysfunction
Diabetes insipidus
Diabetes mellitus
Disseminated intravascular coagulation
Esophageal varices
Fever
Gastrointestinal obstruction
Graft versus host disease
Heart failure
Hemorrhage secondary to cervical cancer
Hemorrhagic cystitis
Hypercalcemia, tumor induced
Hyperkalemia
Hypernatremia
Hypersensitivity reactions to chemotherapy
Hypokalemia
Hypomagnesemia
Hyponatremia
Increased intracranial pressure
Lactic acidosis, type B
Malignant ascites
Malnutrition and cachexia
Pain management: nociceptive and neuropathic
Pathologic fractures
Pulmonary fibrosis
Seizures
Sepsis and septic shock
Sinusoid occlusive syndrome
Spinal cord compression
Superior vena cava syndrome

The following is a list of locations in the body that may be involved in cancer. Primary complications that may be caused by cancer in that area of the body are listed under each disease site. Each primary complication corresponds to a chapter title, where the reader can find necessary information helpful in caring for a client experiencing the complication. The reader is advised that four chapters, "Depression and Anxiety," "End-of-Life Care," "Ethics in Adult Oncology and Critical Care Nursing," and "Spiritual Distress in People with Cancer" provide valuable assistance when working with clients experiencing any type or location of cancer throughout the continuum of care.

ADRENAL GLAND
Hypernatremia
Hyponatremia

BLADDER/KIDNEY
Fever
Hemorrhagic cystitis
Hypercalcemia, tumor induced
Hyperkalemia
Hypernatremia
Hypokalemia
Lambert-Eaton myasthenic syndrome
Malnutrition and cachexia
Pain management: nociceptive and
 neuropathic
Pathologic fractures
Sinusoid occlusive syndrome
Spinal cord compression
Syndrome of inappropriate antidiuretic
 hormone secretion

BREAST
Acute respiratory distress syndrome
Cardiac tamponade and pericardial
 effusions
Cognitive dysfunction
Diabetes insipidus
Disseminated intravascular coagulation
Hepatic encephalopathy
Hypersensitivity reactions to
 chemotherapy
Hypercalcemia, tumor induced
Lactic acidosis, type B
Lambert-Eaton myasthenic syndrome
Malignant ascites

Pain management: nociceptive and
 neuropathic
Pathologic fractures
Pleural effusion
Seizures
Sinusoid occlusive syndrome
Spinal cord compression
Suicidal ideation
Superior vena cava syndrome
Tumor lysis syndrome
Typhlitis in pediatrics

CENTRAL NERVOUS SYSTEM
Cognitive dysfunction
Diabetes insipidus
Diabetes mellitus
Hyponatremia
Increased intracranial pressure
Pain management: nociceptive and
 neuropathic
Pulmonary fibrosis
Seizures
Spinal cord compression
Suicidal ideation
Superior vena cava syndrome
Syndrome of inappropriate antidiuretic
 hormone secretion

CERVIX/UTERINE
Hemorrhagic cystitis
Hemorrhage secondary to cervical cancer
Malignant ascites
Pain management: nociceptive and
 neuropathic
Suicidal ideation

ACUTE CARE
ONCOLOGY
NURSING

ACUTE PANCREATITIS

JEAN ELLSWORTH-WOLK

PATHOPHYSIOLOGICAL MECHANISMS

Acute pancreatitis is an inflammatory process of the pancreas that is caused by the premature activation of pancreatic enzymes. These enzymes are normally secreted in an inactive form for the digestion of fats, carbohydrates, and proteins. The origin of this premature activation can be multifactorial; the cause remains unclear, but obstruction or trauma of the ampulla of Vater of the common bile duct, chronic alcoholism, viral sources, and toxicity caused by other agents have been proposed as causative events. In acute pancreatitis, autodigestion of the pancreatic tissue by proteolytic enzymes (trypsinogen, chymotrypsinogen, proelastase, and phospholipase A) occurs when enzymes are activated in the pancreas rather than in the intestinal lumen (Greenberger & Toskes, 2005). Depending on the degree and extent of pancreatic inflammatory involvement or necrosis, the intensity of disease ranges from mild to severe. Two types of acute pancreatitis can be distinguished morphologically: edematous, or interstitial pancreatitis, and necrotizing pancreatitis (Friedman, 2005; Greenberger & Toskes, 2005).

Edematous or interstitial acute pancreatitis is characterized by interstitial edema, engorgement of capillaries, and dilation of lymphatic vessels. Necrotizing pancreatitis is characterized by pancreatic cell death and may initiate an inflammatory response that extends beyond the pancreas. Surrounding blood vessels may rupture, or the exudate of peritoneal fluid may sequester and become infected, leading to tissue necrosis, peritonitis, shock, and death. Distinction between the two morphologic types is essential for predicting the severity of the course of disease, as well as the outcome. Factors responsible for the transformation of edematous pancreatitis to the necrotizing form are largely unknown (Friedman, 2005; Greenberger & Toskes, 2005).

The pathophysiology of severe pancreatitis can be traced to the extravasation of pancreatic enzymes. These toxic proteolytic enzymes cause widespread chemical inflammation of tissue. As a result, considerable loss and sequestration of protein-rich fluid from the vascular space occurs, leading to hypovolemia, hypotension, and systemic hypoperfusion. Systemic inflammatory response syndrome (SIRS) can occur with the release of systemic inflammatory mediators as a result of pancreatic injury (Greenberger & Toskes, 2005).

Multisystem complications of acute pancreatitis involve almost every organ system and significantly affect the morbidity and mortality associated with this disease. These complications can occur early in the course of the disease or as late as 2 weeks after resolution of the acute phase. The causes of these complications range from enzyme impairment of pancreatic function to pancreatic tissue necrosis (Table 1-1).

Differential diagnosis can be difficult, so it is necessary for the clinician to look at the total picture of physical symptoms, laboratory data, and radiologic tests. The goals of treatment are to rest the pancreas, relieve pain, and maintain intravascular fluid volume.

Table 1-1	COMPLICATIONS OF ACUTE PANCREATITIS	
Complications	**Physiologic Mechanism**	**Symptoms**
Cardiovascular		
Hypotension*	Increased vascular permeability from cytokine release	BP <80/60, dizziness
Central Nervous System		
Encephalopathy	Liver malfunction	Confusion, altered mental status, agitation
Gastrointestinal		
Bleeding	Gastritis, peptic ulcer, Mallory-Weiss tear, pseudocyst rupture or esophageal varices, concomitant liver disease or splenic/portal vein thrombosis	Positive hemoccult, hematemesis, abdominal pain, low Hb/Hct, postural hypotension
Hematologic		
Thrombosis	Vascular stasis	Lower leg pain, erythema,
Coagulation abnormalities	Cytokine release from pancreatic cell death	tenderness, swelling, bruising, petechiae, increased PT and PTT, bleeding from orifices
Metabolic		
Hyperglycemia	Pancreatic malfunction	Anxiety, alteration in mental
Metabolic acidosis	Cytokine release/cell death	status, diaphoresis,
Hypocalcemia	Low parathyroid hormone	fatigue, leg cramps,
Hypomagnesemia*	secretion	nausea and vomiting,
Hypokalemia	Loss of GI secretions through vomiting	polydipsia, polyuria, tetany ($\downarrow$Ca)
Pseudocyst		
	Collection of fluid, tissue, debris, and pancreatic enzymes, caused by blockage, may become infected and develop into abscess	Fever (if abscess), palpable tender LUQ abdomen, abdominal pain
Pulmonary		
Hypoxemia	Cytokine release from	Dyspnea, tachypnea, low
Atelectasis	pancreatic cell death, which	PO_2 levels
Pleural effusion	results in vasodilation,	
Acute respiratory syndrome*	increased vascular permeability, and edema Hypervolemic from fluid replacement (low BP)	
Renal Problems		
Prerenal failure	Intravascular volume depletion	Azotemia, increased BUN/Cr
Acute tubular necrosis	secondary to leakage of fluids in the pancreatic bed	
Septic		
Pancreatic abscess	Infection occurs with	Fever, leukocytosis, shock,
Infected pseudocyst	pancreatic necrosis	organ failure, LUQ
Peritonitis		abdominal pain, elevated C-reactive protein

*Common complications.

BP, Blood pressure; *BUN*, blood urea nitrogen; *Cr*, creatinine; *Hb*, hemoglobin; Hct, hematocrit; *LUQ*, left upper quadrant; *PT*, prothrombin time; *PTT*, partial thromboplastin time.

Management of secondary complications varies according to the organ system involved. The nurse's role is to provide supportive care and to assess for signs and symptoms of complications (see Table 1-1).

EPIDEMIOLOGY AND ETIOLOGY

The annual incidence of acute pancreatitis in the general population is 5 to 10 people per 100,000; thus, the disorder is relatively common (Turner, 2003) and its occurrence has been increasing. Between 1960 and 1980, the incidence of acute pancreatitis has increased 10-fold (Munoz & Katerndahl, 2006). Up to 25% of patients who develop acute pancreatitis have severe or life-threatening complications (Hale, Moseley, & Warner, 2000); within this percentage, between 2% and 10% of events can be fatal (Munoz & Katerndahl, 2006; Despins, 2005). Necrotizing pancreatitis contributes to the occurrence of acute pancreatitis in 3% to 5% of all patients in whom the condition has been diagnosed; a mortality rate of 50% has been reported (Greenberger & Toskes, 2005). The two major causative factors known to be responsible for acute pancreatitis are intake of alcohol and cholelithiasis. Pancreatitis in the oncology patient is likely to be caused by these same factors, but it also can result from direct tumor infiltration into the gland, metastasis to regional lymph nodes producing ductal obstruction, the complication of tumor lysis syndrome, a presenting manifestation of immunoblastic lymphoma, or complications resulting from medical or surgical therapy (Greenberger & Toskes, 2005; Yahanda & Chang, 2005; Yeo et al., 2005; Sinicrope & Levin, 2000). Other causes of pancreatitis include toxins, biliary obstruction, drugs (Box 1-1), hyperparathyroidism, hyperlipidemia, infection, trauma, ischemia, transplant, vasculitis, and autoimmune disorders (Friedman, 2005; Greenberger & Toskes, 2005).

BOX 1-1	**DRUGS ASSOCIATED WITH ACUTE PANCREATITIS**	
Acetaminophen	Furosemide	Phenolphthalein
Amphetamines	Histamine	Procainamide
Azathioprine*	Hydrochlorothiazide	Propoxyphene
Calcium	Indomethacin	Rifampin
Chlorthalidone	Lipids	Salicylates
Cholestyramine	Manganese	Stibogluconate sodium
Cimetidine	Mefenamic acid	Sulfa antibiotics*
Clonidine	Methyldopa	Sulindac
Corticosteroids*	Nitrofurantoin	Tetracycline*
Diazoxide	Opiates	Thiazides*
Enalapril	Pentamidine*	Valproic acid*
Ethacrynic acid	Phenformin	Vitamin D

*Common causes.
Data from Friedman, L. S. (2005). Liver, biliary tract and pancreas. In L. Tierney, S. J. McPhee, & M. A. Papaealis, et al. (Eds.), *Current medical diagnosis and treatment* (pp. 671-674). (44th ed.). New York: Lange Medical Books/ McGraw-Hill; Greenberger, N., & Toskes, P. (2005). Acute and chronic pancreatitis. In D. Kasper, E. Braunwald, & A. Fauci, et al. (Eds.), *Harrison's principles of internal medicine* (pp 1895-1902). (16th ed.). New York: McGraw Hill Medical Publishing Division; Sekimoto, M., Takada, T., & Kawarada, Y., et al. (2006). JPH guidelines for the management of acute pancreatitis: Epidemiology, etiology, natural history, and outcome predictors in acute pancreatitis. *Journal of Hepatobiliary and Pancreatic Surgery 13*:10-24.

RISK PROFILE

Obstruction of the pancreatic ducts: Cholelithiasis caused by gallstones is the most common cause. Other causes of pancreatic duct obstruction include sphincter of Oddi stenosis, impaction of a stone at the ampulla, and occasionally microlithiasis or biliary sludge. In the oncology patient, primary adenocarcinoma of the pancreas is seldom a cause; however, metastases may cause obstruction, and this event is seen in cases of renal cell carcinoma, melanoma, and cancer of the prostate, breast, and lung (Yahanda & Chang, 2005; Yeo et al., 2005).

Alcohol consumption and abuse: The amount of daily consumed alcohol that is estimated to cause pancreatitis is 50 to 150 g (50 g is equivalent to four 12-oz servings of beer with 3% to 5% alcohol content). The average onset of alcohol-related pancreatitis occurs after 4 to 7 years of drinking (Munoz & Katerndahl, 2000).

Chemotherapy and biotherapy: L-asparaginase produces the highest incidence, reportedly with rates as high as 16% (Yahando & Chang, 2005), but numerous chemotherapy and biotherapy agents may be causative (Box 1-2).

Medications: See Box 1-1.

Manipulation of ampulla of Vater/pancreas: Endoscopic retrograde cholangiopancreatography (ERCP), pancreatectomy, splenectomy, trauma, and placement of intrahepatic catheter (Friedman, 2005; Greenberger & Toskes, 2005).

Metabolic abnormalities: Tumor lysis syndrome (TLS), hyperlipidemia, hyperparathyroidism, hypercalcemia, and end-stage renal disease (Friedman, 2005; Yeo et al., 2005; Sinicrope & Levin, 2000).

Infection: Parasitic infection, adenoviruses, mumps, coxsackieviruses, *Staphylococcus*, scarlet fever, hepatitis B, *Campylobacter, Mycoplasma,* rubella, Epstein-Barr virus, cytomegalovirus, and human immunodeficiency virus (HIV) (Sekimoto et al., 2006; Friedman, 2005; Greenberger & Toskes, 2005).

Dietary: High-fat diet (leading to cholelithiasis) and long-term hyperalimentation (biliary sludge) (Sekimoto et al., 2006; Greenberger & Toskes, 2005; Turner, 2003).

Vascular problems: Ischemia, systemic lupus erythematosus and shock states (Friedman, 2005).

Miscellaneous: Post bone marrow transplant, graft-versus-host disease, ectopic pregnancy, pregnancy, ovarian cyst, hypothermia, hereditary pancreatitis, scorpion venom, perforated peptic ulcer, Crohn's disease, and Reye's syndrome (Sekimoto et al., 2006; Friedman, 2005; Greenberger & Toskes, 2005; Yahanda & Chang, 2005; Yeo et al., 2005).

PROGNOSIS

The prognosis is determined through assessment of morphologic involvement, which may be seen as edematous interstitial pancreatitis or necrotizing fulminant pancreatitis. The mechanism of action that determines which form will predominate remains unclear. The edematous interstitial form is usually a mild case that is self-limiting. In 5% to 15%

BOX 1-2	CHEMOTHERAPY/BIOTHERAPY CAUSES OF ACUTE PANCREATITIS

Azathioprine
Bleomycin
Cisplatin
Cyclophosphamide
Cytosine arabinoside
Didanosine
Doxorubicin
Estrogens
5-Fluorouracil

Ifosfamide
Interleukin-2
L-asparaginase
6-mercaptopurine
Methotrexate
Mitomycin-C
Prednisone
Vinblastine
Vincristine

Data from Greenberger, N., & Toskes, P. (2005). Acute and chronic pancreatitis. In D. Kasper, E. Braunwald, & A. Fauci, et al. (Eds.), *Harrison's principles of internal medicine* (pp. 1895-1902). (16th ed.). New York: McGraw Hill Medical Publishing Division; Polovich, M., White, J., & Kelleher, L. (2005). *Chemotherapy and biotherapy guidelines and recommendations for practice.* (2nd ed.). Pittsburgh: ONS Press; Sinicrope, F. A., & Levin, B. (2000). Complications of cancer and its treatment: Gastrointestinal complications. In R. Bast, D. Kufe, & R. Polock, et al. (Eds.), *Cancer medicine* (pp. 1035-1040). (5th ed.). Hamilton, Ontario, Canada: B.C. Decker, Inc.; Yahanda, A. M., & Chang, A. E. (2005). Acute abdomen, bowel obstruction and fistula. In M. Abeloff, J. Armitage, & J. Neiderhuber, et al. (Eds.), *Clinical oncology* (pp. 1030-1031) St. Louis: Elsevier; Yeo, C., Yeo, T., & Hrubcin, R., et al. (2005). Cancer of the pancreas. In V. T. Devita Jr., S. Hellman, & S. A. Rosenberg (Eds.), *Cancer: Principles and practice of oncology* (pp. 1409-1415). (6th ed.). Baltimore: Lippincott Williams & Wilkins.

of all cases, the disease takes the fulminant course (Munoz & Katerndahl, 2006; Despins, 2005). Prognosis can be predicted by the morphologic type and the presence of the following systemic complications:

- Cardiovascular (systolic blood pressure [SBP] less than 80 mm Hg for at least 15 minutes)
- Respiratory (pO_2 less than 60 mm Hg, requiring O_2 longer than 24 hours)
- Renal (serum creatinine greater than 1.4 mg% during hospitalization)
- Sepsislike picture (temperature over 39° C, white blood cell count [WBC] greater than 20,000/mm^3)

With these clinical indicators, a reliable severity of illness scale specific to acute pancreatitis, called Ranson's scale, can be used to predict mortality. A newer and simplified version called the Glasgow (Imrie) criteria is also available for use (Box 1-3) (Sekimoto et al., 2006; Friedman, 2005; Wrobleski, Barth, & Oyen,1999). Within the oncology population, the mortality rate associated with L-asparaginase–induced pancreatitis is 12% (Yahnada & Chang, 2005).

1. **Epigastric pain:** Sudden onset; described as severe, dull or gnawing, knifelike, twisting, and relentless. Walking or lying supine, eating a fatty meal, or drinking alcohol can increase the pain; assuming a sitting or fetal position can ease it. Pain may radiate to either costal margin or may be referred to the lower back.
2. **Nausea and projectile vomiting:** Decreased or absent bowel sounds with distended abdomen, abdominal guarding, and rebound tenderness.

BOX 1-3	SIMPLIFIED GLASGOW (IMRIE) CRITIERIA FOR SEVERITY OF PANCREATITIS

Age over 55 years
Serum white blood cell count greater than 15,000
Glucose greater than 180 mg/dL
Blood urea nitrogen increase greater than 45 mg/dL
PaO_2 less than 60 mm Hg
Albumin less than 3.2 g/dL
Calcium less than 8 mg/dL
Serum lactic dehydrogenase greater than 600 International Units/L

Prognostic Scale (96% accuracy)
Fewer than 3 signs: 1% mortality rate
3-4 signs: 16% mortality rate
5-6 signs: 40% mortality rate
More than 6 signs: 100% mortality rate

PaO_2, Partial pressure of oxygen in arterial blood.
Modified from Wrobleski, D., Barth, M., & Oyen, L. (1999). Necrotizing pancreatitis: Pathophysiology, diagnosis, and acute care management. *AACN Clinical Issues, 10,* 469.

3. **History:** High alcohol consumption, recent alcoholic binge; cholelithiasis, pancreatic manipulation; chemotherapy (Table 1-2), especially L-asparaginase; fever, low grade or higher; diaphoresis; tachycardia; hypotension; tachypnea; anxiety.
4. **Diagnostic Tests:** Plain x-ray film of the abdomen with distended loops of bowel with paralytic ileus over the pancreatic region; chest x-ray film shows pulmonary edema; ERCP abnormalities of the pancreatic duct with obstruction; abdominal computed tomography (CT) scan featuring enlarged indistinct margins of the pancreas, fluid accumulations, and alterations in enhancement patterns.
5. **Laboratory values:** Elevated serum amylase (initially and then normalizes), elevated urine amylase, elevated serum lipase, elevated serum triglycerides, elevated glucose, low calcium, low magnesium, low or high potassium, low albumin, elevated white blood cell count, low hemoglobin and hematocrit, elevated serum creatinine (greater than 1.5 mg), possibly high bilirubin and liver enzymes, prolonged prothrombin time, arterial blood gas (ABG) with hypoxemia, metabolic acidosis, and elevated C-reactive protein.
6. Bruising around the umbilicus (Cullen's sign) and bruising around the loin area (Grey Turner's sign).
7. Ultrasound of abdomen (gallstones).

NURSING CARE AND TREATMENT

Vital signs: Assess for fever, tachycardia, tachypnea, and hypotension.

Pain assessment: Assess for duration (sudden onset), location (epigastric), intensity (scale of 0 to 10; severe, unrelenting), quality (dull, knifelike, twisting), associated factors (radiation to flanks, back), relieving factors (sitting or fetal position), and exacerbating factors (walking or supine position, eating).

Table 1-2 LABORATORY VALUES ASSOCIATED WITH ACUTE PANCREATITIS	
Laboratory Values	**Findings**
ABGs	Hypoxemia, metabolic acidosis
Albumin	Low
Alkaline phosphatase	May be high
Amylase, serum	Initially high (3 × NL) but may normalize
Amylase, urine	High
Bilirubin	May be high
Calcium	Low
Creatinine	May be greater than 1.5 mg%
C-reactive protein	High in pancreatic necrosis
Glucose	High
Lipase, serum	High
Hemoglobin/hematocrit	Low if bleeding
Magnesium	Low
Potassium	Low or high
Prothrombin time	Prolonged
WBC	High

ABGs, Arterial blood gases; *NL*, normal limits; *WBC*, white blood cell count.
Data from Friedman, L. S. (2005). Liver, biliary tract and pancreas. In L. Tierney, S. J. McPhee, & M. A. Papaealis, et al. (Eds.), *Current medical diagnosis and treatment* (pp. 671-674). (44th ed.). New York: Lange Medical Books/McGraw-Hill; Greenberger, N., & Toskes, P. (2005). Acute and chronic pancreatitis. In D. Kasper, E. Braunwald, & A. Fauci, et al. (Eds.), *Harrison's principles of internal medicine* (pp. 1895-1902). (16th ed.). New York: McGraw Hill Medical Publishing Division; Horrell, C. (2000). Pancreatitis. In D. Camp-Sorrell & R. Hawkins (Eds.), *Clinical manual for the oncology advanced practice nurse* (pp. 461-464). Pittsburgh: Oncology Nursing Press.

Hold chemotherapy, biotherapy.

Pain management: Administer opioid (morphine); position patient in knee-to-chest position; offer relaxation techniques to achieve pain control. Intravenous patient-controlled analgesia (PCA) is the preferred modality (Wrobelski et al.,1999).

Abdominal assessment: Distention, Cullen's (bruising around umbilicus) or Grey Turner's sign (bruising around loin area), hypoactive or absent bowel sounds, guarding, and rebound tenderness.

Lung may have crackles, adventitious breath sounds, or decreased chest expansion.

Maintain venous access via peripheral intravenous (IV) or venous access device (VAD).

Antiemetic medications for nausea control.

Laboratory tests: Hallmark laboratory test result is elevated serum amylase and lipase (usually more than 3 times normal) within 24 hours in 90% of all cases; then returns to normal (Friedman, 2005). Many other metabolic changes may be present (see Table 1-2).

Obtain and assess: Chest x-ray (for pleural effusion), abdominal series (for ileus), computed tomography/magnetic resonance imaging (CT/MRI) of abdomen (enlarged indistinct margins of pancreas, fluid accumulation) and ultrasound of pancreas (fluid accumulation, gallstones).

Oxygen therapy if oxygen saturation is low.

Dietary: NPO (withholding of food by mouth), nutritional support; total parenteral nutrition (TPN) or jejunal nasogastric feedings.

Nasogastric (NG) tube to low intermittent suction if patient has gastric distention or is at risk for aspiration.

IV fluid and electrolyte replacement according to deficits (e.g., volume, hypocalcemia, hypokalemia, hypomagnesemia).

Minimize pancreatic stimulation: Bed rest, NPO, anticholinergics.

Antibiotic therapy.

Antianxiety agents.

In shock or if complications arise: Anticipate hemodynamic monitoring, vasopressor therapy, peritoneal lavage, surgical intervention, and renal dialysis.

Oral care every hour if NPO.

Activity: Bed rest in acute phase to maintain comfort and suppress pancreatic stimulation.

Referral to alcohol or drug assessment counselor.

Monitor for signs of pancreatic infection: Persistent pain, prolonged fever, palpable abdominal mass, vomiting, abnormal laboratory results, and radiographic indications of infection such as cyst/fluid accumulation.

EVIDENCE-BASED PRACTICE UPDATES

1. Morphine now is recommended as the pain medication of choice because of its longer half-life, unless the patient has a duct stone (Krumberger, 1999, Wrobleski, 1999).
2. Total enteral nutrition (TEN) beyond the ligament of Treitz, administered within 48 hours of onset of severe acute pancreatitis, may reduce the incidence of total and infectious complications (Despins, 2005; Abou-Assi, Craig, & O'Keefe, 2002; Hale, Mosley, & Warner, 2000; Loan, 2000; Munoz & Katerndahl, 2000; Windsor et al., 1998; Wyncoll, 1998).
3. Withholding of food by mouth has not shown to reduce symptoms, mortality, or hospital stay of patients with acute pancreatitis. However, oral intake should be withheld until the nausea and vomiting have subsided, or when an obstruction is present (Munoz & Katerndahl, 2000).
4. Use of antibiotics in early acute pancreatitis is controversial, but it is recommended in patients with acute necrotizing pancreatitis (Munoz & Katerndahl, 2000; Wyncoll, 1999).

TEACHING AND EDUCATION

Pain management: *Rationale:* Pancreatitis can be a very painful condition; your nurse needs to know when you are in pain and should describe it in terms that the patient is comfortable with.

PCA pump: *Rationale:* You are on this pump so you can administer pain medication. You have some infusing all the time, but if you need more, push this button and it will give you a shot of pain medication. This pump has a safety mechanism so you cannot overdose or administer more than the set amount prescribed.

NPO status/nasogastric tube (if used): *Rationale:* The pain you are having now is the result of your pancreas irritation. Eating and drinking would irritate it. So that your pancreas can rest, you cannot eat or drink anything. It is important that you keep your mouth clean and moist during this time, so use these swabs every hour. Suctioning all fluids out of your stomach decreases pancreas irritation. A tube will go into your nose, down the back of your throat, and into your stomach to suction out the fluid. You will be fed through your IV line or through another tube that will go farther down into your gut (total enteral nutrition).

Tests and procedures: *Rationale:* You may undergo frequent blood and x-ray tests to check the condition of your pancreas and other organs.

Intravenous fluid therapy: *Rationale:* While you cannot eat, you will need fluids to keep you hydrated. You will receive other medications through your IV.

Anxiety: *Rationale:* You may be feeling anxious because of your pain and your illness; this anxiety may make your pain worse, and the pain medication will not be as effective. If you are feeling anxious, relaxation attained by deep breathing, guided imagery, or distraction with TV or music may be helpful, or ask your nurse for anxiety medication.

NURSING DIAGNOSES

1. **Acute pain** related to tissue inflammation or damage
2. **Deficient fluid volume** related to vomiting, NPO status, fever, anorexia, NG suction, vascular fluid leak caused by pancreatic enzyme release
3. **Imbalanced nutrition: less than body requirements** related to anorexia, NPO status, nausea and vomiting, pain, or alteration of digestive enzymes
4. **Impaired gas exchange** related to atelectasis, pleural effusion, or fluid overload from administration or splinting from pain
5. **Anxiety** related to severity of illness, pain, and lack of knowledge regarding illness and cause of pain

EVALUATION AND DESIRED OUTCOMES

1. Pain less than 3 on a 0 to 10 scale. Assess every hour while awake.
2. Blood pressure will be within normal limits (WNL).
3. Renal perfusion will be maintained as evidenced by urine output greater than 30 mL/hr.
4. Lungs are clear to auscultation.

5. Nutritional intake is maintained through TPN or TEN.
6. Serum electrolytes are WNL.
7. Free of signs and symptoms of acute pancreatitis within 7 days.
8. The patient and family are able to verbalize signs and symptoms of complications and the treatment plan.

DISCHARGE PLANNING AND FOLLOW-UP CARE

- Follow up with physician or nurse practitioner office visit within 2 weeks of discharge.
- Call health care provider if symptoms such as fever (as sign of pancreatic abscess), pain, nausea, and vomiting recur.
- Diet modification teaching and supplemental pancreatic enzymes in those with pancreatic damage.
- Referral to alcohol cessation program if alcohol addiction is present or suspected.

REVIEW QUESTIONS

QUESTIONS

1. The hallmark symptom of acute pancreatitis is:
   1. Abdominal pain
   2. Hypotension
   3. Nausea and vomiting
   4. Abdominal distention

2. The underlying pathophysiological mechanism of acute pancreatitis is:
   1. Stimulation of the gallbladder
   2. Blockage of the pancreatic duct
   3. Premature activation of pancreatic enzymes
   4. Increased permeability of intestinal vasculature

3. Initial treatment of acute pancreatitis includes:
   1. TPN, oxygen, and surgical exploration
   2. Analgesia, inhibition of pancreatic enzyme secretion, and fluid replacement.
   3. Invasive monitoring, IV antibiotics, and rest
   4. Needle aspiration of pancreatic enzymes, ventilatory support, and enteral feeding

4. The most urgent complication of acute pancreatitis is:
   1. Immobility
   2. Paralytic ileus
   3. Fluid volume deficit
   4. Pneumonia

5. Complications of acute pancreatitis amenable to surgical intervention include:
   1. Abscess, pseudocyst, and hemorrhage
   2. Pleural effusion
   3. Acute tubular necrosis
   4. Disseminated intravascular coagulation

6. The most useful laboratory test for the early diagnosis of acute pancreatitis is serum:
   1. Lipase
   2. Amylase
   3. Aspartate aminotransferase
   4. Bilirubin

7. The primary cause of acute pancreatitis in cancer patients with the highest morbidity and mortality is:
   1. Malignant transformation of the pancreas
   2. Treatment-induced immunosuppressive state
   3. Radiation toxicity
   4. Treatment with the chemotherapy, L-asparaginase

8. The gold standard diagnostic tool for acute pancreatitis is the abdominal:
   1. CT scan
   2. MRI
   3. MUGA scan
   4. PET scan

9. **A frequent electrolyte imbalance associated with acute pancreatitis is:**
   1. Hypocalcemia and hyperkalemia
   2. Hypermagnesemia and hyponatremia
   3. Hyponatremia and hyperkalemia
   4. Hypokalemia and hypercalcemia

10. **What is the pathobiological mechanism that transforms the edematous mild form of pancreatitis into the necrotizing form?**
    1. Hypotension
    2. Unknown mechanism
    3. Hypoxemia
    4. Pancreatic enzyme activity

ANSWERS

1. *Answer: 1*
   Rationale: The hallmark symptom of acute pancreatitis is epigastric pain described as knife-like, twisting, gnawing, and constant; and it may be referred to the lower back.

2. *Answer: 3*
   Rationale: The inflammation of acute pancreatitis is caused by the premature activation of pancreatic enzymes. This activation can be precipitated by blockage of the pancreatic ducts, alcohol, drugs, viruses, disease conditions, or other miscellaneous causes.

3. *Answer: 2*
   Rationale: The three primary goals in initial management of acute pancreatitis are to treat the cardinal sign of abdominal pain, to maintain blood pressure by through fluid replacement, and to halt secretion of pancreatic enzymes.

4. *Answer: 3*
   Rationale: Fluid volume deficit may have multiple causes and may lead to hypovolemic shock or ARDS.

5. *Answer: 1*
   Rationale: To prevent a fatal outcome, surgical intervention is absolutely necessary in each of these three situations.

6. *Answer: 2*
   Rationale: Serum amylase will be elevated in the early stages of acute pancreatitis and then will normalize.

7. *Answer: 4*
   Rationale: The incidence of acute pancreatitis in patients treated with L-asparaginase is 16%, and the mortality of those who develop it is 12%.

8. *Answer: 1*
   Rationale: The abdominal CAT scan is able to visualize show enlarged indistinct margins of the pancreas, as well as fluid accumulation.

9. *Answer: 4*
   Rationale: Hypokalemia may be present with prolonged vomiting, but serum potassium may be elevated if acute renal failure develops as a systemic complication. Hypercalcemia from hyperparathyroidism is associated with pancreatitis.

10. *Answer: 2*
    Rationale: To date, the underlying mechanism that causes the transformation from edematous pancreatitis to the necrotizing form is unknown.

REFERENCES

Abou-Assi, S., Craig, K., & O'Keefe, S. (2002). Hypocaloric jejunal feeding is better than total parenteral nutrition in acute pancreatitis: Results of a randomized comparative study. *The American Journal of Gastroenterology, 97*(7):2255-2262.

Chernecky, C., & Berger, B. (2004). *Laboratory tests and diagnostic procedures.* Philadelphia: WB Saunders.

Cole, L. (2002). Unraveling the mystery of acute pancreatitis. *Clinical Dimension, 21*(3):86-89.

Despins, L. (2005). Acute pancreatitis: Diagnosis and treatment of a potentially fatal condition. *American Journal of Nursing, 105*(11):54-57.

Friedman, L. S. (2005). Liver, biliary tract and pancreas. In L. Tierney, S. J. McPhee, & M. A. Papaealis, et al. (Eds.), *Current medical diagnosis and treatment* (pp. 671-674). (44th ed.). New York: Lange Medical Books/McGraw-Hill.

Greenberger, N., & Toskes, P. (2005). Acute and chronic pancreatitis. In D. Kasper, E. Braunwald, & A. Fauci, et al. (Eds.), *Harrison's principles of internal medicine* (pp. 1895-1902). (16th ed.). New York: McGraw Hill Medical Publishing Division.

Hale, A., Moseley, M., & Warner, S. (2000). Treating pancreatitis in the acute care setting. *Dimension in Critical Care Nursing, 19*(4):15-22.

Horrell, C. (2000). Pancreatitis. In D. Camp-Sorrell, & R. Hawkins (Eds.), *Clinical manual for the oncology advanced practice nurse* (pp. 461-464). Pittsburgh: Oncology Nursing Press.

Hughes, E. (2004). Understanding the care of patients with acute pancreatitis. *Nursing Standard, 18*(18):45-52.

Krumberger, J. (1999). Ask the experts. *Critical Care Nurse, 19*(2):110-111.

Loan, T. Letters to the editor. *Critical Care Nurse, 20*(1):16.

McArdle, J. (2000). The biological and nursing implications of pancreatitis. *Nursing Standard, 14*(48):46-51.

Munoz, A., & Katerndahl, D. (2006). Diagnosis and management of acute pancreatitis. *American Family Physician, 64*(2):164-174.

Polovich, M., White, J., & Kelleher, L (2005). *Chemotherapy and biotherapy guidelines and recommendations for practice.* (2nd ed.). Pittsburgh: ONS Press.

Sekimoto, M., Takada, T., & Kawarada, Y., et al. (2006). JPH guidelines for the management of acute pancreatitis: Epidemiology, etiology, natural history, and outcome predictors in acute pancreatitis. *Journal of Hepatobiliary and Pancreatic Surgery,* (13):10-24.

Sinicrope, F. A., & Levin, B. (2000). Complications of cancer and its treatment: Gastrointestinal complications. In R. Bast, D. Kufe, & R. Polock, et al. (Eds.), *Cancer medicine* (pp. 1035-1040). (5th ed.). Hamilton, Ontario, Canada: B. C. Decker, Inc.

Turner, B. (2003). Acute pancreatitis: Symptoms, diagnosis and management. *Nursing Times, 99*(46):30-32.

Windsor, A., Kanwar, S., & Li, A., et al. (1998). Compared with parenteral nutrition, enteral feeding attenuates the acute phase response and improves disease severity in acute pancreatitis. *Gut,* (42):431-435.

Wrobleski, D., Barth, M., & Oyen, L. (1999). Necrotizing pancreatitis: Pathophysiology, diagnosis and acute care management. *AACN Clinical Issues, 10*(4):464-477.

Wyncoll, D. (1999). The management of severe acute necrotizing pancreatitis: An evidenced based review of the literature. *Intensive Care Medicine,* (25):146-156.

Yahanda, A. M., & Chang, A. E. (2005). Acute abdomen, bowel obstruction and fistula. In M. Abeloff, J. Armitage, & J. Neiderhuber, et al. (Eds.), *Clinical oncology* (pp. 1030-1031). St. Louis: Elsevier.

Yeo, C., Yeo, T., & Hrubcin, R., et al. (2005). Cancer of the pancreas. In V. T. Devita Jr, S. Hellman, & S. A. Rosenberg (Eds.), *Cancer: Principles and practice of oncology* (pp. 1409-1415). (6th ed.). Baltimore: Lippincott Williams & Wilkins.

ACUTE RESPIRATORY DISTRESS SYNDROME

MERCEDES K. YOUNG

PATHOPHYSIOLOGICAL MECHANISMS

Acute respiratory distress syndrome (ARDS) is a potentially life-threatening syndrome characterized by dyspnea, severe hypoxemias, decreased lung compliance, and diffuse, bilateral pulmonary infiltrates without evidence of left ventricular dysfunction (Hudson et al., 1995). ARDS is acute in onset, frequently developing within 4 to 48 hours, and may persist from days to weeks (Hudson et al., 1995). It can be associated with myriad clinical disorders, including pneumonia, sepsis, aspiration of gastric contents, major trauma, and multiple transfusions of blood products (Sanchez & Toy, 2005; Ware & Matthay, 2000). ARDS can be subclassified as direct or indirect injury to the lungs (Sanchez & Toy, 2005; Ware & Matthay, 2000) (Table 2-1).

Our understanding of the pathophysiologic processes of ARDS has evolved since the early 1960s. ARDS now is understood to be a constellation of pathologic changes characterized by three stages of diffuse alveolar damage (DAD): the exudative phase, the fibroproliferative phase, and the fibrotic phase (Weinacker & Vaszar, 2001; Tomashefski, 2000). However, the extent of ARDS development and the pathogenesis may vary, depending on the different risk factors.

Exudative Phase

Two distinct barriers together make up the alveolar-capillary barrier: the endothelium and the epithelium (Fig. 2.1). The normal alveolar epithelium is composed of two types of cells: flat type I cells, which make up approximately 90% of the alveolar surface area, and cuboidal type II cells, which make up approximately 10% of the alveolar surface area (Ware & Matthay, 2000). These cells are integral to maintenance of the milieu within the lungs. Their functions include surfactant production, ion transport, and proliferation and differentiation after injury (Tomashefski, 2000).

The exudative phase of ARDS is characterized by increased permeability of the alveolar-capillary barrier. The increased permeability results when type I pneumocytes are damaged and slough off, exposing the basement membrane. This allows the influx of protein-rich edema fluid into the airspaces and accumulation of fluid along the alveolar wall, forming a hyaline membrane. As a result, lung volume and pressures increase, causing pulmonary edema and subsequently leading to changes in hydrostatic pressure and, ultimately, impaired diffusion of oxygen (Weinacker & Vaszar, 2001; Tomashefski, 2000). In addition, type II pneumocytes become hyperplastic (Weinacker & Vaszar, 2001). The injury to type II cells results in impaired fluid transport, removal of edema fluid from the alveolar space, and a decrease in surfactant production and turnover (Tomashefski, 2000; Ware & Matthay, 2000).

During the exudative phase of ARDS, neutrophils are recruited to the interstitium in response to cellular adhesion molecules (e.g., selectins and beta-2 integrins) and

Table 2-1	CLINICAL DISORDERS ASSOCIATED WITH THE DEVELOPMENT OF ACUTE RESPIRATORY DISTRESS SYNDROME
Direct Lung Injury	**Indirect Lung Injury**
Common Causes • Pneumonia • Aspiration of gastric contents	**Common Causes** • Sepsis • Severe trauma with shock and multiple transfusions
Less Common Causes • Pulmonary contusion • Fat emboli • Near-drowning • Inhalation injury • Reperfusion pulmonary edema after lung transplantation or pulmonary embolectomy	**Less Common Causes** • Cardiopulmonary bypass • Drug overdose • Acute pancreatitis • Transfusions of blood products

Modified from Ware, L. B., & Matthay, M. A. (2000). Acute respiratory distress syndrome. *New England Journal of Medicine, 342*(18):1334-1349.

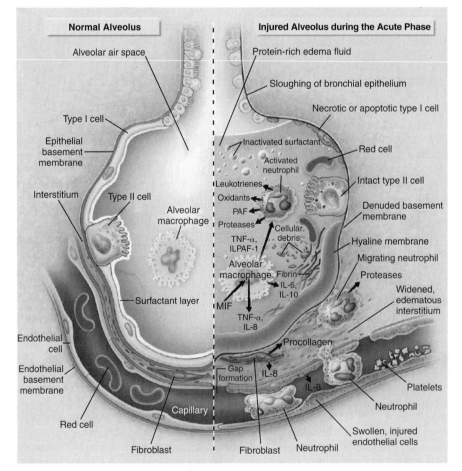

Fig. 2.1 • A normal alveolus *(left)* and an injured alveolus *(right)* in the acute phase of lung injury and acute respiratory distress syndrome. *(Modified from Ware, L. B., & Matthay, M. A. [2000]. Acute respiratory distress syndrome.* New England Journal of Medicine, 342*(18):1334-1349.)*

subsequently are activated by a number of cytokines (e.g., tumor necrosis factor and interleukin-1 [IL-1], IL-6, IL-8, and IL-10) and complement (enzymatic serum proteins), which are thought to induce and sustain an inflammatory response (Weinacker & Vaszar, 2001). Although neutrophils are part of the inflammatory process, they do not play an essential role in overall lung injury, as evidenced by the fact that neutropenic patients can develop ARDS (Mokart et al., 2003). Moreover, the lungs have a reservoir of alveolar and interstitial macrophages. Macrophages not only play an important roll in proinflammatory effects in the lungs, they also have a potentially crucial roll in the antiinflammatory effects and in the resolution of acute lung injury (Pittet et al., 1997).

Furthermore, anticoagulant proteins (protein C and protein S) decrease, and procoagulant proteins (tissue factor) and antifibrinolytic proteins (plasminogen activator inhibitor-1 [PAI-1]) increase. This leads to platelet aggregation and, ultimately, increasing pulmonary vascular resistance. It also contributes to pulmonary hypertension (Bernard, 2005; Weinacker & Vaszar, 2001).

Fibroproliferative Phase

If the exudative phase is sustained, fibroproliferation occurs. This is characterized by the infiltration of fibroblasts and the persistence of inflammation within the interstitium (Weinacker & Vaszar, 2001; Tomashefski, 2000). The type II pneumocytes continue to proliferate and accumulate along the basement membrane, ultimately replacing the type I pneumocytes (Tomashefski, 2000). During this stage, hyaline membranes are no longer formed; instead, the process is complicated by the deposition of collagen by fibroblasts, resulting in thickening of the alveolar walls and, eventually, inhibition of lung compliance (Weinacker & Vaszar, 2001).

Fibrotic Phase

The final stage of ARDS is the fibrotic phase, which is manifested by fibrosis, scarring, and cyst formation (Weinacker & Vaszar, 2001). The lung becomes completely remodeled by sparsely cellular collagenous tissue (Tomashefski, 2000).

EPIDEMIOLOGY AND ETIOLOGY

For decades ARDS went by a plethora of names (e.g., DaNang lung, shock lung, post-traumatic lung) (Bernard et al., 1994). The condition first was described as "acute respiratory distress syndrome" in 1967, in a historic article by Ashbaugh and colleagues in the journal *Lancet* (Ashbaugh et al., 1967). Subsequently, ARDS was frequently referred to as "adult respiratory distress syndrome" to distinguish it from infant respiratory distress syndrome (Ashbaugh et al., 1967). In 1992, the American-European Consensus Committee on ARDS (AECC) was designated to standardize a definition of ARDS and to address the many therapeutic options, as well as prevention of the syndrome in individuals at increased risk (Bernard et al., 1994). This had a positive impact on clinical and epidemiologic research, one that continues to benefit patient survival and overall health-related quality of life (HRQOL) (Heyard et al., 2005; Bernard et al., 1994).

The AECC determined that *acute* rather than *adult* best describes the syndrome because the condition is not strictly limited to adults (Bernard et al., 1994). The AECC also instituted a new term, *acute lung injury* (ALI), to encompass a broader range of pathologic processes; *ARDS* was reserved for the severest end of the spectrum (Bernard et al., 1994). Therefore all patients with ARDS have ALI, but not all patients with ALI have ARDS (Bernard et al., 1994). The criterion for distinguishing between ALI and ARDS is the degree of hypoxemia (Bernard et al., 1994). ALI is defined as a PaO_2/FiO_2 of less than

300 mm Hg; ARDS is defined as a PaO_2/FiO_2 of less than 200 mm Hg (Bernard et al., 1994).

In 1972 the National Institutes of Health (NIH) reported the incidence of ARDS as 75 cases per 100,000 population per year in the United States (Bernard et al., 1994). Subsequent studies have suggested that this may be an overestimation caused by the heterogeneity of underlying disease processes and the lack of a standardized definition. Current estimates range from 1.5 to 8.3 cases per 100,000 (Bernard et al., 1994). Recent prospective studies show promise for accurately gauging the incidence of ARDS because these studies use the criteria established by the AECC, which coincidently reflect the original NIH estimates of the incidence of ARDS (Rubenfeld et al., 2005; Goss et al., 2003). The prevalence of ARDS by procedure is reported as 7.9% for pneumonectomy, 2.96% for lobectomy, and 0.88% for sublobar resection (Dulu et al, 2006).

Since the introduction of ARDS into the medical literature, patient mortality has been estimated to exceed 50% (Ware & Matthay, 2000; Milberg et al., 1995; Suchyta et al., 1997). This is similar to the mortality rate for trauma patients in general (Salim et al., 2006). Advances in supportive care (e.g., changes in the method of mechanical ventilation, early and aggressive use of antibiotics, stress ulcer prophylaxis, and improved nutritional and fluid therapy), as well as early identification of risk factors, have resulted in an overall decrease in the mortality of patients who develop ARDS to about 30% to 36% (Jardin et al., 1999; Milberg et al., 1995). This statistic applies to patients 60 years of age or younger who developed ARDS as a secondary complication of trauma or a noninfectious condition. In this patient group, the overall morality rate for those in the intensive care unit (ICU) dropped from 38% to 30%, and the mortality rate for ARDS patients in the hospital overall dropped from 52% to 37% (Ely et al., 2002; Ware & Matthay, 2000; Milberg et al., 1995). In many studies, local immunosuppression appears to be associated with a good prognosis; however, this does not necessarily apply to neutropenic patients. In fact, several studies suggest an increased mortality in neutropenic patients (57% to 80%) compared with those who are not neutropenic (45%) (Mokart et al., 2003)

RISK PROFILE

The ability to identify patients at risk of developing ARDS is essential to preventing the syndrome and to treating patients earlier, thereby reducing the likelihood of severe complications. Multiple studies have shown that sepsis, whether of pulmonary or non-pulmonary causes, is the leading risk factor for the development of ARDS (18% to 43% of cases) (Stapleton et al., 2005; Fein & Calalang-Colucci, 2000; Hudson et al., 1995). The risk increases if sepsis is coupled with systemic hemodynamic responses, impaired perfusion, or multiple organ failure (Ely et al., 2005; Fein & Calalang-Colucci, 2000; Gattinoni et al., 1994). Research also shows that if sepsis is complicated by prolonged hypotension, disseminated intravascular coagulation (DIC), or shock, the incidence of ARDS increases (Fein & Calalang-Colucci, 2000).

Other factors that have been shown to increase the risk of ARDS include age over 68 years; female gender; severe illness (including chronic obstructive pulmonary disease [COPD], asthma, and bronchitis); malignancies (including malignant lymphoma and acute promyelocytic leukemia) (Kamikura et al, 2006; Larson & Tallman, 2003); opportunistic infections (including adenovirus and vancomycin-resistant enterococcus) (Wallot et al., 2006; Avery et al., 2005); cigarette smoking; chronic alcohol abuse; use of amiodarone (Charles et al., 2006); surgery (including lung resection and pelvic exenteration) (Dulu et al., 2006; Wydra et al., 2006); and treatment-related pulmonary toxicities (e.g., chemotherapeutic agents and radiation) (Hudson et al., 1995; Iribarren et al., 2000).

Patients with oncologic malignancies undergoing treatment with chemotherapy are at an even greater risk of developing ARDS. The pathogenesis is thought to be caused by hemostatic abnormalities, leukocyte activation, and possibly deactivation of alveolar macrophages (Kamikura et al., 2006; Mokart et al., 2003).

PROGNOSIS

Researchers have elucidated a significant proportion of the underlying pathogenicity of ARDS in the hope of finding specific biomarkers that would enhance diagnosis and prognosis and help identify patients at the highest risk of developing the condition (Pittet et al., 1997). As yet, no consistent biomarker has been identified that can be applied to clinical practice.

Nevertheless, our increased knowledge of this complex syndrome allows us to better understand the causes of increased mortality in ARDS patients. Several studies have consistently shown that sepsis coupled with multiple organ failure is the most common cause of death (30% to 50% of cases) (Stapleton et al., 2005; Milberg et al., 1995; Hudson et al., 1995). A correlation exists between sepsis that persists 72 hours or longer after the onset of ARDS and patient survival (Fein & Calalang-Colucci, 2000). In addition, the degree of alveolar-epithelial injury, as well as structural changes, is associated with a higher patient mortality and can be a reliable predictor of overall outcome and HRQOL (Heyard et al., 2005; Ely et al., 2002; Gattinoni et al., 1994).

Patients over age 70 who develop ARDS have a higher mortality rate than patients under age 70 who develop the syndrome, even when gender, multiple organ failure, or sepsis is taken into account. This situation is attributed primarily to the duration of ventilator support. It also may reflect age bias, which can influence the decision on whether to withdraw support or to initiate end-of-life discussions with the families of patients who are likely die (Stapleton et al., 2005; Ely et al., 2002; Suchyta et al., 1997).

Advances also have been made in the treatment options for patients who survive ARDS, prompting clinical research directed at evaluating survivors of ARDS and their HRQOL. These studies have uniformly shown an overall improvement in aspects of physical function at 6 months and 12 months, although with some physical limitations (Heyard et al., 2005; Herritage et al., 2003).

Research suggests that a correlation exists between the degree of pulmonary injury, pre-existing co-morbidities, the duration of the critical illness, and possible treatment-related side effects and the patient's HRQOL (Heyard et al., 2005; Herritage et al., 2003).

PROFESSIONAL ASSESSMENT CRITERIA (PAC)

Clinically ARDS usually occurs in the setting of critical illness. Frequently it reflects the underlying pathology that can co-exist, and it may obscure and possibly delay diagnosis. The first, or acute, phase occurs at the time of injury; symptoms usually develop within 12 to 48 hours of the inciting event (Steinberg & Hudson, 2000). Physical examination findings in this phase most often are minimal. The condition is manifested initially by exertional dyspnea that results in arterial hypoxemia refractory to supplemental oxygen (a classic feature) (Ware & Matthay, 2000). At this point, the chest x-ray findings are not usually diagnostic and can be indistinguishable from those of cardiogenic pulmonary edema (Ware & Matthay, 2000).

Within several hours to days, the latent phase ensues. Bilateral, patchy, ill-defined radiographic infiltrates gradually develop, and fine rales may be auscultated during the physical examination (Steinberg & Hudson, 2000). The latent phase is followed by acute respiratory failure. The patient becomes increasingly dyspneic, tachypneic, and hypoxemic as a result of decreased lung compliance, and diffuse rales can be auscultated. Chest x-ray films show the progression of patchy, coalescing infiltrations (Weinacker & Vaszar, 2001).

The final phase of ARDS is manifested by intrapulmonary shunting that leads to refractory hypoxemia and metabolic and respiratory acidosis. The chest x-ray films show a more reticular pattern, which represents the beginning of fibrosis (Weinacker & Vaszar, 2001).

1. **Vital signs:** Tachypnea, tachycardia, hypertension, chest discomfort, fever
2. **History:** See risk profile.
3. **Hallmark physical signs and symptoms:** Dyspnea
4. **Additional signs and symptoms:** Evidence of respiratory muscle fatigue: intercostal retractions, paradoxical chest and abdominal movement; faint or pronounced rales or cough
5. **Psychosocial signs:** Anxiety
6. **Laboratory values and diagnostic tests:** Early evidence of varying degrees of hypoxemia (generally resistant to oxygen supplementation); respiratory alkalosis, decreased PCO_2; late evidence of arterial metabolic or respiratory acidosis; widened alveolar-arterial gradient; ANC less than 500 neutrophils/mm^3; PaO_2/FiO_2 less than 300 mm Hg for ALI; less than 200 mm Hg for ARDS (Bernard et al., 1994); CXR: initially may be normal, with progression to bilateral pulmonary infiltrates; blood and urine cultures; fluid from bronchoalveolar lavage (reserved for selected patients) shows thioredoxin level greater than 61 ng/mL (Callister et al., 2006).

NURSING CARE AND TREATMENT

Supportive therapy is the basis of treatment for ARDS. It is directed toward identifying and managing pulmonary and nonpulmonary organ dysfunction (Brower et al., 2001). All inciting etiologies should be excluded. In addition, because of the increased mortality related to sepsis, a high index of suspicion should be maintained for potentially treatable infections, and prompt antimicrobial intervention or surgery should be provided as necessary (Ware & Matthay, 2000).

Essential Nursing Care

- Evaluation of chest x-ray films
- Computed tomography (CT) scan evaluation
- Mechanical ventilation
- Blood, urine, and sputum culture evaluations
- Nutritional support
- Intravenous antibiotic intervention
- Arterial blood gas interpretation
- Daily complete blood count and metabolic panel interpretation
- Strict evaluation of intake and output
- Daily weight
- Vital signs at least every 4 hours, assessing for tachypnea, tachycardia, hypertension, fever, and chest pain or discomfort.

Medications

Vasodilators may be considered for patients with mild to moderate pulmonary arterial hypertension, which can develop secondary to hypoxic vasoconstriction, destruction and/or obstruction of the pulmonary vascular bed, and the use of high levels of positive end-expiratory pressure (PEEP). When used to treat the pulmonary arterial hypertension, these drugs (e.g., hydralazine and nitric oxide) may help prevent the development of cardiac dysfunction in some patients (Brower et al., 2001).

Antiinflammatory strategies are thought to diminish the inflammatory response associated with ARDS, thereby reducing the injury caused by proinflammatory molecules. Important studies have suggested that improved clinical outcomes are achieved among patients treated with antiinflammatory agents. However, no drug strategy (e.g., glucocorticoid therapy, antioxidant therapy, prostaglandin agonist/inhibitors, lisofylline, pentoxifylline, and anti-IL-8) has yet been found to improve mortality sufficiently to outweigh the side effects of treatment (Brower et al., 2001).

Lung-protective Ventilatory Strategies

Ventilation with small tidal volumes (6.2 mL/kg rather than 10 to 15 mL/kg) and limited airway pressures may reduce ventilator-associated lung injuries caused by overdistention. These types of injuries (e.g., increased vascular permeability, acute inflammation, alveolar hemorrhage, intrapulmonary shunt, and diffuse radiographic infiltrates) have been seen in many laboratory experiments (ARDS Network, 2000). More important, several studies have shown that the use of lower tidal volumes reduces the number of organ failure–free days and the number of days on ventilatory support; this may account for the substantial decrease in mortality from 40% to 30% (ARDS Network, 2000). In most patients with ARDS, the combination of the fraction of oxygen in the inspired gas (FiO_2) and PEEP is required to support arterial oxygenation (ARDS Network, 2000). However, supportive arterial oxygenation is not without consequences; the clinician must balance the risk of circulatory depression and barotraumas against the risk of hyperoxia (Brower et al., 2001). Nevertheless, some ventilatory strategies can enhance pulmonary gas exchange, improving patient outcomes. These include lung-protective ventilation with higher PEEP, noninvasive positive-pressure ventilation, high-frequency ventilation, tracheal gas insufflation, proportional-assist ventilation, inverse ratio ventilation, and airway pressure release ventilation (Brower et al., 2001).

Hemodynamic Management

Fluid management in patients with ARDS is considered a controversial issue. Some contend that maintaining a negative fluid balance through the use of diuretics and dialysis may improve oxygenation and lung compliance (Brower et al., 2001). However, fluid restriction may worsen the patient's clinical status by reducing cardiac output and tissue perfusion, resulting in nonpulmonary organ dysfunction (Brower et al., 2001). Blood transfusion has been suggested as a way to maintain or support oxygen demand by keeping the hemoglobin concentration at 10 g/dL or higher (Brower et al., 2001).

Vasopressors also have been suggested to help maintain systemic blood pressure (BP) or to increase cardiac output in patients with sepsis (Brower et al., 2001).

Nutritional Support

Nutritional support involves providing adequate nutrients to meet the patient's metabolic needs and to prevent and supplement nutritional deficiencies (Brower et al., 2001). Supplementation can be done either enterally or parenterally, but these supportive measures have their own risks, including infections and intolerance. Emerging data continue to suggest that nutritional immunomodulation can reduce infectious complications, new organ failure, and mechanical ventilation and shorten the hospital stay (Brower et al., 2001).

Surfactant Replacement Therapy

Surfactant replacement therapy has been proposed as a possible treatment on the grounds that it reduces the surface tension at the air-fluid interface of the small airways and alveoli. However, no supportive evidence suggests that surfactant improves arterial oxygenation, shortens the duration of mechanical ventilation, or improves patient survival (Anzueto et al., 1996).

Extracorporeal Gas Exchange

Even with supportive mechanical ventilation, some patients have persistent hypoxemia. Extracorporeal membrane oxygenation (ECMO) was introduced with the goal of improving arterial oxygenation. More recently, extracorporeal carbon dioxide removal (ECCO$_2$R) has been used to remove carbon dioxide and help reduce high respiratory rates and tidal volumes. Overall, research has shown promising outcomes for this new technique; however, no significant increase in patient mortality has been seen (Brower et al., 2001). The use of a pumpless extracorporeal lung-assist device has shown promise (Ruettimann et al., 2006).

Prone positioning has been shown to improve arterial oxygenation and to allow reductions in ventilatory support (e.g., FiO$_2$ and PEEP). However, investigators are unable to predict which patients would benefit most, and to date no supportive studies or standards are available to guide clinicians (Brower et al., 2001).

Ongoing Nursing Assessment

Assess:
- Level of consciousness q1h and PRN
- Respiratory status q1h and PRN
- Skin integrity every shift
- Ventilatory settings q1h and PRN
- Central access q1h and PRN
- Patency of all tubes (e.g., endotracheal tubes, nasogastric tubes, urinary catheters) q1h and PRN

Measure:
- Strict intake and output q1h
- Daily weights
- Vital signs q1h and PRN
- Pulmonary arterial pressure and central venous pressure (CVP) q1h
- Cardiac output/index and systemic vascular resistance q4h and PRN

Send:
- Complete blood count with differential and complete metabolic panel daily
- ABGs PRN
- Blood and urine cultures q72h, or if temperature exceeds 100.4° F (38° C), or with evidence of sepsis

Implement:
- Neutropenic precautions

- Nutritional protocols
- Ventilatory support
- Skin integrity protocols
- Communication of plan with the health care team, patient, and family

EVIDENCE-BASED PRACTICE UPDATES

1. The use of arsenic trioxide in patients with refractory germ cell neoplasms can result in ARDS (Beer et al., 2006).
2. The prevalence of ARDS related to lung procedures is greatest after pneumonectomy (7.9%) (Dulu et al., 2006).
3. Use of a pumpless extracorporeal lung-assist device to remove excess $PaCO_2$ and reduce mechanical stress is beneficial in the treatment of ARDS (Ruettimann et al., 2006).

TEACHING AND EDUCATION

Mechanical ventilator: *Rationale:* Because you are working hard to breathe, you are attached to a breathing machine. This machine will help you breathe by supplying oxygen to your lungs while you heal, until you can breathe for yourself.

Equipment/monitors: *Rationale:* There are a lot of monitors and noises in here. However, this equipment helps us evaluate how you are doing. It can be very confusing and frustrating, but if there is anything you don't understand, please ask us.

Blood samples: *Rationale:* We obtain samples of your blood each day and sometimes more frequently. These samples help us evaluate different aspects of your care, such as how well oxygen is getting to your lungs, your levels of nutrition, and whether you may have an infection.

NURSING DIAGNOSES

1. **Impaired gas exchange** related to underlying pathology of ARDS
2. **Anxiety** related to shortness of breath and fearfulness of death
3. **Imbalanced nutrition: less than body requirements** related to increased metabolic demands of underlying pathology of ARDS
4. **Impaired skin integrity** related to immobility
5. **Acute confusion** related to hypoxemia, dyspnea and respiratory acidosis

EVALUATION AND DESIRED OUTCOMES

1. Improved gas exchange and lung compliance, as evidenced by a decrease in the FiO_2 requirement, improved lung assessment (e.g., decreased rales), improved O_2 sat, decreased heart rate, decreased respiration, and decreased use of accessory muscles.
2. Hemodynamic management of fluid status, as evidenced by consistent daily weights and equal input and output.
3. Adequate nutritional support, as evidenced by maintenance of weight and electrolytes.
4. Adequate skin integrity, as evidenced by absence of pressure ulcers.
5. Adequate antibiotic coverage, as evidenced by absence of fevers and persistently negative blood and urine cultures.

DISCHARGE PLANNING AND FOLLOW-UP CARE

- Follow-up with pulmonary specialist in 1 week for assessment and evaluation of chest x-ray films and laboratory values.
- Baseline pulmonary function test to evaluate functional changes in respiratory status.
- Physical therapy to assist patient in a timely recovery and improve overall quality of life.
- Education of patient regarding symptoms of respiratory tract infections and environmental factors to avoid.

REVIEW QUESTIONS

QUESTIONS

1. ARDS is an acronym for:
   1. Adult respiratory distress syndrome
   2. Adult respiratory disease syndrome
   3. Acute respiratory distress syndrome
   4. Acute rapid distress syndrome

2. The most important risk factor for the development of ARDS is:
   1. Sepsis
   2. Age
   3. Co-morbidities (e.g., COPD, bronchitis, asthma)
   4. Gender

3. The pathogenesis in the early phase of ARDS is described as:
   1. Scarring of the alveolar-epithelial wall caused by deposition of fibrin
   2. Increased permeability of the alveolar- capillary barrier
   3. Rapid influx of protein-rich fluid into the lungs
   4. Overproduction of surfactant by type II pneumocytes

4. ARDS (acute respiratory distress syndrome) is not characterized by the following:
   1. Unilateral diffuse pulmonary infiltrates without evidence of left ventricular dysfunction
   2. Dyspnea
   3. Hypoxemia
   4. Decreased lung compliance

5. Which of the following disorders is directly associated with lung injury in ARDS?
   1. Sepsis
   2. Trauma
   3. Pneumonia
   4. Shock

6. An important predictor of mortality and health-related quality of life (HRQOL) in patients with ARDS is:
   1. Multiple organ failure
   2. Age and multiple organ failure
   3. Degree of alveolar-epithelial injury
   4. Prolonged sepsis

7. A clinical finding in the acute or early phase of ARDS does not include:
   1. Exertional dyspnea
   2. Tachycardia
   3. Bilateral pulmonary infiltrates without evidence of left ventricular dysfunction
   4. Refractory arterial hypoxemia

8. Supportive management of ARDS includes what primary form of treatment?
   1. Mechanical ventilation
   2. Nutritional support
   3. Immunomodulation
   4. Surfactant

9. Which of the following is a mainstay of support for patients with ARDS who require mechanical ventilation?
   1. Tidal volumes of 10 to 15 mL/kg
   2. Tidal volumes of 4 to 6 mL/kg
   3. Prone positioning
   4. Corticosteroids

10. A side effect of traditional mechanical ventilation in patients with ARDS is:
    1. Increased airway pressure, reflecting overdistention of the less affected airways
    2. Alveolar hemorrhage
    3. Intrapulmonary shunting
    4. Acute inflammation

ANSWERS

1. *Answer: 3*
   Rationale: In an article published in 1967 in the journal *Lancet*, Ashbaugh and colleagues described "acute respiratory distress syndrome" (Ashbaugh et al., 1967). ARDS was frequently referred to as *adult respiratory distress syndrome* to distinguish it from infant respiratory distress syndrome (Ashbaugh et al., 1967). However, the AECC resolved that the term *acute* rather than *adult* best describes this syndrome, because it is not strictly limited to adults (Bernard et al., 1994).

2. *Answer: 1*
   Rationale: Multiple studies have shown that sepsis, whether of pulmonary or nonpulmonary causes, is the leading risk factor for the development of ARDS, accounting for 18% to 43% of cases (Stapleton et al., 2005; Fein & Calalang-Colucci, 2000; Hudson et al., 1995). Several studies have consistently documented the fact that sepsis coupled with multiple organ failure is the most common cause of death (30% to 50% of cases) (Stapleton et al., 2005; Milberg et al., 1995; Hudson et al., 1995). A correlation exists between sepsis that persists longer than 72 hours after the onset of ARDS and patient survival (Fein & Calalang-Colucci, 2000).

3. *Answer: 2*
   Rationale: The early, or exudative, phase of ARDS is characterized by increased permeability of the alveolar-capillary barrier. This allows the influx of protein-rich edema fluid into the airspaces and accumulation of fluid along the alveolar wall, forming a hyaline membrane. The result is an increase in lung volume and pressures, which cause pulmonary edema and subsequently lead to changes in hydrostatic pressure, ultimately impairing the diffusion of oxygen (Weinacker & Vaszar, 2001; Tomashefski, 2000).

4. *Answer: 1*
   Rationale: ARDS is a potentially life-threatening syndrome characterized by dyspnea, severe hypoxemias, decreased lung compliance, and diffuse, bilateral pulmonary infiltrates without evidence of left ventricular dysfunction (Hudson et al., 1995).

5. *Answer: 3*
   Rationale: Pneumonia is directly related to the lungs. ARDS can be subclassified as direct or indirect injury to the lungs (Sanchez & Toy, 2005; Ware & Matthay, 2000) (see Table 2-1). It also can be associated with myriad clinical disorders, including sepsis, aspiration of gastric contents, major trauma, and multiple blood-product transfusions (Sanchez & Toy, 2005; Ware & Matthay, 2000).

6. *Answer: 3*
   Rationale: Research has shown that the degree of alveolar-epithelial injury, as well as structural changes, is associated with patient mortality and can be a reliable predictor of overall outcome and HRQOL (Heyard et al., 2005; Ely et al., 2002; Gattinoni et al., 1994).

7. *Answer: 3*
   Rationale: The physical examination findings in the acute or early phase most often are minimal. They are manifested initially by exertional dyspnea, which results in arterial hypoxemia that is refractory to supplemental oxygen (a classic feature) (Ware & Matthay, 2000). Other vital sign abnormalities that may be seen include early compensatory manifestations (e.g., tachycardia, temperature, and hypertension). At this point, chest x-ray findings are not usually diagnostic and can be indistinguishable from those of cardiogenic pulmonary edema (Ware & Matthay, 2000).

8. *Answer: 1*
   Rationale: Lung-protective ventilation is considered the standard for patients with ARDS who require ventilatory support (ARDS Network, 2000). More important, several studies have shown that the use of lower tidal volumes has reduced the number of organ failure–free days and the number of days on ventilatory support; this may account for the substantial decline in mortality, from 40% to 30% (ARDS Network, 2000). The combination of the fraction of oxygen in the inspired gas (FiO_2) and positive end-expiratory pressure (PEEP) is needed for

most patients with ARDS to support arterial oxygenation (ARDS Network, 2000). However, supportive arterial oxygenation is not without consequences, and the clinician must determine how to balance the risk of circulatory depression and barotrauma against the risk of hyperoxia (Brower et al., 2001).

9. *Answer: 2*
Rationale: Ventilation with small tidal volumes (6.2 mL/kg versus 10 to 15 mL/kg) and limited airway pressures can potentially reduce ventilator-associated lung injuries caused by overdistention, which have been seen in laboratory experiments (e.g., increased vascular permeability, acute inflammation, alveolar hemorrhage, intrapulmonary shunt, and diffuse radiographic infiltrates) (ARDS Network, 2000). More important, several

studies have shown that the use of lower tidal volumes has reduced the number of organ failure–free days and the number of days on ventilatory support; this may account for the substantial decrease in mortality, from 40% to 30% (ARDS Network, 2000).

10. *Answer: 1*
Rationale: Ventilation with small tidal volumes and limited airway pressure reportedly has reduced the risk of overall lung injury secondary to overdistention (Brower et al., 2001). In laboratory experiments on animal models, the use of traditional ventilation caused increased pulmonary vascular permeability, acute inflammation, alveolar hemorrhage, intrapulmonary shunt, and diffuse radiographic infiltrates (Brower et al., 2001).

Special thanks to Annmarie Marwitz Kallenbach, RN, BSN, MS, CCRN, TNS, the author of this chapter in the previous edition.

REFERENCES

Acute Respiratory Distress (ARDS) Network. (2000). Ventilation with lower tidal volumes as compared with traditional tidal volumes for acute lung injury and the acute respiratory distress syndrome. The Acute Respiratory Distress Syndrome Network. *New England Journal of Medicine, 342*(18):1301-1308.

Anzueto, A., Baughman, R. P., & Guntupalli, K. K., et al. (1996). Aerosolized surfactant in adults with sepsis-induced acute respiratory distress syndrome. *New England Journal of Medicine, 334*(22):1217-1421.

Artigas, A., Bernard, G. R., & Carlet, J., et al. (1998). The American-European consensus conference on ARDS. *Part 2. Intensive Care Medicine, 24*(4):378-398.

Ashbaugh, D. G., Bigelow, D. B., & Petty, T. L., et al. (1967). Acute respiratory distress in adults. *Lancet, 2*:319-323.

Avery, R., Kalaycio, M., & Pohlman, B., et al. (2005). Early vancomycin-resistant enterococcus (VRE) bacteremia after allogeneic bone marrow transplantation is associated with a rapidly deteriorating clinical course. *Bone Marrow Transplantation, 35*(5):497-499.

Beer, T. M., Tangen, C. M., & Nichols, C. R., et al. (2006). Southwest Oncology Group phase II study of arsenic trioxide in patients with refractory germ cell malignancies. *Cancer, 106*(12):2624-2629.

Bernard, G. R. (2005). Acute respiratory distress syndrome. *American Journal of Respiratory and Critical Care Medicine, 172*(7):798-806.

Bernard, G. R., Artigas, A., & Brigham, K. L., et al. (1994). The American-European consensus conference on ARDS. *American Journal of Respiratory Critical Care Medicine, 149*:818-824.

Brower, R. G., Ware, L. B., & Berthiaume, Y., et al. (2001). Treatment of ARDS. *Chest, 120*(4):1347-1367.

Callister, M. E., Burke-Gaffney, A., & Quinlan, G. J., et al. (2006). Extracellular thioredoxin levels are increased in patients with acute lung injury. *Thorax, 61*(6):521-527.

Charles, P. E., Doise, J. M., & Quenot, J. P., et al. (2006). Amiodarone-related acute respiratory distress syndrome following sudden withdrawal of steroids. *Respiration, 73*(2):248-249.

Dulu, A., Pastores, S. M., & Park, B., et al. (2006). Prevalence and mortality of acute lung injury and ARDS after lung resection. *Chest, 130*(1):73-78.

Ely, E. W., Wheeler, A. P., & Thompson, B. T., et al. (2002). Recovery rate and prognosis in older persons who develop acute lung injury and the acute respiratory syndrome. *Annals of Internal Medicine, 136*(1):25-36.

Fein, A. M., & Calalang-Colucci, M. G. (2000). Acute lung injury and acute respiratory distress syndrome in sepsis and septic shock. *Critical Care Clinics, 16*(2):289-317.

Gattinoni, L., Bombino, M., & Pelosi, P., et al. (1994). Lung structure and function in different stages of severe adult respiratory distress syndrome. *Journal of the American Medical Association, 271*(22):1772-1779.

Goss, C. H., Brower, R. G., & Hudson, L. D., et al. (2003). Incidence of acute lung injury in the United States. *Critical Care Medicine, 31*(6):1607-1611.

Herridge, M. S., Cheung, A. M., & Tansey, C. M., et al. (2003). One-year outcomes in survivors of the acute respiratory distress syndrome. *New England Journal of Medicine, 348*(8):683-693.

Heyard, D. K., Groll, D., & Caeser, M. (2005). Survivors of acute respiratory distress syndrome: Relationship between pulmonary dysfunction and long-term health–related quality of life. *Critical Care Medicine, 33*(7):1549-1556.

Hudson, L. D., Milberg, J. A., & Anardi, D., et al. (1995). Clinical risks for development of the acute respiratory distress syndrome. *American Journal of Respiratory and Critical Care, Medicine, 151*(2, pt 1):293-301.

Hudson, L. D., & Steinberg, K. P. (1999). Epidemiology of acute lung injury and ARDS. *Chest, 116*:74S-82S.

Iribarren, C., Jacobs, D. R., & Sidney, S., et al. (2000). Cigarette smoking, alcohol consumption, and risk of ARDS. *Chest, 117*(1):163-183.

Jardin, F., Fellahi, J. L., & Beauchet, A., et al. (1999). Improved prognosis of acute respiratory distress syndrome 15 years on. *Intensive Care Medicine, 25*:936-941.

Kamikura, Y., Wada, H., & Sasse, T., et al. (2006). Hemostatic abnormalities and leukocyte activation caused by infection in patients with malignant lymphoma during chemotherapy. *Thrombosis Research, 117*(6):671-679.

Larson, R. S., & Tallman, M. S. (2003). Retinoic acid syndrome: Manifestations, pathogenesis, and treatment. *Best Practice & Research Clinical Haematology, 16*(3):453-461.

Milberg, J. A., Davis, D. R., & Steinberg, K. P., et al. (1995). Improved survival of patients with acute respiratory distress syndrome (ARDS): 1983-1993. *Journal of the American Medical Association, 273*(4):306-309.

Mokart, D., Guery, B. P., & Bouabdallah, R., et al. (2003). Deactivation of alveolar macrophages in septic neutropenic ARDS. *Chest, 124*(2):644-652.

Pittet, J. F., Mackersie, R. C., & Martin, T. R., et al. (1997). Biological markers of acute lung injury: Prognostic and pathogenic significance. *American Journal of Respiratory Critical Cars Medicine, 155*(4):1187-1205.

Pugin, P., Verghese, G., & Widmer, M., et al. (1999). The alveolar space is the site of intense inflammatory and profibrotic reactions. *Critical Care Medicine, 27*(2):304-312.

Rubenfeld, G. D., Caldwell, E., & Peabody, E., et al. (2005). Incidence and outcomes of acute lung injury. *New England Journal of Medicine, 353*(16):1685-1693.

Ruettimann, U., Ummenhofer, W., & Rueter, F., et al. (2006). Management of acute respiratory distress syndrome using pumpless extracorporeal lung assist. *Canadian Journal of Anaesthesia, 53*(1):101-105.

Salim, A., Martin, M., & Constantinou, C., et al. (2006). Acute respiratory distress syndrome in the trauma intensive care unit: Morbid but not mortal. *Archives of Surgery, 141*(7):655-658.

Sanchez, R., & Toy, P. (2005). Transfusion related acute lung injury: A pediatric perspective. *Pediatric Blood Cancer, 45*(3):255-284.

Stapleton, R. D., Wang, B. M., & Hudson, L. D., et al. (2005). Causes and timing of death in patients with ARDS. *Chest, 128*(2):525-532.

Steinberg, K. P., & Hudson, L. D. (2000). Acute lung injury and acute respiratory distress syndrome: The clinical syndrome. *Clinics in Chest Medicine, 21*(3):401-407.

Suchyta, M. R., Clemmer, T. P., & Elliott, G. C., et al. (1997). Increased mortality of older patients with acute respiratory distress syndrome. *Chest, 111*:1334-1339.

Tomashefski, J. F. Jr., (2000). Pulmonary pathology of acute respiratory distress syndrome. *Clinics in Chest Medicine, 21*(3):435-466.

Wallot, M. A., Dohna-Schwake, C., & Auth, M., et al. (2006). Disseminated adenovirus infection with respiratory failure in pediatric liver transplant recipients: Impact of intravenous cidofovir and inhaled nitric oxide. *Pediatric Transplantation, 10*(1):121-127.

Ware, L. B., & Matthay, M. A. (2000). The acute respiratory distress syndrome. *New England Journal of Medicine, 342*(18):1334-1349.

Weinacker, A. B., & Vaszar, L. T. (2001). Acute respiratory distress syndrome: Physiology and new management strategies. *Annual Review of Medicine, 52*:221-237.

Wydra, D., Emerich, J., & Sawicki, S., et al. (2006). Major complications following exenteration in cases of pelvic malignancy: A 10-year experience. *World Journal of Gastroenterology, 12*(7):1115-1119.

MALIGNANT ASCITES

DEBORAH MURPHY

PATHOPHYSIOLOGICAL MECHANISMS

Malignant ascites, a collection of fluid in the peritoneum, is a serious prognostic event in the progression of several tumors. These tumors include breast, colorectal, gastric, pancreatic, hepatocellular and gynecologic cancers. Metastatic disease to the liver, peritoneal lining, or lung; testicular cancer; and, less frequently, melanoma, also lead to malignant ascites.

According to Enck (2002), malignant ascites is classified into four categories. The first is peripheral ascites, the most common type, which accounts for approximately 50% of all cases. This type of ascites is the result of mechanical interference with venous or lymphatic drainage at the level of the peritoneal space.

The second type of malignant ascites is central ascites. In this type of ascites, the tumor invades the liver, causing compression of the portal and lymphatic systems. The decreased oncotic pressure in malignant ascites is caused by limited protein intake and a catabolic state caused by the cancer, not by impaired liver protein synthesis. This type of ascites accounts for approximately 20% of all cases of malignant ascites.

The third type of malignant ascites is mixed ascites, in which the tumor is present both in the liver and on the peritoneal surface. This type, which accounts for approximately 20% of all cases of malignant ascites, is the effect of combined central and peripheral ascites.

The fourth and least common type of malignant ascites is chylous ascites. In chylous ascites the tumor infiltrates the retroperitoneal space and causes obstruction of the lymph flow.

Because most patients with malignant ascites survive only about 2 months, treatment should be conservative. Loop diuretics may be helpful for patients with central ascites, because portal hypertension responds well to these drugs. Repeat paracentesis can be effective in providing relief of the symptoms associated with ascites, although the patient is at risk for infections or damage to the visceral peritoneum.

In addition to the presence of a tumor, factors that contribute to the development of malignant ascites include interleukin-2; tumor necrosis factor; vascular endothelial growth factors; lymphatic obstruction, leading to decreased outflow from the peritoneal cavity; and vascular permeability (Itano & Taoka, 2005).

EPIDEMIOLOGY AND ETIOLOGY

Approximately 10% to 15% of ascites cases are caused by intraabdominal malignancies. Ascites caused by cirrhosis of the liver usually results in excessive fluid formation; however, some tumors, particularly ovarian tumors, alter humoral factors that increase capillary leakage of proteins and fluids into the peritoneum is increased (Groenwald et al., 1993; Garrison et al., 1986). Decreased absorption of ascitic fluid by the diaphragmatic or abdominal lymphatics and increased production of capillary fluid are contributing factors in ascites. Increased net filtration results from increases in the capillary surface, capillary permeability, and the protein concentration, leading to an increase in peritoneal oncotic pressure (Tamsma et al., 2001).

Causes of malignant ascites include liver metastases and hepatocellular carcinomas that occlude hepatocellular flow; peritoneal carcinomatosis; a combination of extensive liver metastasis and peritoneal carcinomatosis; malignant lymph node obstruction, with lymph overflow into the peritoneal cavity; and Budd-Chiari syndrome, which develops when a tumor occludes the hepatic vein (Runyon, 1999).

RISK PROFILE

- Lymphoma; melanoma; breast, ovarian, colorectal, gastric, pancreatic, hepatobiliary, testicular, and uterine cancers.

- Extensive liver involvement from metastatic disease; cirrhosis; congestive heart failure; nephrosis with protein wasting; and, infrequently, complications of radiation.

- Pancreatic disease, hepatic encephalopathy, infectious peritonitis, and gut lymphatic or thoracic duct injury can be etiologies of ascites (BC Cancer Agency, 2007).

- **Environment:** Exposure to hepatitis has been speculated to be an environmental risk.

- **Foods:** Nonmalignant causes linked to the formation of ascites include long-term alcohol abuse and a high-sodium diet or increased fluid intake with liver or renal disease.

- **Medications:** Noncompliance with drug regimens in chronic renal or liver disease and complications of chemotherapy can lead to ascites. Herbal preparations that can affect the liver include alfalfa, echinacea, garlic, goldenseal, licorice, red clover, and St. John's wort (Wren & Norred, 2003).

PROGNOSIS

Malignant ascites is an indicator of end-stage disease. Treatment focuses on palliation of symptoms, although effective palliation is difficult to achieve. The mean survival time for patients with malignant ascites is less than 4 months, depending on the underlying cancer. However, with the use of peritoneal drains and intraperitoneal chemotherapy, the survival time is increasing.

PROFESSIONAL ASSESSMENT CRITERIA (PAC)

1. **Initial history and physical examination**: vital signs, weight, abdominal girth, and nutrition. The examiner should record any physical signs and symptoms, such as increased abdominal girth, weight gain, lymphadenopathy, liver enlargement, liver flap, shortness of breath, and edema in the lower extremities. Emotional support plays an important role for those whose prognosis is poor.
2. **Assess baseline laboratory panel**: include a complete blood count, chemistries, liver function, prothrombin and partial thromboplastin times, urinalysis and blood cultures to aid in an overall metabolic view of the patient.
3. **Radiographic studies**: chest and abdominal x-ray films to rule out obstruction and computed tomography (CT) scans to detect any tumor growth or obstruction. Magnetic resonance imagining (MRI) can help identify tumor growth, and ultrasound

studies can be used to determine the depth of the tumor, search for free fluid in the abdomen, or assist in guided needle biopsies. Positron emission tomography (PET) scans can help locate areas of malignancy that cannot be detected by CT scans.

4. **Laboratory values:** Paracentesis should be done, and the peritoneal fluid should be sent for cell count, albumin level, culture, total protein, lactate hydrogenase, carcinoembryonic antigen, cytology, a serum ascites albumin gradient (SAAG), and Gram's staining if infection is suspected.

5. A red blood cell count higher than 20,000/mcL indicates either a traumatic tap or malignancy (Shah, 2006).

6. EGF and sCD44v6 levels are significantly higher in patients with malignant ascites than in those with cirrhotic or tuberculous ascites. VEGF levels are higher in patients with ovarian cancer than in patients with gastric or colon cancer (Dong et al., 2003).

NURSING CARE AND TREATMENT

Elevate head of bed to reduce respiratory compromise and alleviate discomfort

Assess pulse, respiration, blood pressure, and temperature

Monitor for fluid shifts and signs of bacterial peritonitis

Monitor fluid balance through intake and output (I and O) measurements

Assess abdomen and measure girth

Weigh the patient

Assess for lymphadenopathy and lymphedema

Assess for gastroenteral and urologic distress caused by increased abdominal pressure

Monitor function of ascitic drains or shunts if in place

Bed rest

Low-sodium, high-protein, fluid-restricted diet

Diuretic therapy

Serum electrolytes, complete blood count (CBC) daily

Antacids for indigestion as needed

After paracentesis monitor for:
- Hypotension related to hypovolemia or fluid shift
- Infection or peritonitis

After peritoneovenous shunting monitor for:
- Heart failure or pulmonary edema caused by rapid infusion of peritoneal fluid intravascularly
- Disseminated intravascular coagulation caused by procoagulants in ascitic fluid

- Shunt malfunction caused by malposition
- Potential fluid volume deficit and potential electrolyte imbalance caused by increased diuresis
- Infection caused by contamination of the intravascular or intraperitoneal system

Assess:
- Pulmonary status (breath sounds, labor of respirations, oxygen saturation) q4h
- Abdomen for rigidity
- For gastrointestinal/genitourinary (GI/GU) compromise
- Paracentesis site or shunt placement incision for signs of infection daily
- Patient comfort q4h
- Weight pattern to evaluate the effectiveness of interventions
- Patient and family coping on a daily basis

Measure:
- Temperature, respirations, pulse, blood pressure q4h
- I and O q8h
- Weight daily
- Abdominal girth daily
- Urine specific gravity daily

Send:
- CBC, serum electrolytes daily
- Drained ascitic fluid for specific gravity, protein count, cell count, bacteriology, amylase, carcinoembryonic antigen (CEA) (Kehoe, 1991)

Implement:
- Activity restriction
- Low-sodium, high-protein, fluid-restricted diet

The cause of the ascites should be determined based on the patient's history and the physical examination findings. Abdominal paracentesis is performed to determine the etiology of the ascites. Bloody or serosanguineous fluid characterizes malignant ascites. Cirrhotic, nephritic, pancreatic, or cardiac disease results in serous fluid; cloudy fluid is characteristic of infectious peritonitis (Runyon, 1994).

Treatment of malignant ascites is directed toward symptom control. Generally the medical approach is initiated with noninvasive options and proceeds to more invasive treatments as the malignant ascites becomes more refractory.

Management of pain is a priority. Antiemetics and having the patient eat smaller, more frequent meals can relieve abdominal discomfort. Sodium restriction and diuretics can be tried but usually are ineffective.

Peripheral edema and dyspnea are caused by fluid accumulation in the abdomen as a result of poor lymphatic drainage; these symptoms can be managed with paracentesis to drain the fluid.

Initial surgery may be performed to debulk the tumor, but these patients' poor prognosis does not warrant the risk of surgery.

The primary method of treatment for ascites is drainage of the peritoneal fluid. The use of Silastic catheters for peritoneal shunting (e.g., the LeVeen® or the Denver® shunt) has been evolving over the past several decades. The catheters are implanted in the abdominal cavity and tunneled into the superior vena cava to enhance drainage. The Denver® drain is preferred by many surgeons, because it can be pumped manually to prevent clogging (Yarbro et al., 2005). Shunts have been associated with several risk factors, and the current recommendation is to use them only when the ascites proves refractory to other treatments. This is especially true when the patient has ovarian cancer, because in these cases, ascites appears in the early stages and can be controlled with a hysterosalpingo-oophorectomy. Surgical placement of a Silastic catheter into the peritoneal space may relieve the symptoms, but multiple complications can occur, predisposing the shunt to infection, occlusion of flow, or both.

Tube kinking and tip malposition are immediate technical failures. Later failure of the shunt can occur from fibrin clot formation and accumulation of debris at the valve. Leakage of ascitic fluid at the peritoneal site increases the risk of infection.

Removal of approximately 50% of the fluid during catheter placement reduces the potential for fluid overload after shunt placement.

According to Iyenger and Herzog (2002), the Pleurex® drain, which allows external drainage of peritoneal fluid, has been used successfully to control recurrent ascites. Use of the Pleurex drain reduces the risk of infection, because repeated paracentesis is not necessary.

Intraperitoneal administration of chemotherapeutic agents (e.g., doxorubicin, 5-fluorouracil, mitoxantrone, and cisplatin) has reduced the amount of ascitic fluid in patients with ascites (Yarbro et al., 2005). However, infusion of these drugs poses the risk of bleeding, infection, or chemical peritonitis, which can cause significant morbidity.

Biologic response modifiers (e.g., interferon alpha and interleukin-2) have been used with some success to reduce the amount of ascitic fluid. The risks posed by biologic response modifiers include peritoneal fibrosis and abdominal pain.

Radiation therapy is not indicated, other than as part of the treatment regimen for the causative type of cancer.

Loop diuretics and aldosterone-inhibiting diuretics may be prescribed, although their efficacy in malignant ascites is poor compared to their effect in ascites secondary to cirrhosis. A study by Greenway and colleagues (1982) found that high doses of spironolactone (150 to 450 mg/day) reduced the malignant peritoneal effusions in 13 of 15 patients. Additional research is needed to explore high-dose drug therapy further. Use of diuretics should be considered in all patients but should be evaluated on an individual basis (Becker et al., 2006).

Repeat paracentesis may be offered, but complications from frequent abdominal taps can include protein depletion, postural hypotension, and electrolyte abnormalities.

Repeated insertion of a paracentesis catheter into the abdomen can cause infection (Belfort et al., 1990). In most cases an indwelling catheter is inserted to facilitate intermittent drainage of the peritoneal fluid.

A low-sodium, high-protein diet and fluid restrictions may be used, but their efficacy is poor.

EVIDENCE-BASED PRACTICE UPDATES

1. Paracentesis is the key to diagnosis.
2. Intraperitoneal chemotherapy is available to patients who are not expected to respond to systemic or radiation therapy.

3. Peritoneovenous shunts are more valuable for management of nonmalignant ascites than for resistive malignant ascites (Horton, 2001).
4. Intraperitoneal chemotherapy can improve patients' quality of life.
5. Levels of VEGF proteins are higher in patients with ovarian and primary peritoneal carcinoma and can be helpful in differential diagnosis of benign verses malignant ascites (Dong et al., 2003).
6. A SAAG of less than 1:1 is consistent with nonportal hypertensive ascites.
7. Malignant ascites can be distinguished from cirrhotic ascites by the presence of high LDH and cholesterol levels in the peritoneal fluid (D'Auria & Caldwell, 2001).

TEACHING AND EDUCATION

Ascites management: *Rationale:* Your doctors have shared with you that your cancer is causing excess fluid to build up in your belly. This fluid is called *ascites*. Your doctor may try to control the fluid in a number of different ways, including limiting your activity, changing your diet, limiting the amount of fluid you drink, ordering special medications, draining the fluid through a needle, or possibly surgery. Although you may be able to get rid of the extra water through these methods, you may also find that none of these treatments works well. Remember, these treatments are intended to help you feel more comfortable.

Limit activity: *Rationale:* Resting in bed with your head propped up will give your lungs more room to expand. This will help you breathe easier. More rest will also help you get rid of the extra water.

Dietary changes: *Rationale:* Drinking less fluid and eating food without salt may help prevent your body from adding any more fluid. Eating small meals several times a day will help with your indigestion and also help prevent you from feeling so full.

Blood sampling: *Rationale:* Blood samples may be taken as often as every day. These allow us to watch for changes in the minerals in your body. If such changes occur, you may need medication to make sure you feel better.

Monitoring of I and O: *Rationale:* It is important that we measure what you drink and measure your urine to keep your body in balance and to see if the treatments are working.

Abdominal girth and weight: *Rationale:* By measuring around your gut and weighing you, we can see how well the extra fluid (ascites) is coming off.

Treatments: Your doctor has decided to use the following treatment to help your body get rid of the extra fluid.

> **Paracentesis:** *Rationale:* Paracentesis is done to take out some of the fluid (ascites) that is causing you discomfort and making it hard for you to breathe. After a spot on your stomach is numbed, a needle is inserted to drain the fluid.

> **Intracavitary chemotherapy or radiation:** *Rationale:* Chemotherapeutic drugs or a radiation source can be placed directly inside your gut during surgery or through a small tube to try to kill the cancer cells that may be causing the fluid buildup.

Shunt: *Rationale:* In a surgical procedure, a tube can be put inside you that will drain or "shunt" the fluid inside your gut into a vein. This procedure will help your body control the fluid better and may help you feel more comfortable. The tube may have a pump, in which case you will need to push on it to help drain the fluid. Ask your nurse or doctor if this is the kind of tube you will have. They also will show you how to pump the tube.

NURSING DIAGNOSES

1. **Impaired gas exchange** related to the accumulation of ascites with diaphragmatic displacement
2. **Deficient fluid volume** related to drainage or shunting of ascites, osmotic shift with hypoalbuminemia, diuresis with spironolactone or furosemide, increased antidiuretic hormone (ADH)
3. **Risk for activity intolerance** related to respiratory compromise, weakness secondary to anorexia
4. **Anxiety** related to respiratory compromise, physical deterioration, poor prognosis, end-stage disease
5. **Risk for infection** related to indwelling catheter: repeated insertion of a paracentesis catheter, leakage of ascitic fluid at the insertion site

EVALUATION AND DESIRED OUTCOMES

1. Decreased abdominal girth.
2. Improved respiratory status, less-labored breathing.
3. Decreased anorexia, indigestion.
4. Activity, dietary, and fluid restrictions are understood by the patient and caregivers.
5. Patient and significant others show effective coping skills related to the prognosis.

DISCHARGE PLANNING AND FOLLOW-UP CARE

- Long-term assistance with the activities of daily living, depending on the severity of the remaining symptoms.
- Hospice referral, because the prognosis for a patient with this complication often is poor. Under hospice care, the patient and significant others can receive the attention that will help meet their needs during this anxious and stressful time.
- Caregiver teaching about comfort measures, signs of infection, and severe respiratory compromise, all of which may require medical intervention.
- Discussion of advance directives and the patient's wishes with regard to life support. These issues should be addressed early in the course of the disease. If life support decisions have not been made before the patient reaches the terminal stage, the health care provider must initiate and facilitate this discussion. The patient's wishes should be respected and will guide the nurse in giving caregivers appropriate information about comfort measures and when to seek medical intervention. Should the patient choose to decline further medical intervention, the patient and caregivers must be taught what to expect at the end of life (see Chapter 13)
- Continuation of dietary and fluid recommendations, including a high-protein, low-sodium diet.

REVIEW QUESTIONS

QUESTIONS

1. **Malignant ascites is the result of:**
   1. Pulmonary edema
   2. Cardiac insufficiency
   3. Compromised drainage of peritoneal lymphatics
   4. Chemotherapy toxicity

2. **The median survival time for a patient diagnosed with malignant ascites is:**
   1. 4 months
   2. 6 months
   3. 1 year
   4. 5 years

3. **The goal of treatment of malignant ascites is:**
   1. Restoration of previous status/ Karnofsky score
   2. Palliation of symptoms
   3. Absence of micrometastases in the ascitic fluid
   4. Decreased potential for liver failure

4. **The most common treatment options for malignant ascites are diuretics, dietary management, paracentesis, and:**
   1. Peritoneovenous shunting
   2. Intraperitoneal chemotherapy
   3. Intracavitary radiation
   4. Metered-dose inhalers

5. **Nursing assessments of the patient with malignant ascites should include:**
   1. Neurologic integrity
   2. Evaluation of serum uric acid
   3. Pulmonary assessment
   4. Sensory deficits

6. **A nursing diagnosis that could be used for a patient who has malignant ascites is:**
   1. Deficient fluid volume
   2. Acute confusion
   3. Functional urinary incontinence
   4. Impaired swallowing

7. **Nursing interventions for a patient with malignant ascites should include:**
   1. Abdominal assessment and girth measurement
   2. Oxygen therapy
   3. Postural drainage
   4. Placement of a urinary catheter

8. **Patient education regarding malignant ascites should include:**
   1. Elevation of edematous extremities
   2. Valsalva maneuvers
   3. Dietary and activity restrictions
   4. Use of a metered-dose inhaler

9. **Peritoneovenous shunting:**
   1. Is always a successful method of managing ascites
   2. Should be the first line of treatment after malignant ascites is diagnosed
   3. May provide relief of discomfort from ascites if other medical treatments fail
   4. Has few problems after insertion of the shunt

10. **The formation of malignant ascitic fluid is caused by all of the following *except:***
    1. Invasion of the subdiaphragmatic lymphatic channels, resulting in inhibition of fluid drainage
    2. Excessive fluid formation
    3. Increased capillary leakage
    4. Hydrodynamic disequilibrium

ANSWERS

1. *Answer: 3*
   Rationale: Malignant lymph node obstruction causes lymph overflow into the peritoneal cavity.

2. *Answer: 1*
   Rationale: The use of implanted drains and shunts has increased the survival time for these patients. Studies have shown that patients survive 1 to 6 months, and the average survival time is 4 months.

3. *Answer: 2*
   Rationale: Malignant ascites is an indicator of end-stage disease, therefore palliation of symptoms is the goal.

4. *Answer: 1*
   Rationale: Peritoneovenous shunting alleviates the symptoms of ascites.

5. *Answer: 3*
   Rationale: Ascites can cause diaphragmatic displacement, resulting in respiratory compromise.

6. *Answer: 1*
   Rationale: The treatment of ascites usually includes the use of diuretics, which can cause an intravascular fluid volume deficit.

7. *Answer: 1*
   Rationale: Fluid accumulation can be monitored by measuring the abdominal girth and assessing the abdomen.

8. *Answer: 3*
   Rationale: Activity restrictions are important because fatigue and respiratory compromise can be limiting factors for patients with malignant ascites. Dietary recommendations should include small, frequent, low-sodium meals to aid the management of anorexia symptoms, as well as sodium restriction to reduce fluid retention and water weight.

9. *Answer: 3*
   Rationale: A peritoneovenous shunt may relieve ascites, but it should be used only if other treatment methods have failed to alleviate the symptoms.

10. *Answer: 2*
    Rationale: Excessive fluid formation usually is related to cirrhosis of the liver rather than a metastatic disease process.

REFERENCES

BC Cancer Agency. (2007). *Malignant ascites*. In *Telephone consultation protocols*. Retrieved June 30, 2007 from http://www.bccancer.bc.ca/HP/Nursing/References/TelconsultProtocols/default.htm.

Becker, G., Galandi, D., & Blum, H. E. (2006). Malignant ascites: Systematic review and guideline for treatment. *European Journal of Cancer, 42*(5):589-597.

Belfort, M. A., Stevens, P. J., & DeHaek, K. et al. (1990). A new approach to the management of malignant ascites, a permanently implanted abdominal drain. *European Journal of Surgical Oncology, 16*(1):47-53.

D'Auria, S., & Caldwell, S. (2001). Ascites and spontaneous bacterial peritonitis. *Best Practice of Medicine*. Retrieved at www.merck.micromedex.com.

Dong, W., Sun, X., & Yu, B., et al. (2003). Role of VEGF and CD44v6 in differentiating benign from malignant ascites. *World Journal of Gastroenterology, 9*(11):2596-2600.

Enck, R. E. (2002). Malignant ascites. *American Journal of Hospice and Palliative Care, 19*(1):7-8.

Fraught, W., Kirkpatrick, J. R., & Krepart, G. V. et al. (1995). Peritoneovenous shunt for palliation or gynecologic malignant ascites. *Journal of the American College of Surgery, 180*:427-474.

Garrison, R. N., Kaelin, L. D., & Heusser, L. S. et al. (1986). Malignant ascites. Clinical and experimental observations. *Annals of Surgery, 203*(6):644-651.

Greenway, B., Johnson, P. J., & Williams, R. (1982). Control of malignant ascites with spironolactone. *British Journal of Surgery, 69*(8):441-442.

Groenwald, S. L., Frogge, M. H., & Goodman, M., et al. (1993). *Cancer nursing: Principles and practice*. Boston: Jones and Bartlett.

Horton, J. K. (2001). Hospice: Care when there is no cure, *North Carolina Medical Journal, 62*(2):86-90.

Itano, J. K., & Taoka, K. N. (2005). *Core curriculum for oncology nursing*, (4th ed.). St. Louis: Saunders.

Iyengar, T. D., & Herzog, T. J. (2002). Management of symptomatic ascites in recurrent ovarian cancer patients using an intra-abdominal semi-permanent catheter. *American Journal of Hospice and Palliative Care, 19*(1):35-38.

Kehoe, C. (1991). Malignant ascites: Etiology, diagnosis, and treatment. *Oncology Nursing Forum, 18*(3):523-530.

Runyon, B. A. (1994). Care of patients with ascites. *New England Journal of Medicine, 330*(5):337-342.

Runyon, B. A. (1999). Approach to the patient with ascites. In T.O.H.C. *Textbook of gastroenterology* (3rd ed.).

Shah, R. (2006). Ascites. *Medicine*. Retrieved from www.emedicine.com.

Tamsma, J. T., Keizer, H. J., & Meinders, A. E., (2001). Pathogenesis of malignant ascites: Starling's law of capillary hemodynamics revisited. *Annals of Oncology, 12*(10):1353-1357.

Wren, K. R., & Norred, C. L. (2003). *Complementary and alternative therapies*. Philadelphia: WB Saunders.

Yarbro, C. H., Frogge, M. H., & Goodman (6th ed.). Sudbury, MA: Jones and Bartlett.

BRONCHIOLITIS OBLITERANS
(Bronchiolitis Obliterans Organizing Pneumonia)

LAURA MILLIGAN • YVONNE D. MARTIN

PATHOPHYSIOLOGICAL MECHANISMS

Bronchiolitis obliterans organizing pneumonia (BOOP) is a phenomenon that has been studied and documented in the literature since 1901 (Holland et al., 1988). As Ezri and colleagues (1994) stated, it is "a relatively rare disease whose precise prevalence is unknown."

BOOP primarily damages the small conducting airways. The physiologic and radiographic findings are very similar to those of chronic obstructive pulmonary disease (COPD) (King, 1989). King (1989) notes that some of the processes may appear restrictive or both restrictive and obstructive; consequently, bronchiolitis obliterans may be confused with other diffuse infiltrative ventilatory lung disorders. For the purposes of this chapter, bronchiolitis obliterans is discussed as it applies to oncology patients, specifically individuals who have received an allogeneic bone marrow transplant (BMT).

Bronchiolitis obliterans occurs infrequently in patients who have received an allogeneic BMT. It affects approximately 10% of patients with chronic graft versus host disease (GVHD). It also has been identified in patients who received autologous transplants. The disease can present as a mixed restrictive and obstructive process, making diagnosis difficult.

Bronchiolitis obliterans is a pulmonary disease that primarily affects the conductive bronchioles. It is marked by partial or complete obliteration of the bronchiolar lumena either by plugs of granulation tissue or by fibrosis and scarring (Ezri et al., 1994; King, 1989). Bronchiolitis obliterans caused by the deposition of granulation tissue sometimes is referred to as *proliferative bronchiolitis obliterans*. Bronchiolitis obliterans caused by scarring is referred to as *constrictive* or *obstructive bronchiolitis obliterans*.

Proliferative bronchiolitis obliterans is most often characterized by an inflammatory process involving the respiratory bronchioles and alveoli. The resulting defect is restrictive. Understanding the exact defect is important for establishing the prognosis and evaluating the response to treatment. The restrictive, inflammatory defect of proliferative bronchiolitis obliterans is potentially reversible. Obstructive bronchiolitis obliterans, however, is irreversible, because the established fibrosis affects the proximal bronchioles (Ezri et al., 1994).

In the hematology and oncology literature, bronchiolitis obliterans has been described in patients with irradiation pneumonitis (Kaufman & Komorowoski, 1990), amphotericin B toxicity (Roncoroni et al., 1990), autologous BMT (Paz et al., 1992), and allogeneic BMT (King, 1989). Bronchiolitis obliterans occurs in patients who have received hematopoietic stem cell transplants, but it is uncommon. The term *hematopoietic stem cell transplant* (HSCT) has supplanted the previously used term *bone marrow transplant* to reflect the broader range of donor stem cell sources that are now available (e.g., bone marrow, fetal cord blood, and growth factor–stimulated peripheral blood) (Kotloff et al., 2004).

The exact pathogenesis of bronchiolitis obliterans in patients who have received an allogeneic BMT has not been determined. However, Ezri and colleagues (1994), King (1989), and Crawford and Clark (1993) all agree that the presence of chronic GVHD probably affects the development of this pulmonary complication.

Ezri and colleagues (1994) described "enhanced expression of major histocompatibility (MHC) class II antigens on bronchiolar epithelium...associated with cytotoxic T lymphocyte infiltration." The assumption is that this is the initiating factor in a vicious cycle of inflammation and fibrosis. Similarly, King (1989) discusses a "lymphocytic bronchitis, characterized by lymphocyte-associated necrosis of the bronchial mucosa and submucosal glands." In this case, lymphocytic bronchitis is thought to be a pulmonary manifestation of GVHD. King (1989) also discusses two additional theories to explain the pathogenesis of BOOP. Lung biopsies in many BMT patients suspected of having bronchiolitis obliterans have shown marked lymphocyte or plasma cell infiltration of the terminal respiratory bronchioles and obliteration of the bronchiolar lumina with interstitial fibrosis. Chronic GVHD is associated with a fibrosing mechanism in other organs, therefore bronchiolar fibrosis may be an additional manifestation of chronic GVHD. Also, chronic GVHD often contributes to esophageal and sinus disease, which may result in recurrent esophageal aspiration; this could contribute to and further complicate the lung injury.

Crawford and Clark (1993) described a review of 21 BMT patients with pulmonary symptoms. Sixteen of the 21 patients showed small airway involvement with bronchiolitis, only occasionally with fibrinous obliteration of the bronchiolar lumena. The remaining five patients showed evidence only of bronchitis or interstitial pneumonia. This study shows that bronchiolitis obliterans is not always the causative factor for respiratory symptoms in BMT patients.

Paz and colleagues (1992) described the first reported cases of bronchiolitis obliterans in patients who had undergone autologous BMT without demonstrating chronic GVHD. Preparative regimens, the possibility of underlying infection, underlying connective tissue disorder, and an autoimmune response were postulated as possible initiators; however, no clear causative factors were identified in these patients. The important point is that the possibility of bronchiolitis obliterans must be considered in patients who develop clinical signs and symptoms consistent with the disorder after autologous BMT. (See Chapter 14 for further information on GVHD.)

Patients with BOOP usually develop respiratory complaints such as a dry, nonproductive cough; dyspnea on exertion; bibasilar rales and scattered wheezes; and hypoxemia (King, 1989). The chest radiograph may be read as normal or hyperinflated. Most sources report that physical examination is not particularly helpful early in the diagnostic process. Pulmonary function tests and, most likely, lung biopsy are required to confirm the diagnosis.

EPIDEMIOLOGY AND ETIOLOGY

The etiologies implicated in bronchiolitis obliterans include viruses, toxic fume exposure, connective tissue disease, drugs or organ transplantation ("immune" bronchiolitis obliterans), and idiopathic factors (Ezri et al.,1994). The incidence of bronchiolitis obliterans in patients who have undergone allogeneic BMT is approximately 2% to 10% (Paz et al., 1992). As previously mentioned, a few cases have been documented in patients who had received an autologous transplant (Ezri et al, 1994; King, 1989; Crawford & Clark, 1993.)

RISK PROFILE

The following risk factors occur in both adult and pediatric patients. They can be divided into two categories: immunologic risk factors and nonimmunologic risk factors.

Immunologic risk factors:

- GVHD
- Lymphocytic bronchitis/bronchiolitis
- Human leukocyte antigen (HLA) mismatching

Nonimmunologic risk factors:

- Cytomegalovirus (CMV)
- Non-CMV infections (CAP (candida-acquired pneumonia), Influenza)

Cancers: Any malignancy or hematologic disorder for which allogeneic BMT is a treatment option (rare incidence with autologous BMT).

Conditions: Chronic GVHD; treatment of chronic GVHD with methotrexate; (possibly) low serum immunoglobulin level; irradiation pneumonitis; chronic allograft dysfunction after lung transplantation (Pakhale et al., 2005); older age (adults).

Drugs: Methotrexate (for immunosuppression of GVHD), amphotericin B (single case report), amiodarone (Sveinsson et al., 2006).

PROGNOSIS

Patients undergoing BMT are a risk for multiple pulmonary side effects. An accurate differential diagnosis is necessary to establish the prognosis. Once the diagnosis of bronchiolitis obliterans has been established, the prognosis usually is poor. Epler (1988) reported that bronchiolitis obliterans in association with BMT has a poor prognosis and does not respond well to steroid treatment. Fort and Graham-Pole (1990) stated that bronchiolitis obliterans is both irreversible and unresponsive to treatment; bronchiolitis obliterans progresses to recurrent pneumothoraces and hypoxia, which result in death. In a study by Schwarer and colleagues (1992), no identifying infectious component was found in 29 patients who developed late onset pulmonary syndrome (LOPS), and six of the patients (21%) died. According to these researchers, LOPS is the most frequent cause of nonrelapse death in patients 6 months after BMT. In the Schwarer study, the designation *LOPS* included airflow obstruction associated with bronchiolitis obliterans or interstitial lung disease, or both. Paz and colleagues (1992) studied 104 patients who underwent allogeneic BMT; 3.9% developed bronchiolitis obliterans. Crawford and Clark (1993) stated, "The clinical course is variable, but the process usually is fatal in cases with rapidly progressive or severe obstruction."

PROFESSIONAL ASSESSMENT CRITERIA (PAC)

1. **Vital signs:** Normal or elevated temperature; rapid pulse; rapid, dyspneic respiratory rate; normal, elevated or decreased blood pressure

2. **Symptoms, conditions:** Dry, nonproductive cough; wheezing and dyspnea on exertion (DOE); chronic GVHD; infection (e.g., pneumonia, sinusitis)
3. **Hallmark physical signs and symptoms:** Cough, wheeze, DOE despite normal chest radiograph
4. **Additional physical signs and symptoms:** Cachexia
5. **Psychosocial signs:** Anxiety, fear, confusion, exhaustion
6. **Laboratory values:** Elevated WBC (if counts were previously normal) or decreased WBC, with decreased neutrophils and thrombocytopenia. Results vary, depending on other patient factors (e.g., presence of infection, previous bone marrow recovery, or presence of GVHD).; increased BUN; increased creatinine; elevated transaminases (three to six times higher than normal in GVHD); moderately elevated total bilirubin (GVHD); elevated alkaline phosphatase (five to 10 times higher than normal in GVHD); decreased immunoglobulin G (IgG) levels (controversial)
7. **Cultures:** Blood, urine, and sputum cultures positive (with underlying infection) or negative
8. **Diagnostic tests:** Chest radiographs (posteroanterior and lateral) normal, hyperinflated, or diffuse interstitial infiltrates; decreased diffusing capacity; ABGs: hypoxemia, hypocarbia; variable findings with bronchoscopy (depending on underlying infection; positive transbronchial or open lung biopsy; computed tomography (CT) scan of the lung usually not beneficial
9. **Pulmonary function tests:** decreased forced expiratory volume (FEV_1) and flow rates; increased functional residual capacity (FRC); normal total lung capacity (TLC);
10. **Other:** Assess activity tolerance and nutritional status

NURSING CARE AND TREATMENT

Early recognition and treatment of bronchiolitis obliterans is important, because treatment often is ineffective when the disease has reached the late, fibrotic stage (Moore, 2003)

Chemotherapy: Cyclophosphamide—not yet established (Crawford & Clark, 1993).

Medications: Corticosteroids continue to be the drugs of choice for the treatment of BOOP, sometimes in conjunction with cyclosporine.
  Investigation of the immunologic mechanism of GVHD (Epler, 1988)
  Azathioprine
  Tacrolimus and thalidomide—not yet established (Crawford & Clark, 1993)
  Adjunct therapy
  Trimethoprim-sulfamethoxazole
  Penicillin
  IgG (if serum levels are low)
  Bronchodilator (small percentage of users respond)
  Inhaled corticosteroids—not yet established

Immediate nursing interventions

- Monitor respiratory rate, depth, and effort, including use of accessory muscles, nasal flaring, and abnormal breathing patterns.
- Assess pulse, blood pressure, and temperature initially; assess respiratory status q1-2h.
- Apply pulse oximeter.
- Place oxygen and suction equipment at bedside.
- Maintain patient safety.

- Reassure patient that his or her needs will be met.
- Ensure patent IV access.

Anticipated physician prescriptions and interventions

- Arterial blood gases (ABGs)
- Oxygen therapy
- STAT chest radiograph
- High-resolution CT scan (HRCT)
- Transbronchial lung biopsy
- STAT labs: CBC with platelet count, complete
- Metabolic panel, coagulation panel
- Antibiotics
- Pulse oximeter
- Bronchoscopy
- Transbronchial or open lung biopsy
- Initiation of immunosuppressive therapy for chronic GVHD (e.g., corticosteroids, cyclosporine)
- Bronchodilator therapy
- IV replacement of IgG

Ongoing nursing assessment, monitoring, and interventions

Assess:

- Level of consciousness q4h and PRN
- Signs of chronic GVHD (skin, gastrointestinal tract, and liver)
- Signs of infection (bacterial, fungal, or viral)
- Activity tolerance
- Emotional response
- IV site for redness, edema, or pain q4h and PRN

Measure:

- Pulse oximetry q2h and PRN
- Blood pressure, pulse, respiration, and temperature q4h and PRN
- Weight daily

Initiate:

- Oxygen therapy as ordered
- Activity restrictions PRN, as ordered
- Ethical discussions and planning with the patient, family or significant other, and the health care team, as appropriate

EVIDENCE-BASED PRACTICE UPDATES

1. Pegylated filgrastim or rituximab may be causes of BOOP (Macartney et al., 2005).
2. Patients receiving tangential irradiation for breast cancer should be monitored for BOOP (Takai et al., 2006).
3. Patients with lung cancer treated with docetaxel and gemcitabine should be monitored for BOOP (Cobo-Dols et al., 2006).
4. The antirheumatic drug bucillamine can cause BOOP (Kajiya et al., 2006).

TEACHING AND EDUCATION

Chest x-ray films: *Rationale:* An x-ray film of your lungs is taken to assess or evaluate complaints you may have of shortness of breath.

Vital signs: *Rationale:* The nurse will be measuring your blood pressure, pulse, respiratory rate, and temperature frequently to make sure they are not too high or too low.

ABGs: *Rationale:* A blood sample is drawn from the artery in your wrist so that we can determine whether the bloodstream is carrying enough oxygen.

Pulse oximeter placement: *Rationale:* A plastic clip or sticky tape will be placed on your finger so that we can determine whether enough oxygen is present in the bloodstream. The machine beeps because it is monitoring your heartbeat; if an alarm sounds, you should call the nurse.

Oxygen: *Rationale:* To help relieve your shortness of breath, oxygen will be given either through the nostrils or over the nose and mouth.

Activity restriction: *Rationale:* You may need to limit your activity level because of your shortness of breath, and your condition may cause you to tire easily. The nurses will help you with your meals, your bath, and with walking to the bathroom.

IV blood samples: *Rationale:* Blood samples are needed so that we can check the amount of oxygen, as well as blood sugar levels and kidney function. We may need to take several samples; if you have a central line, the blood will be drawn from this line.

Drug therapy—steroids: *Rationale:* You may be started on a drug called a *steroid* to reduce the congestion in your lungs; this will help you breathe better. The steroid may make you feel anxious or may cause swelling; please tell your doctor or nurse if you notice these changes.

Other drugs: *Rationale:* The doctor may start you on other drugs during your treatment. The nurses will explain any new drugs to you; please ask them to explain anything you do not understand.

Pulmonary function tests (PFTs): *Rationale:* We may need to test how well your lungs are working. For this test, you will be asked to breathe into a machine that puts the results on a graph for your doctor to read.

Bronchoscopy: *Rationale:* A tube may need to be placed through your nose and down into your lungs; this tube has a tiny camera on the end that allows the doctor to look at your lungs. The doctor may also take a sample of lung tissue to examine under a microscope. The doctor will give you medicine so that the procedure will not be uncomfortable.

Intensive care unit: *Rationale:* You may need to be transferred to an intensive care unit so that you can be watched more closely by the critical care nurses.

Anticipated patient/family questions and possible answers

Will I get better?
   "It is hard to know at this point. We will be watching you closely to see how your body accepts this treatment."
   "It depends on how you respond to the treatments. Each person responds differently."

How have other people done who have had this same problem?

"Each person responds differently. Some do well, and others have more problems. We will have to evaluate your progress as we go along."

"Everyone is different. Let's concentrate on what we can do to make you better."

Is there anything I can do to make this better?

"The disease will get better if and when your body accepts the treatment. You can help yourself in a number of ways. For example, (1) avoid doing things that make you breathe harder, such as exercise not approved by your doctor; (2) avoid people who have a cold or the flu so that you don't get an infection; (3) eat a healthful diet to help your body fight these problems; (4) do not return to work unless your doctor says it's okay; (5) let your doctor know if you are upset, have trouble sleeping, are unable to eat, feel helpless and out of control, or are just really angry at everyone and everything."

Why do I need to keep repeating these tests?

"We need to see whether your body is accepting the treatment or if changes need to be made that might help things get better."

Why did I get a bone marrow transplant if this was going to happen?

"Treatment for any disease or medical problem carries risks. If you hadn't gotten the bone marrow transplant, your cancer would have come back, and there may have been no way to control it."

"Remember, when you were making the decision to have the bone marrow transplant, we discussed that it was your best option for survival despite possible side effects or problems."

"This condition is a rare complication of bone marrow transplantation. The transplant was necessary to treat your type of cancer. We need to work together to see what we can do to best treat your problems."

NURSING DIAGNOSES

The nursing diagnoses will vary, depending on the specific patient situation. The following are some of the common diagnoses and etiologies.
1. **Activity intolerance** related to dyspnea on exertion secondary to bronchiolitis obliterans
2. **Anxiety** related to acute onset of disease and uncertain outcome
3. **Fatigue** related to exertional dyspnea secondary to bronchiolitis obliterans
4. **Impaired gas exchange** related to restrictive and/or obstructive respiratory dysfunction secondary to bronchiolitis obliterans
5. **Risk for infection** related to suppressed immune system secondary to treatment (e.g., preparative chemotherapy regimen and immunosuppressive agents); also related to injured respiratory system secondary to bronchiolitis obliterans

EVALUATION AND DESIRED OUTCOMES

1. Shortness of breath is relieved within 4 hours.
2. Differential diagnoses are established within 48 hours.
3. Drug therapy is initiated within 2 hours; the need for concomitant antibiotic therapy will be evaluated.
4. Blood and platelet transfusion needs are established within 4 hours and blood products are initiated within 6 hours.

5. The patient in unstable condition is transferred to the ICU within 4 hours if assessment establishes need.
6. Bronchoscopy and PFTs are performed within 24 hours.

DISCHARGE PLANNING AND FOLLOW-UP CARE

The prognosis for patients diagnosed with bronchiolitis obliterans after BMT is usually poor (Ezri et al., 1994; Crawford & Clark, 1993). Although few patients leave the hospital, potential discharge planning needs are outlined below.

Bronchiolitis obliterans patient may need

Oxygen therapy
Enteral or parenteral nutrition to meet increasing nutritional needs.
Home nursing visits, hospice (if bronchiolitis obliterans is progressive), or significant other to manage enteral and parenteral nutritional needs
Short-term intermediate care facility, daily home nursing visits, or trained significant other to administer IV antibiotics or IV IgG, if needed
Custodial caregiver for assistance with activities of daily living
Chaplain or social worker to assist psychosocial adjustment to diagnosis

Anticipated follow-up care may include

Physician office visit within 1 to 2 weeks
PFTs, chest x-ray films, and bronchoscopy monthly if condition continues to deteriorate
CBC and platelet count at outpatient laboratory weekly
Other laboratory tests as appropriate (e.g., liver functions, BUN/creatinine, immunoglobulins)
Evaluation of any signs of infection (cultures)
Home nursing visits (frequency depends on the patient's needs)
   Community oncology nurses who provide care for patients who have had HSCT must be able to recognize treatment-related complications. Each time a patient is seen, the following should be reviewed:
   • Complete medications list
   • Weight
   • Performance status (e.g., Karnofsky score)
   • Routine laboratory work (i.e., CBC with differential, complete metabolic panel, IgG level)

REVIEW QUESTIONS

QUESTIONS

1. **The development of bronchiolitis obliterans is associated with:**
   1. Pneumocystis carinii
   2. GVHD
   3. Tuberculosis
   4. Fungal sepsis

2. **Diagnostic testing for bronchiolitis obliterans includes all of the following *except:***
   1. Pulmonary function tests
   2. ABGs
   3. Echocardiogram (ECHO)
   4. Bronchoscopy

3. **Etiologies implicated in the development of bronchiolitis obliterans include all of the following *except:***
   1. Toxic fume exposure
   2. Bone marrow transplantation
   3. Viral exposure
   4. Electrical shock

4. **Bronchiolitis obliterans results primarily in:**
   1. Restrictive and constrictive lung disease
   2. Only restrictive lung disease
   3. Only constrictive lung disease
   4. Neither restrictive nor constrictive lung disease

5. **Investigational drug therapies for the treatment of bronchiolitis obliterans include which of the following chemotherapeutic agents:**
   1. Methotrexate
   2. Mitoxantrone
   3. Cisplatin
   4. Cyclophosphamide

6. **A nursing diagnosis that is *not* appropriate for a patient with bronchiolitis obliterans is:**
   1. Risk for infection
   2. Impaired gas exchange
   3. Decreased cardiac output
   4. Anxiety

7. **Signs of bronchiolitis obliterans include:**
   1. Cough and dyspnea on exertion
   2. Edema
   3. Decreased transaminases and increased immunoglobulins
   4. Negative lung biopsy

8. **A common risk factor for the development of bronchiolitis obliterans is:**
   1. Allogeneic BMT
   2. High serum IgG levels
   3. Veno-occlusive disease
   4. Lung cancer

9. **A patient evaluated for bronchiolitis obliterans most likely would be taught about which of the following diagnostic procedures:**
   1. Endoscopy
   2. Bone marrow biopsy
   3. Thoracentesis
   4. Bronchoscopy

10. **An expected outcome for a patient diagnosed with bronchiolitis obliterans is:**
    1. Removal of the Foley catheter within 48 hours

2. Insertion of a chest tube within 24 hours
3. Establishment of a differential diagnosis within 48 hours
4. Ambulation in the room three times a day

ANSWERS

1. *Answer: 2*
   Rationale: Bronchiolitis obliterans has been associated with the presence of GVHD in patients who have had an allogeneic or an autologous BMT.

2. *Answer: 3*
   Rationale: An ECHO is done to assess cardiac output, which is not part of the diagnostic testing for bronchiolitis obliterans.

3. *Answer: 4*
   Rationale: Electrical shock has not been implicated in the development of bronchiolitis obliterans.

4. *Answer: 1*
   Rationale: During the disease process, both restrictive and constrictive lung disease develops.

5. *Answer: 4*
   Rationale: Cyclophosphamide has been evaluated as part of the treatment regimen, but definitive results have not yet been established.

6. *Answer: 3*
   Rationale: Cardiac output is not usually altered by bronchiolitis obliterans.

7. *Answer: 1*
   Rationale: Cough and dyspnea on exertion usually are the presenting signs of a patient diagnosed with bronchiolitis obliterans.

8. *Answer: 1*
   Rationale: Allogeneic BMT has been identified as a risk factor because of the high incidence of GVHD in these patients. GVHD has been implicated in the development of bronchiolitis obliterans.

9. *Answer: 4*
   Rationale: Bronchoscopy usually is one of the first diagnostic procedures to be

performed, to rule out infection in patients with new onset respiratory difficulty.

10. *Answer: 3*
Rationale: The differential diagnosis is important for determining the course of treatment and the patient's prognosis.

REFERENCES

Cobo-Dols, M., Gil Calle, S, & Alés Díaz, I., et al. (2006). Bronchiolitis obliterans organizing pneumonia simulating progression in bronchioloalveolar carcinoma. *Clinical & Translational Oncology, 8*(2):133-135.

Crawford, S. W., & Clark, J. G. (1993). Bronchiolitis associated with bone marrow transplantation. *Clinics in Chest Medicine, 14*(4):741-749.

Epler, G. R. (1988). Bronchiolitis obliterans and airways obstruction associated with graft-versus-host disease. *Clinics in Chest Medicine, 9*(4):551-556.

Ezri, T., Kunichezsky, S., & Eliraz, A., et al. (1994). Bronchiolitis obliterans: Current concepts. *Quarterly Journal of Medicine, 87*(1):1-10.

Fort, J. A., & Graham-Pole, J. (1990). Pulmonary complications of bone marrow transplantation. *Bone Marrow Transplantation in Children* (pp. 397-411). New York: Raven Press.

Holland, H. D., Wingard, J. R., & Beschorner, W. E., et al. (1988). Bronchiolitis obliterans in bone marrow transplantation and its relationship to chronic graft-v-host disease and low serum IgG. *Blood, 74*(2):621-627.

Kajiya, T., Koroda, A., & Hokonohara, D., et al. (2006). Radiographic appearance of bronchiolitis obliterans organizing pneumonia (BOOP) developing during bucillamine treatment for rheumatoid arthritis. *American Journal of the Medical Sciences, 332*(1):39-42.

Kaufman, J., & Komorowoski, R. (1990). Bronchiolitis obliterans: A new clinical-pathologic complication of irradiation pneumonitis. *Chest, 97*(5):1243-1244.

King, T. E. Jr. (1989). Bronchiolitis obliterans. *Lung, 167*(2):69-93.

Kotloff, R. M., Ahya, V. N., & Crawford, S. W. (2004). Pulmonary complications of solid organ and hematopoietic stem cell transplantation. *American Journal of Respiratory and Critical Care Medicine, 170*(1):22-48.

Macartney, C., Burke, E., & Elborn, S., et al. (2005). Bronchiolitis obliterans organizing pneumonia in a patient with non-Hodgkin's lymphoma following R-CHOP and pegylated filgrastim. *Leukemia & Lymphoma, 46*(10):1523-1526.

Moore, S. L. (2003). Bronchiolitis obliterans organizing pneumonia: A late complication of stem cell transplantation. *Clinical Journal of Oncology Nursing, 7*(6):659-662.

Pakhale, S. S., Hadjiliadis, D., & Howell, D. N., et al. (2005). Upper lobe fibrosis: A novel manifestation of chronic allograft dysfunction in lung transplantation. *Journal of Heart & Lung Transplantation, 34*(9):1260-1268.

Paz, H. L., Crilley, P., & Patchefsky, A., et al. (1992). Bronchiolitis obliterans after autologous bone marrow transplantation. *Chest, 101*(3):775-778.

Roncoroni, A. J., Corrado, C., & Besuschio, S., et al. (1990). Bronchiolitis obliterans possibly associated with amphotericin B. *Journal of Infectious Diseases, 161*(3):589.

Schwarer, A. P., Hughes, J. M., & Trotman-Dickenson, B., et al. (1992). A chronic pulmonary syndrome associated with graft-versus-host disease after allogeneic marrow transplantation. *Transplantation, 54*(6):1002-1008.

Sveinsson, O. A., Isaksson, H. J., & Guethmundsson, G. (2006). Organizing pneumonia in connection with amiodarone treatment: Case reports and review (Icelandic). *Laeknabladid, 92*(5):385-388.

Takai, Y., Sato, R., & Sugino, K., et al. (2006). A case of cryptogenic organizing pneumonia after postoperative irradiation for breast cancer (Japanese). *Nihon Kokyuki Gakkai Zasshi, 44*(1):55-60.

Cardiac Tamponade and Pericardial Effusions

BRENDA K. SHELTON

PATHOPHYSIOLOGICAL MECHANISMS

Pericardial disease is classified into three categories: pericarditis, pericardial effusion, and pericardial tamponade. The pathophysiologic importance of this constellation of disorders is related to the degree of compromise of cardiac ejection capabilities. *Pericarditis* is defined as inflammation of the pericardium; *pericardial effusion* is excess fluid in the pericardial sac, which reduces venous return and cardiac output; and *pericardial tamponade* is a condition in which pericardial fluid almost completely obstructs venous return and no blood is ejected (Tsolakis et al., 2004). Cardiac arrest, the consequence of pericardial tamponade, reflects the absence of blood in the heart that can be ejected with contraction.

The intrapericardial pressure normally is negative, and the elastic recoil of the pericardial sac permits the heart to fill with blood returning from the venous system. As fluid accumulates in the pericardial space, the pressure becomes more positive and venous return is impaired. As fluid accumulates in the pericardial sac, at a certain point the intrapericardial pressure matches the pressure of returning venous blood, and no blood is allowed to enter the heart. Without returning blood, cardiac output declines, leading to pump failure and cardiac arrest.

In a slowly developing effusion, cardiac ejection failure occurs later, allowing for a larger amount of effusion and a slow onset of what appears to be right heart failure. Most malignant effusions occur slowly and manifest in this manner, notoriously causing higher volume effusions. In the early phases of effusion, venous congestion can cause edema and hepatomegaly. As ventricular filling becomes more impaired, left ventricular output is reduced.

Several physiologic mechanisms can cause additional production of pericardial fluid, abnormal recirculation of fluid, or leakage of other fluids (e.g., blood) into the pericardial space. Pericardial fluid disorders may be infectious, transudative, and hemorrhagic. They may be related to medical disorders, surgery, trauma, or malignancy.

Pericardial effusions are further classified as transudative or exudative by the fluid characteristics (Maisch et al., 2004). Maisch and colleagues (2004) described transudative effusions caused by disorders of capillary permeability as having low LDH and protein levels, a low fluid to serum LDH ratio, and a low serum to fluid protein ratio. Transudative effusions are more commonly associated with nonmalignant effusions, although they may be present when large tumors obstruct recirculation of pericardial fluid.

Exudative effusions occur when an inflammatory stimulus is present. These effusions are characterized by an LDH level greater than 200 units/L, a protein level greater than 35 g/dL, a fluid to serum LDH ratio greater than 0.6, and a fluid to protein ratio greater than 0.3. They are more typical of malignant involvement of the pericardial fluid (Maisch et al., 2004).

EPIDEMIOLOGY AND ETIOLOGY

The incidence and severity of pericardial effusion and tamponade, as well as the prognosis, depend on the etiology and rapidity of onset. Many pericardial effusive disorders are multifactorial, involving both malignant processes and unstable medical conditions. The incidence has been reported as high as 10% to 30% in patients with pericardial involvement of malignancy and large malignant tumors that obstruct pericardial fluid drainage, such as lung cancer (Flounders, 2003). In one study of patients at the end of life, pericardial effusion was associated with an approximate life expectancy of 2 to 8 months (Cullinane et al., 2004). Despite the shortened life expectancy, as many as 95% of patients can expect symptomatic relief with aggressive intervention (Lindenberger et al., 2003). Hemorrhagic effusions are rare in patients with cancer, but they have the most severe prognosis (Flounders, 2003).

RISK PROFILE

Malignancy involving the chest causes pericardial inflammatory responses that may or may not involve the pericardial fluid (Quraishi et al., 2005; Kabukcu et al., 2004).

Malignant invasion or metastases (Suman et al., 2004)
- Bronchogenic cancer (about 80% cases) (Ma et al., 2006; Gowda et al., 2004; Wang et al., 2000)
- Breast cancer, especially invasive ductal cancer involving the inner aspects of the breast (Pokieser et al., 2004)
- Primary lymphomatous involvement of the pericardium (Chaves et al., 2004; Giunta et al., 2004; Nakakuki et al., 2004)
- Renal cell cancer
- Sarcoma—clear cell sarcoma, angiosarcoma (Frankel, 2004; Corso et al., 2003)
- Malignant melanoma
- Mesothelioma (Suman et al., 2004)
- Multiple myeloma (particularly related to amyloidosis) (Abelman et al., 2005; Zeiser et al., 2005; Arat et al., 2002)
- Gastric cancer
- Ovarian cancer
- Sarcoma—osteogenic sarcoma, angiosarcoma (Siddiqui & Al-Diab, 2003)
- Malignant thymoma (Gupta & Mathur, 2003)

Thoracic lymphatic obstruction
- Lymphoma (Giunta et al., 2004; Nakakuki et al., 2004)
- HIV disease (Barbaro, 2003; Gowda et al., 2003)
- Leukemia—especially acute lymphocytic leukemia, chronic lymphocytic leukemia, and chronic myelogenous leukemia (Breccia et al., 2005; Chaves et al., 2004; Kadikoylu et al., 2003; Arya et al., 2002).
- Extramedullary multiple myeloma (Abelman et al., 2005; Zeiser et al., 2005).

Disorders of capillary permeability that occur with high-dose therapy.
- Radiation of at least 3000 cGy involving at least 33% of the heart, heart fractions exceeding 300 cGy per day (Shelton, 2006; Retter, 2002).
- Cyclophosphamide
- Cytosine arabinoside (Gahler et al., 2003)
- Gemcitabine (Vogl et al., 2005)

Disorders of capillary permeability that occur with immune activation therapies.
- Cytokine antitumor agents—interferons, interleukin-2, interleukin -11

- Granulocyte-macrophage hematopoietic growth factor (GM-CSF)
- All-transretinoic acid (ATRA) (Datta & Gerardi, 2003; Larson & Tallman, 2003)
- Imatinib (Breccia et al., 2005)

Nonmalignant medical conditions (Kabukcu et al., 2004).

- Cardiac myxoma
- Autoimmune diseases—myxedema, systemic lupus erythematosus, scleroderma, rheumatoid arthritis (Lin et al., 2003).
- Uremia
- Displaced central venous catheter with fluid infusion (Shields et al., 2003)
- Complications of bone marrow aspiration (Marti et al., 2004)

Infections: Pericardial effusion is particularly common with infections that cause lymphadenopathy of mass effect (Kabukcu et al., 2004; Quraishi et al., 2005; Janoskuti et al., 2003; Levy et al., 2003).

- Bacteria: Actinomyces, *Streptococcus pneumoniae, Citrobacter freundii, Coxiella burnetii, Nocardia* spp., *Serratia* spp. (Janoskuti et al., 2004a; Levy et al., 2003)
- Fungi: *Candida albicans* (Rabinovici et al., 1997).
- Opportunistic organisms: *Legionella pneumophila, Mycoplasma pneumoniae, Mycobacterium tuberculosis,* toxoplasmosis
- Viruses

PROGNOSIS

Pericardial effusion and tamponade usually are indicative of severe, advanced chest malignancy and a poor prognosis. Most patients live less than 1 year after diagnosis of pericardial disease (Cullinane et al., 2004; Bastian et al., 2000), although the severity of the underlying malignancy has been reported to be one of the most important factors for predicting survival (Dosios et al., 2003). Additional predictive factors of a poor outcome are large amounts of pericardial fluid and a diagnosis of HIV infection (Foster, 2000). Patients with a capillary permeability–related disorder have a better prognosis, depending on the reversibility of the etiologic factor.

PROFESSIONAL ASSESSMENT CRITERIA (PAC)

Clinical signs and symptoms

1. The severity of symptoms may reflect the rapidity of onset. Slower developing effusions allow the body to adjust to progressive reductions in venous return, therefore these patients may not become severely symptomatic until several hundred milliliters have accumulated. Sudden pathologies may produce symptoms of tamponade with as little as 50 mL.
2. Dyspnea is the most common presenting symptom of malignancy-related pericardial disease (Chiu et al., 2004; Gibbs et al., 2000).
3. Symptoms of venous congestion from impeded venous return include edema, hepatomegaly, splenomegaly, positive hepatojugular reflex, bilateral jugular venous distention, and increased central venous pressure.
4. Signs and symptoms of increased pericardial pressure include bradycardia/heart block with inspiration, hypotension with narrow pulse pressure (closing the difference between the systolic and diastolic blood pressures), and pulsus paradox (Box 5-1).

| BOX 5-1 | MEASUREMENT OF PULSUS PARADOX |

Clinical Pearls
1. Pulsus paradox is best assessed by the hemodynamic waveform of an arterial line. This allows the variation in blood pressure that occurs on inspiration and expiration to be measured on printed waveforms with graph grid lines.
2. Pulsus paradox is inaccurately assessed by automatic blood pressure devices.
3. The true paradox is determined during inspiration, when venous return is lowest.

Technique
1. Inflate the blood pressure cuff 15 to 20 mm Hg above the systolic pressure.
2. Slowly deflate the cuff until Korotkoff's sounds are heard on expiration (higher systolic pressure) (e.g., 140 mm Hg).
3. Continue to deflate the cuff slowly until sounds are detected equally on inspiration and expiration. During the paradox, sounds may fade on inspiration and return on expiration. When the sounds are equal on inspiration and expiration, note this value (lower systolic pressure) (e.g., 120 mm Hg).
4. Subtract the lower pressure reading from the higher pressure reading to determine the degree of paradox (e.g., 140 − 120 = 20 mm Hg).

Determining the Significance of Findings
1. Paradox greater than 10 mm Hg indicates high thoracic pressure, although it is not specific for pericardial disease.
2. The paradox is more pronounced in patients who have lung masses or who are profoundly dehydrated.

5. Signs of decreased cardiac output include weak, thready distal pulses; cool, clammy extremities; cyanosis; oliguria; and diminished bowel sounds.
6. Pericardial rub is unusual with effusion and tamponade but may be present with pericarditis. It results from inflammation of the visceral and parietal pericardium with displacement of the fluid normally in that space. A rub present with pericardial effusion is related to high-volume effusions with uneven distribution of fluid and the presence of areas without fluid lubrication.
7. Because blood coming from the heart feeds the upper branches of the aortic arch first, patients have better upper extremity pulses than lower extremity pulses.

Radiologic tests

1. The chest x-ray film may show an enlarged cardiac silhouette, and the mediastinum may have a "water bottle" appearance (indicative of accumulation of more than 250 mL fluid). However, the x-ray findings may be inconclusive if the effusion is primarily anteroposteriorly displaced (Goyle & Walling, 2002).
2. A chest computed tomography (CT) scan may show an enlarged cardiac silhouette. It also may differentiate pericardial fluid from a hypertrophied myocardium. If CT scans are done, pericardial disease is more likely to be an incidental finding, because a definitive diagnosis can be made using bedside diagnostic tests.

Other diagnostic tests

1. The two-dimensional echocardiogram is the gold standard for diagnosis of pericardial effusion and tamponade (Spodick, 2003).
   - The echocardiogram will show a fluid layer between the visceral and parietal pericardia, as well as right or left atrial or ventricular collapse, which indicates impending tamponade.

- Right ventricular collapse with impaired filling occurs with severe pericardial effusions.
- When the left ventricle fails to expand and fill with blood, cardiac arrest is imminent.
- The ejection fraction can be estimated and the urgency for treatment can be determined by the results of the echocardiogram.

2. A 12-lead electrocardiogram (ECG) may produce a number of nonspecific findings that, when they occur simultaneously, increase the likelihood that pericardial disease is present.
   - Early changes in pericarditis or small pericardial effusions may include depressed P waves and nonspecific ST changes, although T-wave inversions are less common than with acute myocardial infarction (Kudo et al., 2003; Goyle & Walling, 2002).
   - Early pericarditis is characterized by ST elevations in *all* the precordial ECG leads. Myocardial ischemia however, is an uncommon finding; in a study by Kudo and colleagues (2003), it was detected in fewer than 10% of patients with pericardial effusion.
   - As pericardial effusion develops, the QRS voltage across all leads decreases and an axis deviation may occur. Low voltage is seen in approximately one fourth of patients with pericardial effusion, although its presence does not necessarily predict the volume or severity of the effusion (Kudo et al., 2003).
   - The classic ECG finding associated with impending pericardial tamponade is electrical alternans, in which the R wave alternates between upward and downward deflection. This happens because the heart floats in a fluid casing, causing it to move in relation to the chest wall leads recording its activity (Billakanty & Bashir, 2006; Calkins & Amsterdam, 2004; Goyle & Walling, 2002; Lau et al., 2002).

3. Few laboratory abnormalities are indicative of pericardial disease. None are used to diagnose these disorders, but they may be used to monitor the response to treatment.
   - Pericarditis may produce laboratory results that indicate an inflammatory process, such as elevation of the white blood cell count or the erythrocyte sedimentation rate.
   - Pericarditis may cause an ischemic "troponin leak" that presents as increased serum troponins despite relatively normal CPK levels.
   - Cytopathology of the pericardial fluid may detect malignant cells. This may assist treatment planning, although the yield is low. Combining cytopathology with fluorescence in situ hybridization (FISH) improves the clinical yield of positive pathologic markers (Gornik et al., 2005; Fiegl et al., 2004; Wang et al., 2000).

NURSING CARE AND TREATMENT

Emergency management of symptomatic pericardial effusion or impending pericardial tamponade

1. Administration of high-volume intravenous fluids (150 to 500 mL/hr) as centrally as possible can increase venous pressure above that of the pericardium. Increased venous pressure that exceeds pericardial pressures allows blood to flow into the heart, permitting blood ejection and improving cardiac output.
2. Oxygen therapy should be provided to maximize oxygen delivery to the tissues. The preferred administration is via mask. Assisted ventilation in any way (Ambu bag, endotracheal intubation with mechanical ventilation) changes to a positive pressure mode of ventilation, which will further reduce venous return in an already severely compromised patient (Faehnrich et al., 2003).
3. The patient should be positioned upright to ease dyspnea.

Definitive strategies to remove pericardial fluid

1. Emergency pericardiocentesis is reserved for unique circumstances in which the risk factors are not recognized until tamponade is present. Whenever possible, needle pericardiocentesis should be guided by fluoroscopy or echocardiogram. If rapid validation of the needle's location is not possible, an alligator clamp can be used to link the ECG machine lead and the aspiration needle. If an acute, severe ST elevation occurs when the needle touches the myocardium, the operator can retract the needle fractionally before withdrawing fluid; this helps ensure that pericardial fluid is removed.
2. Pericardial catheter drainage allows for short-term, continuous drainage of the pericardium.
   - This technique allows immediate alleviation of symptoms, assessment of fluid characteristics, and a period of time to reverse the etiologic factors before the catheter is removed.
   - Pericardial catheter drainage is indicated for hemodynamically unstable pericardial effusions. The complication rate is 4% to 17% (Allen et al., 1999).
   - In nonmalignant conditions, the catheter is less likely to be left in the pericardial sac.
   - The catheter may be a hard catheter, similar to a central line, or a soft, Silastic pigtail catheter, such as a long-term indwelling intravenous line.
   - Care of the patient with a pericardial catheter is not well-documented. Impeccable infection precautions are necessary to ensure that catheter-related infection does not occur. A general review of patient care is included in Box 5-2.
   - Recurrence of pericardial effusion is more common with balloon drainage than with insertion of a pericardial window (Allen et al., 1999).
3. Subxiphoid pericardiocentesis performed by video-assisted thoracoscopic surgery (VATS) or an open thoracotomy VATS procedure requires less postoperative recovery time.
   - This procedure, also called a *pericardial window,* involves the insertion of a small patch of screen into the parietal pericardium, allowing excess fluid to drain into the mediastinum instead of accumulating in the pericardial sac.
   - This technique is the safest, most permanent method of fluid drainage. The complication rate is less than 2% (Allen et al., 1999). The procedure is used in patients with a reasonable life expectancy who are hemodynamically stable (Cullinane et al., 2004; Allen et al., 1999).
   - With a malignant effusion, this technique inherently means that malignant fluid is allowed to disperse throughout the thorax; however, it is not considered likely to hasten death.
   - After the procedure, the patient may have a mediastinal chest tube connected to water seal or suction drainage. This tube is placed in the mediastinum and should never have an air leak. As drainage slows, the tube is switched to a water seal setup only and eventually removed.
   - A variation of this procedure performed in patients with both pleural and pericardial effusions is the pleuro-pericardio-peritoneal window, which is used with or without a shunt to internally pump fluid into the peritoneal cavity
   - Talc may be "blown" into the space during the surgery to provide a surgical pleurodesis.

Interventions aimed at treating the cause of effusion

1. Pericarditis is treated with antiinflammatory agents (e.g., salicylic acid 650 mg given orally every 4 hours or ibuprofen 400-600 mg given orally three times daily; dexamethasone 4-10 mg given orally or intravenously three times daily or hydrocortisone 125 mg given intravenously four times daily). Colchicine recently was investigated as a treatment

BOX 5-2	NURSING MANAGEMENT OF A PERICARDIAL CATHETER

Assessment

1. Catheter patency and drainage: Production of continuous small amounts of serous drainage is normal. If the drainage suddenly stops, the patient should be assessed for signs and symptoms of recurrent pericardial effusion. Increased drainage after catheter insertion and initial drainage is rare.
2. Drainage characteristics: Drainage usually is serous or serosanguineous, but it does not usually clot. Amounts normally are less than 100 to 200 mL/day.
3. Exit site: The catheter exit site is assessed for irritation or for drainage that is evidence of infection.
4. Catheter placement: The catheter often is sutured in place, but it can be displaced by sliding out. The length of catheter outside is measured and compared to the baseline every shift. Migration of the catheter outward helps document displacement. Catheter migration into the body occurs less often; it may be indicated by changes in the catheter measurement or by a new onset of dysrhythmias.
5. Evidence of recurrent pericardial effusion/tamponade: If excess pericardial fluid is produced or drainage is blocked, the trapped fluid in the pericardial sac causes recurrent symptoms of effusion and impending tamponade (i.e., bilateral jugular venous distention, pulsus paradox, muffled heart sounds, diminished point of maximal impulse, and reduced extremity pulses). Assessment for the presence or absence of these symptoms may be done every shift; however, this assessment is most important if the drainage is diminished.

Interventions

1. Maintain a sterile, closed, straight drainage system that drains below the level of the heart. No evidence indicates that pericardial drainage can be facilitated (or is safe) by using water seal with suction. Some institutions do not recommend routine emptying of the drainage bag; those that do often recommend exchanging the bag for a new, sterile one when needed.
2. Some institutions advocate sterile catheter flushing with preservative-free normal saline or low-concentration heparin (2 mL or 1:100 concentration) two or three times daily.
3. Use a clear, sterile dressing to facilitate rapid, direct assessment of the exit site. Infection of the pericardial catheter exit site could result in life-threatening endocarditis.
4. Initiate continuous cardiac monitoring for dysrhythmias or ischemia caused by the presence of the catheter.

Reportable Conditions

1. Signs and symptoms of recurrent effusion: pulsus paradox, hypotension with narrow pulse pressure, bilateral jugular venous distention, muffled or absent heart sounds
2. Drainage exceeding 200 mL/day
3. Sudden cessation of drainage
4. Premature ventricular contractions, sudden onset of tachycardia, supraventricular tachycardia
5. Hypotension or pulsus paradox greater than 10 mm Hg

for effusions triggered by inflammatory mechanisms, but the results were inconclusive (Ng et al., 2001).

2. Palliative radiation therapy that includes a portion of the heart can reduce the rate of fluid accumulation. However, it also causes myocyte damage. The usual dose is 100 to 200 cGy daily for 3 to 4 weeks (Shelton, 2006).
3. Antineoplastic chemotherapeutic drugs administered intravenously may slow the rate of growth in some chemosensitive tumors, such as small cell lung cancer and high-grade lymphoma.
4. Instillation of antineoplastic chemotherapeutic drugs into the pericardial sac has been reported to be an effective anticancer therapy. Agents documented as safe to administer

in this manner include cisplatin, mitomycin C, mitoxantrone, and thiotepa (Shelton, 2006; Martinoni et al., 2004; Musch et al., 2003; Siddiqui & Al-Diab, 2003).

5. Instillation of a sclerosing agent into the pericardial sac produces a change in the fluid pH, causing inflammation and adherence of the visceral and parietal pericardia. This technique is used for effusions that recur despite drainage procedures, such as pericardial catheterization or occlusion of a pericardial window (Martinoni et al., 2000).

Supportive care
Pain management

1. Antiinflammatory agents may reduce the chest discomfort more common with pericarditis.
2. Some patients report that sitting up and leaning forward alleviates chest discomfort. This "tripod" position reduces abdominal pressure on the thoracic cavity, making it easier to breathe. It also displaces the heart against the chest wall, reducing mediastinal pressure, and can improve venous return.
3. Pain management is used cautiously in patients with severe hypotension.

Dyspnea management

1. Air hunger, anxiety, and a sense of impending doom, which are characteristic of this disorder, increase oxygen demands in the face of already poor delivery. Dyspnea is the most common clinical finding in pericardial disorders.
2. Morphine is an excellent bronchodilator that can assist in the alleviation of dyspnea. However, its vasodilatory effects can also worsen hypotension in this setting of already impaired venous return and preload (Flounders, 2003).
3. Two components of the patient's perception of the severity of dyspnea are the person's anxiety and fear of death (Chiu et al., 2004). Anxiolytic medications may ease this perception.

Conservation of energy and limitation of myocardial oxygen demands (Flounders, 2003)

1. Divide care into increments to minimize patient effort.
2. Provide assistance with physical care.
3. Provide psychosocial support to reduce anxiety that increases oxygen demands.

EVIDENCE-BASED PRACTICE UPDATES

1. Direct pericardial involvement with malignant infiltration is relatively rare. More pericardial pathologic conditions are related to malignant cytology of the fluid or thoracic lymphatic obstruction. Direct pericardial involvement has been identified with multiple myeloma (Arat et al., 2002) and lymphoma (Giunta et al., 2004).
2. For unexplained reasons, excessive yawning has been associated with pericardial effusion (Krantz et al., 2004).
3. Studies document moderate success and reduced recovery time with placement of a pericardial drain via percutaneous catheter and balloon insertion, compared with the traditional, preferred pericardial window, although the former procedure may have a slightly higher complication rate (Del Barrio et al., 2002; Allen et al., 1999).

TEACHING AND EDUCATION

1. Patient-specific risk factors are defined to help the patient and significant others recognize the potential for this complication in the patient.
2. The ability to recognize the signs and symptoms of early pericardial effusion can prepare the patient and significant others to seek medical attention while the condition can more easily be reversed.
3. The patient and significant others should be taught energy conservation measures. The patient's family role and responsibilities should be explored and modified as necessary. Home health assistance or meals assistance may be helpful.
4. The clinical effects of the treatments for pericardial tamponade may not be immediately evident because of the immediate and dramatic decrease in symptoms such as dyspnea. Procedures such as sclerosing cause permanent constriction of the pericardial sac and some degree of activity intolerance or right heart failure. Patients who are prepared for this potential adverse effect may be better able to understand the need for lifestyle changes.

NURSING DIAGNOSES

1. **Ineffective tissue perfusion:** cardiopulmonary related to fluid in pericardial sac
2. **Ineffective breathing pattern** related to dyspnea
3. **Ineffective tissue perfusion:** cardiopulmonary related to hypotension
4. **Acute pain** related to inflammation
5. **Activity intolerance** related to low cardiac output

EVALUATION AND DESIRED OUTCOMES

1. The patient with clinically symptomatic pericardial effusion will demonstrate immediate return of cardiac perfusion and improved cardiac output once the fluid is removed. A patient in full arrest can return to normal blood pressure and consciousness within minutes of definitive pericardial fluid drainage.
2. The most accurate evaluation for evidence of pericardial effusion and tamponade is a two-dimensional echocardiogram. After definitive treatment or reversal of etiologic factors, periodic echocardiograms may be performed. The frequency will depend on the expected time frame for a treatment response. This could occur within hours of management of the hemopericardium, or months after treatment for lymphatic obstruction.
3. In patients with risk factors for pericardial effusion and tamponade, blood pressures should be taken manually to obtain the most accurate assessment of narrow pulse pressure and pulsus paradox.

DISCHARGE PLANNING AND FOLLOW-UP CARE

- The patient's response to interventions for drainage of excess pericardial fluid should be evaluated, and the patient and his or her significant others should be given a reasonable estimate of how long the patient is likely to remain symptom free.
- Some patients are discharged home with a temporary Silastic pigtail catheter for pericardial drainage. Home care follow-up may be necessary to provide care for the catheter and to assess the patient for fluid reaccumulation.
- Home health assistance may be needed for patients with persistent pericardial effusion after a sclerosing procedure, because these patients are likely to have significant intolerance to physical activity.

- The patient or significant other should be given the name and telephone number of a health care professional whom they can call with questions. The follow-up appointment should be confirmed.

REVIEW QUESTIONS

QUESTIONS

1. **The malignancy most often associated with pericardial effusion and tamponade is:**
    1. Lymphoma
    2. Bronchogenic lung cancer
    3. Renal cell cancer
    4. Breast cancer

2. **The antineoplastic agent most commonly associated with pericardial effusion is:**
    1. Bevacizumab
    2. Cytosine arabinoside
    3. Methotrexate
    4. Oxaliplatin

3. **The most severe pericardial disorder is:**
    1. Pericarditis
    2. Pericardial effusion
    3. Perimyocarditis
    4. Pericardial tamponade

4. **The most definitive diagnostic test to confirm pericardial disease is:**
    1. Chest x-ray film
    2. Chest CT scan
    3. Echocardiogram
    4. 12-lead ECG

5. **The most common symptom of pericardial effusion is:**
    1. Dyspnea
    2. Chest pain
    3. Cyanosis
    4. Confusion

6. **Immediate emergency management to stabilize presumed impending pericardial tamponade is:**
    1. Administration of inotropic agents
    2. Administration of intravenous fluids
    3. Administration of epinephrine
    4. Magnesium bolus infusion

7. **Education for patients at high risk for pericardial effusion includes:**
    1. Instructions for assessing the pulse rate
    2. Strategies to restrict fluid intake
    3. Use of supplemental oxygen therapy
    4. Reportable symptoms of weight gain and edema

8. **Nursing care of a pericardial catheter includes documenting the amount of drainage and correlating it with the patient's symptoms. It also includes:**
    1. Assessing the external catheter markings to make sure the catheter is not displaced
    2. Manually flushing the catheter with heparin to maintain patency
    3. Using a clean dressing technique, because this catheter has a subcutaneous cuff
    4. All of the above

9. **Postoperative nursing care of a patient with a newly placed pericardial window includes:**
    1. Monitoring for an air leak in the chest tube chamber
    2. Carefully maintaining chest tube suction above 20 cm H_2O
    3. Comparing the amount of chest tube drainage with resolution of the symptoms of effusion and tamponade
    4. Observing bleeding precautions because of the anticoagulant therapy

10. **Emergency pericardiocentesis requires which of the following supplies or equipment at the bedside:**
    1. Low continuous suction
    2. 12-lead ECG machine
    3. Petrolatum gauze
    4. Vacuum bottle

ANSWERS

1. *Answer: 2*
    Rationale: The most common malignant

causes of pericardial effusion are malignant diseases involving the mediastinum and its lymph nodes. The most common cancer in this location is lung cancer, and bronchogenic lung cancer is the most centrally located of the subtypes of lung cancer. If lymphoma were a more prevalent malignancy or consistently involved this region, it could surpass bronchogenic cancer as a risk for pericardial disease.

2. *Answer: 2*
Rationale: Although many chemotherapeutic and biologic therapy agents have been associated with fluid retention, only a few have a reported high incidence of pericardial effusion arising from the severe capillary permeability they cause.

3. *Answer: 4*
Rationale: Pericardial diseases are graded according to the severity of cardiac output compromise. In pericardial tamponade, venous return is extremely limited or absent, therefore cardiac output is almost nonexistent. Excess fluid closes the ventricles by means of compression, blocking the inflow of returning venous blood.

4. *Answer: 3*
Rationale: Tests that indirectly measure reduced cardiac activity (e.g. 12-lead ECG) cannot demonstrate the actual presence of pericardial fluid, and radiology tests (e.g., chest x-ray film) cannot demonstrate the effect of the fluid on contractility. An echocardiogram can detect both these pathophysiologic findings.

5. *Answer: 1*
Rationale: Although pericardial effusion involves impaired venous return and cardiac output, the most common symptom is dyspnea. This is thought to be related to the early pathologic conditions of reduced venous return with venous congestion and right heart failure.

6. *Answer: 2*
Rationale: The most immediate physiologic crisis in pericardial tamponade is inadequate cardiac output as a result of low blood volume returning to the right heart. Raising the venous pressure above the pericardial pressures improves venous return, thereby increasing cardiac output. This measure is no longer needed once excess fluid has been removed from the pericardial sac.

7. *Answer: 4*
Rationale: Venous congestion is caused by back pressure from the distended pericardial sac to the venous system. Excess fluid can cause edema and weight gain, which are early clinical findings of pericardial effusion.

8. *Answer: 4*
Rationale: All of the responses are components of basic nursing care of a pericardial catheter.

9. *Answer: 3*
Rationale: The mediastinal chest tube placed after insertion of a pericardial window should not have an air leak. Low suction usually is required for only a short time after surgery. Chest tube drainage should slow after placement of the pericardial window; however, the nurse must be attentive to whether this reflects proper functioning of the new outlet for excess fluid or a recurrence of the pericardial effusion.

10. *Answer: 2*
Rationale: Emergency pericardiocentesis involves blind insertion of a needle between the visceral and parietal pericardia to allow immediate removal of the fluid that is filling that space and impairing venous return to the right heart. The fluid is removed manually, because removal of even small amounts (50 to 150 mL) can either alleviate or cause symptoms. The 12-lead ECG machine, with an alligator clip attachment between the needle and the V1 chest lead, provides an injury ECG tracing when the needle touches the myocardium. This allows the operator to back up the needle a few millimeters before withdrawing fluid, ensuring that pericardial fluid is removed.

REFERENCES

Abelman, W., Virchis, A., & Yong, K. (2005). Extramedullary myeloma representing as a pericardial effusion with tamponade: Two case reports and a further review of 19 cases in the literature. *Leukemia & Lymphoma, 46*:137-142.

Allen, K. B., Faber, L. P., & Warren, W. H., et al. (1999). Pericardial effusion: Subxiphoid pericardiostomy versus pericardial catheter drainage. *Annals of Thoracic Surgery, 67*:437-440.

Arat, M., Ulusoy, V., & Demirer, T., et al. (2002). An unusual presentation of plasma cell dyscrasias: Cardiac tamponade due to myelomatous infiltration. *Leukemia & Lymphoma, 43*(1):145-148.

Arya, L. S., Narain, S., & Thavaraj, V., et al. (2002). Leukemic pericardial effusion causing cardiac tamponade. *Medical Pediatric Oncology, 38*:282-284.

Barbaro, G. (2003). Pathogenesis of HIV-associated heart disease. *AIDS, 17*(Supp. 1):S12-S20.

Bastian, A., Meibner, A., & Lins, M., et al. (2000). Pericardiocentesis: Differential aspects of a common procedure. *Intensive Care Medicine, 26*:572-576.

Billakanty, S., & Bashir, R. (2006). Images in cardiovascular medicine: Echocardiographic demonstration of electrical alternans. *Circulation, 113*(24):e866-e868.

Breccia, M., D'Elia, G. M., & D'Andrea, M., et al. (2005). Pleural-pericardiac effusion as uncommon complication in CML patients treated with imatinib. *European Journal of Haematology, 74*:89-90.

Calkins, J., & Amsterdam, E. (2004). Images in cardiology: Electrical alternans and its resolution in an adult with a large pericardial effusion. *Clinical Cardiology, 27*(12):701.

Chaves, F. P., Quillen, K., & Xu, D. (2004). Pericardial effusion: A rare presentation of adult T-ell leukemia/lymphoma. *American Journal of Hematology, 77*:381-383.

Chiu, T. Y., Hu, W. Y., & Lue, B. H., et al. (2004). Dyspnea and its correlates in Taiwanese patients with terminal cancer. *Journal of Pain and Symptom Management, 28*:123-132.

Corso, R. B., Kraychete, N., & Nardeli, S., et al. (2003). Spontaneous rupture of a right atrial angiosarcoma and cardiac tamponade. *Arquivos Brasileiros de Cardiologia, 81*(6):611-613.

Cullinane, C. A., Paz, I. B., & Smith, D., et al. (2004). Prognostic factors in the surgical management of pericardial effusion in the patient with concurrent malignancy. *Chest, 125*:1328-1334.

Datta, D., & Gerardi, D. A. (2003). Retinoic acid syndrome. *Connecticut Medicine, 67*(9):541-543.

Del Barrio, L. G., Morales, J. H., & Delgado, C., et al. (2002). Percutaneous balloon pericardial window in patients with symptomatic pericardial effusion. *Cardiovascular and Interventional Radiology, 25*(5):360-364.

Dosios, T., Theakos, N., & Angouras, D., et al. (2003). Risk factors affecting the survival of patients with pericardial effusion submitted to subxiphoid pericardiostomy. *Chest, 124*:242-246.

Faehnrich, J. A., Noone, R. B. Jr., & White, W. D., et al. (2003). Effects of positive-pressure ventilation, pericardial effusion, and cardiac tamponade on respiratory variation in transmitral flow velocities. *Journal of Cardiothoracic and Vascular Anesthesia, 17*(1):45-50.

Fiegl, M., Massoner, A., & Haun, M., et al. (2004). Sensitive detection of tumour cells in effusions by combining cytology and fluorescence in situ hybridisation. *British Journal of Cancer, 91*(3):558-563.

Flounders, J. A. (2003). Cardiovascular emergencies: Pericardial effusion and cardiac tamponade. *Oncology Nursing Forum On-Line Exclusive, 30*(2). Retrieved June 2, 2005, from www.ons.org/xp6/ONS/Library.xml/ONSPublications.xml/ONF.xml/ONF2003?M.

Foster, E. (2000). Pericardial effusion: A continuing drain on our diagnostic acumen. *The American Journal of Medicine, 00*(2):169-170.

Frankel, K. M. (2004). Malignant pericardial effusions. *Chest, 126*(5):1713.

Gahler, A., Hitz, F., & Hess, U., et al. (2003). Acute pericarditis and pleural effusion complicating cytarabine chemotherapy. *Onkologie, 26*(4):348-350.

Gibbs, C. R., Watson, R. D., & Singh, S. P., et al. (2000). Management of pericardial effusion by damage: A survey of 10 years' experience in a city centre general hospital serving a multiracial population. *Postgraduate Medical Journal, 76*:809-813.

Giunta, R., Cravero, R. G., & Granata, G., et al. (2004). Primary cardiac T-cell lymphoma. *Annals of Hematology, 83*(7):450-454.

Gornik, H. L., Gerhard-Herman, M., & Beckman, J. A. (2005). Abnormal cytology predicts poor prognosis in cancer patients with pericardial effusion. *Journal of Clinical Oncology, 23*(22):5211-5216.

Gowda, R. M., Khan, I. A., & Mehta, N. J., etal. (2003). Cardiac tamponade in patients with human immunodeficiency virus disease. *Angiology 54*(4):469–474.

Gowda, R. M., Khan, I. A., & Mehta, N. J., et al. (2004). Cardiac tamponade and superior vena cava syndrome in lung cancer: A case report. *Angiology, 55*(6):691-695.

Goyle, K. K., & Walling, A. D. (2002). Diagnosing pericarditis. *American Family Physician, 66*(9):1695-1702.

Gupta, K., & Mathur, V. S. (2005). Diagnosis of pericardial disease using percutaneous biopsy: Care report and literature review. *Texas Heart Institute Journal, 30*(2):130-133.

Janoskuti, L., Lengyel, M., & Fenyvesi, T. (2004). Cardiac actinomycosis in a patient presenting with acute cardia tamponade and a mass mimicking pericardial tumour. *Heart, 90*:27-28.

Kabukcu, M., Demircioglu, F., & Yanik, E., et al. (2004). Pericardial tamponade and large pericardial effusions: Causal factors and efficacy of percutaneous catheter drainage in 50 patients. *Texas Heart Institute Journal, 31*(4):398-403.

Kadikoylu, G., Onbasili, A., & Barutca, S., et al. (2003). A symptomatic pericardial effusion in chronic myelogenous leukemia. *Leukemia & Lymphoma, 44*(4):723-725.

Krantz, M. J., Lee, J. K., & Spodick, D. H. (2004). Repetitive yawning associated with cardiac tamponade. *American Journal Cardiology, 94*:701-702.

Kudo, Y., Yamasaki, F., & Doi, T., et al. (2003). Clinical significance of low voltage in asymptomatic patients with pericardial effusion free of heart disease. *Chest, 124*:2064-2067.

Larson, R. S., & Tallman, M. S. (2003). Retinoic acid syndrome: Manifestations, pathogenesis. *Best Practices in Research in Clinical Haematology, 16*(3):453-461.

Lau, T. K., Civitello, A. B., & Hernandez, A., et al. (2002). Cardiac tamponade and electrical alternans. *Images in Cardiovascular Medicine, 29*(1):66-67.

Levy, P. Y., Corey, R., & Berger, P., et al. (2003). Etiologic diagnosis of 204 pericardial effusions. *Medicine, 82*(6):385-391.

Lin, C. T., Liu, C. J., & Lin, T. K., et al. (2003). Myxedema associated with cardiac tamponade. *Japanese Heart Journal, 44*(3):447-450.

Lindenberger, M., Kjellberg, M., & Karlsson, E., et al. (2003). Pericardiocentesis guided by 2-D echocardiography: The method of choice for treatment of pericardial effusion. *Journal of Internal Medicine, 253*(4):411-417.

Ma, T. S., Hayes, T. G., & Levine, G. N., et al. (2006). Malignant pleural/pericardial effusion with tamponade and life-threatening reversible myocardial depression in a case of an initial presentation of lung adenocarcinoma. *Cardiology, 105*(1):30-33.

Maisch, B., Seferović, P. M., & Ristić, A. D., et al. (2004). Guidelines on the diagnosis and management of pericardial diseases. *European Heart Journal, 25*:587-610.

Marti, J., Anton, E., & Valenti, C. (2004). Complications of bone marrow biopsy. *British Journal of Haematology, 124*(4):557-558.

Martinoni, A., Cipolla, C. M., & Cardinae, D., et al. (2004). Long-term results of intrapericardial chemotherapeutic treatment of malignant pericardial effusions with thiotepa. *Chest, 126*(5):1412-1416.

Martinoni, A., Cipolla, C. M., & Civelli, M., et al. (2000). Intrapericardial treatment of neoplastic pericardial effusions. *Herz, 25*(8):787-793.

Musch, E., Gremmler, B., & Nitsch, J., et al. (2003). Intrapericardial instillation of mitoxantrone in palliative therapy of malignant pericardial effusion. *Onkologie, 26*(2):135-139.

Nakakuki, T., Masuoka, H., & Ishikura, K., et al. (2004). A case of primary cardiac lymphoma located in the pericardial effusion. *Heart Vessels, 19*(4):199-202.

Ng, T., Gatt, A., & Pagliuca, A., et al. (2001). Colchicine: An effective treatment for refractory malignant pericardial effusion. *Acta Haematologica, 104*:217-219.

Pokieser, W., Cassik, P., & Fischer, G., et al. (2004). Malignant pleural and pericardial effusion in invasive breast cancer: Impact of the site of the primary tumor. *Breast Cancer Research and Treatment, 83*:139-142.

Quraishi, A. R., Khan, A. A., & Kazmi, K. A., et al. (2005). Clinical and echocardiographic characteristics of patients with significant pericardial effusion requiring pericardiocentesis. *Journal of the Pakistan Medical Association, 55*(2):66-70.

Rabinovici, R., Szewczyk, D., & Ovadia, P., et al. (1997). Candida pericarditis: Clinical profile and treatment. *Annals of Thoracic Surgery, 63*:1200-1204.

Retter, A. S. (2002). Pericardial disease in the oncology patient. *Heart Disease, 4*(6):387-391.

Shelton, B. K. (2006). Pericarditis/pericardial effusion/pericardial tamponade. In D. Camp-Sorrell, & R. A. Hawkins (Eds.), *Clinical manual for the advanced oncology nurse* (pp. 369-383). (2nd ed.). Pittsburgh: Oncology Nursing Society.

Shields, L. B., Hunsaker, D. M., & Hunsaker, J. C. III. (2003). Iatrogenic catheter-related cardiac tamponade: A case report of fatal hydropericardium following subcutaneous implantation of a chemotherapeutic injection port. *Journal of Forensic Science, 48*(2):414-418.

Siddiqui, N., & Al-Diab, A. I. (2003). Intrapericardial chemotherapy for the management of neoplastic cardiac tamponade. *Saudi Medical Journal, 24*(5):526-528.

Spodick, D. H. (2003). Acute cardiac tamponade. *New England Journal of Medicine, 329*(7):684-690.

Suman, S., Schofield, P., & Large, S. (2004). Primary pericardial mesothelioma presenting as pericardial constriction: A case report. *Heart, 90*(1):e4.

Tsang, T. S., Seward, J. B., & Barnes, M. E., et al. (2000). Outcomes of primary and secondary treatment of pericardial effusion in patients with malignancy. *Mayo Clinic Proceedings, 75*(3):248-253.

Tsang, T. S., Enriquez-Sarano, M., & Freeman, W. K., et al. (2002). Consecutive 1127 therapeutic echocardiographically guided pericardiocenteses: Clinical profile, practice patterns, and outcomes spanning 21 years. *Mayo Clinic Proceedings, 77*(5):429-436.

Tsolakis, E. J., Charitos, C. E., & Mitsibounas, D., et al. (2004). Cardiac tamponade rapidly evolving toward constrictive pericarditis and shock as a first manifestation of noncardiac cancer. *Journal of Cardiac Surgery, 19*:134-135.

Vogl, D. T., Glatstein, E., & Carver, J. R., et al. (2005). Gemcitabine-induced pericardial effusion and tamponade after unblocked cardiac irradiation. *Leukemia & Lymphoma, 46*(9):1313-1320.

Wang, P. C., Yang, K. Y., & Chao, J. Y., et al. (2000). Prognostic role of pericardial fluid cytology in cardiac tamponade associated with non-small cell lung cancer. *Chest, 118*(3):744-749.

Zeiser, R., Hackanson, B., & Bley, T. A., et al. (2005). Unusual cases in multiple myeloma and a dramatic response in metastatic lung cancer: Case 1. Multiple myeloma relapse presenting as malignant pericardial effusion. *Journal of Clinical Oncology, 23*(1):230-231.

CAROTID ARTERY RUPTURE

CATHERINE SARGENT

PATHOPHYSIOLOGICAL MECHANISMS

A general understanding of the anatomy is helpful for understanding what occurs with a carotid artery rupture (CAR). The carotid arteries run parallel to the jugular vein on each side of the neck. Their primary role is to supply blood to the head and neck regions. The common carotid artery on the right arises from the brachiocephalic artery, and the left common carotid artery arises directly from the aortic arch. The common carotid arteries then bifurcate into the internal and external carotids on either side of the neck. At the site of the bifurcation is an area in which the arterial walls are naturally thin; this is an area of increased risk. The external carotid artery supplies blood to the neck, face, jaw, scalp, and base of the skull. It also supplies blood to the frontal part of the brain, where thinking, speech, personality, and sensory and motor function reside. The internal carotid supplies blood to the rest of the brain and the cranial nerves, affecting the ophthalmic, anterior, and middle cerebral arteries.

Four primary causes of hemorrhage are associated with CAR (Johnson, 2003): (1) tumor hemorrhage secondary to tumor neovascularity; (2) tumor erosion or vascular laceration of the external carotid branch; (3) formation of a pseudoaneurysm secondary to tumor erosion and/or radiation therapy to the head and neck region; and (4) acute major vessel rupture secondary to formation of a pseudoaneurysm or tumor erosion. The mechanism by which erosion develops is related to the drying process that occurs when the carotid artery is exposed to the environment, either during surgery or secondary to tumor exposure. Surgery also can result in edema formation and decreased lymphatic and/or venous drainage, which may increase the risk of CAR.

EPIDEMIOLOGY AND ETIOLOGY

CAR occurs in 3% to 4% of patients who undergo head and neck surgery, and it accounts for about 10% of deaths from advanced cancer (Warren et al., 2002). Death is caused by exsanguination, with the patient dying within minutes of hypovolemic shock.

RISK PROFILE

- Cancers
  - Head and neck cancer
  - Thyroid cancer
  - Lymphoma in cervical areas
- Most patients now undergo modified neck dissection, which reduces the exposure of the carotid artery secondary to protection of the sternocleidomastoid muscle. However, if a radical neck dissection is required, the outer layer of the carotid is exposed, resulting in desiccation and weakness.

59

- Infection, either from the tumor or the surgical site, can lead to poor wound healing, resulting in flap necrosis, fistula formation, and/or hematoma.
- Neck irradiation, either neoadjuvant or high-dose radiation (more than 60 Gy), can be a risk factor.
- Malnourishment, especially low serum levels of protein, iron, and vitamin C, contributes to poor wound healing.
- Middle to older age (i.e., 50 years or older), especially with significant weight loss, poses a risk.
- Co-morbidities can contribute to poor wound healing and wound breakdown. These may include:
  - History of diabetes mellitus
  - History of general arteriosclerosis
  - Renal disease
  - Hypothyroidism
  - Protein calorie malnutrition

PROGNOSIS

No mortality statistics are available for CAR. However, the prognosis for this patient population is extremely poor. Those who survive a rupture often are left with a neurologic deficit of varying degrees, which occurs as a result of arterial disruption of brain dysfunction.

PROFESSIONAL ASSESSMENT CRITERIA (PAC)

1. **Vital signs**
   - Pulse—rapid and weak
   - Respirations—tachypneic, dyspneic
   - Blood pressure—systolic blood pressure less than 90 mm Hg, or 20 mg Hg below baseline; or pulse pressure less than 20 torr
   - Central venous pressure (CVP)—less than 2 mm Hg
2. **Medical history**
   - Wound infection or dehiscence (or both)
   - History of cardiovascular or renal disease
   - Hypothyroidism
   - Diabetes
   - Malnourished state
3. **Physical signs and symptoms**
   - Slow or mild bleeding from the wound, flap site, mouth, or tracheotomy (may be seen 12 to 24 hours before the actual rupture)
   - Sternal or high epigastric pain, often several hours before rupture
   - Enlargement or increased tenderness of the neck
   - Cough with sputum that may or may not be blood tinged
   - Pulsation in or on top of the mass
   - Reduced temporal pulse on the same side as the tumor
   - Visual changes—blurred or double vision
   - Neurologic changes—diminished level of consciousness

4. **Psychosocial signs**
   - Anxiety
   - Fear of bleeding or dying (or both)
   - Restlessness
   - Irritability
5. **Laboratory values**
   - Hemoglobin—decreased
   - Hematocrit—decreased
   - White blood cell count—elevated if infection is present
6. **Diagnostic tests**
   - CBC, comprehensive metabolic profile, PT/PTT
   - Electrocardiogram
   - Pulse oximetry (over 95% is normal for an adult) (Upile et al., 2005)
   - Duplex scan to detect narrowing of the carotids
   - MRI to help detect nodal fixation to the carotids
   - Bilateral imaging of the carotids and vertebral arteries—to help detect bleeding sites and determine the integrity of the circle of Willis in the brain (Johnson, 2003)

NURSING CARE AND TREATMENT

Prerupture care

1. Make sure the call bell is within the patient's reach.
2. Ensure multiple large-diameter IV access routes at all times for fluid resuscitation and blood infusion.
3. Type and cross-match and screen for multiple units of blood in case rupture occurs.
4. Keep oxygen setup with pulse oximetry available and ready in the room.
5. Keep suction setup available and ready in the room.
6. Provide antibiotic therapy if infection is present.
7. Perform wound care using wet to dry dressing.
8. Obtain nutrition consult to enhance would healing.
9. Discuss code status with the patient and significant others in case a rupture occurs.
10. Ensure ready access to emergency equipment and body substance isolation equipment (i.e., gowns, gloves, goggles) should rupture occur.
11. Assess for signs and symptoms of subtle "herald" bleeding from nose, mouth, tracheostomy site, tumor site, and/or wound (Potter, 2005).
12. Obtain laboratory tests, specifically a CBC, to detect unnoted chronic herald bleeding and poor nutritional status (Upile et al., 2005).
13. Provide humidified air to reduce crusting of the wound and to decrease cough.
14. Monitor intake and output to ensure adequate hydration.
15. Keep the head of the bed elevated at least 30 degrees at all times.
16. Refer the patient to social worker/case manager for emotional support and assistance with finances, power of attorney, and home care or hospice care.

Emergency care

(Box 6-1 lists the contents of a carotid rupture precautions box.)
1. With a gloved hand, apply digital pressure directly to the rupture site.
   - If the external carotid has ruptured, position the patient supine with the head turned toward the rupture.
   - If the internal carotid has ruptured, nothing can be done to prevent aspiration.
2. Notify the physician immediately and call a code situation.

BOX 6-1	**CAROTID RUPTURE PRECAUTIONS**

Box of gloves	About 5 L of normal saline or lactated Ringer's solution
Goggles	Oxygen setup and tubing
Face masks and shields	Sterile dressings
Gowns	Dark, absorbent towels
Suction equipment	Medications: midazolam (sedation/anxiety), morphine (pain)
Cuffed tracheotomy tube	Syringes
Red trash bags	

Data from Potter, E. (2005). *The management of carotid artery rupture related to the terminal care of head and neck cancer patient: information and guidelines.* Retrieved March 8, 2006, from www.bahnon.org.uk; and Frawley, T., & Begley, C. (2005). Causes and prevention of carotid artery rupture. *British Journal of Nursing, 14*(22):1198-1202.

3. Hang normal saline or lactated Ringer's solution and infuse as quickly as possible to reduce the risk of hypovolemic shock.
4. Obtain blood products on an emergency basis.
5. Administer a high concentration of oxygen.
6. Notify the operating room of the emergent need for surgery. Maintain digital pressure on the site until the vessels are exposed.
7. Suction oral or tracheal secretions and bleeding (Frawley & Begley, 2006).
8. Provide emotional support to the patient and significant others (Potter, 2005). Frequently the patient is awake and alert when the rupture occurs.
9. Administer antianxiety or analgesic medications (Frawley & Begley, 2005; Potter, 2005).
   - Midazolam 2.5 to 7.5 mg IV, administered over 30 to 60 seconds. This drug is a short-acting benzodiazepine that can cause anterograde amnesia and can cross the blood-brain barrier (Frawley & Begley 2006).
   - Morphine 4 to 10 mg IV, administered over 4 to 5 minutes, to reduce the patient's distress and suffering.
10. In some cases placing the patient in the Trendelenburg position helps continue the supply of blood to the brain.

Postrupture care

1. A patient who survives the rupture is managed postoperatively in the intensive care unit until the person's condition stabilizes.
   - Assess level of consciousness every hour and as needed.
   - Perform neurologic assessment for motor and sensory deficits every hour and as needed.
   - Assess the incision for bleeding every 5 min × 6, then every 30 min × 4, then hourly.
   - Monitor vital signs and oxygen saturation via pulse oximetry every hour and as needed.
   - Obtain CBC and complete metabolic profile every 6 h for 24 hours.
   - Obtain arterial blood gases as ordered by the physician.
   - Assess patency of airway and suction PRN.
2. Assess for possible signs and symptoms of hemorrhage, because patient is at increased risk of rebleeding.
3. If the patient did not survive the carotid artery rupture, provide bereavement care to the significant others; if they wish it, contact their clergy member.

Medical treatment

1. Traditionally, if the danger was identified and the condition caught before a rupture occurred, the patient underwent ligation of the carotid artery, endarterectomy, radiation therapy, and/or a graft.
   - These treatments do not necessarily eliminate the risk of CAR.
   - Radiation therapy may be used to shrink the tumor mass. However, as the mass shrinks, it may tear or open a previously sealed hole in the artery, causing rupture. For this reason, fractionation of radiation is done over a period of 6 to 7 weeks.
   - Carotid endarterectomy increases the risk of cranial nerve palsy, hematoma, pulmonary emboli, and myocardial infraction.
2. Endovascular treatments, such as carotid stents or coils, are an alternative for patients thought to be high risk for surgery or occlusions (Kim et al., 2006; Warren et al., 2002).
   - Placement of carotid coils is more invasive than placement of carotid stents.
   - Carotid coils are used to stop bleeding. Like a Chinese finger trap, the coil tightens as it expands.
3. Balloon occlusion may be used as a temporary measure in carefully selected cases.

EVIDENCE-BASED PRACTICE UPDATES

1. Infection is a major predisposing risk factor for carotid artery rupture (Upile et al., 2005).
2. Postoperative complications such as fistula formation, wound breakdown, wound necrosis, infection, and tumor recurrence almost always precede and are major risk factors for exposure of the carotid artery, ultimately leading to rupture. However, tissue coverage of the carotid artery is not a major element of carotid rupture prevention in patients with head and neck cancer.
3. CAR can occur at any time in any patient with head and neck cancer (Frawler & Begley, 2005).
4. Nurses play an essential role in the early detection and recognition of CAR. Providing early and aggressive nutritional support, promoting wound healing, and detecting and treating infection all can reduce the risk of rupture (Frawler & Begley, 2005; Upile et al., 2005).

TEACHING AND EDUCATION

1. **Explain why the carotid artery rupture could occur.** *Rationale:* Since you had surgery and radiation therapy to remove the cancer in your neck, one of the major blood vessels in your neck, called the *carotid artery*, may become weakened. If the artery wall becomes too weak, it can break down, causing considerable bleeding. If the bleeding is not stopped quickly enough, you could bleed to death.
2. **Instruct the patient and significant others in how to apply digital pressure** (Johantgen, 1998). *Rationale:* If bleeding should occur, apply fingertip pressure directly over the site to reduce blood loss. This pressure must be maintained until the doctor can tie off the artery to stop the bleeding.
3. **Teach the patient and significant others the signs and symptoms of an impending rupture.** *Rationale:* Any signs of bleeding, no matter how small, should be reported immediately to the doctor or nurse, who can assess whether you are at risk for carotid artery rupture.
4. **List the equipment the patient should have on hand in case a rupture occurs at home** (Potter, 2005):
   - Several dark-colored towels to mask the true amount of bleeding

- Gloves and gown
- Suction machine (if possible)
- Red trash bag (for dark colored towels)

5. Make sure the patient and significant others know how to call for emergency assistance and arrange transport to hospital.

NURSING DIAGNOSES

1. **Ineffective tissue perfusion** of cerebral and cardiopulmonary areas related to hemorrhage
2. **Ineffective airway clearance** related to hemorrhage into oropharynx or compression of the trachea
3. **Anxiety** related to poor prognosis and high risk of death
4. **Acute pain** related to tumor infection, fistula formation, and/or tumor
5. **Fear** related to bleeding and/or dying from carotid artery rupture

EVALUATION AND DESIRED OUTCOMES

1. Risk of hemorrhage will be prevented or controlled so that the patient does not die of exsanguination.
2. The patient will have a normal neurologic outcome or minimal neurologic deficit after surgery.
3. Laboratory values, especially hemoglobin and hematocrit, will stabilize and return to normal levels within 48 hours, and pulse oximetry or ABGs will show oxygen at greater than 90% saturation within 20 minutes.
4. If the patient and significant others have decided against emergency measures for resuscitation, the patient will die a calm and peaceful death.

DISCHARGE PLANNING AND FOLLOW-UP CARE

- Have a frank and open discussion with the patient and family about the prognosis for carotid artery rupture.
- Educate the patient and significant others about the signs of a pending carotid artery rupture, reportable symptoms (e.g., slow oozing from the wound site), and how to initiate emergency procedures.
- If emergency procedures are not desired, educate the patient and significant others about how to help the patient have a peaceful death.
- Educate the patient and significant others about how to manage wound care and/or how to arrange daily home visits from visiting nurses or hospice care.
- Remind the patient and significant others to schedule a follow-up visit to the physician's office within 1 to 2 weeks after discharge.
- Advise the patient and significant others that follow-up care should include a weekly complete blood count.
- Advise the patient and significant others that daily home nursing visits should be arranged for wound care management.

REVIEW QUESTIONS

QUESTIONS

1. **Carotid artery rupture is most likely to occur if the patient has a history of:**
   1. Hypertension
   2. Receiving chemotherapy
   3. Metastatic disease
   4. Radical neck surgery and radiation therapy

2. **The initial goal of therapy for patients with carotid artery rupture is to:**
   1. Prevent infection
   2. Improve nutritional status
   3. Control hemorrhage
   4. Control pain

3. **The incidence of CAR in patients who have head and neck cancer is:**
   1. 1% to 2%
   2. 3% to 4%
   3. 5% to 8%
   4. Over 10%

4. **After surgery, all of the following may further weaken the carotid artery** *except:*
   1. Infection at the tumor or surgical site
   2. Formation of a fistula
   3. Tumor invasion into the arterial wall
   4. Chemotherapy

5. **The initial intervention for rupture of the carotid artery is:**
   1. Place the patient in the Trendelenburg position
   2. Apply digital pressure directly to the area of rupture
   3. Administer oxygen at 4 L
   4. Hang 2 units of packed red blood cells

6. **In treating a sudden carotid artery rupture, all of the following interventions should be performed** *except:*
   1. Administration of antiemetics and pain medications
   2. Fluid resuscitation
   3. Maintaining a calm atmosphere
   4. Maintaining airway and cerebral perfusion

7. **Patient education about the potential for carotid artery rupture should include:**
   1. Mouth care
   2. Factors that may increase nausea
   3. Prognostic information, should rupture occur
   4. Activity restrictions

8. **Dark-colored towels are recommended for use during a rupture because:**
   1. They help mask the true amount of bleeding.
   2. They are more absorbent than light-colored towels.
   3. They can show how much bleeding is occurring.
   4. They are softer and can give the patient comfort.

9. **All of the following equipment should be part of the carotid rupture precautions box** *except:*
   1. Gloves and gowns
   2. About 5 L of D5W and red bags
   3. Suction and a Yankauer catheter
   4. Dark, absorbent towels and about 5 L of normal saline

10. **A patient who does not want emergency intervention if a rupture occurs should:**
    1. Receive emergency care anyway
    2. Be provided nutritional support
    3. Be allowed to die with dignity and comfort
    4. Receive fluid resuscitation

ANSWERS

1. *Answer: 4*
   Rationale: Both neck surgery and radiation therapy are known risk factors for CAR.

2. *Answer: 3*
   Rationale: If hemorrhage is not controlled immediately, the patient will exsanguinate and die within a matter of minutes.

3. *Answer: 2*
   Rationale: The incidence of carotid artery rupture in patients who have been

diagnosed with cancer of the head and neck is 3% to 4%.

4. *Answer: 4*
   Rationale: All these factors weaken the artery wall or increase its exposure to air except chemotherapy.

5. *Answer: 2*
   Rationale: Applying direct pressure to the site of the rupture is critical for reducing the danger of exsanguination.

6. *Answer: 1*
   Rationale: Maintaining a patent airway and supporting cerebral perfusion are the primary goals. Administration of antiemetics is unnecessary during a rupture. Antianxiety and pain medications, as well as a calm environment, can help keep the patient calm and comfortable. Fluid resuscitation helps minimize the risk of hypovolemic shock.

7. *Answer: 3*
   Rationale: A frank and open discussion of the risk of carotid artery rupture should be held with the patient and significant others, so that they can make an informed decision about care to be provided if a rupture occurs.

8. *Answer: 1*
   Rationale: Dark-colored towels can help mask the true amount of bleeding, which is especially important if the rupture occurs while the patient is at home.

9. *Answer: 2*
   Rationale: All of the supplies should be part of the carotid precautions box except D5W. Normal saline or lactated Ringer's solution is the fluid of choice for resuscitation.

10. *Answer: 3*
    Rationale: The patient should be allowed to die with dignity and comfort, because the prognosis for CAR is poor, and treatment is not without consequences. Emergency care does not promote either dignity or comfort.

REFERENCES

Frawley, T., & Begley, C. (2006). Caring for people with carotid artery rupture. *British Journal of Nursing*, 15(1):24-28.

Frawley, T., & Begley, C. (2005). Causes and prevention of carotid artery rupture. *British Journal of Nursing*, 14(22):1198-1202.

Johantgen, M. (1998). Carotid artery rupture. In C. Chernecky, & B. Berger (Eds.), *Advanced and critical care oncology nursing* (pp. 97-105). Philadelphia: WB Saunders.

Johnson, M. H. (2003). Carotid blowout syndromes. *Endovascular Today*, January/February, 15.

Kim, H., Lee, D., & Kim, H., et al. (2006). Life-threatening common carotid artery blowout: Rescue treatment with a newly designed self-expanding covered nitinol stent. *British Journal of Radiology*, 79:226-231.

Potter, E. (2005). *The management of carotid artery rupture related to the terminal care of head and neck cancer patient: information and guidelines*. Retrieved March 8, 2006, from www.bahnon.org.uk.

Upile, T., Triardis, S., & Kirkland, P., et al. (2005). The management of carotid artery rupture. *European Archives of Otorhinolaryngology*, 262:555-560.

Warren, F., Cohen, J., & Nesbit, G., et al. (2002). Management of carotid "blowout" with endovascular stent grafts. *Laryngoscope*, 112:428-433.

COGNITIVE DYSFUNCTION

NANCY JO BUSH

PATHOPHYSIOLOGICAL MECHANISMS

Impairment of cognitive function can have a profound effect on the quality of life of cancer survivors. *Cognitive function* is a multidimensional concept that describes the brain's transcription of information necessary to direct behavior and decision making (Muscari, 2006a; Jansen et al., 2005b). Cognitive disorders can occur as a result of dysfunctions in brain anatomy or physiology caused by injury, degenerative disease, neoplasms, arterial or infectious processes, metabolic or nutritional conditions, and medications or substance abuse (Barry, 2002).

Normal, healthy brain function involves the domains of attention and concentration, learning and memory, psychomotor and visuospatial skills, manual dexterity, language, and intelligence (Table 7-1) (Muscari, 2006a; Jansen et al., 2005a). The processes of brain functioning are so interrelated that impairment in one domain unavoidably affects another (Jansen et al., 2005b). Symptoms of cognitive dysfunction can range on a continuum from decreased concentration and short-term memory loss to confusion and delirium. Mild cognitive dysfunction can be misdiagnosed as a psychological problem, such as anxiety or depression. Cognitive dysfunction is associated with a poorer prognosis and difficult patient management issues (Walch et al., 1998). Impairments in learning, memory, focus, and concentration have negative effects on the patient's quality of life, relationships, and safety. Negative effects may include poor job performance, academic difficulties, poor self-esteem, and altered social relationships. Most important are the risk to the patient's safety (e.g., unable to remember medication schedules) and problems with taking care of children (e.g., inability to multitask) (Staat & Segartore, 2005).

EPIDEMIOLOGY AND ETIOLOGY

Multiple factors contribute to cognitive dysfunction in cancer patients. These can be classified as *direct/disease-related factors* and *indirect/treatment-related factors* (Muscari, 2006a; O'Shaughnessy, 2003). Disease-related factors include primary tumors of the central nervous system and brain metastases. Primary brain tumors often cause diffuse cognitive dysfunction or focal deficits related to the site of the tumor (Walch et al., 1998). Frontal lobe tumors have been associated with behavioral symptoms such as emotional lability, apathy, poor judgment, and socially inappropriate behaviors. Temporal lobe tumors have been associated with mania or depressed mood, irritability or anxiety, and seizures. Tumors in the parietal lobe have been associated with sensory abnormalities (e.g., agraphesthesia [loss of tactile recognition]) and motor problems (e.g., apraxias [motor abnormalities]). Occipital tumors have been associated with visual problems such as hemianopsia (loss of half of the visual field in both eyes) (Walch et al., 1998). Even though few research studies have focused on cognitive dysfunction related to primary brain tumors, the findings of these studies can help health care providers use the site of the tumor or metastasis in the brain as a guide for assessment of possible cognitive deficits.

Table 7-1	DOMAINS OF COGNITIVE FUNCTION
Domain	Cognitive Function
Attention	Attention enables the brain to decipher relevant information while ignoring information that is irrelevant or distracting. The three types of attention are *selective attention* (ability to focus), *sustained attention* (concentration), and *directed attention* (ability to multitask).
Concentration	Concentration is the ability to focus and sustain attention.
Learning	Learning is the process of acquiring new information.
Memory	Memory is the retention of learned information by repetition. The two types of memory are *short-term memory* (brief, working memory) and *long-term memory* (semantic memory) that contains the knowledge that is learned and remembered.
Psychomotor	Psychomotor function is the motor function responsible for motor performance, speed, strength, and coordination of movement; includes manual dexterity.
Visuospatial	Visuospatial function is the ability to process visual information about where objects are in space; it is necessary to perform manual tasks.
Language	Language processing involves comprehending and communicating verbal and written symbols to express thoughts, follow directions, and be in relationships with others.
Intelligence	Also referred to as *executive function*, the intelligence domain involves higher order cognitive processing such as initiation, planning, judgment, and decision making.

Data from Jansen, C., Miaskowski, C., & Dodd, M., et al. (2005a). Chemotherapy-induced cognitive impairment in women with breast cancer: A critique of the literature. *Oncology Nursing Forum, 32:*329-342; and Jansen, C., Miaskowski, C., & Dodd, M., et al., (2005b). Potential mechanisms for chemotherapy-induced impairments in cognitive function. *Oncology Nursing Forum, 32:*1151-1161.

Other direct/disease-related factors that contribute to cognitive dysfunction are age, intelligence, and educational level (Muscari, 2006a). Cognitive decline is expected as adults age and may be exacerbated by the decline in hearing and sight. Normal, expected cognitive changes among the elderly must be differentiated from disease- or treatment-related cognitive impairment, psychiatric diagnoses (e.g., depression and anxiety), dementia (Muscari, 2006a; Smith & Buckwalter, 2006), and delirium (Bond et al., 2006; Boyle, 2006). Although not yet investigated in the oncology population, *cognitive reserve,* or the baseline intelligence quotient (IQ), may be a protective mechanism against brain trauma (Muscari, 2006a).

Indirect/treatment-related factors that contribute to cognitive dysfunction can be classified according to (1) the adverse effects of treatment modalities (e.g., radiation, chemotherapy, biologic response modifiers) and (2) indirect factors, including the metabolic, endocrinologic, and nutritional abnormalities that commonly occur with malignancies or as side effects of treatment and primary psychiatric co-morbidities. Radiation therapy to treat metastatic disease or used prophylactically puts patients at risk for cognitive impairment. Variables that contribute to neurotoxicity include the dose of radiation, the volume of tissue irradiated, and the number of treatments (Walch et al., 1998). Adverse effects of radiation therapy include cerebral edema, demyelination, leukoencephalopathy, and radiation necrosis (Walch et al., 1998). Assessing the true impact of radiotherapy on cognitive function is difficult, because problems arise with following patients long term and differentiating between progression of CNS disease and the negative effects of radiotherapy (Muscari, 2006a). Patients who receive high doses of cranial radiation while undergoing high-dose chemotherapy may be at greatest risk (Walch et al., 1998).

Cognitive impairment caused by chemotherapeutic agents often is referred to as *chemo brain* or *chemo clutter* (Muscari, 2006a; Jansen et al., 2005b; Staat & Segatore, 2005; Walch et al., 1998). Most research on chemotherapy-related cognitive dysfunction has involved patients treated for breast cancer. As many as 50% of these patients reported mental changes, such as difficulties with memory, thinking, and concentration (Muscari, 2006a; Jansen et al., 2005a; Staat & Segatore, 2005). The impairment has been described as subtle, mild to moderate changes that can last as long as 10 years after treatment (Staat & Segatore, 2005).

A review of the literature investigating chemotherapy-induced cognitive impairment in women treated for breast cancer (Jansen et al., 2005a) provided a comprehensive analysis of the cognitive domains that may be impaired by the neurotoxicity of chemotherapy. Three hypothetical mechanisms for neurotoxicity have been postulated: direct neurotoxicity, inflammatory or immunologic responses, and microvascular invasion (Staat & Segatore, 2005; Saykin et al., 2003). Neurotoxicity has been described as including encephalopathy, leukoencephalopathy, cytokine-induced inflammatory response, cerebellar symptoms and, most often, chemotherapy-induced anemia and chemotherapy-induced menopause (Jansen et al., 2005b; Walch et al., 1998).

The direct impact of certain chemotherapeutic agents has been described (Table 7-2), but drawing definitive conclusions is difficult because of the numerous drug combinations and schedules (Walch et al., 1998) and the need for valid, reliable, and sensitive neuropsychological tests (Jansen et al., 2005a). Agents such as cyclophosphamide, doxorubicin, methotrexate, and 5-fluorouracil have been reported to correlate with dysfunction, especially in doses that enable the drug to cross the blood-brain barrier (Jansen et al., 2005b; Staat & Segatore, 2005). High-dose, intensive chemotherapy regimens, combination chemotherapy and radiation protocols, and bone marrow transplantation may also exacerbate short- and long-term cognitive dysfunction. Pre-existing neurologic abnormalities (e.g., cerebral atrophy, brain metastases) and variables such as gender (e.g., hormonal differences) and age (e.g., normal cognitive decline in the elderly) compound the difficulty of drawing definitive conclusions about treatment-related neuropsychological effects (Muscari, 2006a; Walch et al. 1998). Interestingly, subjective complaints do not always seem to correlate with objective tests of cognitive function (Statt & Segatore, 2005).

Additional indirect effects that exacerbate cognitive impairment in patients with cancer are listed in Box 7-1. Common adverse effects of the disease and its treatment, such as infection, fever, and vitamin and nutritional deficiencies, may also contribute to cognitive loss. Deficiencies in estrogen and progesterone (e.g., chemotherapy-induced menopause and estrogen-blocking medications) have been shown to have deleterious effects on attention, learning, and memory (Muscari, 2006a; Staat & Segatore, 2005). Research has shown that anemia (e.g., a hemoglobin level less than 12 g/dL in women and less than 13 g/dL in men) has a deleterious effect on cognitive function (Muscari, 2006a; Cunningham, 2003); administration of epoetin alfa or darbepoetin to patients with a hemoglobin level less than 10 g/dL may have a neuroprotective effect (Cunningham, 2003). In addition, concurrent use of medications such as antiemetics and antidepressants may adversely affect cognitive ability, and the negative effect of substance abuse must not be overlooked.

RISK PROFILE

- Benign or malignant tumors of the brain or metastases to the brain
- Elderly patients who have concurrent, expected age-related changes in sight, hearing, and sensory input, degenerative diseases (e.g., Alzheimer's disease), or arterial insufficiency (cerebral vascular accident or vascular dementia)

Table 7-2	EXAMPLES OF CHEMOTHERAPY-RELATED COGNITIVE DYSFUNCTION
Chemotherapeutic Agent	**Dysfunction**
Cyclophosphamide	Can cross the blood-brain barrier.
	Causes reversible visual blurring, dizziness, and confusion when administered in high doses.
Doxorubicin	Combination of doxorubicin and cyclosporine may increase doxorubicin levels in the brain, possibly leading to encephalopathy.
	Doxorubicin-induced cardiac toxicity may lead to cerebral ischemia or infarct.
5-Fluorouracil (5-FU)	Easily crosses the blood-brain barrier; highest concentrations in the cerebellum.
	Causes accumulation of neurotoxic metabolites.
	Individuals with a genetic deficiency in the enzyme needed to break down 5-FU (dihydropyrimidine dehydrogenase) are at greater risk for neurotoxicity.
	Cerebellar symptoms of neurotoxicity include ataxia, vertigo, diplopia, and limb incoordination.
Methotrexate (MTX)	Intrathecal MTX causes neurotoxicity; effects can range from memory and concentration deficits to progressive dementia.
	Acute encephalopathy with confusion, altered behavior, and disorientation have occurred with high doses of intravenous MTX.
Paclitaxel	Commonly causes peripheral neuropathies.
	In rare cases causes encephalopathy and seizures.
L-asparaginase	Causes cerebral toxicities by inducing metabolic changes.
	Causes altered level of consciousness, confusion, depression, personality changes, and hallucinations.
Ifosfamide	Metabolite chloroacetaldehyde causes direct CNS damage.
	Causes altered level of consciousness, ataxia, seizures, encephalopathy, CNS dysfunction.
High-dose interleukin-2	Causes dose-related cognitive changes.
	Causes disorientation, impaired attention, psychomotor slowing, and aphasia.
Interferon alpha	Causes psychomotor slowing and impaired memory, speech, and concentration.
	Causes permanent deficits in memory and motor coordination; frontal lobe executive function deficits have been reported.
Glucocorticosteroids	Reduces cerebral blood flow, impairs the blood-brain barrier.
	Causes personality changes, "steroid psychosis."

Data from Jansen, C., Miaskowski, C., & Dodd, M., et al. (2005b). Potential mechanisms for chemotherapy-induced impairments in cognitive function. *Oncology Nursing Forum, 32*:1151–1161; Staat, K., & Segartore, M. (2005). The phenomenon of chemo brain. *Clinical Journal of Oncology Nursing, 9*:713–721; and Walch, S. E., Ahles, T. A. & Saykin, A. J. (1998). Neuropsychologic impact of cancer and cancer treatments. In J. C. Holland (Ed.), *Psycho-oncology* (pp. 500-505). New York: Oxford University Press.

- Estrogen and progesterone deficiency related to chemotherapy-induced or natural menopause
- Disease- or treatment-induced anemia
- Nutritional deficiencies in folic acid, thiamine, and nicotinic acid
- Infectious processes and fever
- Electrolyte imbalances (e.g., hypercalcemia)
- Alcohol or controlled substance abuse
- Concurrent psychiatric illnesses, such as depression and anxiety, treated with antidepressants, or associated symptoms, such as sleep disorders

BOX 7-1	DIRECT AND INDIRECT MECHANISMS OF COGNITIVE DYSFUNCTION

Direct Mechanisms
• Primary CNS malignancies
• CNS metastases

Indirect Mechanisms
• Tumor type
• Chemotherapeutic agents
• Anemia
• Metabolic abnormalities
• Endocrinologic abnormalities
• Nutritional deficiencies
• Infection/fever
• Medications
• Advancing age
• Gender
• Depression or anxiety
• Sleep disorders

*Data from Cunningham, R. S. (2003). Anemia in the oncology patient: Cognitive function in cancer. *Cancer Nursing, 26*(Suppl. 6):38S-42S; Muscari, E. (2006a). Cognitive impairment in cancer. In R. M. Carroll-Johnson, L. M. Gordon, & N. J. Bush (Eds.), *Psychosocial nursing care along the cancer continuum* (pp. 191-201). Pittsburgh: Oncology Nursing Society; and O'Shaughnessy, J. (2003). Chemotherapy-related cognitive dysfunction in breast cancer. *Seminars in Oncology Nursing, 19* (Suppl. 2):17–24.

• Chemotherapeutic agents (i.e., type of drug and dosage, duration of treatment, combination protocols)
• Radiation therapy (i.e., localization of treatment, duration of treatment, number of fractionated doses)

PROGNOSIS

The associated risks and the incidence of cognitive dysfunction for patients undergoing cancer treatment require further investigation. However, emerging research has confirmed the existence of treatment-induced impairments and the negative impact on the patient's quality of life (Jansen et al., 2005a; Staat & Segatore, 2005). The symptoms of cognitive dysfunction are extremely distressing to both the patient and the family, and the devastating and demoralizing impact of these dysfunctions must not go unrecognized (Staat & Segatore, 2005). Neuropsychological changes can persist only during treatment, for a short time after treatment stops, or for many years after treatment, as is the case with patients who undergo bone marrow transplantation (Walch et al., 1998).

The prognosis is influenced by the patient's intelligence and educational level before diagnosis; by the patient's age and gender; and by treatment variables, such as the chemotherapeutic drug used and the dosage, the radiation dose and fractionation schedule, and the intensity, duration, and combination of treatment protocols. The prognosis also is influenced by any concurrent neuropsychiatric illnesses, such as depression and anxiety.

PROFESSIONAL ASSESSMENT CRITERIA (PAC)

1. Ensure the patient's physical safety and that of any dependent children. Patients with cognitive impairment can have problems with memory, understanding and

following directions, multitasking, and so forth. Ask the patient if she is having any trouble carrying out activities of daily living or caring for her young children or elderly family members. Ask her if her job performance has been negatively affected during or after treatment, and if so, in what way. This is especially important for professionals in high-risk professions, such as airline pilots (Staat & Segatore, 2005).

2. All patients undergoing cancer treatment should be assessed for cognitive impairment before and during treatment and also at follow-up appointments. The assessment should include thorough evaluation of both direct/disease-related factors and indirect/treatment-related factors (Muscari, 2006a; O'Shaughnessy, 2003). Observational assessment may be the most appropriate and sensitive method of screening for cognitive dysfunction (Staat & Segatore, 2005; O'Shaughnessy, 2003). If cognitive impairment is not reported directly by the patient or family, nurses can look for certain signs during each routine history and physical examination. These signs include repetition of questions, difficulty following conversation or directions, searching for words, or inability to remember sequences of events. The patient may say she has withdrawn from social activities she once enjoyed out of embarrassment because she recognizes the behaviors associated with the cognitive changes. Family members may report that the patient is unable to carry out activities of daily living, such as finances or housework, or meals go unattended (Muscari, 2006a).

3. Available systematic screening tools (e.g., the High Sensitivity Cognitive Screen and the Executive Interview) are valid and easy to administer in the clinical practice setting (O'Shaughnessy, 2003). The Mini-Mental State Examination (MMSE), adapted from a more extensive cognitive mental status examination, is user friendly in the clinical setting (Muscari, 2006b). These tools are not diagnostic measures, but they can help clinicians appropriately refer patients for more thorough neuropsychological testing if needed.

4. Differential diagnosis for cognitive impairment must include a thorough assessment of medical conditions that may contribute to or exacerbate dysfunction (Muscari, 2006a). These conditions include uncontrolled symptoms related to the disease and treatment, such as trauma, infection, or stroke. Impaired metabolic status (e.g., electrolyte imbalance) and conditions such as hypercalcemia can contribute to confusion. Other medical factors may include anemia, nutritional deficiencies, hormonal abnormalities, and substance abuse, to name a few. Differential diagnosis also must consider organic CNS involvement (e.g., brain metastasis), delirium, and dementia.

5. Delirium is a syndrome of altered cognition, attention, and behavior that results from pathophysiologic disturbances of the central nervous system (Bond et al., 2006). Delirium is a *medical* problem, not a psychological one, but early symptoms often are misdiagnosed as anxiety, depression, anger, or psychosis (Breitbart et al., 1998). Delirium is a common disorder of the elderly that affects as many as 80% of hospitalized patients (Muscari, 2006b). As many as 90% of patients in the terminal stage of cancer have delirium in the final weeks of life (Bond et al., 2006). Variables that increase the risk of delirium in a patient with cancer include age, advanced disease, co-morbid illnesses, and pre-existing cognitive impairment (Bond et al., 2006). Unfortunately, little research has been done on delirium in older patients with cancer, a situation that has contributed to misdiagnosis and lack of early identification that could reduce symptoms (Boyle, 2006). *Delirium* is defined as an acute organic brain syndrome involving a change in level of consciousness and cognitive function (thinking, perception, and memory) that develops over a short period (American Psychiatric Association, 2000). This onset of acute confusion often signifies a worsening of the primary illness or

a complication of treatment. The etiology of delirium is multifactorial, especially in older patients and the terminally ill (Box 7-2) (Boyle, 2006; Musari, 2006b). Assessment should focus on the patient's clinical situation in the 48 hours before the symptoms developed (e.g., an older, postoperative patient with cancer with pain, fever, and multiple medications) (Boyle, 2006). The hallmark features of delirium include impaired cognition, disturbance in consciousness, sudden onset of or fluctuating symptoms, and sleep-wake cycle alterations (Boyle, 2006). Symptoms of delirium usually become worse at night and are accompanied by hyperactivity (Muscari, 2006b). Delirium is a medical emergency, and a diagnosis of delirium should be considered in any patient who experiences an acute onset of agitation, impaired cognitive function, or a change in level of consciousness (Kuebler et al., 2006; Muscari, 2006b; Breitbart et al., 1998). Pharmacologic agents, specifically drugs with central anticholinergic CNS effects and those that can cross the blood-brain barrier, are the most common causes of acute delirium (Boyle, 2006). Dysfunctional cognition in a delirious patient hinders communication between the patient and family members and between the patient and health care personnel. This compromises reliable symptom assessment, counseling, and active patient participation in the therapeutic decision-making process.

6. *Dementia*, a global loss of cognitive and intellectual functioning, is an important risk factor for delirium; however, it is a distinctly different form of cognitive impairment (Box 7-3) (Muscari, 2006b; Smith & Buckwalter, 2006). Dementia may be the result of different diseases (e.g., Parkinson's disease, Huntington's disease, AIDS, and Alzheimer's disease), but all these diseases have common symptoms. Dementia that is truly oncologic is disease- or treatment-related involvement of the brain and spinal cord (e.g., radiation therapy for brain metastases) (Muscari, 2006b). Differential diagnosis is important, because changes in cognition caused by medications, treatment, delirium, or mood states such as depression and anxiety may trigger dementia-like syndromes that are treatable. Dementia also has a behavioral component, such as apathy, withdrawal, and paranoia; sleep changes; and wandering (Smith & Buckwalter, 2006).

7. The psychosocial impact of cognitive impairment on the patient, family, and primary caregiver is immeasurable. For patients who have insight into their cognitive changes, the fear of losing control and losing their dignity can be devastating, putting the patient at risk for anxiety, depression, and suicide ideation (Muscari, 2006b). Even patients who suffer from dementia often have insight into their declining mental faculties, which compounds the emotional impact of their impending losses. Short-term

BOX 7-2	ASSESSMENT FOR UNDERLYING CAUSES OF DELIRIUM, AGITATION, AND CONFUSION

Drugs (especially psychotropics)
Electrolyte or glucose abnormality
Liver failure
Ischemia or hypoxia
Renal failure
Impaction of stool
Urinary tract (or other) infection
Metastasis to the brain

From Storey, P. (1994). Symptom control in advanced cancer. *Seminars in Oncology, 21*:748-753.

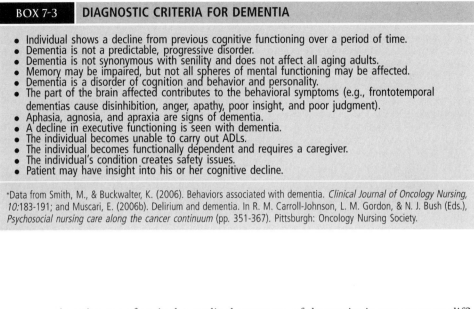

*Data from Smith, M., & Buckwalter, K. (2006). Behaviors associated with dementia. *Clinical Journal of Oncology Nursing, 10*:183-191; and Muscari, E. (2006b). Delirium and dementia. In R. M. Carroll-Johnson, L. M. Gordon, & N. J. Bush (Eds.), *Psychosocial nursing care along the cancer continuum* (pp. 351-367). Pittsburgh: Oncology Nursing Society.

memory impairment often is the cardinal symptom of dementia; it progresses to diffi-culty carrying out ADLs and becoming functionally dependent on others. Caregiver strain is very common with dementia, as is the emotional trauma of losing the loved one gradually with cognitive decline. The rapid onset of delirium and its symptoms can be frightening and overwhelming to a family that is not aware of what is happening to their loved one. Health care professionals also may become frustrated and angry with a delirious patient who is negative or hostile or who displays impulsive behaviors (Muscari, 2006b).

NURSING CARE AND TREATMENT

1. Nursing interventions for cognitive dysfunction should be directed toward patient safety, identification of underlying etiologies, symptom management, and psychological support for the patient and family (Boyle, 2006).
2. Identify patients at risk for cognitive dysfunction related to disease or treatment, espe-cially elderly individuals with co-morbid illness, age-related sensory deprivation, and dementia. Monitor laboratory values, evaluate adverse effects of medications, monitor nutrition and hydration, and assess for anemia, pain, and fever (Boyle, 2006).
3. Protect decision making on the patient's behalf (e.g., ensure informed consent) when the patient is incapacitated or cognitively impaired. This may require repeated educational sessions with assistance from family members to make sure the patient understands treatment protocols or clinical research findings (Muscari, 2006b). Patients must also be well informed of the risks and benefits associated with treatments, including the risk of cognitive impairment, so that they can make informed decisions and are prepared (O'Shaughnessy, 2003). Special attention must be paid to elderly patients, who may also have deficits in sight and hearing.
4. Symptom management of conditions that may contribute to or exacerbate cognitive dysfunction includes appropriate treatment for pain, fatigue, anemia, chemotherapy-induced menopause, sleep disorders, depression, and anxiety (Muscari, 2006b; O'Shaughnessy, 2003). The most commonly reported and most distressing side effect

of chemotherapy is fatigue. Physical fatigue and mental fatigue negatively affect cognitive function and diminish the quality of life (Jansen et al., 2005b).

5. Provide the patient and family with tools and resources to empower the patient who has memory loss or attention deficits. These may include visual aids, written medication profiles with daily or weekly prefilled medication trays, calendars dated for follow-up appointments, calculators, and so forth (Muscari, 2006b).

6. Administer pharmacotherapeutic agents that may provide neuroprotection (e.g., erythropoietin) or that reduce the adverse effects of chemotherapy that exacerbate cognitive impairment (e.g., venlafaxine [Effexor] for the mood and sleep disorders caused by chemotherapy-induced menopause), or medications that support attention and memory (e.g., the psychostimulant methylphenidate [Ritalin]).

7. Emotional and psychosocial support is imperative for the cognitively impaired patient and the patient's caregiver. Validate the patient's experiences so that the person does not feel as if he is "going crazy." Assure the patient that impairment in certain cognitive domains does not lead to dysfunction in all domains, nor does it contribute to the development of dementia. Tailoring informed consent to the specific risks as determined by the tumor site, the treatment modalities, and the patient's educational level, hormonal status, and age can reduce anxiety and apprehension about "the worst." (Muscari, 2006b).

8. Help the patient identify activities that will support her independence and quality of life. As mentioned, cognitive rehabilitation has not been studied in oncology patients, but interventions developed for other patient groups (e.g., those with dementia) can be applied (Walch et al., 1998). First, identify and validate the patient's deficits. Then provide alternative solutions for problem solving that will help ease the patient's fear and frustration (Muscari, 2006b). For example, if a patient is struggling with attention problems, encourage her to schedule additional time when learning a new task or to take rest periods during a stressful workday; this helps her *reframe* her deficits and feel in control of her cognitive challenges.

9. Symptomatic and supportive measures to reduce agitation, anxiety, and disorientation are of utmost importance in treating patients with delirium. These measures range from providing a safe, nonstimulating, familiar environment to pharmacologic management with haloperidol, the drug of choice in the treatment of delirium in the terminally ill (Brietbart et al., 1998). Psychosocial assessment of the effect of delirium and of end of life care on the family is a priority. Terminal restlessness is a form of delirium that may occur in the last days or hours before death, and it is emotionally challenging for the family (Itano & Taoka, 2005). The term *acute confusional state* has also been used to describe this syndrome (National Cancer Institute, 2007).

EVIDENCE-BASED PRACTICE UPDATES

1. The National Coalition for Cancer Survivorship (NCCS) recognizes cognitive impairment as a significant challenge for cancer survivors (Ferrell & Dow, 1997).

2. Each of the major forms of cancer therapy poses a risk for neuropsychological impairment (Walch et al., 1998).

3. Cognitive disorders and delirium are neuropsychiatric syndromes that occur frequently in patients with cancer, particularly in those with advanced disease. The incidence ranges from 28% to 48% in hospitalized and hospice patients with advanced cancer; approximately 90% of these patients experience delirium in the hours to days before death (National Cancer Institute, 2007).

4. Cognitive dysfunction, especially delirium, is negatively associated with physiologic consequences such as falls and fractures. It also interferes with hydration, nutrition,

medication administration, completion of treatment, and the patient's ability to recognize and articulate symptoms. These sequelae ultimately affect the patient's quality of survival (Boyle, 2006).

TEACHING AND EDUCATION

1. **Teach the patient and family about the possible adverse effects of the disease or treatment on cognitive function.** *Rationale:* This is a part of informed consent
2. **Instruct the patient in self-care strategies.** *Rationale:* These strategies will help reframe deficits and reduce feelings of powerlessness (Box 7-4).
3. **Validate the patient's fears and concerns about therapy-related changes in the cognitive domains.** *Rationale:* This will normalize feelings and give reassurance that the patient is not "losing his mind."
4. **Educate family caregivers of patients in the terminal stages of illness about the prodromal signs of delirium: confused thinking, difficulty concentrating, perceptual distortions, and behavioral changes, such as anxiety, restlessness, irritability, mood disturbance, insomnia, and hypersensitivity to light and noise** (Boyle, 2006). *Rationale:* Knowing what to expect helps families to prepare for the changes in the patient's mental status.

NURSING DIAGNOSES

1. **Risk for injury** related to poor mental judgment
2. **Powerlessness** related to loss of decision making capacity
3. **Self-care deficit** related to altered judgment
4. **Acute confusion** related to metabolic disturbance
5. **Impaired home maintenance** related to confusion

BOX 7-4   SELF-CARE STRATEGIES TO ENHANCE COGNITIVE FUNCTIONING

Mental Strategies
- Keep your expectations realistic (i.e., reframe).
- Break down big projects into smaller, simpler components.
- Organize and prioritize tasks.
- Avoid multitasking.
- Establish a routine.
- Reduce work stressors.
- Work in a quiet environment.
- Keep lists, calendars, and memory cards.
- Exercise your brain (e.g., read, do crossword puzzles).

Physical Strategies
- Exercise to increase your strength and reduce stress.
- Pace your activities.
- Get adequate sleep and rest periods.
- Avoid stimulants such as caffeine and nicotine.
- Wear glasses and/or hearing aids if necessary.
- Look into relaxation therapy or guided imagery.

Psychosocial Strategies
- Inform health care providers of your deficits.
- Ask for help if you feel overwhelmed.
- Stay socially active with friends and family.
- Consider joining a support group.

Modified from Staat, K. & Segartore, M. (2005). The phenomenon of chemo brain. *Clinical Journal of Oncology Nursing,* 9:713-721.

EVALUATION AND DESIRED OUTCOMES

1. The patient will be safe from self-harm.
2. Cognitive dysfunction will be diagnosed and treated.
3. Delirium will be diagnosed and treated.
4. Education and emotional support will be provided to the patient so that the person does not feel as if he or she is "going crazy."
5. The patient will express a sense of control and self-efficacy.
6. The patient will verbalize quality of life and a sense of hope.
7. A family systems approach will be carried out for psychosocial assessment and interventions to prevent caregiver strain.
8. The patient will be able to identify self-help strategies that will optimize cognitive functioning and reduce frustration.

DISCHARGE PLANNING AND FOLLOW-UP CARE

- Continuity of care between inpatient care, ambulatory care, and home care will be planned, with medication instructions and follow-up instructions clearly delineated using supportive tools (e.g., prefilled medication trays, calendars, memory cards).
- Arrangements for home care or a visiting nurse will be made when needed, especially for elderly patients who may have both cognitive and sensory deficits. A home assessment will be arranged for safety and management if appropriate.
- Hospice will be arranged for patients with advanced cancer, and the family will be educated about the prodromal symptoms of delirium.

REVIEW QUESTIONS

QUESTIONS

1. **Which of the following has been associated with an increased risk for cognitive dysfunction:**
   1. Chemotherapy-induced anemia
   2. Decreased liver function
   3. Chronic renal failure
   4. Neutropenic fever

2. **All of the following may contribute to cognitive impairment** *except:*
   1. Advanced age
   2. Chemotherapy-induced menopause
   3. Estrogen hormone replacement
   4. Infection with fever

3. **You are caring for a patient with mild cognitive dysfunction. She tells you that she is having difficulty completing her tasks at work, and she feels frustrated. Your best response is:**
   1. "You just need to try harder."
   2. "You've been working throughout chemotherapy, what's the problem now?"
   3. "If you wanted to complete the tasks, you'd focus more attention on them."
   4. "Can you describe what tasks you are having trouble with and maybe we can discuss some possible solutions."

4. **A common side effect of chemotherapy that has also been shown to exacerbate cognitive dysfunction is:**
   1. Anorexia
   2. Nausea
   3. Fatigue
   4. Diarrhea

5. **An important nursing intervention when caring for a patient with delirium is:**
   1. Using restraints to ensure the patient's safety
   2. Providing a calm environment
   3. Barring family visitors
   4. Turning out the lights in the room

6. **Which of the following is the preferred neuroleptic for managing delirium:**
   1. Haloperidol
   2. Gabapentin
   3. Phenobarbital
   4. Phenytoin

7. **An important distinction between delirium and dementia is that delirium involves:**
   1. Associated depression
   2. Impaired level of consciousness
   3. A rapid onset
   4. Disorientation

8. **Your patient has been informed that she may suffer from chemotherapy-related cognitive changes, and she expresses her distress at this possibility. Your best response is:**
   1. "Focus on the challenges of getting through chemotherapy."
   2. "It may comfort you to know that other patients experience the same symptoms, and there are self-care strategies and skills you can learn that are helpful."
   3. "Cognitive impairment is nothing compared to facing a life-threatening illness."
   4. "Don't dwell on the worst case scenarios of chemotherapy."

9. **The population of patients at highest risk for complications related to cognitive impairment is:**
   1. The socially disadvantaged
   2. The withdrawn and isolated
   3. The elderly
   4. Patients undergoing radiation therapy

10. **Your elderly patient comes into the clinic for his follow-up appointment. He is slightly confused and does not remember that he is undergoing chemotherapy today. Which of the following behaviors alerts you to his increased risk for cognitive impairment:**
    1. When you ask him if he took his required pretreatment dexamethasone, he states that he does not remember and he dumps all his medicine bottles on your desk.

2. He tells you that it is difficult for him to remember which day he has chemotherapy, so he appreciates the phone call to remind him.
3. He is slightly irritable and complains that he has been in the waiting room for over an hour.
4. He tells you that he has been feeling sad the last few weeks "for no reason at all."

ANSWERS

1. *Answer: 1*
   Rationale: Chemotherapy-induced anemia may contribute to cognitive dysfunction with symptoms such as poor concentration, memory problems, and difficulty with attention (Cunningham, 2003).

2. *Answer: 3*
   Rationale: Advancing age, menopause, and infection with fever can all contribute to cognitive impairment. Estrogen deficiency has been associated with cognitive decline (e.g., impaired learning and verbal memory) in healthy postmenopausal women or in women who have experienced natural or surgical menopause (Staat & Segatore, 2005; O'Shaughnessy, 2003). Hormonal replacement therapy (HRT) with estrogen may serve a protective function, but research findings remain inconclusive, and HRT is not recommended for women with a history of estrogen receptor–positive breast cancer (Staat & Segatore, 2005).

3. *Answer: 4*
   Rationale: Well-meaning caregivers can worsen patient anxiety and frustration by telling the person to "just try harder." Supportive interventions include helping the patient to problem-solve and to break down tasks into smaller steps while at the same time providing reassurance (Smith & Buckwalter, 2006).

4. *Answer: 3*
   Rationale: The most commonly reported and most distressing side effect of chemotherapy is fatigue. Physical fatigue and mental fatigue negatively affect cognitive function and diminish the

quality of life (Jansen et al., 2005b). Patients have said that they are "too tired to think."

5. *Answer: 2*
   Rationale: Supportive measures to reduce agitation, anxiety, and disorientation are of utmost importance in treating the patient with delirium. These measures include providing a safe, nonstimulating, and familiar environment. Patients with delirium are sensitive to extremes of activity and noise. A well-lit room with reduced stimuli is advised, and family visits are encouraged to increase the patient's sense of security and familiarity (Boyle, 2006). Sedation for severe agitation is preferable over restraints, which should be used only to prevent injury (Breitbart et al., 1998).

6. *Answer: 1*
   Rationale: Haloperidol is the drug of choice because it is a high-potency dopamine-blocking agent, it has no active metabolites, and it can be administered by mouth, intravenously, or intramuscularly. Haloperidol also has a less sedative effect than phenothiazine neuroleptics (Boyle, 2006).

7. *Answer: 3*
   Rationale: Dementia is slow to develop, whereas delirium is sudden in onset. Cognitive changes with dementia are progressive and irreversible, whereas the symptoms of delirium wax and wane and are more prominent at night and in the dark (Boyle, 2006; Muscari, 2006b). Disorientation as to time and place occurs in delirium and fluctuates in severity. Disorientation in dementia increases as the disease progresses (Boyle, 2006). Symptoms of depression may mimic dementia or early delirium, and depression is an important differential

diagnosis. The patient with dementia may also become depressed, especially early in the disease if the person has insight into the cognitive losses.

8. *Answer: 2*
   Rationale: Patients should be informed of both the risks and the benefits of chemotherapy, including the possibility of cognitive impairment. It is important to validate the patient's concerns, at the same time offering reassurance that self-care strategies can enhance cognitive function if deficits occur (Boyle, 2006; Muscari, 2006b).

9. *Answer: 3*
   Rationale: The elderly are at greatest risk for complications related to cognitive impairment, because advancing age is associated with changes in sight and hearing, as well as age-related dementia, co-morbid illnesses, and other risks for cognitive dysfunction, such as endocrinologic, metabolic, nutritional, and vascular insufficiency (Boyle, 2006).

10. *Answer: 1*
    Rationale: Pharmacologic agents are the most common cause of acute confusion and cognitive dysfunction, especially in older patients, who experience age-related changes in drug absorption, distribution, metabolism, and excretion (Boyle, 2006). Most likely this patient is being treated with multiple drugs to combat disease and chemotherapy-related sequelae (e.g., dexamethasone, antiemetics, and possibly benzodiazepines for anxiety and opioids for pain). He therefore is at increased risk for cognitive impairment caused by polypharmacy and the likelihood of drug interactions or his own reactions to the drugs (e.g., steroid-induced psychosis) (Boyle, 2006)

REFERENCES

American Psychiatric Association. (2000). *Diagnostic and statistical manual of mental disorders.* (4th ed., text rev.). Washington, D.C.: The Association.

Barry, P. D. (2002). *Mental health and mental illness.* (7th ed.). Philadelphia: Lippincott.

Bond, S. M., Neelon, V. J., & Belyea, M. J. (2006). Delirium in hospitalized older patients with cancer. *Oncology Nursing Forum, 33*:1075-1083.

Boyle, D. A. (2006). Delirium in older adults with cancer: Implications for practice and research. *Oncology Nursing Forum, 33*:61-78.

Breitbart, W., Jaramillo, J. R., & Chochinov, H. M. (1998). Palliative and terminal care. In J. C. Holland, (Ed). *Psycho-oncology* (pp. 437-449). New York: Oxford University Press.

Cunningham, R. S. (2003). Anemia in the oncology patient: Cognitive function in cancer. *Cancer Nursing, 26*(Suppl. 6):38S-42S.

Ferrell, B. R., & Dow, K. H. (1997). Quality of life among long-term cancer survivors. *Oncology, 11:*565-576.

Itano, J. K, & Taoka, K. N. (2005). *Core curriculum for oncology nursing* (pp. 117-118). (4th ed.). St. Louis: Elsevier.

Jansen, C., Miaskowski, C., & Dodd, M. (2005a). Chemotherapy-induced cognitive impairment in women with breast cancer: A critique of the literature. *Oncology Nursing Forum, 32:*329-342.

Jansen, C., Miaskowski, C., & Dodd, M., et al. (2005b). Potential mechanisms for chemotherapy-induced impairments in cognitive function. *Oncology Nursing Forum, 32:*1151-1161.

Kuebler, K. K., Heidrich, D. E., & Vena, C., et al. (2006). Delirium, confusion, and agitation. In B.R. Ferrell, & N. Coyle (Eds.), *Textbook of palliative nursing* (pp. 401-420). (2nd ed.). New York: Oxford University Press.

Muscari, E. (2006a). Cognitive impairment in cancer. In R. M. Carroll-Johnson, L. M. Gordon, & N. J. Bush (Eds.), *Psychosocial nursing care along the cancer continuum* (pp. 191-201). Pittsburgh: Oncology Nursing Society.

Muscari, E. (2006b). Delirium and dementia. In R. M. Carroll-Johnson, L. M. Gordon, & N. J. Bush (Eds.), *Psychosocial nursing care along the cancer continuum* (pp. 351-367). Pittsburgh: Oncology Nursing Society.

National Cancer Institute (2007). Cognitive disorders and delirium PDQ. Retrieved December 12, 2007, from http://www.cancer.gov/cancertopics/pdq/supportivecare/delirium/healthprofessional.

O'Shaughnessy, J. (2003). Chemotherapy-related cognitive dysfunction in breast cancer. *Seminars in Oncology Nursing, 19*(Suppl. 2):17-24.

Saykin, A. J., Ahles, T. A., & McDonald, B. C. (2003). Mechanisms of chemotherapy induced cognitive disorders: Neuropsychological, pathophysiological, and neuroimaging perspectives. *Seminars in Clinical Neuropsychiatry, 8:*201-216.

Smith, M., & Buckwalter, K. (2006). Behaviors associated with dementia. *Clinical Journal of Oncology Nursing, 10:*183-191.

Staat, K., & Segartore, M. (2005). The phenomenon of chemo brain. *Clinical Journal of Oncology Nursing, 9:*713-721.

Walch, S. E., Ahles, T. A., & Saykin, A. J. (1998). Neuropsychologic impact of cancer and cancer treatments. In J. C. Holland, (Ed). *Psycho-oncology* (pp. 500-505). New York: Oxford University Press.

DEPRESSION AND ANXIETY

NANCY JO BUSH

PATHOPHYSIOLOGICAL MECHANISMS

The diagnosis and treatment of cancer almost invariably, and understandably, evoke in patients fear of the unknown and sadness over physical and psychosocial losses. Most often, both the patient and family members experience these emotions at specific transition points along the cancer trajectory: diagnosis, treatment, recurrence, and progressive illness. Even in patients in long-term remission and those considered survivors, fears of recurrence and disabilities caused by cancer treatment can continue to cause feelings of uncertainty and anguish.

The National Comprehensive Cancer Network (NCCN) chose the word *distress* to characterize the psychosocial nature of the cancer experience (NCCN, 2007). The NCCN defines *distress* as a multifactorial, unpleasant experience that is emotional, psychological, social, or spiritual in nature. Distress can occur at any point along the cancer continuum and can range from normal feelings of vulnerability, fear, and sadness to disabling conditions such as clinical depression, anxiety and panic, isolation, and existential or spiritual crises (NCCN, 1999). Basing its framework on the *Diagnostic and Statistical Manual of Mental Disorders*, fourth edition, text revision (DSM-IV-TR) (APA, 2007), the NCCN identified the seven psychosocial disorders most often seen in patients with cancer: dementia and delirium (cognitive changes), substance abuse—related disorder, personality disorder, and (those discussed in this chapter) adjustment disorder, mood disorder, and anxiety disorder.

The state of feeling sad is often referred to as "depression," and the state of fear or apprehension about a perceived threat often is referred to as "anxiety." Yet, both depression and anxiety can range from an acute, transient distress to a major psychiatric illness. Depression and anxiety are common emotional responses to cancer, and these two diagnoses often coexist. The *intensity*, *duration*, and *extent* to which these symptoms interfere with the patient's ability to function differentiate a depressive or anxiety disorder from normal emotional responses to chronic illness (Pasacreta et al., 2006; Bowers & Boyle, 2003). Depression and anxiety consist of a cluster of psychological and physiologic symptoms that, if recognized, often respond to treatment but if unrecognized interfere with coping and quality of life. Untreated depression places the patient at risk for suicide; this makes diagnosis and treatment imperative (see Chapter 45).

Depression has been defined as a more intense and debilitating version of sadness (Bowers and Boyle, 2003) and as a complex, progressive, neurologic-cognitive response to loss or deprivation (Lovejoy et al., 2000b). The neurophysiology of depression involves an imbalance of neurotransmitters (i.e., dopamine, norepinephrine, and serotonin [5-HT]) in the mood-sensitive areas of the brain (the limbic system, basal ganglia, and hypothalamus) (Townsend, 2004; Bowers & Boyle, 2003; Lovejoy et al., 2000a; Keltner et al., 1998). A decrease in neurotransmitters, particularly serotonin, negatively affects homeostasis throughout the body, causing cognitive, behavioral, and systemic symptoms (Box 8-1). It is important to note that depressive disorders are biologic in nature (Barry, 2002) and

| BOX 8-1 | CRITERIA FOR MAJOR DEPRESSIVE EPISODE |

Five or more of the following symptoms must be present during the same 2-week period and must represent a change from previous functioning; at least one of the symptoms must be depressed mood or loss of interest or pleasure.

1. Depressed mood most of the day, nearly every day, as indicated by either subjective report (e.g., feels sad or empty) or objective report by others (e.g., appears tearful).
2. Markedly diminished interest or pleasure in all, or almost all, activities most of the day, nearly every day (e.g., withdrawn).
3. Significant weight loss while not dieting, or weight gain (e.g., a change of more than 5% of body weight in a month), or a decrease or increase in appetite nearly every day.
4. Insomnia or hypersomnia nearly every day.
5. Psychomotor agitation or retardation nearly every day (e.g., irritable mood).
6. Fatigue or loss of energy nearly every day.
7. Feelings of worthlessness or excessive or inappropriate guilt nearly every day.
8. Diminished ability to think or concentrate, or indecisiveness, nearly every day.
9. Recurrent thoughts of death (not just fear of dying), recurrent suicidal ideation without a specific plan, or a suicide attempt or a specific plan for committing suicide.

Data from American Psychiatric Association (APA). (2000). *Diagnostic and statistical manual of mental disorders.* (4th ed., text rev.). Washington, D.C.: The Association.
Physical symptoms of depression may mirror symptoms caused by cancer and its treatment; assessment, therefore, should focus on mood and psychological changes in the patient with cancer.

that symptoms reflect a progressive derangement of underlying neurologic circuits (Lovejoy et al., 2000b). A person does not choose to be depressed. Stressful experiences can "burn out" neurologic circuits in the brain; or, as in the case of hereditary depression, neurotransmitter systems may fail first, contributing to responses of sadness and ineffective coping when the individual is faced with stressful situations, such as cancer (Lovejoy et al., 2000b).

Anxiety has been defined as severe apprehension or worry, and although it is a normal response to stressful events such as cancer, anxiety becomes a pathologic condition if it persists and interferes with the patient's ability to function (Noyes et al., 1998). Fear is a normal affective response to the *real* threat of a cancer diagnosis or treatment, whereas anxiety is the affective response to a *perceived* threat or danger. Therefore fear is the *cognitive appraisal* that cancer is a threat to well-being, and anxiety is the *emotional response* to that cognitive appraisal (Beck & Emery, 1985). Thus fear and anxiety are interrelated. Fear leads to the stress response of fight or flight; in contrast, anxiety reduces the individual's ability to act. Severe anxiety can cause a patient with cancer to feel emotionally paralyzed (Stein, 2004; Wolman, 1994). The physical symptoms of anxiety are associated with the autonomic response, and the psychological symptoms are associated with feelings of apprehension and impending doom (Box 8-2). Individuals with a history of generalized anxiety disorder may experience a re-emergence or intensification of symptoms with the development of cancer. If the person has a history of post-traumatic stress disorder, that condition also may be reactivated, and specific phobias and claustrophobia (i.e., fear of enclosed places) may interfere with cancer treatment (Marrs, 2006; Noyes et al., 1998).

EPIDEMIOLOGY AND ETIOLOGY

Emotional distress is a normal response to the threat of cancer at the time of diagnosis, relapse, treatment failure, and other transitional points along the cancer continuum.

BOX 8-2	SYMPTOMS OF GENERALIZED ANXIETY DISORDER

Apprehension: Excessive and uncontrolled worry about a real or perceived threat to personal safety.

Motor tension: Muscle tension, aches or soreness, restlessness, trembling or feeling shaky, easily fatigued.

Autonomic hyperactivity: Palpitations, shortness of breath or feeling smothered, sweating, dizziness, dry mouth, gastrointestinal distress, flushing, trouble swallowing or lump in throat.

Vigilance: Scanning the environment, exaggerated startle response, difficulty concentrating or going blank, difficulty falling asleep or staying asleep, and irritability.

Data from American Psychiatric Association (APA). (2000). *Diagnostic and statistical manual of mental disorders.* (4th ed., text rev.). Washington, D.C.: The Association; and Noyes et al., (1998). Anxiety disorders. In J. C. Holland (Ed.). *Psycho-oncology* (pp. 548-563). New York: Oxford University Press.

According to surveys of the cancer population, 20% to 40% of patients show a significant level of distress, such as depression and anxiety; however, significantly, fewer than 10% of patients with these conditions are identified and referred for psychosocial assistance (NCCN, 2007). Characteristic emotional responses to cancer and its treatment may include initial shock and disbelief, periods of turmoil with mixed symptoms of anxiety and depression, irritability, and disruption of daily patterns such as appetite and sleep. Most patients with cancer have fears about a painful death, changes in body image and function, and becoming disabled and dependent. However, the level of psychological distress that accompanies these fears depends on a number of factors.

The incidence of cancer-related depression increases with the acuity and chronicity of the illness (Albright & Valente, 2006; Lovejoy et al., 2000b). Depression is strongly correlated with unmanaged pain in the cancer population (Breitbart & Payne, 1998; Massie & Popkin, 1998). Patients with cancer have a higher than average risk for depression, and the incidence of depression in these patients is significantly higher than in the general population (Albright & Valente, 2006). Anxiety is closely associated with other psychiatric states and may also occur as a response to pain, fatigue, or metabolic side effects, heightening the patient's feelings of helplessness and hopelessness, which contribute to depression (Bush, 2006b; Noyes et al., 1998).

Depression and anxiety may also be caused by specific medications (e.g., corticosteroids), and certain cancer diagnoses (e.g., pancreatic carcinoma) have been associated with depressive symptoms. Organic factors, such as tumor involvement of the central nervous system, may also contribute to cognitive deficits and mood disorders such as depression (Massie & Popkin, 1998). The phase, duration, and intensity of cancer treatment may challenge the patient's ability to cope and diminish the person's quality of life (Schreier & Williams, 2004).

The risk of psychiatric illness in response to cancer is greater if the patient has a personal or family history of depression or anxiety before diagnosis. Individuals who have had a major depressive episode are at increased risk of recurrent depression, and the risk of suicide is higher for a person who has made a previous attempt (Albright & Valente, 2006; APA, 2000). Other variables that may increase the patient's risk for depression and anxiety are the individual's normal personality traits and coping styles before diagnosis. Individuals who have a negative or pessimistic outlook on life are more prone to depressive states; the cancer validates their negative world view (Albright & Valente, 2006).

Research has shown that avoidant and passive styles of coping, such as helplessness and hopelessness, also correlate with poor disease outcomes (Bush, 2006a). If a person has a history of pre-existing trait anxiety (a personality characteristic), the normal fear and anxiety associated with the disease and treatment may be heightened and may manifest more frequently (state anxiety) (Gorman et al., 2002; Noyes et al., 1998). Patients with trait anxiety are more prone to developing anticipatory nausea and vomiting before chemotherapy, and patients with a history of generalized anxiety disorder, such as panic attacks, may suffer more intense anxiety with the cancer experience than the general population (Bush, 2006b; Noyes et al., 1998).

Other contributing factors for psychological distress during the cancer experience include gender, developmental life stage, cultural and socioeconomic dimensions, and social support. In the general population, rates of depression vary across the life span, and the rates demonstrate gender differences. The lifetime prevalence of clinical depression is approximately twice as high in women as in men (Kornstein & McEnany, 2000). Various theories have proposed both a biologic and a social basis for this gender difference. Women have differences in brain structure and function, different genetic factors, and hormonal fluctuations across the reproductive life span that increase their vulnerability to depression. Cancer treatments, such as certain chemotherapeutic agents, may also contribute to depression by placing a woman in premature, unnatural menopause. Psychosocial factors that increase a woman's risk for depression include gender differences in socialization, roles, coping styles, and economic and social status (Kornstein & McEnany, 2000).

Men experience symptoms of depression similar to those seen in women, but they are less likely to identify or report depressive moods because they fear stigmatization, loss of job security, or loss of health insurance benefits (Porche, 2005). It also is important to note that depression in men manifests differently; men are more apt to engage in coping efforts such as using alcohol and drugs, submerging themselves in work-related activities, or acting out reckless and risky behaviors. A grave concern is that suicide can be either a symptom or a consequence of depression, and in the United States, men are four times more likely than women to succeed at committing suicide (Porche, 2005) (see Chapter 45).

Geriatric depression is a widespread health problem in the United States, affecting at least 1 in 6 patients seen in general medical practice. This is an important problem that must be addressed, particularly in the cancer population, because cancer is the second leading cause of death in individuals over age 55 (Itano & Taoka, 2005; Reynolds & Kupfer, 1999; Boyle et al., 1992;). The incidence of significant depression in later life increases to about 25% for those with chronic illnesses such as cancer, especially if the person suffers from cognitive impairment (Albright & Valente, 2006; Reynolds & Kupfer, 1999) (see Chapter 7). The elderly also have the highest suicide rate of any age group because of rising rates among Caucasian men age 85 or older (Reynolds & Kupfer, 1999).

Depression rates differ among females and males and among the young and the elderly. Therefore the developmental life stage, cultural and socioeconomic factors, and social support all affect the risk and rates of depressive episodes. Cancer may strike at any point in the life cycle, be treated and stay in remission for years, and then recur unexpectedly. Childhood survivors live with the fear of possible secondary malignancies related to their primary treatments (e.g., female survivors of Hodgkin's disease may develop breast cancer as a result of mantle radiation). At each stage of psychological growth a person must resolve inherent developmental tasks or challenges, and cancer can disrupt emotional development and the resolution of life goals (Bush, 2006a; Barry, 2002). Studies have found that with regard to fertility, threats to physical health, finances, and employment, young people with cancer have greater adjustment problems and a poorer quality of life than older persons with the disease (Bush, 2006a; Barsevick et al., 2000). Yet the elderly may be less apt to recognize and report depressive symptoms because of the physical and social losses that have accumulated throughout their life span; for example, bereavement grief in the elderly increases their risk of chronic depression. Also, signs among the elderly are more complex because many in this age group have co-morbid diseases, and telltale symptoms may be mixed with dementia, anxiety, and alcohol or benzodiazepine use or may manifest in psychotic forms (Reynolds & Kupfer, 1999).

Social support is a significant variable believed to be positively associated with a patient's ability to cope and adapt to the stress of cancer (Bush, 2006a). Social support includes the community of family, friends, church, and larger social systems, such as culture. Social support can provide emotional support by helping the patient evaluate the cancer experience as less threatening, by helping the patient problem solve and make decisions, and by assisting with physical supportive measures. Social support includes the health care professionals who care for the patient through diagnosis, inpatient hospitalization, ambulatory outpatient clinics, and in the home. In evaluating social support, it is important to determine how the patient *perceives* his or her social support; that is, is communication between the patient and significant others open and supportive or closed and restricted (Hudek-Knezevic et al., 2002)? Special populations, such as minorities and the elderly, have less access to continuity of care and social support systems; this contributes to feelings of isolation and powerlessness, which ultimately can lead to depression and anxiety. Depression can also be undiagnosed or misdiagnosed in certain cultural and ethnic groups as a result of stereotypes about the groups' expected behaviors and because of language barriers between health care providers and the patient (Albright & Valente, 2006; Faysman & Oseguera, 2002).

RISK PROFILE

- Personal or family history of psychological illness
- Inadequate symptom management, particularly pain
- Severity of illness and poor prognosis
- Prolonged, intensive treatment modalities
- Medications, including specific chemotherapeutic agents
- Co-morbid medical conditions, especially organic CNS disease
- Developmental life stage, gender, and family and social roles
- Personality characteristics of pessimism, perceived loss of personal control
- Concurrent or cumulative personal and family crises and loss
- Perceived or actual loss of social support systems

PROGNOSIS

Depression and anxiety are common mood states in patients confronting the stress of cancer and its treatment. These symptoms of distress are responsive to pharmacologic, psychological, and social treatments aimed at reduce the patient's emotional suffering. This suffering should not be viewed as an unavoidable consequence of cancer (Massie & Popkin, 1998) but should be evaluated and treated promptly to bring about relief. Depression worsens the prognosis for medical illnesses such as cancer, and the worst consequence of untreated major depressive disorder (MDD) is suicide (Albright & Valente, 2006; Ballenger et al., 1999). Patients with a history of previous suicidal attempts are at higher risk for repeated attempts (Albright & Valente, 2006).

PROFESSIONAL ASSESSMENT CRITERIA (PAC)

1. Ensure the patient's physical safety. Patients with depression and other mood disorders can develop suicidal tendencies (see Chapter 45). Ask the patient if there is a personal or family history of depression and suicide attempts. Ask the patient, "Have you ever had thoughts about hurting yourself?" All depressed patients should be assessed for the risk of suicide by direct questioning about suicidal thinking and impulses. If the patient has an active plan for suicide or if significant risk factors exist, refer the patient immediately to a mental health specialist such as a psychiatric nurse practitioner, psychologist, or psychiatrist (Sharp, 2005).

2. All patients experiencing cancer should be assessed for depressed mood and co-existing anxiety. The assessment should include a thorough consideration of the medical, endocrinologic, neurologic, situational, and developmental risk factors (Itano & Taoka, 2005; Massie & Popkin, 1998). Simple, straightforward questions can be used to identify a patient's emotional outlook, such as, "Are you feeling sad, blue, or depressed?" "Are you sleeping poorly?" "Have you lost energy or do you suffer from unexplained fatigue?' "Do you worry too much?" and "Have you lost interest and pleasure in activities that you usually enjoy?" (Ballenger et al., 1999; Reynolds & Kupfer, 1999).

3. Differential diagnosis for depression and anxiety must include a thorough assessment of medical conditions that may contribute to or exacerbate psychosocial distress (Albright & Valente, 2006). This includes uncontrolled symptoms related to the disease and treatment such as unmanaged pain and unrelenting fatigue. Metabolic status (e.g., electrolyte imbalances) can contribute to confusional states such as delirium and must be differentiated from depression and anxiety. Depression may be an outcome of chronic alcohol intake or substance abuse, and anxiety may reflect withdrawal of both (Albright & Valente, 2006). Other medical factors may include anemia, hypothyroidism or hyperthyroidism, and nutritional deficiencies of vitamin B_{12} and folate (Van Fleet, 2006). The differential diagnosis must consider organic central nervous system involvement (e.g., brain metastasis) and medications, including chemotherapeutic agents that can contribute to depression (e.g., corticosteroids, vinblastine, vincristine, interferon, procarbazine, and asparaginase).

4. The standard for diagnosing psychopathology is the *Diagnostic and Statistical Manual of Mental Disorders*, fourth edition, text revision (DSM-IV-TR) (APA, 2000). The primary DSM-IV-TR symptoms for major depression are depressed mood and/or loss of interest or pleasure in almost all activities most of the day, nearly every day, persisting for a 2-week period and associated with physical and psychological symptoms. Differentiating the many physical manifestations of cancer and treatment-related symptoms from the DSM-IV-TR diagnostic criteria for clinical depression make the assessment challenging, (e.g., fatigue, weight loss or gain, anorexia, insomnia or hypersomnia). Therefore use of the DSM-IV-TR criteria for diagnosing depression in patients with cancer is controversial (Van Fleet, 2006; Bowers & Boyle, 2003). Assessment for depression in the patient with cancer should focus on risk factors for depression and psychological symptoms that affect appearance, behavior, and cognition, which are a change from the patient's previous level of functioning (e.g., flat affect, slowed speech, crying, labile emotions, pessimism, guilt, hopelessness, and problems with concentrating and decision making). Depending on the major symptoms present, the common disorders classified by the DSM-IV-TR are adjustment disorders with depressed mood, anxiety or mixed anxiety and depressed

mood, and mood disorder with depressive features due to cancer (Itano & Taoka, 2005; Massie & Popkin, 1998).

5. Symptoms of distress that require further evaluation in the patient with cancer include excessive worries and fears, excessive sadness, unclear thinking, despair and hopelessness, severe family problems, and spiritual crises (NCCN, 2007). The NCCN has formulated standards of care for psychosocial management of the patient with cancer (see the section Evidence-Based Practice Updates), as well as algorithms outlining assessment, treatment, and management guidelines. Creative approaches to psychosocial distress have been discussed in the literature and can be implemented across settings. At the Johns Hopkins Cancer Center, a trained volunteer administers the Brief Symptom Inventory (BSI) to all new patients in the waiting room. At the University of Wisconsin Comprehensive Cancer Center in Madison, patients undergoing chemotherapy are screened for common psychiatric disorders and then referred to a cancer psychologist or psychiatric nurse practitioner for further evaluation and counseling. At Memorial Sloan-Kettering, a "distress thermometer," similar to the 0 to 10 graphic rating scale for pain, has been implemented. The patient is shown the visual thermometer and asked, "How would you rate your feelings of distress today, on a scale of 0 to 10?" Studies have shown that patients who indicate a mark or verbalize a score above 5 have symptoms in need of intervention (NCCN, 2007; Madden, 2006; NCCN, 1999).

6. The Agency for Health Care Policy and Research (AHCPR) (1993) has developed a practical guide for the management of depression in adults. This guide provides an overview of both the general population and the medically ill patient. It is an excellent resource for health care practitioners across all care settings. Other diagnostic tools for evaluating mood disorders are available for clinical and research use. Common examples include the Brief Symptom Inventory (BSI), the Common Problems Checklist (CPCL), the Profile of Mood States (POMS), the Beck Depression Inventory (BDI), the Beck Anxiety Inventory (BAI), the Hospital Anxiety and Depression Scale, and the Hamilton Rating Scale for Depression (Madden, 2006; Bowers & Boyle, 2003; Zabora et al., 2003). For initial diagnosis in the clinical setting, a thorough intake history, physical examination, and psychosocial assessment are appropriate and effective. A single-item screening question, such as, "Do you feel low in mood or depressed?" has the benefit of being simple and efficient and begins a dialog that is nonthreatening to both the patient and the nurse (Bowers & Boyle, 2003; Chochinov et al., 1997).

NURSING CARE AND TREATMENT

1. If the depression or anxiety is caused by a medical condition or a drug, the underlying problem must be identified and treated initially. After the underlying problem has been treated, the patient is again assessed for mood disorder before treatments specific for depression or anxiety, or both, are started (NCCN, 2007; Itano & Taoka, 2005; Massie & Popkin, 1998).

2. At the initial assessment, the intake process (i.e., clinical history and interview) is an excellent tool for obtaining information about the patient's psychosocial status, symptoms, and disability related to depressed mood or anxiety. Including a family member or significant other in the intake process can be beneficial, because many patients are unaware of changes in their behavior and affect or may minimize their disability for fear of being stigmatized. Recording of the patient's initial complaints should be followed with a thorough review of systems and a physical examination. If no cause or associated factors are identified for the symptoms of depression or anxiety, the patient should

be diagnosed with a primary mood disorder, referred if necessary, and appropriate treatment should be started. When generalized anxiety disorder coexists with major depression, treatment first should be directed toward managing the depression (AHCPR, 1993).

3. Treatment for depression and anxiety should involve a multimodality approach: pharmacologic management, individual or family psychotherapy, cognitive and behavioral interventions, and complementary therapies such as relaxation and guided imagery (NCCN, 2007; Ikano & Taoka, 2005). A combination of antidepressant medication and psychotherapy often proves effective in medically ill patients (Pasacreta et al., 2006).

4. Distress management should proceed as follows: (1) psychosocial distress should be identified, monitored, documented, and treated promptly at all stages of disease; (2) educational and training programs should be implemented to ensure that all health care professionals have the knowledge and skills to assess, manage, and refer patients with psychosocial distress; and (3) patients and families should be informed that management of psychosocial distress is a primary goal of the medical team, and they should be referred appropriately to psychosocial services in the treatment center and community (NCCN, 2007).

5. Pharmacologic management of depression should be initiated first because antidepressant therapy often treats coexisting anxiety effectively. The antidepressants most often used in patients with cancer are the selective serotonin reuptake inhibitors (SSRIs), tricyclic antidepressants (TCAs), psychostimulants, and monamine oxidase inhibitors (MAOIs) (Table 8-1) (Massie & Popkin, 1998). A stigma often is associated with depression and pharmacotherapy, therefore it is important to educate the patient and family about depression and the therapeutic benefits of antidepressants. Education should include the expected time frame for therapeutic effectiveness of the medication, the dose escalation, and side effects. Once a patient has recovered from a depressive episode, the antidepressant should be continued for another 6 months to preserve remission and prevent relapse (Moore, 2006).

6. *Principles of antidepressant drug therapy*: Drugs must be individually tailored to the patient's age, health history, and symptoms, and close attention must be paid to the drug's side effect profile. The drug and dosage may need to be adjusted for the elderly, for patients with liver disease, and for patients with a history of seizure activity. Medications for treating depression are categorized according to their pharmacologic mechanisms. For example, the SSRIs are selective for serotonin, which means that more serotonin becomes available at all presynaptic and postsynaptic receptors. The specific physiologic workings of each medication contribute to its antidepressant efficacy, but also to its adverse effects. Serotonin-mediated side effects may include agitation, gastrointestinal disturbance, and sexual dysfunction. The SSRIs often are the medication of choice because of their low side effect profile and their low overdose potential. They also are the drug of choice for patients who have symptoms of both depression and anxiety (Van Fleet, 2006; Bowers & Boyle, 2003; Stahl, 1998).

Consideration of drug efficacy and differences in adverse effects is clinically important. For example, before recent advances were made in antidepressant medications, the TCAs were the drugs of choice in oncology patients. Amitriptyline (Elavil) was prescribed for its sedative properties and its effectiveness in managing pain and relieving severe depression. However, because the TCAs block cholinergic, alpha-adrenergic, and histamine receptors, they contribute to drowsiness, dizziness, dry mouth, constipation, hypotension, and the risk of cardiac arrhythmias (Van Fleet, 2006; Bowers & Boyle, 2003; Stahl, 1998). Antidepressants may also be chosen for their proven effectiveness against other treatment-related side effects that may contribute to depression and anxiety. For example, venlafaxine (Effexor) has proven to diminish mood swings and hot flashes in patients

Table 8-1   ANTIDEPRESSANT MEDICATIONS

Class	Drug Name	Dosing Information	Indications for Use (Includes Off-Label Use)	Side Effects Profile
Selective serotonin reuptake inhibitors (SSRIs)	Fluoxetine (Prozac) Sertraline (Zoloft) Paroxetine (Paxil) Fluvoxamine (Luvox)	20-80 mg by mouth daily 50-200 mg by mouth daily 20-50 mg by mouth daily 50-150 mg by mouth twice a day	First-line agent for depression alone or in combination with anxiety	Agitation, sleep disturbance, sexual dysfunction, and gastrointestinal disturbance. Patient may become refractory to clinical benefit.
Tricyclic antidepressants (TCAs)	Citalopram (Celexa) Amitriptyline (Elavil) Nortriptyline (Pamelor) Desipramine (Norpramin) Clomipramine (Anafranil) Imipramine (Tofranil)	20-60 mg by mouth daily 50-150 mg by mouth at bedtime 50-150 mg by mouth at bedtime 100-300 mg by mouth in the morning 150-250 mg by mouth at bedtime 150-300 mg by mouth at bedtime	First-line agent for depression, neuropathic pain syndrome, or insomnia	Dry mouth, blurred vision, drowsiness, hypotension, dizziness, and risk of cardiac arrhythmias
Serotonin and norepinephrine reuptake inhibitor	Venlafaxine (Effexor)	37.5-75 mg by mouth three times a day	Enhanced therapeutic effect on dual neurotransmitters with dose escalation; fewer drug interactions than SSRIs	Agitation, insomnia, weight loss, sexual dysfunction, and hypertension
Serotonin antagonist reuptake inhibitors	Nefazodone (Serzone) Trazodone (Desyrel)	100-300 mg by mouth twice a day 50-100 mg by mouth two or three times a day	Indicated in SSRI nonresponders and those unable to tolerate SSRIs; effective for treatment of depression in association with agitation, anxiety, and sleep disturbance	Hypersomnia; difficult to manage in patients who have difficulty with medication adherence
Norepinephrine-dopamine reuptake inhibitor	Bupropion (Wellbutrin)	100 mg by mouth three times a day	Treatment of SSRI nonresponders; preferred in patients with hypersomnia or cognitive slowing; good for patients concerned about sexual dysfunction	Overstimulation agitation, insomnia, nausea, and seizures

Continued

Table 8-1	ANTIDEPRESSANT MEDICATIONS—cont'd			
Class	Drug Name	Dosing Information	Indications for Use (Includes Off-Label Use)	Side Effects Profile
Noradrenergic-specific serotonergic antidepressant (NaSSA)	Mirtazapine (Remeron)	15-45 mg by mouth at bedtime	Severe depression, SSRI side effect burden, or nonresponders; good for use with anxiety and insomnia disturbances	Weight gain, sedation, cognitive slowing, and motor disturbance
Monoamine oxidase inhibitors (MAOIs)	Phenelzine (Nardil)	15-30 mg by mouth three times a day	Second-line therapy for patients with atypical or refractory depression	Must strictly follow dietary restrictions (avoid tyramine-rich foods); high incidence of drug-drug interactions
	Tranylcypromine (Parnate)	15-30 mg by mouth twice a day		
Psychostimulants	Methylphenidate (Ritalin)	2.5-30 mg by mouth every morning and at noon	First-line therapy alone or in combination with alternate agent for severe depression or in patients with limited life expectancy; onset of action is 24 to 48 hours	Hypertension, anxiety, agitation, confusion, and risk of arrhythmias and hepatic dysfunction; potential for tolerance or addiction
	Dextroamphetamine (Dexedrine)	2.5-30 mg by mouth every morning at noon		
	Pemoline (Cylert)	37.5-75 mg by mouth every morning and at noon		

From Bowers, L., & Boyle, D. A. (2003). Depression in patients with advanced cancer. *Clinical Journal of Oncology Nursing, 7*:281-288.

with breast cancer who experience treatment-induced menopause. It also is effective against neuropathic pain. Combination therapy may be initiated to provide a broader spectrum of coverage or when the patient does not respond to SSRIs. Pain pathways are mediated by serotonin and norepinephrine, therefore a selective norepinephrine reuptake inhibitor (e.g., bupropion [Wellbutrin]) may be combined with a similar drug that has serotonin properties (e.g., venlafaxine [Effexor]) to treat a patient with severe depression who also requires pain management (Sharp. 2005).

7. Benzodiazepines are used most often for anxiety in both the medical and psychiatric settings. The dosage should be modified for the elderly, in patients with liver disease, and if the patient is concurrently taking an antidepressant. This class of drugs is also effective for treating insomnia, chemotherapy-related nausea and vomiting, and treatment-related fears (e.g., before bone marrow aspiration). Lorazepam (Ativan) often is the drug of choice because its short half-life is unaffected by liver disease, age, or concurrent use of an SSRI. The amnestic effects of lorazepam may be beneficial for patients who experience anticipatory nausea and vomiting with chemotherapy; however, the drug may be contraindicated in patients who suffer from chemotherapy-related cognitive dysfunction, or "chemo brain" (see Chapter 7). Longer-acting benzodiazepines, such as clonazepam (Klonopin), are effective for panic disorders or generalized anxiety disorders, but they must be used cautiously in the elderly (Pasacreta et al., 2006).

8. *Psychostimulants* (e.g., methylphenidate [Ritalin]) play a role in the treatment of depression because of their rapid onset and ability to improve energy levels and mood, as well as concentration and attention span (Van Fleet, 2006). Psychostimulants are also effective in pain management because they counteract opioid-induced sedation and improve mood (Pasacreta et al., 2006). Side effects include insomnia, tachycardia, and agitation, therefore these drugs may exacerbate anxiety associated with depression.

9. Nonpharmacologic management of depression and anxiety includes psychotherapy using cognitive behavioral therapy (CBT). Any patient with severe depression or suicide ideation should be referred for psychiatric evaluation and pharmacotherapy. Patients who are immobilized by sadness, fear, or anxiety find it very difficult to engage in CBT until the medication takes effect. CBT approaches to treatment are well accepted and have shown proven positive outcomes. Underlying CBT is the goal of helping patients cognitively "reframe" their negative and hopeless perceptions with realistic and positive perceptions (Lovejoy et al., 2000b). Techniques used for CBT include guided imagery and relaxation, psychoeducation, music or art therapy, and scheduling pleasurable and distracting activities, such as exercise or gardening, to reduce stress. Guided imagery and relaxation can reduce the patient's fear of treatments such as MRI scanning and radiation therapy. Psychoeducational approaches provide patients with knowledge to help them in problem solving and decision making, thereby increasing their sense of control and competency. I Can Cope is an example of an effective psychoeducational approach.

Integrative oncology is the use of complementary therapies to treat pain, anxiety, and mood disturbance (Deng & Cassileth, 2005; Kwekkeboom, 2003; Kocsis, 2000). Interventions such as music and art therapy, acupuncture, mind-body techniques, massage, aromatherapy, and self-hypnosis have been shown to improve physical and mental health. It has been said that because cancer is a life-threatening diagnosis and the treatment regimens often elicit an emotional stress response, or reaction to danger, the disease promotes a persistent anxiety reaction, along with feelings of isolation, hopelessness and helplessness. Therefore interventions require a holistic and existential perspective (Sloman, 2002) and a multimodality approach.

EVIDENCE-BASED PRACTICE UPDATES

1. Twenty-five percent of patients with cancer suffer from depression (NIMH, 2002).
2. People with depression have poorer outcomes from physical illness and its treatment (Albright & Valente, 2006; NIMH, 2002).
3. Individuals with cancer, their family members, and even their health care providers often misinterpret the symptoms of depression, mistaking them for the inevitable accompaniments of cancer. Consequently, the depression is neither diagnosed nor treated in most patients with cancer (Albright & Valente, 2006; NIMH, 2002).
4. A personal history of depression increases the risk of recurrent episodes, and depression increases the risk of suicide (Albright & Valente, 2006).
5. Prescription antidepressants generally are well tolerated and safe for patients being treated for cancer (NIMH, 2002). They are most effective when used in combination with psychotherapy, support groups, or complementary therapies (Pasacreta et al., 2006; Bowers & Boyle, 2003; Deng & Cassileth, 2005; Lovejoy et al., 2000a and 2000b; Massie & Popkin, 1998).
6. Anxiety and depressive symptoms commonly coexist. The anxiety seen in patients with cancer is accompanied by greater autonomic hyperactivity (Noyes et al., 1998) and can exacerbate depression, pain, and other symptoms (Bush, 2006b).
7. Depression and anxiety negatively affect a patient's ability to cope with and adapt to the stress of cancer and its treatment (Bush, 2006a), decrease the patient's quality of life and response to treatment (NCCN, 2007), and may reduce survival (NIMH, 2002).

TEACHING AND EDUCATION

1. **In the clinical management of depression, the AHCPR guidelines suggest that patient and family education include the points presented in Box 8-3.** *Rationale:* The response to and effectiveness of treatment depends on the cooperative effort of the patient, family, and practitioner (AHCPR, 1993).
2. **Educate the patient and family members about the expected emotional reactions to a cancer diagnosis (e.g., shock and disbelief).** *Rationale:* This normalizes the patient's and family's feelings and gives them permission to share.
3. **Educate the patient and family about the signs and symptoms of anxiety and depression, the risk factors, and the professional resources available to them.** *Rationale:* Family may be instrumental in identifying symptoms and encouraging the patient to recieve help.
4. **Educate the patient about preventive measures, such as nutrition, exercise, and good sleep habits, in addition to open communication with health care providers and family members about his or her feelings and emotions.** *Rationale:* Physical well-being may contribute to general psychological health. Expression of emotion can reduce tension.
5. **Explain to the patient what is involved in appointments, treatments, examinations, follow-up, and so forth.** *Rationale:* This will help to reduce the person's fears and anxiety.
6. **Involve both the patient and family in decision making and problem solving with regard to the disease and its treatment.** *Rationale:* This helps the patient and family increase their sense of control, autonomy, and self-esteem.
7. **Educate the patient about any medications prescribed (i.e., name, purpose, dosage, route, frequency, and common side effects).** *Rationale:* This helps the patient avoid medication errors.
8. **Teach the patient nonpharmacologic strategies to control anxiety (e.g., relaxation and guided imagery) and encourage the patient to engage in enjoyable activities (e.g., gardening).** *Rationale:* These nonpharmacologic strategies may assist in diminishing feelings of sadness.

| BOX 8-3 | **POINTS FOR PATIENT AND FAMILY EDUCATION ABOUT DEPRESSION** |

- Depression is a medical illness, not a character defect or weakness.
- Recovery is the rule, not the exception.
- Treatments are effective, and many treatment options are available. An effective treatment can be found for nearly every patient.
- The aim of treatment is complete symptom remission; that is, not just getting better, but getting and staying well.
- The risk of recurrence is significant: 50% after one episode, 70% after two episodes, and 90% after three episodes.
- The patient and family should be alert for early signs and symptoms of recurrence and seek treatment early if depression returns.

From U. S. Department of Health and Human Services, Public Health Service, Agency for Health Care Policy and Research (AHCPR). (1993). *Depression in primary care: Detection, diagnosis, and treatment.* (AHCPR Publication No. 93–0552). Rockville, MD: U. S. Government Printing Office.

NURSING DIAGNOSES

1. **Ineffective coping** related to complex life changes
2. **Anxiety** related to uncertain future
3. **Disturbed thought processes** related to medications
4. **Powerlessness** related to disease progression
5. **Complicated grieving** related to cumulative losses

EVALUATION AND DESIRED OUTCOMES

1. The patient will be safe from self-harm.
2. Depression will be diagnosed and treated.
3. Anxiety will be diagnosed and treated.
4. Symptom management, significantly pain, will be effectively treated.
5. The patient will express a sense of control and self-efficacy.
6. The patient will verbalize quality of life and a sense of hope.
7. A family systems approach will be carried out for psychosocial assessment and interventions.
8. Referral to appropriate interdisciplinary team members will be carried out.
9. Pharmacotherapy and/or psychotherapy will be carried out when appropriate.
10. The patient and family will be able to identify available social systems and resources to support coping.

DISCHARGE PLANNING AND FOLLOW-UP CARE

- Continuity of care across inpatient care, ambulatory care, and home care is planned, and all members of the multidisciplinary team are informed.
- Follow-up appointments with the oncologist, psychiatrist, psychiatric nurse practitioner, and other necessary team members are planned and clearly identified.
- Resources needed by the patient and family to meet health care needs are planned and arranged (e.g., visiting nurse, transportation to appointments).
- Psychosocial resources are identified (e.g., I Can Cope, Wellness Community), and their use is encouraged, along with local cancer support groups for patients and family.

- The patient identifies self-care activities to reduce anxiety and depression and to promote effective coping (e.g., relaxation exercises, guided imagery, physical exercise, and hobbies such as gardening).

REVIEW QUESTIONS

QUESTIONS

1. Which of the following symptoms would most likely indicate depression in the patient with cancer:
   1. Anorexia
   2. Weight loss
   3. Unclear thinking
   4. Sleep disturbances

2. Which of the following assessment criteria takes priority when caring for a cancer patient with depression:
   1. Unrelenting pain
   2. Anger
   3. Delirium
   4. Suicidal ideation

3. Your patient states that her feelings of sadness and hopelessness are a sign of personal weakness. All of the following responses are both supportive and educative except:
   1. "Depression is a medical illness, not a sign of character defect or weakness."
   2. "Feeling sad and hopeless can initially be a normal response to cancer."
   3. "Wait and see, you will feel better in no time."
   4. "Let's talk further about your feelings to determine why you may be feeling this way."

4. Your patient was admitted with a recent diagnosis of breast cancer that has metastasized to the bone and brain. She is showing symptoms of depression, including tearfulness, flat affect, and inability to concentrate. Your initial intervention is:
   1. Initiate antidepressant medication to control symptoms
   2. Treat the underlying medical disorder of CNS metastasis
   3. Request a psychiatric consultation
   4. Inform the patient that what she is feeling is normal

5. Which of the following is the best tool the oncology nurse can use at the bedside to assess the patient for depression and anxiety:
   1. Beck Depression Inventory
   2. Profile of Mood States
   3. Single-item screening question
   4. DSM-IV-TR

6. Your patient appears very anxious and inquires about his next doctor's visit for his first chemotherapy treatment. Which response would be most supportive to help alleviate the patient's fear:
   1. "Chemotherapy is not your enemy; it is to try and cure you."
   2. "It is very normal to feel anxious about chemotherapy. Let me tell you what to expect."
   3. "Everyone is scared of chemotherapy, but everyone survives."
   4. "Didn't the doctor already review the treatment with you?"

7. In an assessment for anxiety and depression, which of the following criteria are important causes to determine:
   1. Alcohol and substance abuse
   2. Insomnia and hypersomnia
   3. Anorexia and weight loss
   4. Hopelessness and helplessness

8. Which of the following factors places your patient with cancer at a higher risk for major depression:
   1. Lack of social support
   2. Male gender and middle age
   3. Personal history of depression
   4. Family history of alcoholism

9. Which of the following symptoms is the least characteristic of anxiety:
   1. Flat affect
   2. Irritability
   3. Inability to focus
   4. Rapid speech

10. **In caring for a patient with depression or anxiety, the most appropriate nursing intervention is:**
    1. Allowing the patient private time in a dark, quiet room to contemplate
    2. Cheering up the patient by encouraging long visits from family and friends.
    3. Encouraging the patient to take an active role in the plan of care
    4. Disturbing the patient only when absolutely necessary

ANSWERS

1. *Answer: 3*
   Rationale: Physical manifestations of cancer and treatment may mirror some of the diagnostic criteria for clinical depression. Symptoms of depression that require further evaluation in the patient with cancer include excessive worries and fears, excessive sadness, unclear thinking, despair and hopelessness, severe family problems, and spiritual crises (NCCN, 2007).

2. *Answer: 4*
   Rationale: Too often health care providers assume that psychological distress is normal for the patient confronting cancer, and they overlook its significant impact. Patients with cancer have a higher rate of depression than the general population, and depressive states place patients with cancer at a higher risk for suicide (Albright & Valente, 2006).

3. *Answer: 3*
   Rationale: Telling the patient that she will feel better in no time does not acknowledge the patient's emotions, nor does it provide the patient with support to continue sharing her concerns. This response is closed-ended communication; it inadvertently indicates disinterest to the patient, and it does not allow the practitioner to further assess the possibility of major depression.

4. *Answer: 2*
   Rationale: The symptoms your patient is experiencing may be related to tumor involvement of the central nervous system. This medical condition should be treated first, most likely with steroids and radiation therapy. Once the patient's conditioned has been treated and stabilized, a further assessment and evaluation of depressive symptoms should be carried out before pharmacologic interventions.

5. *Answer: 3*
   Rationale: Structured clinical interviews using formalized tools such as the DSM-IV-TR and others are valuable for psychiatric evaluation and in research settings. However, they can be time-consuming and rigorous, especially for patients with advanced illness (Bowers & Boyle, 2003). The single-item screening question, such as, "Have you been feeling sad or blue?" can be very effective for allowing the nurse to open dialog with the patient for a more thorough psychosocial assessment.

6. *Answer: 2*
   Rationale: Fear and anxiety result from a perceived threat or apprehension about the unknown. Educating the patient about what to expect when undergoing examinations (e.g., MRI scanning) or new treatments (e.g., cycle one of chemotherapy) helps the patient regain a sense of control over the cancer and its treatment (Stephenson, 2006). A simple explanation of what the patient may expect allows the person to ask further questions and gives the nurse the opportunity to assess what the patient understands so far and what the patient still needs to learn. Prioritizing education is important, especially when the patient is experiencing anxiety (e.g., overwhelming anxiety is common at diagnosis); therefore only as much information as the patient can handle should be initially provided (Stephenson, 2006). A high level of anxiety at the start of treatment has been shown to negatively affect overall quality of life, and studies have shown that psychological distress does not diminish over the course of treatment (Schreier & Williams, 2004)

7. *Answer: 1*
   Rationale: An excessive alcohol intake, the use of illicit drugs, or abuse of prescription medications can cause or

complicate major depression or anxiety disorders (AHCPR, 1993). Individuals experiencing the symptoms of depression or anxiety often self-medicate with alcohol or drugs in an attempt to alleviate their symptoms. Answers 2, 3, and 4 are symptoms of depression.

8. *Answer: 3*
Rationale: A personal history of major depression increases the risk of recurrent depression significantly (AHCPR, 1993), although lack of social support or alcoholism can be contributing factors. Depression rates are higher in women than men.

9. *Answer: 1*
Rationale: Symptoms such as flat affect, indifference, and withdrawal are related to depression. Symptoms of anxiety are caused by arousal of the autonomic nervous system and include signs of facial tension, as well as the symptoms listed in answers 2, 3, and 4.

10. *Answer: 3*
Rationale: Patients with depression may feel helpless and hopeless, and if anxiety coexists, they may feel overwhelmed by what is happening to them. Encouraging the patient to take an active role in the plan of care and educating the person so that he or she can make informed decisions empowers the patient, allowing him or her to feel more in control and independent. Patients experiencing depression may become withdrawn, therefore interventions 1 and 4 would increase the risk of isolation. If anxiety coexists with the patient's depression, intervention 2 may further overwhelm the patient with false reassurance and exacerbate feelings of fatigue.

REFERENCES

Albright, A. V., & Valente, S. M. (2006). Depression and suicide. In R. M. Carroll-Johnson, L. M. Gordon, & N. J. Bush (Eds.), *Psychosocial nursing care along the cancer continuum* (pp. 241-260). Pittsburgh: Oncology Nursing Society.

American Psychiatric Association (APA) (2000). *Diagnostic and statistical manual of mental disorders.* (4th ed., text rev. ed.). Washington, D.C: The Association.

Ballenger, J. C., Davidson, J. R. T., & Lecrubier, Y., et al. (1999). Consensus statement on the primary care management of depression from the International Consensus Group on Depression and Anxiety. *Journal of Clinical Psychiatry, 60*(Suppl. 7):54-61.

Barry, P. D. (2002). *Mental health and mental illness.* (7th ed.). Philadelphia: Lippincott.

Barsevick, A. M., Much, J., & Sweeney, C. (2000). Psychosocial responses to cancer. In C. H. Yarbro, M. H. Frogge, & M. Goodman, et al. (Eds.), *Cancer nursing: Principles and practice* (pp. 1529-1549). (5th ed.). Sudbury, MA: Jones and Bartlett.

Beck, A. T., & Emery, G. (1985). *Anxiety disorders and phobias: A cognitive perspective.* New York: Basic Books.

Bowers, L., & Boyle, D. A. (2003). Depression in patients with advanced cancer. *Clinical Journal of Oncology Nursing, 7*:281-288.

Boyle, D. M., Engelking, C., & Blesch, K., et al. (1992). *Oncology Nursing Society position paper on cancer and aging: The mandate for oncology nursing.* Pittsburgh: Oncology Nursing Society.

Breitbart, W., & Payne, D. K. (1998). Pain. In J. C. Holland, (Ed), *Psycho-oncology* (pp. 451-467). New York: Oxford University Press.

Bush, N. J. (2006a). Coping and adaptation. In R. M. Carroll-Johnson, L. M. Gordon, & N. J. Bush (Eds.), *Psychosocial nursing care along the cancer continuum* (pp. 61-88). Pittsburgh: Oncology Nursing Society.

Bush, N. J. (2006b). Anxiety and the cancer experience. In R. M. Carroll-Johnson, L. M. Gordon, & N. J. Bush (Eds.), *Psychosocial nursing care along the cancer continuum* (pp. 205-221). Pittsburgh: Oncology Nursing Society.

Chochinov, H. M., Wilson, K. G., & Enns, M., et al. (1997). "Are you depressed?" Screening for depression in the terminally ill. *American Journal of Psychiatry, 154*:674-676.

Deng, G., & Cassileth, B. R. (2005). Integrative oncology: Complementary therapies for pain, anxiety, and mood disturbance. *CA: A Cancer Journal for Clinicians, 55*:109-116.

Faysman, K., & Oseguera, D. (2002). Cultural dimensions of anxiety and truth telling. *Oncology Nursing Forum, 29*:757-759.

Gorman, L. M., Raines, M. L., & Sultan, D. F. (2002). *Psychosocial nursing for general patient care.* (2nd ed.). Philadelphia: F. A. Davis.

Hudek-Knezevic, J., Kardum, I., & Pahljina, R. (2002). Relations among social support, coping, and negative affect in hospitalized and nonhospitalized cancer patients. *Journal of Psychosocial Oncology, 20*(2):45-63.

Itano, J. K., & Taoka, K. N. (2005). *Core curriculum for oncology nursing.* (4th ed.). St. Louis: Elsevier.

Keltner, N. L., Folks, D. G., & Palmer, C. A., et al. (1998). *Psychobiological foundations of psychiatric care.* St. Louis: Mosby.

Kocsis, J. H. (2000). New strategies for treating chronic depression. *Journal of Clinical Psychiatry, 61*(Suppl. 11):42-45.

Kornstein, S. G., & McEnany, G. (2000). Enhancing pharmacologic effects in the treatment of depression in women. *Journal of Clinical Psychiatry, 61*(Suppl. 11):18-27.

Kwekkeboom, K. L. (2003). Music versus distraction for procedural pain and anxiety in patients with cancer. *Oncology Nursing Forum, 30*:433-440.

Lovejoy, N. C., Tabor, D., & Deloney, P. (2000a). Cancer-related depression. Part II. Neurological alterations and evolving approaches to psychopharmacology. *Oncology Nursing Forum, 27*:795-808.

Lovejoy, N. C., Tabor, D., & Matteis, M., et al. (2000b). Cancer-related depression. Part I. Neurologic alterations and cognitive-behavioral therapy. *Oncology Nursing Forum, 27*:667-678.

Madden, J. (2006). The problem of distress in patients with cancer: More effective assessment. *Clinical Journal of Oncology Nursing, 10*:615-619.

Marrs, J. (2006). Stress, fears, and phobias: The impact of anxiety. *Clinical Journal of Oncology Nursing, 10*:319-322.

Massie, M. J., & Popkin, M. K. (1998). Depressive disorders. In J. C. Holland, (Ed), *Psycho-oncology* (pp. 518-540). New York: Oxford University Press.

Moore, S. (2006). Depression management during cancer treatment. *Oncology Nursing Forum, 33*:33-35.

National Institute of Mental Health (NIMH). (2002). *Older adults: Depression and suicide facts.* Retrieved October 21, 2006, from http://www.nimh.nih.gov/publicat/elderlydepsuicide.cfm.

NCCN. (1999). NCCN practice guidelines for the management of psychosocial distress. National Comprehensive Cancer Network Proceedings. *Oncology,* 13(5A):113-147.

NCCN (2007). *NCCN practice guidelines in oncology.* v.1.2007. Distress management. Retrieved December 12, 2007, from http://www.nccn.org/professionals/physician_gls/PDF/distress.pdf.

Noyes, R., Holt, C. S., & Massie, M. J. (1998). Anxiety disorders. In J. C. Holland, (Ed), *Psycho-oncology* (pp. 548-563). New York: Oxford University Press.

Pasacreta, J. V., Minarik, P. A., & Nield-Anderson, L. (2006). Anxiety and depression. In B. R. Ferrell, & N. Coyle (Eds.), *Textbook of palliative nursing* (pp. 375-399). (2nd ed.). New York: Oxford University Press.

Porche, D. J. (2005). Depression in men. *Nurse Practitioner, 1*:138-139.

Reynolds, C. F., & Kupfer, D. J. (1999). Depression and aging: A look to the future. *Psychiatric Services, 50*:1167-1172.

Schreier, A. M., & Williams, S. A. (2004). Anxiety and quality of life of women who receive radiation or chemotherapy for breast cancer. *Oncology Nursing Forum, 31*:127-130.

Sharp, K. (2005). Depression: The essentials. *Clinical Journal of Oncology Nursing, 9*:519-525.

Sloman, R. (2002). Relaxation and imagery for anxiety and depression control in community patients with advanced cancer. *Cancer Nursing, 25*:432-435.

Stahl, S. M. (1998). Selecting an antidepressant by using mechanism of action to enhance efficacy and avoid side effects. *Journal of Clinical Psychiatry, 59*(Suppl. 18):23-29.

Stein, D. J. (2004). *Clinical manual of anxiety disorders.* Washington, D.C.: American Psychiatric Publishing.

Stephenson, P. L. (2006). Before the teaching begins: Managing patient anxiety prior to providing education. *Clinical Journal of Oncology Nursing, 10*:241-245.

Townsend, M. C. (2004). *Essentials of psychiatric mental health nursing.* (3rd ed.). Philadelphia: F. A. Davis.

U. S. Department of Health and Human Services, Public Health Service, Agency for Health Care Policy and Research (AHCPR). (1993). *Depression in primary care: Detection, diagnosis, and treatment.* (AHCPR Publication No. 93–0552). Rockville, MD: U. S. Government Printing Office.

Van Fleet, S. (2006). Assessment and pharmacotherapy of depression. *Clinical Journal of Oncology Nursing, 10*:158-161.

Wolman, B. B. (1994). Defining anxiety. In B. B. Wolman, & G. Stricker (Eds.), *Anxiety and related disorders: A handbook* (pp. 3-10). New York: John Wiley.

Zabora, J. R. (1998). Screening procedures for psychosocial distress. In J. C. Holland, (Ed), *Psycho-oncology* (pp. 653-661). New York: Oxford University Press.

Zabora, J. R., Loscalzo, M. J., & Weber, J. (2003). Managing complications in cancer: Identifying and responding to the patient's perspective. *Seminars in Oncology Nursing, 19*:1-9.

CHAPTER 9

DIABETES INSIPIDUS

JENNIFER U. VARMA

PATHOPHYSIOLOGICAL MECHANISMS

Diabetes insipidus (DI) is a disorder of urinary concentration caused by a temporary or chronic deficiency of or insensitivity to vasopressin, or antidiuretic hormone (ADH). This condition leaves the kidneys (specifically the renal collecting ducts and tubules) unable to conserve water. The result is excretion of large volumes of dilute or hypotonic urine and excessive thirst (polydipsia) (Fig. 9.1). (Arvanitis & Pasquale, 2005; Wong & Verbalis, 2002)

ADH, which is produced in the supraoptic and paraventricular nuclei of the hypothalamus, controls water balance. The serum water content is measured by serum osmolality (a normal value is 285 to 295 mmol/kg). From the hypothalamus ADH is transported through nerve fibers in neurosecretory granules to the posterior pituitary gland, where it is stored. When released, it travels to the kidneys, where it causes the renal tubules to concentrate the urine and return excess water to the bloodstream. If a person starts to become dehydrated, the anterior pituitary signals the posterior pituitary to release ADH and signals the kidneys to reabsorb free water (Urden et al., 2006; Arvanitis & Pasquale, 2005; Ropper & Brown, 2005; South-Paul et al., 2004; Wong & Verbalis, 2002).

EPIDEMIOLOGY AND ETIOLOGY

DI is an uncommon disorder that affects 3 of 100,000 people in the general population and about 1% of patients suffering from head injury (Arvanitis & Pasquale, 2005). These patients are unable to conserve free water and therefore excrete large volumes of dilute urine (polyuria). They also are excessively thirsty, particularly for ice-cold water (polydipsia), which reflects the body's attempt to maintain osmolality. Polyuria and polydipsia can lead to dehydration and resulting hypernatremia (Adam, 1997).

DI can be categorized into several types, including central DI (hypothalamic, pituitary, cranial neurogenic, or neurohypophyseal), nephrogenic DI (renal), gestagenic DI (pregnancy), and dipsogenic DI (psychogenic).

Patients who have *central DI*, the most common type, do not secrete or produce enough ADH in response to osmotic or nonosmotic stimuli, and the result is dilute urine. This usually is caused by damage to the hypothalamus or the posterior pituitary; although a secondary cause may be related to an idiopathic or primary cause (Suarez, 2004; Graham & Lantos, 2002). Primary causes of central DI may include idiopathic or genetic mutations. Secondary causes (most often the cause) may include head trauma, infection, tumors, hypoxic brain tissue injury, and infiltrative systemic disease (see the section, Risk Profile) (Graham & Lantos, 2002; Wong & Verbalis, 2002). Patients affected with central DI generally respond well to medical treatment involving the administration of desmopressin or exogenous ADH and fluid replacement.

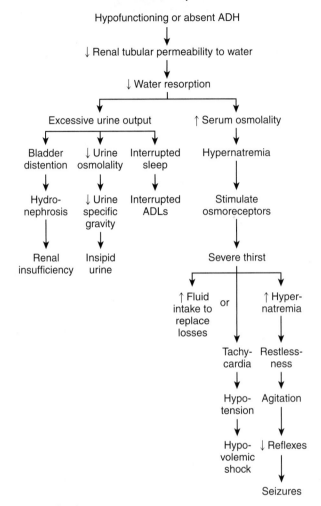

Fig. 9.1 • Pathophysiology of diabetes. *(From Urden L. D., Stacy, K. M., & Lough, M. E. [2006]. Thelan's critical care nursing: Diagnosis and management. [5th ed.]. St. Louis: Mosby.)*

Nephrogenic DI (NDI) occurs as a result of renal unresponsiveness to ADH. This impairs the kidneys' ability to concentrate urine and reabsorb water. Most water reabsorption occurs in the collecting ducts at the V_2 receptors; however this process continues with the transfer and transport of sodium chloride in the loop of Henle. In nephrogenic DI, ADH does not increase water permeability or concentrate urine. The cause may be underlying kidney disease or possibly a drug-related reaction. Patients with nephrogenic DI have normal ADH levels and therefore do not respond to desmopressin or exogenous ADH therapy. They are best treated with therapies that target the underlying condition (Greenspan & Gardner, 2004; Wong & Verbalis, 2002).

Gestagenic DI is associated with a pregnancy that is complicated by pre-eclampsia or hepatic dysfunction. It develops as a result of increased levels of vasopressinase, an enzyme that destroys circulating endogenous vasopressin. The enzyme does not affect synthetic vasopressin, therefore these patients respond well to treatment with desmopressin. The condition usually resolves within 10 days after delivery (Fitzgerald, 2006). However, the mother then has a higher risk of developing diabetes.

Dipsogenic DI is a condition seen in the psychiatric population as a result of an excessive intake of water (usually more than 20 L of fluid per day). This type of DI may be due to illness or to side effects (e.g., dry mouth) caused by anticholinergic or antipsychotic medications (Arvanitis & Pasquale, 2005; Adam, 1997).

RISK PROFILE

Oncology: Primary tumors include glioma, hypothalamic hamartoma, hypothalamic tumors, germinoma, meningioma, lymphoma, craniopharyngioma, granular cell tumor (choristoma), large chromophobe adenomas, pinealoma, Rathke's cleft cyst, massive pituitary tumors that invade the pituitary stalk, and multiple myeloma. Metastatic pituitary lesions and metastatic tumors originating in the lung or breast, leukemic infiltration, and a history of brain irradiation put a patient at risk of developing DI (Ropper & Brown, 2005; Vance, 2003; Wong & Verbalis, 2002). Table 9-1 lists the causes of central and nephrogenic DI.

Genetics: Nearly 90% of patients with congenital NDI are males with X-linked recessive NDI, with mutations of the AVPR2 gene (Bichet, 2006). Other mutations include the AQP2 gene.

PROGNOSIS

Although the outcome depends on the underlying pathologic condition, DI, when treated, does not cause severe problems or reduce life expectancy. Life expectancy largely depends on the underlying cause. Acute DI can be treated in the hospital with medication, fluid and electrolyte replacement, and treatment of the underlying cause, a process that may take days to weeks. Patients with chronic DI are treated on an outpatient basis for control of symptoms and for monitoring of serum sodium levels, other electrolytes, and fluid status (Fitzgerald, 2006).

PROFESSIONAL ASSESSMENT CRITERIA (PAC)

The diagnosis of DI should be considered in patients who have large volumes of urine output, excessive thirst, and nocturia. Excessive thirst and nocturia are found only in responsive patients; therefore serum laboratory values, as well as intake and output, must be closely monitored in the high-risk unresponsive patient. Neurologic signs may include a change in the level of consciousness, restlessness, weakness, confusion and, in severe cases, convulsion caused by sodium and other electrolyte imbalances. Responsive patients may complain of a dry tongue and mouth. Cardiovascular signs are consistent with dehydration and may include hypotension, tachycardia, azotemia, and increased temperature as a result of fluid volume loss and disruption of the hypothalamus. Patients who are dehydrated may have poor skin turgor, sunken eyes, dry mucous membranes, fatigue,

Table 9-1 CAUSES OF CENTRAL AND NEPHROGENIC DIABETES INSIPIDUS	
Causes of Central DI	**Causes of Nephrogenic DI**
Idiopathic	Familial causes
Familial causes	• X-linked nephrogenic DI (most common in males)
• Wolfram syndrome, or DIDMOAD (DI + DM + optic atrophy + deafness); rare genetic autosomal recessive mutation of WFS1 gene encoding	**Renal disease**
	• Polycystic kidney disease
	• Chronic pyelonephritis
Trauma	• Medullary cystic disease
• Head injury, especially basilar skull fracture	• Sickle cell nephropathy
Autoimmune causes	• Sarcoidosis
Causes in surgical patients	• Chronic renal failure
• Brain tumors (especially pituitary adenomas and metastatic pituitary lesions)	• Multiple myeloma
	• Analgesics
• Intracerebral hemorrhage	• Sjögren's syndrome
• Ruptured aneurysm	**Medications**
Infection	• Lithium
• Meningitis	• Demeclocycline
• Tuberculosis	• Methoxyflurane anesthesia
• Syphilis	• Foscavir
• Encephalitis	• Cidofovir
Anoxic encephalopathy	• Aminoglycosides
Ischemia	• Vinblastine
• Shock	• Rifampin
• Cardiac arrest	• Valproic acid
• Sheehan's syndrome	**Metabolic causes**
• Sickle cell disease	• Chronic hypokalemia
Granulomatous causes	• Chronic hypocalcemia
• Neurosarcoidosis	• Protein starvation
• Langerhans' cell histiocytosis	
• Letterer-Siwe disease	
• Hand-Schüller-Christian disease	

Data from Greenspan, F. S., & Gardner, D. G. (2004). *Basic and clinical endocrinology.* (7th ed.). Columbus, OH: McGraw Hill Companies; Lemarie, X., Corne, P., & Jonquet, O. (2006). Transient central diabetes insipidus during valproic acid poisoning (French). *Annales Francaises d'Anesthesie et de Reanimation* 25(5):525-527; Smith, C. J., Crock, P. A., & King, B. R., et al. (2004). Phenotype-genotype correlations in a series of Wolfram syndrome families. *Diabetes Care, 27(8):*2003-2009; South-Paul, J. E., Matheny, S. C., & Evelyn, L. L. (2004). *Current diagnosis and treatment in family medicine.* Columbus, OH: McGraw-Hill Companies; Urden, L. D., Stacy, K. M., & Lough, M. E. (2006). *Thelan's critical care nursing: Diagnosis and treatment.* (5th ed.). St. Louis: Mosby; and Vance, M. L. (2003). Perioperative management of patients undergoing pituitary surgery. *Endocrinology and Metabolism Clinics of North America,* 32:355-365.

lethargy, headache, and irritability. Nocturia and polyuria (urine output greater than 30 mL/kg/day) are classic signs of DI, along with polydipsia (fluid ingestion ranging from 2 to 20 L/day) (Fitzgerald, 2006; Ropper & Brown, 2005; Barkley & Myers, 2001).

Diagnostic findings

1. Urine hyposmolarity (less than 150 to 200 mOsm/L) as a result of dilute urine
2. Serum hyperosmolarity (greater than 300 mOsm/L) as a result of dehydration
3. Low specific gravity (1.001 to 1.005) as a result of decreased urine concentration
4. Sodium level normal or above normal (greater than 145 mEq/L) as a result of dehydration
5. A water deprivation test is performed by making the patient NPO and stopping IV fluids; a normal result is decreased urinary output and increased urine osmolality.
6. Monitoring of serum glucose, BUN, and creatinine

7. Potassium and calcium levels are assessed initially, because hypokalemia and hyper-calcemia cause polyuria.
8. A 24-hour urine collection can be obtained for measurement of volume and the cre-atinine level.
9. If central DI is suspected, a desmopressin (vasopressin or ADH) challenge test can be prescribed.
   - During this test, an initial dose of 5 to 10 mcg of intranasal desmopressin (or 1 mcg of subcutaneous or intravenous desmopressin) is administered. Strict measurement of urine volume is done for 12 hours before and 12 hours after administration.
   - If minimal or no response is seen, the dose of desmopressin can be doubled.
   - In patients who respond, a distinct reduction in polyuria and thirst is seen.
10. If nephrogenic DI is suspected, the serum vasopressin level can be measured; with NDI this usually is elevated.
11. If brain lesions or head trauma is suspected, imaging of the brain with CT and MRI should be considered. (Fitzgerald, 2006; Morton et al., 2005; Ropper & Brown, 2005; Bakerman, 2002; Barkley & Myers, 2001).

Management

1. Replace fluids.
   - May initially be provided with 0.9% saline to restore volume despite hypernatremia; consider D5W if minimal effect on serum glucose is expected.
2. Treat the underlying cause.
3. Central or gestagenic DI:
   - Administer desmopressin/DDAVP.
     - Parenteral: 1-4 mcg IV, IM, or SC q12-24h
     - Oral: 0.1 and 0.2 mg tablets given in a starting dose of 0.05 mg BID; may increase to a maximum of 0.4 mg q8h
     - Intranasal: 0.05-0.1 mL (100 mcg/mL solution) q12-24h
   - For patients with partial preservation of ADH, chlorpropamide, clofibrate, or carba-mazepine can be used to stimulate the release of ADH.
   - Hydrochlorothiazide 50-100 mg daily, along with a potassium supplement, may pro-duce a partial response.
4. Nephrogenic DI:
   - Indomethacin 50 mg orally q8h or combined with hydrochlorothiazide
   - Diuretic therapy with thiazides may be effective and should be given in combination with a potassium supplement.
   - A high-salt diet may be helpful for individuals with chronic NDI.
5. Dipsogenic DI:
   - Psychotherapy for patients with compulsive water drinking.
   - Avoidance of thioridazine and/or lithium if these are causative agents (Fitzgerald, 2006; Morton, et al., 2005; Arvanitis & Pasquale, 2005; Adam, 1997)

NURSING CARE AND TREATMENT

Fluid replacement and strict monitoring of fluid balance.

Daily weights.

Strict intake and output.

Skin and mouth care.

Precautions for confused patients and those at risk for seizures.

Frequent neurologic assessments up to q1h but usually q4h.

Vital signs: especially assess for hypotension and elevated temperature.

IV access: peripheral or prepare for central line insertion.

Preparation for prescriptions, such as frequent laboratory draws and urine assessments, administration of fluids and medications.

Monitoring for signs and symptoms of sinusitis with use of intranasal medications.

Patient and family education about disease process and management.

Discharge planning, including medication instruction and teaching.

Monitoring for medication side effects, including elevated liver enzymes, gastrointestinal upset, facial flushing, headache, sinusitis, and nasal irritation.

Management of constipation and diarrhea.

EVIDENCE-BASED PRACTICE UPDATES

1. A formula can be used to estimate water deficit (Arvanitis & Pasquale, 2005):

   Current water deficit $= 0.6 \times$ Premorbid lean body weight $\times [1 - (140/\text{serum NA(mEq/L)})]$

2. Enhanced imaging can be done to visualize pituitary abnormalities and anticipate the need to treat the patient for conditions such as DI (Vance, 2003).
3. Advances in medicine targeted at kidney disease may aid in the diagnosis and treatment of nephrogenic DI (Fitzgerald, 2006; Greenberg, 2001).
4. Wolframin localization is in the endoplasmic reticulum (Philbrook, et al., 2005).
5. A 16-bp depletion is a mutation in Italian patients with Wolfram syndrome (Lombardo, et al., 2005).
6. Arab families may have a mutation for congenital ND on the AVPR2 and AQP2 genes (Carroll, et al., 2006).
7. A mutation for male infant nephrogenic DI has been found on the V2R gene, with mutations on R137C and R137L (Gitelman, et al., 2006); a mutation also is known to exist on R137H.

TEACHING AND EDUCATION

1. **Medications (desmopressin):** *Rationale*: You are taking this medication because your body's normal water balance system is not functioning properly. Antidiuretic hormone is not being produced or your body is not responding to it, so it is replaced in the form of desmopressin. You should contact your healthcare provider if you develop fatigue, drowsiness, confusion, headaches, or seizures while taking this medication as these may indicate the need for a medication adjustment. Your body will respond to this medication by holding on to water. Therefore, you should not be urinating as frequently and should not be feeling as thirsty.
2. **Dosage adjustments of chemotherapy or other medications:** *Rationale*: Certain medications and chemotherapeutic agents may cause an imbalance in the body's normal

water balance system. If a certain medication or chemotherapeutic agent is the cause, this may need to be adjusted or changed.

3. **Blood and urine samples:** *Rationale*: Frequent blood and urine samples may be taken during your hospital stay to monitor the levels of sodium and water in your body. Medications and fluids will be administered based on the test results.

4. **Placement of an intravenous (IV) catheter:** *Rationale*: An IV line will be placed into a vein to provide access to your blood stream. Through this IV, we may be able to collect blood samples and will be able to administer IV fluids and medications as needed.

5. **Indwelling urinary catheter:** *Rationale*: A catheter will be placed inside your bladder to enable accurate measurement of your urine; a very important measurement for one with altered sodium levels.

6. **Replacement of fluids:** *Rationale*: Fluids need to be replaced throuth your IV or through oral intake. Since this is a disease of water imbalance, prevention of dehydration is crucial.

7. **Clinical symptoms and signs suggestive of hyponatremia (low sodium level) or hypernatremia (high sodium level):** *Rationale*: Treatment of hyponatremia and hypernatremia are necessary and will help you feel better. If your sodium level is too high or too low, you may experience lethargy, weakness, confusion, mood changes, muscle cramps or twitching, seizures, nausea, vomiting, extreme thirst, rapid heart peat, palpitations, or dizziness. You need to notify your healthcare provider if you experience any of these symptoms.

NURSING DIAGNOSES

1. **Risk for deficient fluid volume** related to active fluid loss or regulatory failure
2. **Effective therapeutic regimen management** related to complexity of therapeutic regimen
3. **Fatigue** related to sleep deprivation or sleep disturbance
4. **Acute confusion** related to electrolyte imbalance
5. **Deficient knowledge** related to disease state and management plan

EVALUATION AND DESIRED OUTCOMES

1. Water deficit and fluid status will be corrected within 72 hours in acute cases.
2. Further water loss will be prevented within 72 hours in acute cases.
3. Electrolyte imbalances will be corrected within 72 hours in acute cases.
4. Vital signs will be maintained within a normal range within 24 to 48 hours in acute cases.
5. The patient will acquire an understanding of the underlying cause, disease process, and treatment before discharge.
6. The patient and family will verbalize an understanding of the signs and symptoms of disease progression, including dehydration and overhydration.
7. In chronic cases, the patient and family will have an understanding of the treatment process and of the signs and symptoms of worsening disease.
8. The patient will return to baseline sleep patterns before discharge.

DISCHARGE PLANNING AND FOLLOW-UP CARE

- In-home nursing, physical therapy, and occupational therapy visits as appropriate.
- Follow-up with physicians (e.g., surgeon, primary care physician, endocrinologist, nephrologist) 1 to 2 weeks after discharge.
- Patient education in medication and fluid balance.
- Outpatient laboratory testing and diagnostic imaging as appropriate.
- Dietary and fluid management.

- Patient given written instructions on when to notify the physician and/or report to the emergency department.
- Patient given nutritional information to manage constipation and diarrhea.

REVIEW QUESTIONS

QUESTIONS

1. **In a patient with DI, which of the following is the main cause of hypernatremia:**
   1. Sodium retention
   2. Sodium excretion by the kidneys
   3. Loss of waters
   4. Dilutional effects

2. **Which of the following is the most likely cause of nephrogenic DI:**
   1 Excessive water intake
   2 Basilar skull fracture
   3 Chronic lithium use
   4 Damage to the pituitary stalk

3. **In general, DI is a condition characterized by:**
   1. Polyuria, dehydration, and increased serum osmolality
   2. Hypernatremia, polyuria, and increased urine specific gravity
   3. Polyuria, hyponatremia, and decreased serum osmolality
   4. Hypernatremia, polyphagia, and increased serum osmolality

4. **In a postoperative craniotomy patient, which of the following may be signs and symptoms of developing DI:**
   1. Decreased urine output and hypothermia
   2. Increased urine output and hyperthermia
   3. Hypertension and hypothermia
   4. Bradycardia and hyperthermia

5. **Which laboratory finding would you expect in a postoperative craniotomy patient who is developing DI:**
   1. Urine specific gravity of 1.004
   2. Serum osmolality of 195
   3. Serum sodium of 133
   4. Urine osmolality of 225

6. **Which of the following medications may be used to manage chronic central DI and nephrogenic DI:**
   1. DDAVP
   2. Desmopressin
   3. Thiazide diuretics
   4. Indomethacin

7. **Central DI results from:**
   1. Increased production of ADH
   2. Decreased production of ADH
   3. Increased renal responsiveness to ADH
   4. Decreased renal responsiveness to ADH

8. **The urine specific gravity is decreased in DI because of:**
   1. Fluid loss
   2. Decreased serum calcium
   3. Increased serum sodium
   4. Decreased urinary concentration

9. **Which of the following conditions puts a pregnant woman at risk of developing DI:**
   1. Pre-eclampsia
   2. Renal dysfunction
   3. Preterm labor
   4. Abruption of the placenta

10. **Acute central DI best responds to:**
    1. Fluid replacement and sodium supplementation
    2. Fluid restriction and DDAVP administration
    3. High-salt diet and administration of hydrochlorothiazide
    4. Fluid replacement and DDAVP administration

ANSWERS

1. *Answer: 3*
   Rationale: Dehydration is the main cause of an increased sodium level

2. *Answer: 3*
   Rationale: Answer choices 1, 2, and 4 are causes of central DI.

3. *Answer: 1*
Rationale: Patients with DI are dehydrated as a result of excess water loss; they therefore have an increased serum osmolality (increased concentration).

4. *Answer: 2*
Rationale: Urine output is increased as a result of excessive water loss, and the patient may become hyperthermic from dehydration.

5. *Answer: 1*
Rationale: Urine specific gravity is decreased because of the dilute status of the urine. Serum osmolality is increased (not decreased) secondary to dehydration, therefore the serum sodium level is decreased. Urine osmolality is decreased, not increased

6. *Answer: 3*
Rationale: Thiazide diuretics result in increased water and sodium reabsorption.

7. *Answer: 2*
Rationale: Central DI is caused by decreased production of ADH.

8. *Answer: 4*
Rationale: The urine is very dilute, which is reflected by a low specific gravity.

9. *Answer: 1*
Rationale: Mothers with pre-eclampsia and hepatic dysfunction are at increased risk of developing DI.

10. *Answer: 4*
Rationale: The standard of care for central DI is fluid replacement and administration of DDAVP.

REFERENCES

Adam, P. (1997). Evaluation and management of diabetes insipidus. *American Family Physician, 55*(6):2146-2154.

Arvanitis, M. L., & Pasquale, J. L. (2005). External causes of metabolic disorders. *Emergency Medicine Clinics of North America, 23*(3):827-841.

Bakerman, S. (2002). *ABCs of interpretive laboratory data.* (5th ed.). Scottsdale, AZ: Interpretive Laboratory Data.

Barkley, T. W., & Myers, C. M. (2001). *Practice guidelines for acute care nurse practitioners.* Philadelphia: W. B. Saunders.

Bichet, D. G. (2006). Nephrogenic diabetes insipidus (review). *Advances in Chronic Kidney Failure, 13*(2): 96-104.

Carroll, P., Al-Mojalli, H., & Al-Abbad, A., et al. (2006). Novel mutations underlying nephrogenic diabetes insipidus in Arab families. *Genetics in Medicine, 8*(7):443-447.

Diabetes Insipidus Foundation. (2003). *What is diabetes insipidus?* Retrieved June 22, 2006, from http://www.diabetesinsipidus.org/

Fitzgerald, P. A. (2006). *Current medical diagnosis and treatment.* (46th ed.). Columbus: OH: McGraw Hill Companies.

Gitelman, S. E., Feldman, B. J., & Rosenthal, S. M. (2006). Nephrogenic syndrome of inappropriate antidiuresis: A novel disorder in water balance in pediatric patients. *American Journal of Medicine, 119*(Suppl. 1):S54-S58.

Graham, D. I., & Lantos, P. L., (Eds.). (2002). *Greenfield's neuropathology.* (7th ed.). New York: Arnold Publishers.

Greenberg, M. S. (2001). *Handbook of neurosurgery.* (5th ed.). Lakeland: Greenberg Graphics.

Greenspan, F. S., & Gardner, D. G. (2004). *Basic and clinical endocrinology.* (7th ed.). Columbus: McGraw Hill Companies.

Lombardo, F., Chiurazzi, P., & Hortnagel, K., et al. (2005). Clinical picture, evolution and peculiar molecular findings in a very large pedigree with Wolfram syndrome. *Journal of Pediatric Endocrinology, 18*(12):1391-1397.

Morton, P. G., Fontaine, D., & Hudak, C. M., et al. (2005). *Critical care nursing: A holistic approach.* (8th ed.). Philadelphia: Williams, & Wilkins.

Perkins, R. M., Yuan, C. M., & Welch, P. G. (2006). Dipsogenic diabetes insipidus: Report of a novel treatment strategy and literature review. *Clinical & Experimental Nephrology, 10*(1):63-67.

Philbrook, C., Fritz, E., & Weiher, H. (2005). Expressional and functional studies of Wolframin, the gene function deficient in Wolfram syndrome, in mice and patient cells. *Experimental Gerontology, 40*(8-9): 671-678.

Ropper, A. H., & Brown, R. H. (2005). *Adams and Victor's principles of neurology.* (8th ed.). Columbus: McGraw-Hill Companies.

South-Paul, J. E., Matheny, S. C., & Evelyn, L. L. (2004). *Current diagnosis and treatment in family medicine.* Columbus, OH: McGraw-Hill Companies.

Su, D. H., Liao, K. M., & Chen, H. W., et al. (2006). Hypopituitarism: A sequela of severe hypoxic encephalopathy. *Journal of the Formosan Medical Association, 105*(7):536-541.

Suarez, J. I. (2004). *Critical care neurology and neurosurgery.* Totowa: NJ: Humana Press.

Urden, L. D., Stacy, K. M., & Lough, M. E. (2006). *Thelan's critical care nursing: Diagnosis and treatment.* (5th ed.). St. Louis: Mosby.

Vance, M. L. (2003). Perioperative management of patients undergoing pituitary surgery. *Endocrinology and Metabolism Clinics of North America, 32*(2):355-365.

Wong, L. L., & Verbalis, J. G. (2002). Systemic diseases associated with disorders of water homeostasis. *Endocrinology and Metabolism Clinics of North America, 31*(1):121-140.

DIABETES MELLITUS

TIMOTHY L. WREN • KATHLEEN R. WREN

PATHOPHYSIOLOGICAL MECHANISMS

Diabetes mellitus (DM) is a disease in which altered carbohydrate metabolism leads to high blood glucose levels (Huether & Tomky, 1998). DM has several causes and can be categorized into several types (Table 10-1). DM also frequently occurs with other diseases and conditions, such as hypertension, metabolic syndrome, cardiac disease (Nathan et al., 2005) and vascular disease (Ganne et al., 2007).

Type 1 Diabetes

Type 1 diabetes appears to arise from a complex genetic and environmental interaction that causes an individual's immune system to attack and destroy pancreatic beta cells. Pancreatic beta cells are responsible for insulin secretion. As beta cells are destroyed, insulin production diminishes. However, more than 75% of the beta cells must be destroyed before hyperglycemia occurs. When all the beta cells have been destroyed, insulin production ceases, and insulin must be supplied from an alternative (outside) source.

Hyperglycemia causes an increased osmotic load in the blood vessels. Fluid transfers from the tissues or cells (area of lower osmotic pressure) to the blood vessels (area of higher osmotic pressure). This causes tissue cell dehydration and increased vascular volume. The kidneys respond to increased vascular volume by excreting additional fluid into the urine. This leads to increases in the volume and frequency of urination, a condition called *polyuria*.

With hyperglycemia, the renal tubules cannot reabsorb all the glucose, which is "spilled" into the urine. Glucose is a large molecule that takes fluid with it, leading to increased volume and frequency of urination. Electrolytes are excreted along with the large volume of fluid in the urine, and the result is severe electrolyte imbalances.

Even though the bloodstream has an overabundance of glucose, without insulin the glucose does not enter the cell. The cell is starving and in dire need of an energy source, therefore fatty acids are released and metabolized. During this process, ketones develop, leading to ketoacidosis, a severe metabolic condition (Table 10-2).

Type 2 Diabetes

Type 2 diabetes is caused by a not well understood interaction of genetic and environmental factors. Hyperglycemia in type 2 diabetes results from insulin resistance in the tissues. As tissues progressively decrease their response to a given concentration of insulin, less glucose enters the cell and therefore remains in the bloodstream. In response, pancreatic beta cells increase insulin secretion, raising the insulin level in the bloodstream. At a critical point, pancreatic beta cells are unable to increase insulin secretion any further in an attempt to counter the lack of tissue response to insulin, and hyperglycemia occurs. This process usually occurs slowly, over a prolonged period, and many people with type 2 diabetes are not even aware that they have developed the disease.

Table 10-1	CAUSES OF INCREASED BLOOD GLUCOSE LEVELS
Diabetes Type	**Cause**
Type 1	Destruction of pancreatic beta cells, leading to reduced and finally no insulin secretion by the pancreas.
Type 2	Increased resistance of body tissues and cells to the action or actions of insulin.
Type 3	Possible new type of diabetes; described as a decrease in the secretion of brain insulin, which may be important for the survival of brain cells.
Type 4	Interference in insulin production, insulin secretion, blood glucose level regulation, or tissue sensitivity to the action or actions of insulin as a result of genetic, pancreatic, or hormonal problems. Several herbals and medications also can increase blood glucose levels.
Gestational	Increased resistance of body tissues and cells to the action or actions of insulin as a result of the hormones of pregnancy.
Stress response	Hormones released by the body in response to stressors (cortical hormones, epinephrine, norepinephrine) increase the release of glucose stores from the liver and muscle through glycolysis. These hormones also cause the manufacture of glucose from noncarbohydrate sources (e.g., proteins) through gluconeogenesis. Stressors that activate the stress response can be physical or emotional and may include invasive surgeries, traumatic injuries, taking an examination/test, or public speaking.

Until the later stages of type 2 diabetes, varying amounts of insulin secretion allow some glucose to be transported into the cell for energy. Therefore fatty acids are not mobilized as an alternative energy source, nor is ketoacidosis a common complication. Instead, glucose continues to increase in the bloodstream, reaching levels of 600 mg/dL and higher, resulting in extremely high osmotic levels. This is called hyperglycemic hyperosmolar nonketotic (HHNK) coma. During HHNK, as a result of the very high serum glucose levels, fluid shifts from the tissues and is excreted in the urine (polyuria), further increasing osmotic levels. The degree of cognitive dysfunction (confusion, coma) is related to the dehydration and the osmotic level.

Gestational Diabetes

Gestational diabetes occurs during pregnancy and involves tissue resistance to insulin, as in type 2 diabetes. During pregnancy, placental growth hormone, placental lactogen, cortisol, and progesterone levels increase, leading to insulin resistance in the tissues. Insulin resistance progressively increases throughout the second and third trimesters. When the pancreas is unable to increase insulin secretion to overcome the continually increasing insulin resistance of the tissues, blood glucose levels rise. Gestational diabetes usually resolves after delivery. However, these mothers often develop type 2 diabetes later in life.

Table 10-2	LABORATORY VALUES FOR DIABETIC KETOACIDOSIS IN ADULTS	
Measurement	**Normal Serum Level**	**Serum Level in Ketoacidosis**
Glucose	70-100 mg/dL	350+ mg/dL
Ketone bodies	0.3-2.0 mg/dL	20+ mg/dL
Bicarbonate (HCO_3^-)	22-26 mEq/L	5 mEq/L
Chloride (Cl^-)	97-107 mEq/L	90 mEq/L
PH	7.35-7.45	7.0 or lower
Anion gap	12-20 mEq/L	Over 20 mEq/L

From Chernecky, C. C., & Berger, B. J. (2008). *Laboratory tests and diagnostic procedures.* (5th ed.). St. Louis: Elsevier.

Medications

Several prescription and over-the-counter medications, as well as herbal preparations and supplements, affect blood glucose levels (Tables 10-3 and 10-4). Medications that increase blood glucose levels may cause hyperglycemia and diabetes: they include corticosteroids (prednisone, dexamethasone), stress hormones (cortisol, epinephrine), sex hormones (androgens, estrogens), stimulants (ephedrine, amphetamines), some antipsychotics (clozapine, olanzapine), and the chemotherapeutic agent L-asparaginase.

Table 10-3	EFFECTS OF CERTAIN HERBS AND SUPPLEMENTS ON BLOOD GLUCOSE LEVELS
Herb or Supplement	**Effect on Blood Glucose Level**
Ackee	Decrease
Agrimony	Decrease
Aloe gel	Decrease
Alpha lipoic acid	Decrease
Annatto	Increase
Astragalus	Decrease
Banaba	Decrease
Bean pod	Decrease
Bilberry	Decrease
Bitter melon	Decrease
Black mulberry	Decrease
Black psyllium	Decrease
Black tea	Increase or decrease
Blond psyllium	Decrease
Blue cohosh	Increase
Blueberry	Decrease
Bugleweed	Decrease
Burdock	Decrease
Cassia cinnamon	Decrease
Chanca piedra	Decrease
Chinese cucumber root	Decrease
Chromium	Decrease
Cinnamon bark	Decrease
Cocoa	Increase
Coffee	Increase or decrease
Cola nut	Decrease
Corn silk	Decrease
Country mallow	Increase
Cowhage	Decrease
Cumin	Decrease
Damiana	Decrease
Dandelion	Decrease
Devil's claw	Increase
Devil's club	Decrease
Ephedra	Increase
Eucalyptus dried leaf	Decrease
Fenugreek	Decrease
Flaxseed	Decrease
Fo-ti	Decrease
Ginger	Decrease
Ginkgo leaf	Increase or decrease

Continued

Table 10-3	EFFECTS OF CERTAIN HERBS AND SUPPLEMENTS ON BLOOD GLUCOSE LEVELS—cont'd
Herb or Supplement	**Effect on Blood Glucose Level**
Ginseng (American, panax, Siberian)	Decrease
Glycomannam	Decrease
Glucosamine hydrochloride	Increase
Glucosamine sulfate	Increase
Goat's rue	Decrease
Green tea	Increase or decrease
Guar gum	Decrease
Guarana	Increase or decrease
Gymnema	Decrease
Horse chestnut	Decrease
Hydrazine sulfate	Decrease
Juniper	Decrease
Kudzu	Decrease
Lycium	Decrease
Madagascar periwinkle	Decrease
Marijuana	Decrease
Maitake mushroom	Decrease
Marshmallow	Decrease
Melatonin	Increase
Myrrh	Decrease
N-acetyl glucosamine	Increase
Niacin (niacinamine, vitamin B3)	Increase
Olive leaf	Decrease
Olive oil	Decrease
Onion	Decrease
Ribose	Decrease
Sage	Decrease
Solomon's seal	Decrease
Spinach	Decrease
Stevia	Decrease
Stinging nettle	Decrease
Vanadium	Decrease
Xanthan gum	Decrease

EPIDEMIOLOGY AND ETIOLOGY

Each year since 1997, the number of new diabetic cases has increased nationwide (CDC, 2007a). In 2004 alone, approximately 1.4 million adults were newly diagnosed with the disease (CDC-e, 2007a). The Centers for Disease Control and Prevention (CDC, 2005) estimate that 21 million Americans have diabetes, and an additional 41 million are prediabetic (CDC, 2005b). Prediabetes manifests as impaired glucose tolerance or impaired fasting glucose. The incidence of diabetes increases with advancing age, with most cases attributable to type 2 diabetes. However, although the incidence of diabetes increased for all age groups from 1997 to 2004 (CDC-c), the largest increase occurred among individuals age 18 to 44 (45%).

RISK PROFILE

Type 2 diabetes occurs almost twice as often in African Americans and one and a half times as often in Hispanics as in Caucasians (CDC, 2007b). Native Americans by far are the

Table 10-4	EFFECTS OF PRESCRIPTION AND OVER-THE-COUNTER MEDICATIONS ON BLOOD GLUCOSE LEVELS
Medication	**Effect on Blood Glucose Level**
Allopurinol	Decrease
Androgens	Increase
Ascorbic acid (vitamin C)	Increase
Aspirin	Decrease
Betamethasone	Increase
Clofibrate	Decrease
Clozapine	Increase
Cortisone	Increase
Estrogens	Increase
Dexamethasone	Increase
Guanethidine sulfate	Decrease
Haloperidol	Increase
Heparin	Increase
Hydrocortisone	Increase
Isoniazid	Decrease
L-asparaginase	Increase
Levodopa	Increase
Metaproterenol	Increase
Methylprednisolone	Increase
Olanzapine	Increase
Phenylephrine	Increase
Phenytoin	Increase
Prednisolone	Increase
Prednisone	Increase
Pseudoephedrine	Increase
Triamcinolone	Increase

ethnic group most highly at risk. More than one fourth of Native American adults living in the southeastern United States (27.8%) have diabetes (CDC, 2005a). Family history, advancing age (over 40), and gestational diabetes are uncontrollable risk factors for type 2 diabetes. However, hypertension, obesity, and lack of exercise are modifiable risk factors. Recent research has found genetic risk factors for diabetes: for type 2, these are human INS (insulin) gene promoter (Karaca et al., 2007), genes TCF7L2 (Owen & McCarthy, 2007) and CDKAL1 (Steinthorsdottir et al., 2007), and a mutant 128R allele of the E-selectin gene (Abu-Amero et al., 2007); for gestational diabetes, the genetic risk factor is a INS-VNTR class III gene (Litou et al., 2007).

PROGNOSIS

Even though it is underreported, diabetes is the sixth leading cause of death in the United States. People with diabetes are twice as likely to die of heart disease and stroke and one and one half times more likely to have hypertension (CDC, 2005a). The incidence of retinopathy, nephropathy, and neuropathies is significantly higher in the diabetic population (CDC, 2005a), and these conditions are worsened by periods of poorly controlled serum glucose levels (−Diabetic control study, Genuth, 2006). Diabetes is the major contributing factor in new cases of blindness, end-stage renal disease, and nontraumatic lower limb amputations. The CDC's National Center for Chronic Disease Prevention and Health Promotion estimates the death risk for individuals with diabetes to be twice that of the nondiabetic population (CDC, 2005c). Recent research has revealed racial and gender disparities among Medicare patients treated for diabetes mellitus; Caucasians appear to receive better treatment than African Americans, and women receive less intensive cholesterol treatment than men (Chou et al., 2007).

PROFESSIONAL ASSESSMENT CRITERIA (PAC)

1. **Fasting blood glucose test (FBG):** 100 mg/dL to less than 126 mg/dL indicates prediabetes; 126 mg/dL or higher indicates diabetes (ADA, n. d.; WHO, 2007).
2. **Oral glucose tolerance test (OGTT):** 140 mg/dL to less than 200 mg/dL indicates prediabetes; 200 mg/dL or higher indicates diabetes (ADA, n. d.; WHO, 2007).
3. **Nonfasting plasma glucose measurement:** 200 mg/dL or higher indicates diabetes (ADA, n. d.; WHO, 2007).
4. **Glycosylated hemoglobin (HgbA$_{1c}$):** 6% or higher is considered abnormal in most laboratories. This test is not usually used for diagnostic purposes, but rather to monitor blood glucose control over the past 90 days. An HgbA$_{1c}$ of less than 6.5% to 7% is considered good glycemic control (Genuth, 2006).
5. Polyuria
6. Polydipsia
7. Polyphagia
8. Unexplained weight loss
9. Increased incidence of recurrent infections (especially fungal or urinary tract infections)
10. Poor wound healing
11. **Visual changes:** Retinopathy develops in patients with type 1 diabetes who have vascular endothelial growth factor A (VEGFA) variants (Al-Kateb et al., 2007).
12. Unexplained foot wound or ulcer
13. Neuropathy
14. History of gestational diabetes or large for gestational age (LGA) fetus
15. Family history of diabetes
16. Long-term steroid use
17. Chemotherapy with L-asparaginase
18. History of co-morbidities (e.g., myocardial infarction, stroke, neuropathy, hypertension, obesity, Cushing's disease, cystic fibrosis, elevated cholesterol levels, fatty liver, chronic pancreatitis)
19. **Haptoglobin (Hp) genotype:** Test for Hp-2-2, because patients with diabetes who have this genotype are at significant risk of developing nephropathy, retinopathy, and cardiovascular disease (Nakhoul et al., 2007).

NURSING CARE AND TREATMENT

1. **Assess for diabetic ketoacidosis (DKA):** Moderate to severe DKA can be a life-threatening emergency, and treatment must be started immediately (i.e., insulin and IV fluid therapy).
2. Measure serum glucose levels q1-2h as indicated.
3. Measure urinary ketone levels.
4. Maintain IV access.
5. Monitor cognitive status and assess q1-2h.
6. Measure ABGs if level of ketoacidosis and patient's status indicate the need.
7. Measure intake and output (I&O) hourly.

8. Administer oral hypoglycemic agents or insulin therapy as indicated by patient's status.
9. Obtain hypoglycemic treatment agents (i.e., IV or oral dextrose-containing solutions or tablets).
10. **Physical assessment:** peripheral neurologic status, vision, circulation and intactness of lower limbs, prayer sign, abdominal pain. (NOTE: To assess the prayer sign, have the patient place the palms together with the elbows flexed, as if preparing to offer prayer or grace. Check the proximal and distal joints of the fingers to see whether the patient can bring the palms and digits together, touching one other. Prolonged periods of high blood glucose can lead to a joint stiffening syndrome, and patients who are unable to approximate the palms and digits may have this syndrome. This joint stiffening occurs throughout the body and can affect structures such as the temporomandibular joint [TMJ] and the spinal vertebrae.)
11. **Obtain a diet and nutritional consultation:** A high dietary intake of fiber has beneficial effects on metabolic control in patients with type 2 diabetes (Hinata et al., 2007).
12. Use hyperbaric oxygen treatments to heal lower extremity lesions, especially those with a Wagner grade of 3 or higher (Fife et al., 2007).
13. Significant improvements in systolic blood pressure and HgbA$_{1c}$ results are seen in patients who receive individualized interventional care rather than basic interventional care (Hiss et al., 2007).

EVIDENCE-BASED PRACTICE UPDATES

1. Intensive glucose control in patients with type 1 diabetes reduces the risk of stoke or cardiovascular disease by 50% (Nathan et al., 2005; UKPDS Group, 1998; "The Effect Of", 1993).
2. Early implementation of intensive glucose control in patients with type 1 diabetes continues to reduce cardiovascular-related complications, even if the patient does not continue intensive glucose control therapy, because of a phenomenon called *metabolic memory* (Nathan et al., 2005).
3. Patients with type 2 diabetes who consistently keep their endocrinology appointments show better adherence to an intensive glucose control regimen (Rhee et al., 2005).
4. The use of sliding scale insulin therapy to treat hyperglycemia in hospitalized patients should be discontinued, because it allows hyperglycemia to occur before treatment is started. Instead, frequent blood glucose monitoring and an insulin drip should be implemented, with the goals of maintaining normoglycemia and preventing hyperglycemia (AACE, 2006).
5. Microvascular complications are reduced in patients with type 1 or type 2 diabetes who follow intensive glucose control guidelines ("The Effect Of", 1993).
6. Exubra, the first noninjectable insulin, works similar to short-acting injectable insulins in lowering blood glucose levels in patients with type 1 or type 2 diabetes. Patient satisfaction was higher with the noninjectable insulin (Laustsen, 2007).
7. Blocking the actions of interleukin-1 reduces pancreatic beta cell damage in patients with type 1 or type 2 diabetes (Rother, 2007).
8. Vascular abnormalities and coronary artery disease are common complications in type 2 diabetes. Recent evidence supports the use of the more invasive coronary bypass grafting technique, rather than percutaneous coronary revascularization, for the treatment of some types of coronary artery disease in individuals with type 2 diabetes (Srikanth & Deedwania, 2007).
9. Hypertension is both a complication and a risk factor in type 2 diabetes. The treatment and control of hypertension should be a priority, along with blood glucose control and lifestyle changes, in the health care management of patients with type 2 diabetes (Srikanth & Deedwania, 2007).

10. Yalin and colleagues (2007) have identified specific genotypes associated with an increased risk of the development of type 2 diabetes. Genetic identification of individuals with an increased risk may be the first step toward preventing type 2 diabetes by targeting treatment on lifestyle changes.

11. A new blood serum test for both type 1 and type 2 diabetes has been identified. Plasma levels of IR alpha increase with hyperglycemia, possibly making it a better indicator of blood glucose control than $HgbA_{1c}$ (Xia et al., 2007).

12. Administration of specially treated beta cells protects against the development of type 1 diabetes in mice. Further study is needed to determine whether this treatment may also be useful in the prevention and treatment of type 1 diabetes in humans.

13. Admission $HgbA_{1c}$ measurements predict the risk of mortality and length of stay for patients with type 2 diabetes who are admitted for sepsis (Gornik et al., 2007). As an indicator of blood glucose control, $HgbA_{1c}$ measurements provide an indication of diabetes control. Individuals with diabetes who stringently control their blood glucose levels have a decreased incidence and severity of many diabetic complications, such as coronary artery disease, renal failure, and retinopathy ("The Effect Of," 1993).

TEACHING AND EDUCATION

Medications: *Rationale*: It is important to take your medications as prescribed and as indicated by your blood glucose measurements. Diabetes medications are a lifetime treatment.

Medications: *Rationale*: Many herbal preparations, supplements, and over-the-counter and prescription medications affect blood glucose levels (see Tables 10-3 and 10-4). You should disclose to and discuss with your health care provider all medications, herbal preparations, and supplements that you are taking.

Blood glucose testing: *Rationale*: For intensive therapy regimens, you need to test your blood glucose levels two to four times daily, depending on the type of diabetes you have and the medications you need. Under special circumstances, such as illness, you may need to check your blood glucose level more frequently. Blood glucose monitoring is done through finger or arm punctures using monitoring kits specially designed for use at home.

Nutrition: *Rationale*: It is important for you to follow the diet plan prescribed for you by your doctor or dietician. People with diabetes who are undergoing chemotherapy need special monitoring of their nutritional status to ensure an adequate intake despite possible problems such as nausea, vomiting, lack of appetite, inability to eat, oral or gastric upset, and so forth.

Prevention of infection: *Rationale*: It is important for you to monitor your skin integrity and circulation, especially in your lower limbs. You also need to check your temperature every day or any time you feel overly warm (feverish).

Foot care: *Rationale*: You must be extremely careful to keep your toenails trimmed to a moderate length. The best course is to have a foot specialist or podiatrist care for your feet and toenails.

Web sites for information: *Rationale*: A number of Web sites can provide you with important information about diabetes: the American Diabetes Association (www.diabetes.org), Joslin Diabetes Center (www.joslin.harvard.edu), National Diabetes Information Clearinghouse (NDIC) (http://diabetes.niddk.nih.gov), and the American Association of Clinical Endocrinologists (http://www.aace.com).

NURSING DIAGNOSES

1. **Risk for imbalanced nutrition: less than body requirements** related to inability to absorb glucose because of insulin deficit (typically seen in type 1 diabetes)
2. **Risk for imbalanced nutrition: more than body requirements** related to excessive intake/obesity (typically seen in type 2 diabetes)
3. **Risk for infection** related to impairment of white blood cell activity caused by hyperglycemia
4. **Impaired tissue integrity** related to peripheral vascular changes as a complication of diabetes
5. **Deficient fluid volume** related to active fluid loss during polyuria

EVALUATION AND DESIRED OUTCOMES

1. Fasting blood glucose levels will be within target range.
2. $HgbA_{1c}$ will be 6.5% to 7% or lower.
3. Patient will self-administer insulin in accordance with therapeutic goals.
4. Patient will perform at-home monitoring of blood glucose levels at least four times daily.
5. Patient's daily food intake will be consistent with therapeutic goals.

DISCHARGE PLANNING AND FOLLOW-UP CARE

- Arrange follow-up visit to physician's office 1 to 2 weeks after discharge to discuss glucose control and medications.
- Instruct patient to call health care provider immediately if blood sugar level is higher than 300 mg/dL or urinary ketones are 3+ or higher.
- Arrange follow-up visit with dietician 1 to 2 weeks after discharge to discuss diet plan.
- Schedule office visit with ophthalmologist for thorough eye examination.
- Obtain MedicAlert identification badge for diabetes diagnosis.
- Inform other health care providers (e.g., the dentist) of diabetic condition.
- Follow-up $HgbA_{1c}$ in 30 to 90 days, as determined by the physician.
- Consult assigned diabetic case manager for assistance in obtaining diabetic supplies.

REVIEW QUESTIONS

1. Your patient is having bowel resection surgery this morning because of a mass seen on colonoscopy. You would expect to _____ of the patient's morning dose of insulin.
   1. Hold the morning dose
   2. Give the full dose
   3. Give a partial dose
   4. Give more than usual

2. While taking the vital signs of your newly diagnosed patient with diabetes, you discover a stash of candy bars on the bedside table. You ask about them and learn that the patient has been snacking on the candy bars. The most appropriate nursing response is:
   1. "You are killing yourself with those candy bars."
   2. "We can never eat any candy bars when we are diabetic."
   3. "An occasional candy bar may be okay if you cover it in your meal plan."
   4. "Would you like to talk about all the changes that are going on in your diet as you cope with diabetes?"

3. **Your patient tells you that even when she is sick from chemotherapy, she still takes her full dose of insulin. Your response should be:**
   1. "You should adjust your insulin dose based on your finger stick blood sugars and what you are eating."
   2. "That is correct; you should take your full insulin dose always."
   3. "When you are sick, you should hold your insulin because you are not eating."
   4. "You should not get sick this time from the chemotherapy, so do not worry about it."

4. **Your newly diagnosed patient with diabetes tells you that as long as she covers what she eats with the insulin, she can eat whatever she wants. Your response to this should be:**
   1. "You are right."
   2. "No, you can only eat nonsweet foods."
   3. "People with diabetes who are trying to keep tight control of their blood sugar should eat regular, balance meals."
   4. "Sugars are always bad for people who have diabetes."

5. **A patient with diabetes is at greater risk for renal damage associated with some types of chemotherapy because of the:**
   1. effect insulin has on cancer tissues
   2. renal damage often associated with diabetes
   3. inability of the bladder to remove toxins
   4. associated peripheral vascular problems

6. **As you teach patients with diabetes about foot care, you emphasize the importance of protecting their feet because:**
   1. Patients with diabetes often get athlete's foot.
   2. Patients with diabetes have no blood flow to their toes.
   3. Patients with diabetes often have associated neuropathies that diminish sensory perception of pain.

   4. Any wound on the foot is far from the central circulation, and this distance results in decreased oxygen to foot tissues.

7. **You are caring for an oncology patient, for whom high-dose steroids are part of the chemotherapy regimen. You would expect the patient's blood sugar levels to:**
   1. Remain the same
   2. Decrease slightly
   3. Decrease drastically
   4. Increase

8. **Your patient is scheduled to have surgery this morning for a right mastectomy related to cancer. The patient also has diabetes and wears an insulin pump. What should you do with the pump when the patient goes to surgery:**
   1. Remove it; it is an electrical hazard in the operating room.
   2. Do nothing with it.
   3. Have the patient increase the pump's basal rate to counter the effects of the stress of surgery.
   4. Switch the patient's insulin delivery system to an intravenous drip.

9. **Your patient has type 2 diabetes that has required only oral therapy before this hospitalization. The patient now needs insulin therapy, and he is worried about taking insulin at home. You should tell the patient:**
   1. "At times, during stressful periods, some patients with diabetes need insulin injections. Often, once the stress is over, insulin injections can be reduced and even discontinued."
   2. "You will always need insulin injections now that you have started taking insulin injections; there is no turning back."
   3. "You will need to check with your doctor to see why you need to take insulin injections while you are in the hospital."
   4. "You have developed antibodies to your oral medication. You will need to discontinue your oral medication for 2 weeks and take insulin. After this time, you can

return to your oral medication for blood glucose control."

10. **A patient who has diabetes is lethargic and appears almost drunk. You would anticipate that:**
    1. The patient has had a stroke.
    2. The patient may be hypoglycemic.
    3. The patient's blood glucose level needs to be measured.
    4. The patient is just acting out; tell the patient to straighten up.

ANSWERS

1. *Answer: 3*
   Rationale: While the patient may be NPO for surgery, he is still in need of a basal amount of insulin to cover the early needs of surgical stress.

2. *Answer: 4*
   Rationale: A person newly diagnosed with diabetes may find all the changes overwhelming; a chance to review and reinforce teaching is the best choice.

3. *Answer: 1*
   Rationale: A person with diabetes who is sick still needs insulin, but the amount will vary depending on the individual's food intake. Insulin should never be stopped completely, even if the person is sick, because ketoacidosis can occur, resulting in a life-threatening event.

4. *Answer: 3*
   Rationale: For patients with diabetes who are trying to establish a healthy lifestyle, a regular, balanced diet is the best way to help maintain blood sugar control.

5. *Answer: 2*
   Rationale: IPatients with diabetes often already have poor renal function as a result of microvascular complications in the kidney caused by hyperglycemia.

6. *Answer: 3*
   Rationale: Patients with diabetes who have associated complications such as peripheral neuropathy and poor circulation are at greater risk of developing a foot or toe injury that can become serious.

7. *Answer: 4*
   Rationale: Because of their glucocorticoid actions, steroids can cause blood glucose levels to increase.

8. *Answer: 4*
   Rationale: The patient's insulin delivery method should be changed to an intravenous method, because insulin absorption from subcutaneous sites can vary widely during anesthesia and surgery.

9. *Answer: 1*
   Rationale: The need for insulin, even in individuals with type 2 diabetes, may arise with stress, such as an illness or surgery. Often these individuals can return to prestress blood glucose control measures as they recover from the source of the stress.

10. *Answer: 2*
    Rationale: Low blood sugar (hypoglycemia) often causes a person to act in a slow, lethargic, drunkenlike manner. Glucose must be administered immediately, rather than taking the time to first obtain a blood glucose measurement.

REFERENCES

Abu-Amero, K. K., Al-Mohanna, F., & Al-Boudari, O. M., et al. (2007). The interactive role of type 2 diabetes mellitus and E-selectin S128R mutation on susceptibility to coronary heart disease. *BMC Medical Genetics, 8*:35.

Al-Kateb, H., Mirea, L., & Xie, X., et al. (2007). Multiple variants in vascular endothelial growth factor (VEGFA) are risk factors for time to severe retinopathy in type 1 diabetes: The DCCT/EDIC Genetics Study. *Diabetes, 56*(8):2161-2168.

American Association of Clinical Endocrinologists (AACE). (2006). *Inpatient diabetes and glycemic control: A call to action.* Retrieved December 21, 2006, from http://www.diabetes.org/uedocuments/InpatientDMGlycemicControlPositionStmt02.01.06.rev.pdf.

American Diabetes Association (ADA). (n. d.). *How to tell if you have pre-diabetes.* Retrieved August 15, 2007, from http://www.diabetes.org/pre-diabetes/pre-diabetes-symptoms.jsp.

Centers for Disease Control and Prevention, National Center for Chronic Disease Prevention and Health Promotion (CDC-*b*). *Prediabetes manifests as impaired glucose tolerance or impaired fasting glucose.* Retrieved December 11, 2007 from www.cdc.gov/diabetes/faq/prediabetes.htm.

Centers for Disease Control and Prevention, National Center for Chronic Disease Prevention and Health Promotion (CDC-*e*). (2005a). *National diabetes fact sheet.* Retrieved August 13, 2007, from http://www.cdc.gov/diabetes/pubs/estimates.htm.

Centers for Disease Control and Prevention, National Center for Chronic Disease Prevention and Health Promotion (CDC-*f*). (2007a). *Age-adjusted incidence of diagnosed diabetes per 1000 population aged 18-79 years, by sex, United States, 1997-2004.* Retrieved August 13, 2007, from http://www.cdc.gov/diabetes/statistics/incidence/fig4.htm.

Centers for Disease Control and Prevention. National Center for Chronic Disease Prevention and Health Promotion (CDC-*d*). (2007b). *Age-adjusted incidence of diagnosed diabetes per 1000 population aged 18-79 years, by race/ethnicity, United States, 1997-2004.* Retrieved August 13, 2007, from http://www.cdc.gov/diabetes/statistics/incidence/fig6.htm.

Centers for Disease Control and Prevention, National Center for Chronic Disease Prevention and Health Promotion (CDC-*c*). (2007c). *Incidence of diagnosed diabetes per 1000 population aged 18-79 years, by age, United States, 1997-2004.* Retrieved August 13, 2007, from http://www.cdc.gov/diabetes/statistics/incidence/fig3.htm.

Centers for Disease Control and Prevention, National Center for Chronic Disease Prevention and Health Promotion (CDC-*a*). (2007d). *Annual number (in thousands) of new cases of diagnosed diabetes among adults aged 18-79 years, United States, 1997-2004.* Retrieved August 13, 2007, from http://www.cdc.gov/diabetes/statistics/incidence/fig1.htm.

Centers for Disease Control and Prevention (CDC). (2005b). *National diabetes fact sheet: General information and national estimates on diabetes in the United States.* Retrieved December 21, 2006, from http://www.cdc.gov/diabetes/pubs/factsheet.htm.

Chou, A. F., Brown, A. F., & Jensen, R. E., et al. (2007). Gender and racial disparities in the management of diabetes mellitus among Medicare patients. *Women's Health Issues, 17*(3):150-161.

Fife, C. E., Buyukcakir, C., & Otto, G., et al. (2007). Factors influencing the outcome of lower-extremity diabetic ulcers treated with hyperbaric oxygen therapy. *Wound Repair & Regeneration, 15*(3):322-331.

Ganne, S., Arora, S. K., & Dotsenko, O., et al. (2007). Hypertension in people with diabetes and the metabolic syndrome: Pathophysiologic insights and therapeutic update. *Current Diabetes Report, 7*(3):208-217.

Genuth, S. (2006). Insights from the Diabetes Control and Complications Trial/Epidemiology of Diabetes Interventions and Complications Study on the use of intensive glycemic treatment to reduce the risk of complications of type 1 diabetes. *Endocrinology Practice, 12*(Suppl. 1):34-41.

Gornik, I., Gornik, O., & Gasparovic, V. (2007). HbA1c is an outcome predictor in diabetic patients with sepsis. *Diabetes Research & Clinical Practice, 77*(1):120-125.

Hinata, M., Ono, M., & Midorikawa, S., et al. (2007). Metabolic improvement of male prisoners with type 2 diabetes in Fukushima Prison, Japan. *Diabetes Research & Clinical Practice, 77*(2):327-332.

Hiss, R. G., Armbruster, B. A., & Gillard, M. L., et al. (2007). Nurse care manager collaboration with community-based physicians providing diabetes care: A randomized controlled trial. *Diabetes Educator, 33*(3):493-500.

Huether, S., & Tomky, D. (1998). Alterations of hormonal regulation. In K. L. McCance, & S. E. Huether (Eds.), *Pathophysiology: The biologic basis for disease in adults and children.* St. Louis: Mosby.

Karaca, M., Durel, B., & Languille, L., et al. (2007). Transgenic expression of human INS gene in Ins1/Ins2 double knockout mice leads to insulin underproduction and diabetes in some male mice. *Frontiers in Bioscience, 12*:1586-1593.

Laustsen, G.. (2007). A new breakthrough in diabetes treatment. *The Nurse Practitioner, 32*(4):12-14.

Litou, H., Anastasiou, E., & Thalassinou, L., et al. (2007). Increased prevalence of VNTR III of the insulin gene in women with gestational diabetes mellitus (GDM). *Diabetes Research & Clinical Practice, 76*(2):223-228.

Nakhoul, F. M., Miller-Lotan, R., & Awaad, H., et al. (2007). Hypothesis: Haptoglobin genotype and diabetic nephropathy. *Nature: Clinical Practice Nephrology, 3*(6):339-344.

Nathan, D. M., Cleary, P. A., & Backlund, J. Y., et al. (2005). Diabetes Control and Complications Trial/ Epidemiology of Diabetes Interventions and Complications (DCCT-EDIC) Study Research Group:

Intensive diabetes treatment and cardiovascular disease in patients with type 1 diabetes. *New England Journal of Medicine, 353*(25):2643-2653.

Owen, K. R., & McCarthy, M. I. (2007). Genetics of type 2 diabetes. *Current Opinion in Genetics & Development, 17*(3):239-244.

Rhee, M. K., Slocum, W., & Ziemer, D.C., et al. (2007). Patient adherence improves glycemic control. *Diabetes Educator, 31*(2):240-250.

Rother, K. (2007). Focus on research: Diabetes treatment—bridging the divide. *New England Journal of Medicine, 356*(15):1499-1501.

Srikanth, S., & Deedwania, P. (2007). Management of coronary artery disease in patients with type 2 diabetes mellitus. *Current Cardiology Reports, 9*(4):264-271.

Steinthorsdottir, V., Thorleifsson, G., & Reynisdottir, I., et al. (2007). A variant in CDKAL1 influences insulin response and risk for type 2 diabetes. *Nature: Genetics, 39*(6):770-775.

The effect of intensive treatment of diabetes on the development and progression of long-term complications in insulin-dependent diabetes mellitus: The Diabetes Control and Complications Trial (DCCT). (1993). *New England Journal of Medicine, 329*(14):977-986.

UKPDS Group. (1998). Effect of intensive blood glucose control with metformin on complications in overweight patients with type 2 diabetes. *Lancet, 352*(9131):854-865.

World Health Organization (WHO). (2007). *Surveillance: Definition, diagnosis and classification of diabetes mellitus and its complications.* Retrieved August 30, 2007, from http://www.who.int/diabetes/publications/en/

Xia, C. Q., Peng, R., & Qiu, Y., et al. (2007). Transfusion of apoptotic beta cells induces immune tolerance to beta-cell antigens and prevents type 1 diabetes in NOD mice. *Diabetes, 56*(8):2116-2123.

Yalin, S., Hatungil, R., & Tamer, L., et al. (2007). N-acetyltransferase 2 polymorphisms in patients with diabetes mellitus. *Cell Biochemistry & Function, 25*(4):407-411.

Disseminated Intravascular Coagulation (DIC)

BRENDA K. SHELTON

PATHOPHYSIOLOGICAL MECHANISMS

DIC is a secondary disorder that occurs as a result of tissue injury, inflammation, or abnormal regulatory mechanisms (Fig. 11.1) (Mercer et al., 2006; Toh & Downey, 2005; Geiter, 2003; Messmore & Wehrmacher, 2002; Levi & de Jonge, 2000). Inflammatory cytokines thought to contribute to the development of DIC include tumor necrosis factor and interleukin-6 (Furlong & Furlong, 2005; Levi & de Jonge, 2000). Endothelial injury activates monocytes and endothelial cells, causing them to produce and express tissue factor that stimulates thrombin (Toh & Downey, 2005; Messmore & Wehrmacher, 2002).

The International Society on Thrombosis and Haemostasis defines DIC as "[an] acquired syndrome characterized by the intravascular activation of coagulation with loss of localization arising from different causes. It can originate from and cause damage to the microvasculature sufficiently severe to produce organ dysfunction" (Angstwurm et al., 2006; Voves et al., 2006; Taylor et al., 2001). DIC is also known as *consumption coagulopathy* and *defibrination syndrome* (Kanwar et al., 2006; Leung, 2006a).

The clinical stimulus for DIC originally was thought to be multifactorial. The disorder now is known to be caused almost exclusively by extrinsic factor (Factor VII, tissue factor, tissue plasminogen activator) (Mercer et al., 2006; Leung, 2006b; Toh & Downey, 2005; Levi & de Jonge, 2000).

Increased thrombin generation leads to widespread intravascular deposition of this protein, causing thrombotic occlusion of midsize and small vessels (Leung, 2006b).

Impairment of mechanisms to prevent coagulation and inadequate fibrinolysis exacerbate the thrombotic process. Normal anticoagulant regulatory processes, such as tissue factor platelet inhibitor (TFPI), antithrombin III, and activated protein C, are impaired (Mercer et al., 2006; Furlong & Furlong, 2005).

Simultaneous use and subsequent depletion of platelets and clotting factors, as a consequence of the ongoing coagulation, may result in thrombocytopenia, reduced fibrinogen levels, and severe bleeding (Leung, 2006b).

Most patients have thromboses, and a minority of patients have acute hemorrhage despite thrombocytopenia (Hambleton et al., 2002).

The pathophysiology of cancer-related DIC may have some unique characteristics. Solid tumor malignancies can express tumor-associated procoagulants, such as cancer procoagulant (CP) (Kanwar et al., 2006; Leung, 2006a; Hambleton et al., 2002). Tumors are major stimulants of tissue injury and the extrinsic pathway, making them one of the major causes of both acute and chronic DIC. Because the brain contains large amounts of tissue factor, DIC and other procoagulant activity are common in patients with primary brain tumors, brain metastases, or brain injury and in those who have had brain surgery.

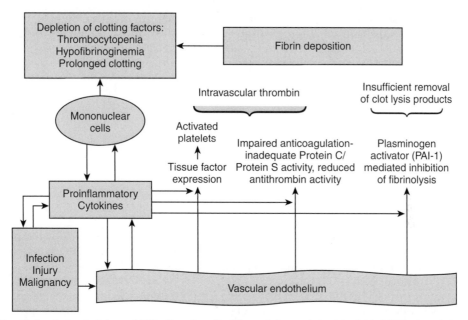

Fig. 11.1 • Pathophysiology of DIC. *(Data from Hambleton, J., Leung, L. L., & Levi, M. (2002). Coagulation: Consultative hemostasis. Hematology, 1:335–352; Levi, M. (2005). Disseminated intravascular coagulation. Critical Care Clinics, 21:449–467; Messmore, H. L., & Wehrmacher, W. H. (2002). Disseminated intravascular coagulation: A primer for primary care physicians. Postgraduate Medicine, 111(3). Retrieved August 3, 2007, from http://www.postgradmed.com/issues/2002/03_02/messmore.htm.)*

EPIDEMIOLOGY AND ETIOLOGY

The incidence of DIC likely is underreported because of its similarity to bleeding arising from other causes. The incidence in hospitalized adults is reported to be 1% (Leung, 2006a). In a study of hospitalized children, the overall incidence was 1.12% (Oren et al., 2005). The incidence of DIC in sepsis is thought to exceed 30% to 50%, but other coagulopathic abnormalities make concrete diagnosis of this disorder difficult (Furlong & Furlong, 2005). Patients with cancer have clearly identifiable tissue injury stimuli, and the reported incidence of DIC in patients with solid tumors or hematologic malignancies is 10% to 15% (Leung, 2006b).

RISK PROFILE

The most common etiology of DIC is sepsis (Duran & Tannock, 2006; Leung, 2006b; Oren et al., 2005; Hambleton et al., 2002).

- Although DIC has been associated with all microbes (bacteria, fungi, protozoa, and viruses), bacteria are the most common etiologic organisms (Leung, 2006b), and of these, gram-negative bacteria are the most common causes.
- Specific organisms with a pronounced risk for causing DIC include *meningococci, Staphylococcus aureus, Streptococcus pneumoniae,* and *Clostridium perfringens* (Kanwar et al., 2006; Leung, 2006b).
- Factors that accentuate the DIC pathophysiologic process include endotoxin damage to the endothelium, shock-induced tissue damage, and impaired hepatic perfusion that impedes clearance of activated clotting proteins (Leung, 2006b).

Severe tissue injury that stimulates widespread clotting by means of activation of Factor VII or the release of tissue material is the second most common cause of DIC in the following patient populations (Duran & Tannock, 2006; Hambleton et al., 2002):
- Traumatic injury (particularly brain injury that results in high levels of tissue factor [Leung, 2006b])
- Burns
- Major surgeryj
- Renal failure
- Severe pancreatitis (Toh & Downey, 2005)

Obstetric complications can be a factor in the development of DIC. The presence of the "foreign" fetus has been known to trigger inflammatory and immunologic processes, causing autodestruction of tissue. Leakage of a thromboplastin-like substance from the placenta is another proposed mechanism by which obstetric disorders cause DIC (Hambleton et al., 2002). Eclampsia and hemolytic syndrome are inflammatory processes, and placenta abruptio causes life-threatening hemorrhage.

Solid tumor malignancies provide a constant level of tissue injury, triggering abnormal clotting stimuli. They have long been associated with the development of DIC and are the third most common cause of this disorder (Duran & Tannock, 2006; Schlaeppi et al., 2006; Levi, 2001; Sallah et al., 2001).
- Approximately 10% to 15% of all patients with metastatic solid tumor malignancies have evidence of DIC (Duran & Tannock, 2006).
- Prostate cancer has been reported with greater predominance than many other tumors. The theory is that the prostate is rich in urokinase, which is released when this organ is injured, resulting in tissue injury and microvascular hemorrhage.
- Metastatic malignant melanoma has been associated with extensive soft tissue injury and release of tissue thromboplastin (Schlaeppi et al., 2006).

Hematologic malignancies can be a catalyst for DIC.
- Both at diagnosis and after treatment, as many as 15% of patients with acute leukemia show abnormal results on coagulation laboratory tests that are indicative of DIC (Duran & Tannock, 2006). For many of these patients, DIC remains subclinical; however, it is still an omnipresent, serious risk for thrombosis, bleeding, or multiorgan failure (Barbui & Falanga, 2001; Chojnowski et al., 1999).
- Patients with leukemia or lymphoma and high fibrinogen levels have a poorer prognosis than those with low fibrinogen levels (Wada et al., 2003).
- Acute myelogenous leukemia, M3 subtype (acute progranulocytic leukemia [APL]) is the most common hematologic malignancy to present with DIC. The less differentiated progranulocytes contain granules filled with procoagulants, which cause excessive clotting when undergoing lysis (Yanada et al., 2006; Barbui & Falanga, 2001).
- Acute lymphoblastic leukemia, B cell subtype, when associated with a high bone marrow blast count (Smith et al., 2006) is a catalyst for DIC.

Hemoglobinemia or hemoglobinuria caused by hemolysis can cause DIC.
- Primary hematologic disorders that cause hemolysis, such as paroxysmal nocturnal hemoglobinuria (PNH), can give rise to DIC (Furlong & Furlong, 2005).
- Intravenous immunoglobulin (anti-D IVIg) used to treat immune thrombocytopenia purpura has been reported to cause fatal DIC (Gaines, 2005).
- Vascular necrosing disorders, such as giant hemangioma, can cause DIC (Furlong & Furlong, 2005).

Vascular disorders (e.g., vasculitis, major vascular trauma, large vascular aneurysms, and giant hemangiomas) can cause local inflammation and activation of coagulation (Hambleton et al., 2002).

Severe hepatic failure may result in DIC (Leung, 2006b; Hambleton et al., 2002).

Toxic or immunologic reactions can cause DIC, such as snakebite, recreational drug use, transfusion reactions, organ transplant rejection, exacerbation of autoimmune disorders (e.g., systemic lupus erythematosus, rheumatoid arthritis), tuberculosis, osteomyelitis, heat stroke, and amphetamine overdose (Kanwar et al., 2006; Leung, 2006b; Furlong & Furlong, 2005; Hambleton et al., 2002; Messmore & Wehrmacher, 2002).

PROGNOSIS

The syndrome of disseminated intravascular coagulation may present in an acute and fulminant state, for which the prognosis for full recovery is unlikely but survival is approximately 50%. Factors associated with a poor outcome include advanced age, severity of underlying disease, and severity of hemostatic abnormalities (Leung, 2006a). The most important prognostic variable is the ability to correct the underlying disorder (Kanwar et al., 2006; Leung, 2006a); meningococcal infection, for example, has an extremely high mortality rate (60% to 80%) (Leung, 2006a).

In children, DIC frequently is associated with sepsis and organ failure, bleeding rather than thrombosis, and a mortality rate over 75% (Oren et al., 2005; Vincent & De Backer, 2005).

Chronic DIC occurs with a persistent, low-level coagulation stimulus, such as the presence of a tumor in the abdomen. The clotting stimulus produces abnormal thromboses, exemplified by hypercoagulability and a high risk for clotting complications such as pulmonary emboli or upper extremity thromboses. However, the patient does not have the rapid, uncontrolled hemorrhage seen in the acute form of DIC (Leung, 2006b; Messmore & Wehrmacher, 2002).

DIC is an independent predictor of mortality in patients with sepsis or severe trauma (Sivula et al., 2005; Hambleton et al., 2002).

PROFESSIONAL ASSESSMENT CRITERIA (PAC)

1. Thromboses in the microvasculature are early and common clinical findings. It is generally accepted that thromboses are manifested as organ failure (Mercer et al., 2006; Vincent & De Backer, 2005).
2. Hemorrhage, initially from small vessels but later more globally, manifests as the coagulation factors are depleted by microcirculatory clotting. Initial bleeding is mucosal and also is seen around intravenous lines or from wounds and skin injuries. As the disorder progresses, bleeding from larger vessels becomes evident.
3. Intracranial hemorrhage is the most common cause of early mortality in DIC, followed by multiorgan failure (Leung, 2006a).
4. *Purpura fulminans* is a condition of severe, subcutaneous hemorrhagic lesions that spread and are most often associated with a sepsis etiology (Kanwar et al., 2006). These patients have a higher risk for mortality (Furlong & Furlong, 2005).
5. DIC may present with a wide range of clinical findings (Table 11-1). The acute and fulminant form of the disorder (referred to as *bleeding DIC*), in which activation of fibrinolysis is the predominant feature, is well known in the critical care area. Bleeding DIC is more likely to be related to sepsis or obstetric complications, tissue injury, and acute progranulocytic leukemia (Duran & Tannock, 2006). Chronic, or low-grade, DIC is more common in patients with mild to moderate continuous tissue injury, such as those with mucin-producing tumors (e.g., adenocarcinoma).

Table 11-1	**SIGNS AND SYMPTOMS OF DIC**	
Body System	Thrombotic Symptoms/ Complications	Hemorrhagic Symptoms/ Complications
Neurologic/sensory	Confusion/disorientation Ischemic stroke	Unilateral weakness, papillary changes Intracranial hemorrhage
Respiratory	Persistent dry cough Pulmonary emboli	Alveolar hemorrhage Hemoptysis Pleural effusion/hemothorax
Cardiovascular	Myocardial infarction Trousseau's syndrome (superficial migratory thrombophlebitis) Nonbacterial thrombotic endocarditis	Pericardial effusion
Renal	Acute renal failure Oliguria	Hematuria
Gastrointestinal	Bowel infarction Jaundice from hepatic obstruction	Gastrointestinal hemorrhage (hematochezia, hematemesis, melena)
Musculoskeletal	Joint pain Severe muscle pain	Joint swelling and limited motion Swollen, hard muscle/compartment syndrome
Integumentary/ mucosal	Acral cyanosis Skin necrosis of limbs	Ecchymoses Epistaxis Gangrene Gingival bleeding Hemorrhagic bullae Petechiae Wound bleeding
Endocrine	Adrenal infarction/insufficiency	Adrenal hemorrhage/insufficiency Metrorrhagia
Hematologic	Jaundice from hemolysis	N/A

Data from Furlong, M. A., & Furlong, B. R. (2005). Disseminated intravascular coagulation. Retrieved January 24, 2007, from www.medscape.com/files/emedicine/disseminated-intravascular-coagulation/; Leung, L. L. K. (2006a). Clinical features, diagnosis, and treatment of disseminated intravascular coagulation in adults. Retrieved January 24, 2007, from www.UpToDate.com; Levi, M., & de Jonge, E. (2000). Current management of disseminated intravascular coagulation. *Hospital Practice, 35*(8):59-66; and Geiter, H., Jr. (2003). Disseminated intravascular coagulation. *Dimensions in Critical Care Nursing, 22*(3):108-114.

6. Clinically, DIC is very similar to some other clotting and bleeding phenomena. Disorders that must be ruled out include hemolysis, elevated liver enzymes, low platelets (HELLP) syndrome, idiopathic purpura fulminans, primary fibrinolysis, thrombotic thrombocytopenic purpura–hemolytic uremic syndrome (TTP-HUS), and vitamin K deficiency. The primary tool for differential diagnosis is a laboratory test that shows excess production of thrombin (Leung, 2006a; Furlong & Furlong, 2005).
7. Laboratory coagulation tests (Cauchie et al., 2006; Song et al., 2006; Toh & Downey, 2005; Geiter, 2003; Taylor et al., 2001) (Table 11-2).
   • A variety of laboratory diagnostic tests show abnormal results with DIC, but some are more sensitive or specific than others. Because of the lack of specificity of most readily available laboratory tests, several researchers have attempted to develop a scoring system to confirm the diagnosis of DIC.
     • Three scoring systems have been devised to predict the diagnosis of DIC. Two of the Japanese systems are more sensitive for overt DIC, the other is helpful for indicating candidates for early intervention. The scoring systems are the Japanese Association

Table 11-2 DIAGNOSTIC TESTS FOR DIC

Diagnostic Test	Normal Values	Indicative of DIC
Platelet count	150,000-400,00/mm^3	Decreased
Fibrinogen level	200-400 mg/dL	Decreased or low normal
Prothrombin time (PT)	11-15 seconds	Prolonged
Prothrombin time Internationalized Ratio (INR)	1.0-1.2 X normal	Higher ratio
Partial thromboplastin time (PTT)	60-70 seconds	Prolonged
Fibrin degradation products (FDPs)/Fibrin split products (FSPs)	< 10 mcg/mL	Increased
Firbin d-dimer	< 50 mcg/dL	Increased
Anti-thrombin III level	80%-120%	Decreased
Protein C level	72-1425	Decreased
Schistocytes of peripheral blood smear	Absent	Present
Bilirubin level	0.1-1.2 mg/dL	Increased
Blood urea nitrogen (BUN)	0.1-0.7 mg/dL	Increased

Data from Geiter, H., Jr. (2003). Disseminated intravascular coagulation. *Dimensions in Critical Care Nursing,* *22*(3):108-114; Furlong, M. A., & Furlong, B. R. (2005). Disseminated intravascular coagulation. Retrieved January 24, 2007, from www.medscape.com/files/emedicine/disseminated-intravascular-coagulation/; Leung, L. L. K. (2006b). Clinical features, diagnosis, and treatment of disseminated intravascular coagulation in adults. Retrieved January 24, 2007, from www.UpToDate.com; Levi, M., & de Jonge, E. (2000). Current management of disseminated intravascular coagulation. *Hospital Practice, 35*(8):59-66; and Toh, C., & Downey, C. (2005). Back to the future: Testing in disseminated intravascular coagulation. *Blood, Coagulation and Fibrinolysis, 16*:535–542.

for Acute Medicine (JAAM) system, the Japanese Ministry of Health and Welfare (JMHW) system, and the International Society on Thrombosis and Haemostasis (ISTH) system (Cauchie et al., 2006; Gando et al., 2006; Taylor et al., 2001).

- All three systems require that a potential risk factor or etiologic factor be identified before the patient's laboratory values can be scored.
- The most prevalent of the three systems is the ISTH scoring system (Table 11-3) (Taylor et al., 2001). The major difference between the Japanese systems and the ISTH system is that the latter does not require bleeding or organ failure for a diagnosis of DIC. Rather, it is based entirely on laboratory test results. The ISTH system also does not account for the percentage decrease from baseline, as do the Japanese scoring systems (Cauchie et al., 2006; Gando et al., 2006).
- Four clinical criteria drive the diagnosis of DIC:
  - Procoagulant activation and evidence of clot formation
  - Fibrinolytic activation (accelerated clot lysis)
  - Consumption of inhibitory factors
  - Evidence of organ damage from microvascular injury and clotting

Table 11-3 DIC SCORING SYSTEMS*

Laboratory Test	0	1	2	3
Platelet count/mm^3	> 100,000	> 50,000	< 50,000	
D-dimer mcg/mL	< 1		1-5	> 5
Fibrinogen g/L	> 1	< 1		
Prothrombin index%	> 70	40-70	< 40	

From Taylor, F. B., Toh, C. H., & Hoots, W. K., et al. (2001). Towards a definition, clinical and laboratory criteria and a scoring system for disseminated intravascular coagulation. *Thrombosis and Haemostasis, 86*:1327-1330.
*All scoring systems require the presence of a risk factor for DIC before the laboratory test results can be evaluated.

- The defining test for DIC generally is accepted to be validation of excessive production of thrombin.
  - Although evident in thrombin formation, fibrinogen levels are not extremely sensitive, because they may begin at higher than normal levels as a result of inflammatory stimuli, and the rate of reduction is inconsistent (Wada et al., 2003).
  - The thrombin time is extremely sensitive to minor changes in thrombin and therefore not sensitive; however, it is prolonged with DIC.
- Clinical significance is unlikely without evidence of excessive fibrinolysis.
  - Excessive fibrinolysis is best determined by the presence of excessive fibrin degradation products (FDPs). Measurement of FDPs has been described as the only reliable diagnostic test for DIC in patients with progranulocytic leukemia (Yanada et al., 2006).
  - Fibrinogen d-dimer is an antigen formed from the lysis of plasmin that is cross-linked inside the clots (Chernecky & Berger, 2004). This antigen is also present in other clotting disorders, such as deep vein thrombosis and pulmonary embolism. A monoclonal antibody that binds to this antigen often is used in conjunction with measurement of FDPs to enhance the specificity of the diagnosis (Furlong & Furlong, 2005).
- Thrombocytopenia occurs early in the pathophysiologic process of DIC, reflecting massive platelet aggregation that precedes excess fibrin clot formation. Unfortunately, many patients at risk for DIC have other risk factors for thrombocytopenia, and it is not always reflective of the presence of DIC (Levi & de Jonge, 2000; Yanada et al., 2006). Platelet counts that are 50% of baseline are considered diagnostic for DIC in the absence of other presumed etiologies (Geiter, 2003; Toh & Downey, 2005).
- The prothrombin time (PT) is abnormally prolonged in DIC but not specific for the disorder.
- The partial thromboplastin time (PTT) is not a consistent reflection of DIC; it may be either normal or prolonged (Furlong & Furlong, 2005).
- Laboratory evidence of deficiency of endogenous coagulation inhibitors is apparent, but many laboratories do not have the facilities to perform these tests (Leung, 2006a; Mercer et al., 2006; Toh & Downey, 2005; Levi & de Jonge, 2000). The values are:
- Decreased protein C
- Decreased protein S
- Consistently decreased antithrombin III (this synthetic substrate assay test is not readily available in all practice settings) (Furlong & Furlong, 2005).
- Research-based laboratory tests hold promise for the future but are not yet readily available (Toh & Downey, 2005; Levi et al., 2002). They include:
- Soluble fibrin monomer complexes (SFMC)
- Lipoprotein C–reactive protein (LP-CRP) complexes (MDA slope 1 and Flag A2)
- Plasma Factor XIII activity levels: These values are more predictive of overt DIC and correlate well with other common laboratory parameters (Song et al., 2006).
- Prothrombin fragment (F1 + 2) enzyme-linked immunosorbent assay (ELISA): This test demonstrates Factor X activation (Furlong & Furlong, 2005; Barbui & Falanga, 2001).
- Thrombin-antithrombin complex (TAT) (Barbui & Falanga, 2001)
- Fibrinopeptide A (FPA): A breakdown product of fibrinogen, FPA indicates thrombin activity. This finding is abnormal in 88% of patients with DIC, but the test is not readily available from all laboratories (Furlong & Furlong, 2005; Barbui & Falanga, 2001).
- Plasminogen activator inhibitor (PAI-1) (Mercer et al., 2006)
- Some laboratory tests reflect the hemolysis that occurs as blood cells are sheared or damaged by the intravascular clots. These include an elevated bilirubin, elevated

blood urea nitrogen (BUN), and schistocytes on a blood smear (Leung, 2006b; Furlong & Furlong, 2005; Geiter, 2003).

NURSING CARE AND TREATMENT

1. Identify and treat the underlying cause as soon as possible. The success of all other treatment measures may depend on removal of the stimulus for excess clotting (Mercer et al., 2006; Schlaeppi et al., 2006; Labelle & Kitchens, 2005; Geiter, 2003; Bick, 2002; Messmore & Wehrmacher, 2002).
2. Maintain vascular volume so that hyperviscosity does not contribute to the microvascular clotting process (Geiter, 2003).
3. Avoid vasoconstriction so that organ perfusion is not further compromised by constricted vessels and poor blood flow (Geiter, 2003).
4. Avoid invasive procedures, surgery, and other factors that enhance risk of bleeding.
5. If the disease is detected early, low-level anticoagulation is recommended.
   - Heparin is administered as a low-dose, continuous infusion (about 50 to 300 units/hr) if the primary manifestations are thrombotic and in progranulocytic leukemia (Leung, 2006a; Mercer et al., 2006; Geiter, 2003; Bick, 2002).
   - Administration of antithrombin III concentrates has had mixed clinical results (Kienast et al., 2006; Leung, 2006a; Mercer et al., 2006; Geiter, 2003; Bick, 2002; Levi et al., 2002; Levi & de Jonge, 2000;)
   - Protein C concentrates have been used in the management of DIC related to meningococcemia, in which acquired protein C deficiency is clearly associated with DIC, because meningococcemia has such a high mortality rate (Leung, 2006a; Mercer et al., 2006).
6. If the patient is actively bleeding, implement measures to stop the bleeding while awaiting resolution of the underlying microvascular process (Levi et al., 2006).
   - Localized bleeding can be treated with topical agents. These agents minimally disrupt the microvascular processes and are recommended as first-line management of mild bleeding until the causes of the excess clotting have been reversed. Table 11-4 describes some local hemostatic treatments.
   - Blood component replacement may be necessary if bleeding is excessive. In active bleeding diathesis, coagulation products are commonly used despite the underlying initial pathophysiology of clotting. Some disagreement exists over whether transfusions are appropriate in asymptomatic patients (Mercer et al., 2006). Some new coagulation products and fractions (e.g., activated protein C and Factor VII concentrate) are now more readily available and are thought to better target the coagulation deficits. Obtaining unusual blood components (e.g., cryoprecipitate, Factor VI concentrate, antithrombin III) may require approval by Blood Bank physicians (Levi et al., 2006).
     - Indications for platelet replacement therapy include an asymptomatic platelet count less than $20,000/mm^3$, or a platelet count less than $50,000/mm^3$ with serious bleeding (Leung, 2006a).
     - Fresh frozen plasma is administered to patients with asymptomatic fibrinogen levels < 50 mg/dL.
   - Activated Factor VIIa has been used in a number of severe hemorrhagic conditions, such as hemophilia, severe trauma, and intracranial hemorrhage. It has been used off-label for life-threatening hemorrhage in DIC (Mercer et al., 2006).
7. Patients with DIC associated with acute progranulocytic leukemia may show immediate improvement in the DIC with administration of the tumor cell–differentiating agent all-transretinoic acid (ATRA) (Leung, 2006a; Yanada et al., 2006).

Table 11-4 MANAGEMENT OF DIC

Management Strategy	Specific Agents	Administration Guidelines
Local treatment of bleeding	Avitene	Apply to skin and mucous membrane bleeding sites as needed. Do not forcefully remove after clotting has occurred, as it may restart bleeding. Warm saline rinsing may remove excess superficial clotted blood.
	Gelfoam	Cut square approximate size of puncture site that is bleeding. Apply with prolonged pressure over the site. Do not remove, allowing to loosen as skin heals or rinse off with saline.
	Surgicel	Apply strip of oxidized cellulose across bleeding area (works well with abrasions that have multiple small bleeding sites). Cover and apply pressure. Allow to remain until rinses off easily with saline.
	Topical thrombin	Use pill crusher to create a powder for application or reconstitution with sterile water, or leave as crystals to apply to bleeding sites. Apply dry substance to bleeding sites, applying pressure to assist adherence. If bleeding is inside an orifice (e.g., nasal), the powder can be reconstituted into a liquid and instilled into bleeding area.
Blood component therapy	Activated Factor VIIa	Obtained with approval of blood bank physician. Usually distributed in 30-50 mg increments for intravenous push administration. Observe for hypersensitivity reactions. Follow-up with prothrombin time (PT) testing.
	Antithrombin III concentrate	Use should be considered in some patients, no real statistical significant benefits.
	Cryoprecipitate (CRYO)	Prepared from 1 unit of FFP thawed at $40°$ C. Precipitate refrozen in 10-15 mL of plasma and stored at $-18°$ C or colder for 1 year. Dosage calculation based on amount of fibrinogen in 1 unit of cryoprecipitate, the plasma volume, and the desired increment. Dosing frequency based on clinical and laboratory response. Hypersensitivity risks similar to those of FFP.
	Fresh frozen plasma (FFP)	Administered in increments of units (volume obtained from one donor). Contains all clotting factors except Factor VIII that is destroyed during freezing process. Requires advance notice to thaw product ($\sim$ 1 hour). Usually administered in increment of 2, 4, or 6 units. Monitor for hypersensitivity reactions. Fibrinogen levels are monitored for efficacy.

Table 11-4 MANAGEMENT OF DIC—cont'd		
Management Strategy	**Specific Agents**	**Administration Guidelines**
	Platelets	Administered in increments of units (volume obtained from one donor). Contains platelets suspended in small amount of plasma. Usually administered in 4, 6, 10, 12 unit increments. Hypersensitivity reactions are common, and patients may require acetaminophen and histamine blockers to abrogate reactions. Post-platelet counts are drawn approximately 1 hours after infusion to determine efficacy.
	Red blood cells (RBCs)	Red blood cells do not directly assist coagulation but are administered to support blood volume to replace lost cells from bleeding diathesis.
Anticoagulants	Heparin	
	Argatroban	Thrombin inhibitor/anticoagulant. Administered as IV infusion. **Must be diluted 100-fold before infusion in 0.9% NaCl, D$_5$W, or lactated Ringer's solution to provide a final concentration of 1 mg/mL.** Rate of administration is based on body weight at 2 mcg/kg/min (e.g., 50-kg pt infuse at 6 mL/hr). Proposed as an alternative to heparin. Has a high affinity for clot-bound-thrombin that may enhance beneficial effects in DIC.
	Activated Protein C	Administered to patients with sepsis and organ failure as a 96 hour infusion dosed 24 mcg/kg/hour. Can cause excessive bleeding, so careful monitoring of hemorrhage is necessary.
	Defibrotide	Decreases thrombin generation, increases prostacyclen, and inhibits deposition of fibrin and collagen, which leads to reduction of fibrosis. Average active dose is 25 mg/kg/day, but the general recommendations are 800 mg IV daily for 7-8 days to prevent thromboembolism, 400-1200 mg/day for treatment of thromboembolism, and up to 60 mg/kg/day for prevention or management of hepatic veno-occlusive disease.
Procoagulants/agents that slow or block fibrinolysis (administered in carefully controlled circumstances where bleeding is clearly more severe than thromboses.)		

8. Supportive care includes pain relief, positioning for comfort, skin care, and minimization of bleeding risks.

EVIDENCE-BASED PRACTICE UPDATES

1. Traditionally DIC was thought to result from activation of both the intrinsic and extrinsic coagulation pathways. We now recognize that almost all thrombin formation is the result of extrinsic factor activation of tissue Factor VII (Leung, 2006b; Hambleton et al., 2002). This may have significant implications for the development of effective treatment modalities.
2. Recently discovered pathophysiologic mechanisms indicate a multiphase process that requires individualized treatment, depending on whether the clinical presentation is primarily thrombotic or hemorrhagic. Other factors that must be considered in the choice of treatment include the patient's age, the etiology of the DIC, the site or severity of thrombosis or hemorrhage, and hemodynamic stability (Bick, 2002).
3. Diagnosis of DIC historically has been difficult because of a lack of uniformity in findings and because DIC covers a spectrum of chronic to fulminant disease. New diagnostic scoring systems to identify overt or nonovert DIC have recently been established and have a reported 91% accuracy. Some scoring systems also reflect the prognosis and 28-day mortality (Angstwurm et al., 2006; Cauchie et al., 2006; Voves et al., 2006; Hambleton et al., 2002).
4. New, molecular-targeted microscopy may aid the development of methods for evaluating the microvessel inflammation and microthrombi associated with DIC (Norman, 2005).
5. Activated protein C is both an anticoagulant and an antiinflammatory agent that has been licensed for use in the reversal of organ dysfunction related to severe sepsis. It has not been indicated for specific treatment of DIC, but the theoretical benefit is being explored (Leung, 2006a; Toh & Downey, 2005; Geiter, 2003; Levi et al., 2002; Levi & de Jonge, 2000). One large trial showed a greater risk reduction for death in septic patients with DIC as opposed to those without DIC (38% versus 18%) (Dhainaut et al., 2004).
6. Tissue factor pathway inhibitor (rTFPI), an endogenous inhibitor of coagulation, has been administered in some trials, but data are limited, and no benefit has been proven (Mercer et al., 2006)

TEACHING AND EDUCATION

1. Interventions that help health care providers maximize tissue perfusion: wearing covers/clothing, maintaining fluid intake, temperature management
2. Topical and local management of bleeding
3. **Web sites for information:**
   - www.nlm.nih.gov/medlineplus/ency/article/000573.htm
   - www.umm.edu/ency/article/000573.htm
   - www.clevelandclinicmeded.com/diseasemanagement/hematology/platelet/table2.htm
   - www.fda.gov/cber/blood/dicigiv.pdf

NURSING DIAGNOSES

1. **Ineffective tissue perfusion**, peripheral or cardiopulmonary, related to thromboses
2. **Ineffective tissue perfusion**, gastrointestinal or cerebral, related to hemorrhage
3. **Deficient fluid volume** related to hemorrhage
4. **Impaired tissue integrity** related to petechiae, ecchymoses, or localized bleeding
5. **Disturbed sensory perception**, kinesthetic/visual, related to pain and/or visual disturbances resulting from bleeding

EVALUATION AND DESIRED OUTCOMES

1. Serum coagulation parameters are monitored frequently in patients with DIC, with the goal returning these values to normal. The specific test used depends partly on the patient's primary diagnosis and pre-existing abnormalities.
   - In patients with previously normal platelet counts, the blood platelet count test is used, because it is the most sensitive to subclinical clotting.
   - In patients with abnormal baseline platelet counts, the fibrinogen level is followed for trends, although the level may begin higher than normal and never drop below normal.
   - Although previously thought to be the most definitive tests, fibrin degradation products and d-dimer are now used in conjunction with at least one other coagulation test (platelet count or fibrinogen level).
2. Evidence of abnormal bleeding or clotting is a clinical indicator of continuing DIC.

DISCHARGE PLANNING AND FOLLOW-UP CARE

- After acute DIC resolves, minimal follow-up care should be needed.
- Unresolved thrombotic complications, such as visual disturbances, bowel ischemia, or renal insufficiency, may require referral and follow-up by specialists.
- Patients with low-grade or chronic DIC should be referred to a hematologist for evaluation, follow-up, and treatment as needed (Furlong & Furlong, 2005).
- Chronic DIC often causes chronic, low-level blood component consumption. Periodic transfusions usually are required.
- A long-term complication of DIC is distal vascular occlusion that leads to soft tissue necrosis, which can result in limb amputation.

REVIEW QUESTIONS

QUESTIONS

1. **Which medical-surgical disorder places the patient at greatest risk for the development of DIC?**
    1. Blunt trauma to the lower legs
    2. Gastrointestinal bleeding with estimated blood loss of 300 to 500 mL and mild hypotension
    3. Meningococcemia
    4. Acute myocardial infarction

2. **The hematologic malignancy most commonly associated with DIC is:**
    1. Multiple myeloma
    2. Burkitt's lymphoma
    3. Acute lymphocytic leukemia
    4. Acute progranulocytic leukemia

3. **Our most current knowledge of the pathophysiology of DIC suggests that the most significant factor activation that leads to excess thrombin formation is:**
    1. Factor V
    2. Factor VII
    3. Factor VIII
    4. Factor XIII

4. **The prognosis associated with acute DIC syndrome includes an expected mortality of approximately:**
    1. 20%
    2. 30%
    3. 50%
    4. 80%

5. **The most common cause of early death in patients with DIC is:**
    1. Bowel infarction
    2. Hypoxemia
    3. Multiorgan failure
    4. Intracranial hemorrhage

6. **The diagnostic test most sensitive for and indicative of overt DIC is:**
    1. Low platelet count
    2. Low fibrinogen level

3. Elevated fibrin degradation products
4. Prolonged prothrombin time

7. **A major clinical goal in the treatment of DIC is to:**
   1. Avoid vasoconstriction
   2. Administer blood components to prevent factor deficiency
   3. Treat all bleeding as noninvasively as possible (local/topical interventions)
   4. Hyperoxygenate to reduce tissue hypoxemia

8. **Medications that may be used to treat DIC include all of the following except:**
   1. Heparin
   2. Antithrombin
   3. Reteplase (Retavase)
   4. Activated protein C

9. **A common long-term complication of DIC is:**
   1. Autoimmune hemolytic anemia
   2. Amputation
   3. Lymphedema
   4. Hepatic failure

10. **The highest nursing priority for a patient with DIC is:**
    1. Immunoglobulin monitoring
    2. Neurologic protection
    3. Protection of the skin and mucous membranes
    4. Maintenance of tissue perfusion

ANSWERS

1. **Answer: 3**
   Rationale: Disorders associated with DIC usually involve considerable tissue injury. Patients with infectious complications caused by certain virulent organisms, such as meningococci, are at highest risk of developing DIC.

2. **Answer: 4**
   Rationale: Both solid tumor malignancies and hematologic malignancies place patients at risk for DIC; together they are the third highest etiology of the disorder. Malignant conditions that put patients at greatest risk for DIC include progranulocytic leukemia, metastatic cancer, brain tumors (primary or metastatic), and adenocarcinomas (mucin producing).

3. **Answer: 2**
   Rationale: A new pathophysiologic finding is that the most significant trigger of DIC is tissue activator (also known as Factor VII), the primary component of the extrinsic coagulation pathway.

4. **Answer: 3**
   Rationale: Chronic forms of DIC are associated with a very low mortality rate, and highly virulent infections can have a mortality rate as high as 80%. However, the average mortality with acute DIC is approximately 50%.

5. **Answer: 4**
   Rationale: Although DIC is primarily a thrombotic disorder, the most deadly complications are hemorrhagic. Early bleeding indicates a poor prognosis. Among these patients, the most common cause of death is intracranial hemorrhage. Late deaths are more likely to be caused by organ failure.

6. **Answer: 3**
   Rationale: Before laboratory tests can be evaluated for possible DIC, a clinical risk factor must be present. No one test is definitive, but evidence of thrombin production and excessive fibrinolysis are considered hallmarks of the disorder. Because both thrombocytopenia and hypofibrinogenemia are inconsistent indicators of thrombin production due to inflammatory interference, elevated fibrin degradation products, as an indicator of excess lysis, may be the most helpful and specific diagnostic test.

7. **Answer: 1**
   Rationale: Patients with DIC have subclinical thromboses, which are the primary pathophysiologic manifestation of the disease. Treatments to reduce thromboses and improve microvascular blood flow are most important. The key objectives are to prevent dehydration and vasoconstriction. Blood components are replaced only if the patient is symptomatic or severely depleted.

8. **Answer: 3**
   Rationale: Because DIC is a primary thrombotic disorder, heparin,

antithrombin (also known as antithrombin III), and activated protein C are administered to reduce clots. Reteplase is a potent fibrinolytic, but it is not used for DIC because of its high risk of bleeding.

9. Answer: 2
Rationale: Thrombotic occlusion of vessels is likely to result in a variety of thrombotic ischemic complications. One of the most

common is distal vascular occlusion that leads to peripheral soft tissue necrosis, necessitating amputation.

10. Answer: 4
Rationale: Because DIC is a systemic clotting disorder, all organs benefit from maintenance of tissue perfusion. Organ-specific interventions protect only one aspect of the affected organs.

REFERENCES

Angstwurm, M. W., Dempfle, C, & Spannagl, M. (2006). New disseminated intravascular coagulation score: A useful tool to predict mortality in comparison with Acute Physiology and Chronic Health Evaluation II and logistic organ dysfunction scores. *Critical Care Medicine, 34*(2):314-320.

Barbui, T., & Falanga, A. (2001). Disseminated intravascular coagulation in acute leukemia. *Seminars in Thrombosis and Hemostasis, 27*(6):593-604.

Bick, R. L. (2002). Disseminated intravascular coagulation: A review of etiology, pathophysiology, diagnosis, and management: Guidelines for care. *Clinical and Applied Thrombosis/Hemostasis, 8*(1):1-31.

Cauchie, P., Cauchie, C., & Boudjeltia, K., et al. (2006). Diagnosis and prognosis of overt disseminated intravascular coagulation in a general hospital: Meaning of the ISTH Score System, fibrin monomers, and lipoprotein-C–reactive protein complex formation. *American Journal of Hematology, 81*(6):414-419.

Chernecky, C., & Berger, B (2004). *Laboratory tests and diagnostic procedures.* (4th ed.). Philadelphia: W. B. Saunders.

Chojnowski, K., Wawrzyniak, E., & Trelinski, J., et al. (1999). Assessment of coagulation disorders in patients with acute leukemia before and after cytostatic treatment. *Leukemia & Lymphoma, 36*(1-2):77-84.

Dhainaut, J. F., Yan, S. B., & Joyce, D. E., et al. (2004). Treatment effects of drotrecogin alfa (activated) in patients with severe sepsis with or without disseminated intravascular coagulation. *Journal of Thrombosis & Haemostasis, 2*(11):1924-1933.

Duran, I., & Tannock, I. F. (2006). Disseminated intravascular coagulation as the presenting sign of metastatic prostate cancer. *Journal of General Internal Medicine, 21*(11):C6-C8.

Furlong, M. A., & Furlong, B. R. (2005). *Disseminated intravascular coagulation.* Retrieved January 24, 2007, from www.medscape.com/files/emedicine/disseminated-intravascular-coagulation/.

Gaines, A. R. (2005). Disseminated intravascular coagulation associated with acute hemoglobinemia or hemoglobinuria following Rh(0)(D) immune globulin intravenous administration for immune thrombocytopenia purpura. *Blood, 106*(5):1532-1537.

Gando, S., Iba, T., & Eguchi, Y., et al. (2006). A multicenter, prospective validation of disseminated intravascular coagulation diagnostic criteria for critically ill patients: Comparing current criteria. *Critical Care Medicine, 34*(3):625-631.

Geiter, H. Jr. (2003). Disseminated intravascular coagulation. *Dimensions in Critical Care Nursing, 22*(3):108-114.

Hambleton, J., Leung, L. L., & Levi, M. (2002). Coagulation: Consultative hemostasis. *Hematology, 1*:335-352.

Kanwar, V. S., Galardy, P. J., & Grabowski, E. (2006). *Consumption coagulopathy.* Retrieved January 25, 2007, from www.emedicine.com/ped/topic473.htm.

Kienast, J., Juers, M., & Wiedermann, C. J., et al. (2006). Treatment effects of high-dose anti-thrombin without concomitant heparin in patients with severe sepsis with or without disseminated intravascular coagulation. *Journal of Thrombosis and Haemostasis, 4*(1):90-97.

Labelle, C. A., & Kitchens, C. S. (2005). Disseminated intravascular coagulation: Treat the cause, not the lab values. *Cleveland Clinics Journal of Medicine, 72*(5):383-385, 390.

Leung, L. L. K. (2006a). *Clinical features, diagnosis, and treatment of disseminated intravascular coagulation in adults.* Retrieved January 24, 2007, from www.UpToDate.com.

Leung, L. L. K. (2006b). *Pathogenesis and etiology of disseminated intravascular coagulation.* Retrieved January 24, 2007, from www.UpToDate.com.

Levi, M. (2001). Cancer and DIC. *Haemostasis, 31*(Suppl. 1):47-48.

Levi, M., & de Jonge, E. (2000). Current management of disseminated intravascular coagulation. *Hospital Practice, 35*(8):59-66.

Levi, M., de Jonge, E, & Meijers, J. (2002). The diagnosis of disseminated intravascular coagulation. *Blood Reviews, 16*(4):217-223.

Levi, M., de Jonge, E, & van der Poll, T. (2006). Plasma and plasma components in the management of disseminated intravascular coagulation. *Best Practice and Research Clinical Haematology, 19*(1): 127-142.

Mercer, K. W, Macik, B. G, & Williams, M. E. (2006). Hematologic disorders in critically ill patients. *Seminars in Respiratory and Critical Care Medicine, 27*(3):286-296.

Messmore, H. L., & Wehrmacher, W. H. (2002). Disseminated intravascular coagulation. A primer for primary care physicians. *Postgraduate Medicine, 111*(3). Retrieved August 3, 2007, from http://www.post-gradmed.com/issues/2002/03_02/messmore.htm.

Norman, K. (2005). Techniques: Intravital microscopy—a method for investigating disseminated intravascular coagulation? *Trends in Pharmacology Science, 26*(6):327-332.

Oren, H., Cingoz, I., & Duman, M., et al. (2005). Disseminated intravascular coagulation in pediatric patients: Clinical and laboratory features and prognostic factors influencing survival. *Pediatric Hematology Oncology, 22*(8):679-688.

Sallah, S., Wan, J. Y., & Nguyen, N. P., et al. (2001). Disseminated intravascular coagulation in solid tumors: Clinical and pathologic study. *Thrombosis and Hemostasis, 86*(3):828-833.

Schlaeppi, M. R., Korte, W., & von Moos, R, et al. (2006). Successful treatment of acute disseminated intravascular coagulation in a patient with metastatic melanoma. *Onkologie, 29*(11):531-533.

Sivula, M., Tallgren, M., & Pettila, V. (2005). Modified score for disseminated intravascular coagulation in the critically ill. *Intensive Care Medicine, 31*(9):1209-1214.

Smith, A., Das, P., & O'Reilly, J., et al. (2006). Three adults with acute lymphoblastic leukemia and DIC. *Cancer Genetics and Cytogenetics, 66*(1):86-88.

Song, J. W., Choi, J. R., & Song, K. S., et al. (2006). Plasma factor XIII activity in patients with disseminated intravascular coagulation. *Yonsei Medical Journal, 47*(2):196-200.

Taylor, F. B., Toh, C. H., & Hoots, W. K., et al. (2001). Towards a definition, clinical and laboratory criteria and a scoring system for disseminated intravascular coagulation. *Thrombosis and Haemostasis, 86*(5):1327-1330.

Toh, C. H., & Downey, C. (2005). Back to the future: Testing in disseminated intravascular coagulation. *Blood, Coagulation and Fibrinolysis, 16*(8):535-542.

Vincent, J. L., & De Backer, D. (2005). Does disseminated intravascular coagulation lead to multiple organ failure? *Critical Care Clinics, 21*(3):469-477.

Voves, C., Wuillemin, W. A., & Zeerleder, S. (2006). International Society on Thrombosis and Haemostasis: Score for overt disseminated intravascular coagulation predicts organ dysfunction and fatality in sepsis patients. *Blood Coagulation and Fibrinolysis, 17*(6):445-451.

Wada, H., Moi, Y., & Okabayashi, K., et al. (2003). High plasma fibrinogen level is associated with poor clinical outcome in DIC patients. *American Journal of Hematology, 72*(1):1-7.

Yanada, M., Matsushita, T., & Suzuki, M., et al. (2006). Disseminated intravascular coagulation in acute leukemia: Clinical and laboratory features at presentation. *European Journal of Haematology, 77*(4):282-287.

Dyspnea and Airway Obstruction

CYNTHIA C. CHERNECKY • LIBBY MONTOYA

PATHOPHYSIOLOGICAL MECHANISMS

Dyspnea, a symptom, and airway obstruction, a sign, are most notably associated with primary lung cancer and metastatic disease (Torres-Carranza et al., 2006; Le 2005; Wickham, 2002; Chernecky & Shelton, 2001; Jones et al., 2001; Chernecky Sarna, 2000, Chernecky, 2004). In the clinical setting, *dyspnea* is commonly defined as shortness of breath, difficulty breathing, breathlessness, or a tight throat. It is a subjective symptom that often is not assessed, or considered of little relevance, and poorly managed.

The gold standard for assessment is patient self-reporting. In children, the parent or caregiver report, a change in the child's level of activity, and changes in vital signs are the usual indicators. Dyspnea can be a problem for patients on ventilators (Bergbom-Engberg et al., 1989), and it also is common in pathological processes such as obesity, chronic obstructive pulmonary disease (COPD), anemia, anxiety, cachexia, and heart failure. Therapy-induced dyspnea can result from surgical thoracotomy, radiation-caused fibrosis of the lungs, and chemotherapy-related pulmonary and cardiac toxicities. Dyspnea in the cancer patient is usually multifactorial and includes symptom clusters (Esper & Heidrich, 2005), and affects the patient's quality of life through decreasing physical and social functioning.

The two subcategories of dyspnea are dyspnea at rest and dyspnea with activity (also known as *dyspnea on exertion*). Once the type of dyspnea has been identified, it is quantified in time and/or relation to activity and impact on quality of life. Dyspnea is a predictor of an increased likelihood of hospital death rather than death at home. It is the one symptom that causes the greatest distress for caregivers. Dyspnea causes loss of physical stamina, therefore activities such as shopping, getting the mail, bathing, grooming, and dressing can become difficult, if not impossible. This change in activity status can lead to anger, helplessness, frustration, and depression. In particular, a fear of dying arises, because the patient feels like "I cannot breathe." This feeling of drowning as a result of air hunger is real and should be discussed with the patient and caregiver at the appropriate time.

Airway obstruction is the occlusion of the airway passage that begins in the nose and ends in the lungs. Occlusions can be partial or complete. The diagnosis usually begins with the patient complaining of difficulty breathing, having something stuck in the throat, having a hard time breathing, or being winded. The result is a cycle of air hunger, lowering oxygen concentration, and anxiety. Interventions are started to break the cycle, and some interventions are provided immediately.

EPIDEMIOLOGY AND ETIOLOGY

The incidence of dyspnea is 21% to 90% in all cancer patients, with a predominance of 80% in patients with lung cancer. The incidence of airway obstruction is 30% (Chan et al.,

Table 12-1 CANCEROUS AND NONCANCEROUS CAUSES OF DYSPNEA*	
Cancerous Causes	**Noncancerous Causes**
Aortic tumor	Aberrant thymic tissue (infant) (Shah et al., 2001)
Head and neck cancer (esophagus, nares, oral	AIDS
cavity, pharynx, salivary gland, sinuses,	Anaphylaxis
tongue, tonsils, trachea)	Cachexia
Hodgkin disease	COPD
Lung	Cystic cervical thymus (infant)
Lymphoma	Diaphragmatic excursion problem
Non-Hodgkin lymphoma	GERD
	Heart disease or failure
	Hypophosphatemia
	Hypersensitivity reaction
	Lung reduction surgery
	Neuromuscular abnormalities
	Obesity
	Pleural effusion
	Pneumonia
	Pneumothorax
	Pulmonary emboli
	Sarcoidosis
	Superior vena cava syndrome (SVCS)
	Thoracic scoliosis
	Thyroid toxicosis
	Tobacco use history
	Tuberculosis (TB)

*Cancer treatment modalities also can cause airway obstruction.

2002) to 75% (Shohat et al., 2004). Dyspnea can take weeks to months to develop, and the onset often is gradual. Airway obstruction can be immediate or gradual in onset and result in either partial or complete obstruction. Both cancerous and noncancerous conditions can cause dyspnea and airway obstruction (Tables 12-1 and 12-2).

RISK PROFILE

- Primary cancers of the lung, head, or neck (especially the esophagus), lymphoma, or metastasis to the lung.
- Superior vena cava syndrome (see Chapter 46), right-side heart failure, obesity, COPD, pneumonia, anemia, or anxiety.
- Radiation therapy to the lungs, endotracheal intubation (Chen et al., 2005), administration of narcotics (Byard & Gilbert, 2005), or laser ablation (Skoulas & Kountakis, 2003).
- History of tobacco use or exposure to asbestos (Dudgeon et al., 2001), radon (Carta et al., 2001), or Agent Orange (Pavuk et al., 2005).
- **Pediatric population:** Space-occupying lesions (e.g., metastatic tumors); tumor-associated effusions and infections (e.g., pneumonia or after an aspiration procedure); or severe skeletal or neuromuscular impairments that interfere with respiration (Kane & Himelstein, 2002). About 50% to 60% of all patients with T-cell acute lymphoblastic leukemia have a mediastinal mass; this is also a frequent finding in patients with Hodgkin's or non-Hodgkin's lymphoma (Howard et al., 2006).

Table 12-2 CANCEROUS AND NONCANCEROUS CAUSES OF AIRWAY OBSTRUCTION*	
Cancerous Causes	**Noncancerous Causes**
Acute lymphoblastic leukemia: T cell with mediastinal mass (in child) (Howard et al., 2006)	Adenoids
B-cell lymphoma	Pseudotumor caused by motor vehicle air bag injury (Alaani et al., 2005)
Burkitt's lymphoma (Choo et al., 2005)	Juvenile angiofibroma
Chordoma (in child) (Tao et al., 2005)	Juvenile hyaline fibromatosis
Head and neck cancer: adenoid cystic carcinoma, chondrosarcoma (nasal), craniopharyngioma, ectomesenchymoma (nose), esophageal, nares, olfactory neuroblastoma, oropharynx histiocytoma, salivary gland (Mehra & Woessner, 2005), sinuses, thyroid, tongue, tracheal paraganglioma	Narcotic administration, morphine (Byard & Gilbert, 2005)
	Papilloma (in child)
	Papillomatous tissue during CO_2 laser treatment
	Postendotracheal tube/tracheostomy stricture
	Pseudotumor of lung
Hodgkin disease	Rheumatoid arthritis (Haben et al., 2005)
Lung	Superior vena cava syndrome (SVCS)
Meningioma (extracranial)	Thyroid goiter
Multiple myeloma	Tonsillitis
Non-Hodgkin lymphoma	Vocal cord paralysis with fixed stenosis
Ovarian (Tasci et al., 2005)	
Plasmacytoma	
Renal metastasis (Torres-Carranza et al., 2006)	
Schwannoma	

*Cancer treatment modalities also can cause airway obstruction.

PROGNOSIS

The prognosis depends on the cause of the dyspnea or airway obstruction and the effectiveness of treatment. For dyspnea, structured nursing programs are effective for patients with lung cancer (Moore et al., 2002; Bredin et al., 1999; Sarna, 1998; McCorkle et al., 1989). These interventions have not been tested in the pediatric population. For airway obstruction, effective treatments include radiation therapy, surgery, endoscopic laser ablation (Venuta et al., 2002), photodynamic therapy (Jones et al., 2001), and stenting (Chan et al., 2002). With metastatic disease, only palliative treatment is possible.

PROFESSIONAL ASSESSMENT CRITERIA (PAC)

1. Inspect and assess for cyanosis, tachypnea, stridor (See & Olopade, 2005), dyspnea (Ayers & Lappin, 2004), shortness of breath, use of accessory muscles, and capillary refill longer than 3 seconds.
2. **Assess for hypoxemia:** PaO_2 less than 92% and/or abnormal ABGs; unexplained respiratory alkalosis may be an early sign of sepsis and can progress to metabolic acidosis (Lynch, 2006).
3. Measure dyspnea on a 0 to 10 scale, with 0 being no dyspnea and 10 being severe dyspnea. Measures should be compared from one assessment to the next assessment. Note whether dyspnea occurs at rest and with exertion. The Visual Analogue Scale (Corner et al., 1995) and the numeric rating scale (Gift & Narsavage, 1998) have been validated for use in adults, and the Dalhousie Dyspnea Scale has been validated for use

in children age 8 or older (McGrath et al., 2005). Consider using terms and phrases such as *shortness of breath, tight throat, difficulty breathing, breathlessness,* and *labored breathing* to enhance the patient's understanding of dyspnea.

4. Assess vital signs for hypotension, dyspnea, tachycardia, tachypnea, stridor, chest pain, and fever (for pulmonary infection).

5. Auscultate the lung fields for crackles, adventitious breath sounds, and bilateral inequality; visually assess for decreased or unequal chest expansion and decreased diaphragmatic excursion.

6. Observe for anxiety, restlessness, and change in level of consciousness. Asking the patient to rate his or her anxiety on a 0 to 10 scale (0 meaning "no anxiety" and 10 meaning "the worst anxiety I could ever have") may be useful for assessing anxiety and its severity.

7. Obtain and assess a chest x-ray film (CXR) for obstruction (Fig. 12.1, *A*), pleural effusion, or other abnormalities (Chernecky & Berger, 2004). The lateral view (Fig. 12.1, *B*) can allow a gross estimate of the degree of airway compromise by a mediastinal mass (Guillerman et al., 2005).

8. Obtain and assess a computed tomography (CT) scan and/or endobronchial ultrasound (EBUS) scan (Chernecky & Berger, 2004). CT (Fig. 12.2) is considered the most accurate imaging modality for detecting airway compromise (Guillerman, 2005).

9. **Obtain and assess laboratory test and biopsy results** (Chernecky & Berger, 2004): WBC total and differential to assess for neutropenia; RBCs, hematocrit, and hemoglobin to assess for anemia (Lynch, 2006); electrolytes; lung or other biopsy.

10. Obtain pulmonary function tests and assess for restrictive or obstructive disease. In patients with cancer, this is indicated by decreases in:
    - Total lung capacity (TLC)
    - Diffusion capacity (DLCO)
    - Forced vital capacity (FVC)
    - Forced expiratory volume in 1 second (FEV_1)
    - $FEV_1/FVC\%$
    - Residual volume (RV)
    - Peak expiratory flow (PEF)
    - Forced expiratory reserve (FER)

11. Obtain sputum for culture and sensitivity.

12. **Assess for right-side heart failure/cor pulmonale:** ECG changes (Chernecky et al., 2006), CVP changes, dependent peripheral edema, fatigue, nausea, anorexia, weight gain, hepatomegaly, jugular vein distention (JVD), positive hepatojugular (HJ) reflex, systolic or diastolic murmur, prominent S2, polyuria at night, and ascites.

NURSING CARE AND TREATMENT

1. For airway obstruction, consider preparing the patient for high-dose brachytherapy (Allison et al., 2004), chemotherapy, surgical resection, stenting (Allison et al., 2004), tracheotomy, or intubation; or, in the case of lung cancer, for YAG laser therapy (Venuta et al., 2002). Also prepare the patient for diagnostic tests (e.g., EBUS or CT scanning of the chest) (Herth et al., 2003).

2. For dyspnea, prepare the patient for use of medications (steroids, morphine, bronchodilators, anxiolytic agents), inhalation therapy (metered-dose inhaler, nebulized morphine, furosemide, or fentanyl citrate or IPPB), and oxygen therapy (Chernecky, 2005). Theophyllines have not been shown to be effective in treating dyspnea in patients with lung cancer, as they have in patients with COPD.

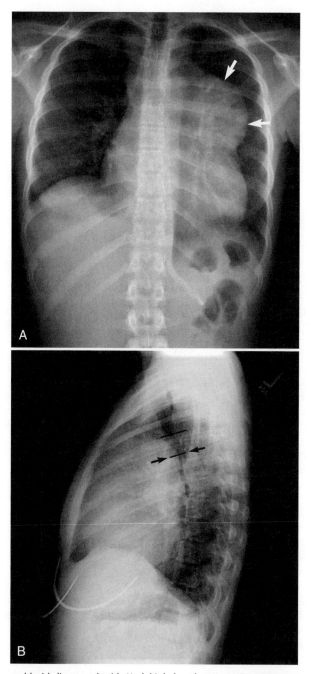

Fig. 12.1 ● A 15-year-old girl diagnosed with Hodgkin's lymphoma. **A,** Anteroposterior chest x-ray film shows a large mediastinal mass (*arrows*). **B,** Lateral chest x-ray film shows compression of the distal trachea (*arrows*) by the mediastinal mass. From Guillerman, R. P., Braverman, R. M., & Parker, B. R. (2006). Imaging studies in the diagnosis and management of pediatric malignancies. In P. A. Pizzo & P. G. Poplack. *Principles and practice of pediatric oncology.* (5th ed.). Philadelphia: Lippinocott Williams & Wilkins.

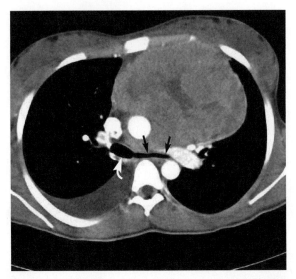

Fig. 12.2 • The same patient as in Fig. 12.1, *A.* The CT image shows marked compression of the left mainstem bronchus *(straight arrow)* compared to the normal-caliber right mainstem bronchus *(curved white arrow).* From Guillerman, R. P., Braverman, R. M., & Parker, B. R. (2006). Imaging studies in the diagnosis and management of pediatric malignancies. In P. A. Pizzo & P. G. Poplack. *Principles and practice of pediatric oncology.* (5th ed.). Philadelphia: Lippinocott Williams & Wilkins.

3. For patients with non-small cell lung cancer, prepare the patient for photodynamic therapy (PDT) to help relieve airway obstruction and dyspnea (Jones et al., 2001).

4. Elevate the head of the bed to high Fowler's position to relieve airway obstruction and dyspnea in patients with tumors that are not interthoracic. For patients with interthoracic tumors, placing the good lung down may increase ventilation. The nurse and patient may need to evaluate various patient positions to maximize air exchange and facilitate mobilization of secretions.

5. Obtain and interpret O_2 saturation values (signs of hypoxia include restlessness, dyspnea, anxiety, and cyanosis).

6. Administer oxygen to treat hypoxia and high-dose corticosteroids (over 100 mg/day or 1 mg/kg) for inflammation. The use of air blowing through the nose has been shown to be effective in reducing dyspnea (Philip et al., 2006).

7. In adults, maintain venous access via a peripheral IV line with an 18-gauge needle or use a venous access device (VAD). For children, use a peripheral venous device that is age appropriate in size.

8. Administer low-dose morphine sulfate and/or an anxiolytic agent for anxiety and dyspnea.

9. Encourage the use of diaphragmatic breathing or pursed-lip breathing, which uses the lips as a mild resistor to prolong exhalation. This increases airway pressure, delaying compression of the airway and minimizing air trapping.

10. Activity: bed rest with bathroom privileges as tolerated; may gradually increase activity, with planned rest periods, as dyspnea resolves.

11. Use relaxation techniques such as imagery or music therapy to reduce anxiety (Gift et al., 1992).

12. Consider whether uncontrolled coughing that leads to dyspnea may be controlled with cough suppressants (dextromethorphan or opioids).

13. Consider whether dyspnea related to anemia may be improved by transfusion of packed red blood cells.

14. Consider the use of antibiotic therapy to treat bacterial pneumonia.
15. Provide referral to clinical nurse specialist, home health nurse, hospice, social worker, and/or respiratory therapist as appropriate.

EVIDENCE-BASED PRACTICE UPDATES

Review of the literature reveals an impressive lack of recent evidence-based reports. In many studies, the term *breathlessness* is used instead of *dyspnea* (Froggatt & Walford, 2005; Johnson & Moore, 2003; Hoyal et al., 2002; Krishnasamy et al., 2001; Bredin et al., 1999; Connolly & O'Neill, 1999; Corner et al., 1996). Breathlessness is presented as a symptom commonly seen in advanced cancer and is described as the subjective sensation of an uncomfortable awareness of breathing or difficulty breathing (Corner et al., 1996). It is seen as a complex symptom involving physical, psychological, emotional, and functional factors (O'Driscoll et al., 1999).

A consensus statement issued by the American Thoracic Society (ATS) in 1999 is a great step forward in defining and understanding the symptom of dyspnea. The statement defines dyspnea as a symptom "generally applied to sensations experienced by individuals who complain of unpleasant or uncomfortable respiratory sensations," and it includes other phrases such as *difficulty breathing, breathlessness, labored breathing, uncomfortable breathing, awareness of breathing distress* and *air hunger* (ATS, 1999). The statement also says that a symptom can be described only by the person experiencing it, and it explains the differences between a respiratory sensation, the neural activation that results from stimulation of a peripheral receptor, and perception (i.e., the reaction of a sentient individual to the sensation).

1. Intervention strategies were implemented by nurses for patients with lung cancer who experienced breathlessness. Interventions included breathing retraining, relaxation techniques, and weekly goal setting. Outcomes were assessed on visual analog scales to rate breathlessness, the functional capacity scale to assess ability to walk distances and climb stairs, and a checklist to determine difficulty with activities of daily living (ADLs). Hospital anxiety and depression scales also were used. Improvements in median scores on all measures were observed in the intervention group, with the exception of depression, compared to the control group in which scores remained the same or worsened (Bredin et al., 1999; Corner et al., 1996).
2. For therapy to be effective, it is important that nurses understand the nature and impact of breathlessness from the perspective of the patient experiencing it (Krishnasamy et al 2001; Bredin et al., 1999; Connolly and O'Neill, 1999; O'Driscoll et al., 1999; Corner et al., 1995).
3. Interventions considered as complementary and alternative medicine have also produced improvement in breathlessness. Acupuncture, acupressure, muscle relaxation, and breathing retraining, combined with coping strategies, have been shown to reduce breathlessness and increase functional capacity, which enhances the quality of life (Pan et al., 2000).

TEACHING AND EDUCATION

Dyspnea: *Rationale:* Oxygen may be necessary to make you less short of breath and help your heart pump easier. You should keep your activity level to a minimum. Also, you may find some relaxation techniques, such as guided imagery or music therapy, to be helpful.

Anxiety: *Rationale:* When you are short of breath, you sometimes feel anxious and restless, which can push you into a cycle of more anxiety and shortness of breath. To break this cycle, try using guided imagery, watching TV or listening to music, or taking medicine, all of which may help.

Pursed-lip breathing: *Rationale:* A simple technique can slow your respiratory rate, prolong exhalation, and increase airway pressures to prevent small airway collapse. Inhale through your nose, then form your lips as if you are going to blow out a candle or blow on a hot liquid to cool it, and then exhale slowly through your mouth.

Diaphragmatic breathing: *Rationale:* This breathing technique helps reduce stress and increase relaxation. Locate your diaphragm by placing your hand on your upper abdomen; then, concentrate on moving your hand with each inhalation, rather than expanding your chest wall. This technique can be combined with pursed-lip breathing for more control.

Tests and procedures: *Rationale:* You may need x-ray films or other types of scans of your chest or head and neck areas. A tube may need to be placed in your mouth or into your midneck to help you breathe easier. This tube may be attached to a machine that helps you breathe better. You may need an intravenous access, so that we can give you medicines and/or chemotherapeutic drugs through your veins, or a venous access device, through which we can administer drugs and also take blood samples.

Tumor treatment: *Rationale:* You may need surgery, radiation therapy, and/or chemotherapy to shrink your cancer or get rid of it.

Web sites for information:
- American Lung Association: www.lungusa.org (telephone: 1-800-LUNGSUSA)
- American Cancer Society: www.cancer.org
- American Thoracic Society: www.thoracic.org
- Oncology Nursing Society: www.ons.org

NURSING DIAGNOSES

1. **Ineffective airway clearance** related to mechanical obstruction
2. **Impaired gas exchange** related to V/Q mismatch, tumor obstruction, tumor infiltration, and/or edema
3. **Ineffective tissue perfusion**, cardiopulmonary, related to compromised blood flow secondary to pulmonary fibrosis, hypoxia, and/or anxiety
4. **Decreased cardiac output** related to increased pulmonary vascular resistance
5. **Activity intolerance** related to dyspnea and/or obstruction

EVALUATION AND DESIRED OUTCOMES

1. Dyspnea and anxiety will be rated less than 3 on a 0 to 10 scale.
2. O_2 saturation will be greater than 92%.
3. No adventitious lung sounds or congestion will be present.
4. ECG and diagnostic findings (e.g., CXR/CT/EBUS) will be within normal limits.
5. The patient's heart rate, respiratory rate, and blood pressure will return to baseline.
6. The patient will have increased functional capability (i.e., ADLs) without dyspnea.

DISCHARGE PLANNING AND FOLLOW-UP CARE

- Home oxygen via tube or mask as prescribed
- Home health nursing visits for assessment of pulmonary and airway status for 1 to 2 months; may involve tracheotomy or ventilator tube care

- Follow-up visit to physician's office 1 to 2 weeks after discharge; discuss pulmonary rehabilitation program as an option
- Follow-up chest x-ray film, PFTs, and/or ABGs every 2 to 3 months for 1 year, then every 6 months or as determined
- Instruct patient to call the health care provider immediately if dyspnea is rated higher than 3 on a 1 to 10 scale and for any airway obstruction, unusual swelling of the hands or feet, weight gain exceeding 3 pounds in 1 week, heart palpitations, chest discomfort, and increased shortness of breath

REVIEW QUESTIONS

QUESTIONS

1. **In a patient with airway obstruction, the priority nursing diagnosis is:**
   1. Activity intolerance
   2. Ineffective tissue perfusion
   3. Decreased cardiac output
   4. Ineffective airway clearance

2. **Knowledge that will increase the patient's control over the dyspnea is:**
   1. Diaphragmatic and pursed-lip breathing
   2. Explanation of a packed red blood cell transfusion
   3. Explanation of the purpose of bronchodilator therapy
   4. Results of the CT scan

3. **A desired outcome in the management of dyspnea is:**
   1. Adventitious breath sounds
   2. Copious, thin, watery secretions
   3. Improved ability to perform ADLs
   4. Tachypnea

4. **Medications used to treat dyspnea in patients with lung cancer include all of the following** *except:*
   1. Bronchodilators
   2. Morphine
   3. Steroids
   4. Theophylline

5. **In assessing a patient with dyspnea, which of the following is** *not* **indicative of hypoxia:**
   1. Anxiety
   2. Dyspnea
   3. Restlessness
   4. Urinary retention

6. **The most accurate diagnostic modality for determining airway obstruction is:**

   1. Bronchoscopy
   2. Chest CT scan
   3. Forced vital capacity
   4. Total lung capacity

7. **In caring for a patient with airway obstruction, an important nursing intervention is to:**
   1. Ambulate frequently, with increasing distance each time
   2. Maintain the temperature in the room over 85° F or 29° C
   3. Position the patient flat in bed
   4. Prepare the patient for intubation or tracheostomy

8. **Discharge teaching for a patient with dyspnea or airway obstruction includes:**
   1. Bed rest with no physical activity
   2. Diet high in sodium
   3. Notify the physician if you rate your dyspnea higher than 3 on a scale of 1 to 10
   4. Return to the physician's office in 6 to 8 weeks

9. **An oncology patient at high risk for airway obstruction is one who has been diagnosed with which type of cancer:**
   1. Gastric
   2. Head and neck
   3. Ovarian
   4. Prostate

10. **To make sure that therapy is effective in patients with breathlessness, the most important thing the nurse can do is:**
    1. Accept the premise that all patients will eventually succumb to respiratory arrest

2. Formulate a plan to be used exactly by each patient
3. Involve family caregivers in the therapy
4. Understand the nature and impact of breathlessness on the individual patient

ANSWERS

1. **Answer: 4**
   Rationale: Airway clearance is always the first priority, because the other problems are related to the lack of oxygen caused by the obstruction. Once the obstruction has been cleared, oxygenation will improve and the other problems will resolve.

2. **Answer: 1**
   Rationale: Breathing techniques, as well as relaxation techniques, which the patient can initiate as needed, can provide a sense of control over the dyspnea.

3. **Answer: 3**
   Rationale: Improved ability to perform ADLs represents a lower oxygen demand for greater activity, whereas the other options reflect a greater oxygen demand.

4. **Answer: 4**
   Rationale: Although effective in patients with COPD, theophylline has not proved effective in treating dyspnea associated with lung cancer.

5. **Answer: 4**
   Rationale: Urinary retention is unrelated to hypoxia, whereas anxiety, dyspnea, and restlessness reflect behavioral and respiratory signs.

6. **Answer: 2**
   Rationale: Forced vital capacity and total lung capacity, which are measured during pulmonary function studies, may be affected by airway obstruction, and bronchoscopy may allow visualization of the obstruction. However, a chest CT scan provides the most accurate and comprehensive information about an airway obstruction.

7. **Answer: 4**
   Rationale: Intubation or tracheostomy may be required to establish a patent airway. Ambulation, a warm room, and a flat position will all increase the oxygen requirement in a compromised patient.

8. **Answer: 3**
   Rationale: If dyspnea progresses to a rating higher than 3, further intervention by the physician may be required. A diet high in sodium will result in fluid retention, and lack of physical activity will decrease conditioning, both of which increase the need for oxygen. The usual return to the physician's office is 1 to 2 weeks after discharge.

9. **Answer: 2**
   Rationale: Head and neck malignancies, especially the nasal, esophageal, laryngeal, tongue, and thyroid types, frequently occur with airway obstruction.

10. **Answer: 4**
    Rationale: In their 1995 study on breathlessness in lung cancer patients, Corner and colleagues demonstrated the importance of understanding the unique effects of breathlessness in each patient.

REFERENCES

Alaani, A., Hogg, R., & Warfield, A. T., et al. (2005). Air bag injury as a cause of inflammatory myofibroblastic pseudotumour of the subglottic larynx progressing to myositis ossificans. *Acta Oto-Laryngologica, 125*(6):674-677.

Allison, R., Sibata, C., & Sarma, K., et al. (2004). High-dose-rate brachytherapy in combination with stenting offers a rapid and statistically significant improvement in quality of life for patients with endobronchial recurrence. *Cancer Journal, 10*(6):368-373.

American Thoracic Society (ATS). (1999). Dyspnea: Mechanisms, assessment, and management—a consensus statement. American Thoracic Society. *American Journal of Respiratory & Critical Care Medicine, 159*(1):321-340.

Ayers, D. M. M., & Lappin, J. (2004). Act fast when your patient has dyspnea. *Nursing, 34*(7):36-41.

Bergbom-Engberg, I., & Haljamae, H. (1989). Assessment of patients' experience of discomforts during respirator therapy. *Critical Care Medicine, 17*(10):1068-1072.

Bredin, M., Corner, J., & Krishnasamy, M., et al. (1999). Multicentre randomized controlled trial of nursing intervention for breathlessness in patients with lung cancer. *British Medical Journal, 318*(7188):901-904.

Byard, R. W., & Gilbert, J. D. (2005). Narcotic administration and stenosing lesions of the upper airway: A potentially lethal combination. *Journal of Clinical Forensic Medicine, 12*(1):29-31.

Carta, P., Aru, G., & Manca, P. (2001). Mortality from lung cancer among silicotic patients in Sardinia: An update study with 10 more years of follow up. *Occupational & Environmental Medicine, 58*(12):786-793.

Chan, K. P., Eng, P., & Hsu, A. A., et al. (2002). Rigid bronchoscopy and stenting for esophageal cancer causing airway obstruction. *Chest, 122*(3):1069-1072.

Chen, S. H., Hsu, J. C., & Chen, C. H., et al. (2005). Airway obstruction by a metastatic mediastinal tumor during anesthesia. *Chang Gung Medical Journal, 28*(4):258-263.

Chernecky, C. (2004). Respiratory/dyspnea. In C. G. Varricchio, T. B. Ades, P. S. Hinds, & M. Pierce (Eds.), *A cancer source book for nurses.* (8th ed.). (pp. 407-414). Atlanta, GA: American Cancer Society.

Chernecky, C., & Berger, B. (2004). *Laboratory tests and diagnostic procedures.* Philadelphia: W.B. Saunders.

Chernecky, C., Garrett, K., & Hodges, B., et al. (2006). *ECGs and the heart.* (2nd ed.). St. Louis: Mosby.

Chernecky, C., & Sarna, L. (2000). Pulmonary toxicities of cancer therapy. *Critical Care Nursing Clinics of North America, 12*(3):281-295.

Chernecky, C., & Shelton, B. (2001). Pulmonary complications in patients with cancer. *American Journal of Nursing, 101*(5):24A-24H.

Choo, S. P., Lim, D. W., & Lo, C. P., et al. (2005). Variable problems in lymphomas: CASE 1. Burkitt's lymphoma presenting with central airway obstruction. *Journal of Clinical Oncology, 23*(31):8112-8113.

Connolly, M., & O'Neill, J. (1999). Teaching a research-based approach to the management of breathless-ness in patients with lung cancer. *European Journal of Cancer Care, 8*(1):30-36.

Corner, J., Plant, H., & A'Hein, R., et al. (1996). Nonpharmacological intervention for breathlessness in lung cancer. *Palliative Medicine, 10*(4):299-305.

Corner, J., Plant, H., & Warner, L. (1995). Developing a nursing approach to managing dyspnea in lung cancer. *Industrial Journal of Palliative Nursing, 1*(1):5-10.

Dudgeon, D. J., Kristjanson, L., & Sloan, J. A., et al. (2001). Dyspnea in cancer patients: Prevalence and associated factors. *Journal of Pain and Symptom Management, 21*(2):95-102.

Esper, P., & Heidrich, D. (2005). Symptom clusters in advanced illness. *Seminars in Oncology Nursing, 21*(1):20-28.

Froggatt, C., & Walford, C. (2005). Developing advanced clinical skills in the management of breathlessness: Evaluation of an educational intervention. *European Journal of Cancer Care, 8*(1):37-43.

Gift, A. G., Moore, T., & Soeken, K. (1992). Relaxation to reduce dyspnea and anxiety in COPD patients. *Nursing Research, 41*(4):242-246.

Gift, A. G., & Narsavage, G. (1998). Validity of the numeric rating scale as a measure of dyspnea. *American Journal of Critical Care, 7*(3):200-204.

Guillerman, R. P., Braverman, R. M., & Parker, B. R. (2005). Imaging studies in the diagnosis and manage-ment of pediatric malignancies. In P. A. Pizzo, & D. G. Poplack (Eds.), *Principles and practice of pediatric oncology.* (5th ed.). (pp. 205-236). Philadelphia: Lippincott, Williams & Wilkins.

Haben, C. M., Chagnon, F. P., & Zakhary, K. (2005). Laryngeal manifestation of autoimmune disease: Rheumatoid arthritis mimicking a cartilaginous neoplasm. *Journal of Otolaryngology, 34*(3):203-206.

Herth, F., Ernst, A., & Schulz, M., et al. (2003). Endobronchial ultrasound reliably differentiates between airway infiltration and compression by tumor. *Chest, 123*(2):458-462.

Howard, S. C., Ribeiro, R. C., & Pui, C. H. (2006). Acute complications. In C. H. Pui, (Ed.), *Childhood leukemias.* (2nd ed.). (pp. 719-720). New York: Cambridge University Press.

Hoyal, C., Grant, J., & Chamberlain, F., et al. (2002). Improving the management of breathlessness using a clinical effectiveness program. *International Journal of Palliative Nursing, 8*(2):78-87.

Johnson, M., & Moore, S. (2003). Research into practice: The reality of implementing a non-pharmacolo-gical breathlessness intervention into clinical practice. *European Journal of Oncology Nursing, 7*(1):33-38.

Jones, B. U., Helmy, M., & Brenner, M., et al. (2001). Photodynamic therapy for patients with advanced non-small-cell carcinoma of the lung. *Clinical Lung Cancer, 3*(1):37-41.

Kane, J. R., & Himelstein, B. P. (2002). Palliative care in pediatrics. In A. M. Berger, R. K. Portenoy, & D. E. Weissman (Eds.), *Principles and practice of palliative care and supportive oncology.* (2nd ed.). (pp. 1044-1061). Philadelphia: Lippincott, Williams & Wilkins.

Krishnasamy, M., Corner, J., & Bredin, M., et al. (2001). Cancer nursing practice development: Understanding breathlessness. *Journal of Clinical Nursing, 10*(1):103-108.

Le, B. H., & Rosenthal, M. A. (2005). Small cell lung cancer with tracheal obstruction. *Internal Medicine Journal, 35*(8):490.

Lynch, M. P. (2006). Dyspnea. *Clinical Journal of Oncology Nursing, 10*(3):323-326.

McCorkle, R., Benoliel, J., & Donaldson, G., et al. (1989). A randomized clinical trial of home nursing care for lung cancer patients. *Cancer, 64*(6):1375-1382.

McGrath, P. J., Pianosi, P. T., & Unruh, A. M., et al. (2005). Dalhousie dyspnea scales: Construct and content validity of pictorial scales for measuring dyspnea. *BMC Pediatrics, 33*(5):33.

Merha, P. K., & Woessner, K. M. (2005). Dyspnea, wheezing, and airway obstruction: Is it asthma?. *Allergy & Asthma Proceedings, 26*(4):319-322.

Moore, S., Corner, J., & Haviland, J., et al. (2002). Nurse led follow up and conventional medical follow up of patients with lung cancer: Randomized trial. *British Medical Journal, 325*(7373):1145-1151.

O'Driscoll, M., Corner, J., & Barley, C. (1999). The experience of breathlessness in lung cancer. *European Journal of Cancer Care, 8*(1):37-43.

Pan, C. X., Morrison, R. S., & Ness, J., et al. (2000). Complementary and alternative medicine in the management of pain, dyspnea, and nausea and vomiting near the end of life: A systematic review. *Journal of Pain & Symptom Management, 20*(5):374-387.

Pavuk, M., Michalek, J. E., & Schecter, A., et al. (2005). Did TCDD exposure or service in Southeast Asia increase the risk of cancer in Air Force Vietnam veterans who did not spray Agent Orange?. *Journal of Occupational & Environmental Medicine, 47*(4):335-342.

Philip, J., Gold, M., & Milner, A., et al. (2006). A randomized, double-blind, crossover trial of the effect of oxygen on dyspnea in patients with advanced cancer. *Journal of Pain & Symptom Management, 32*(6):541-550.

Sarna, L. (1998). Effectiveness of structured nursing assessment of symptom distress in advanced lung cancer. *Oncology Nursing Forum, 25*(6):1041-1048.

See, C. Q., & Olopade, C. O. (2005). An unusual cause of stridor and progressive shortness of breath. *Chest, 128*(3):1874-1877.

Shah, S. S., Lai, S. Y., & Ruchelli, E., et al. (2001). Retropharyngeal aberrant thymus. *Pediatrics, 108*(5):E94.

Shohat, I., Berkowicz, M., & Dori, S., et al. (2004). Primary non-Hodgkin's lymphoma of the sinonasal tract. *Oral Surgery, Oral Medicine, Oral Pathology. Oral Radiology, and Endodontics, 97*(3):328-331.

Skoulas, I. G., & Kountakis, S. E. (2003). Endotracheal tube obstruction: A rare complication of laser ablation of recurrent laryngeal papillomas. *Ear, Nose, & Throat Journal, 82*(7):504-506.

Tao, Z. Z., Chen, S. M., & Liu, J. F., et al. (2005). Paranasal sinuses chordoma in a pediatric patient: A case report and literature review. *International Journal of Pediatric Otorhinolaryngology, 69*(10):1415-1418.

Tasci, S., Kovacs, A., & Leutner, C., et al. (2005). Patients with malignancy requiring urgent therapy: CASE 1. Central airway obstruction as first presentation of ovarian cancer. *Journal of Clinical Oncology, 23*(27):6791-6793.

Torres-Carranza, E., Garcia-Perla, A., & Infante-Cossio, P., et al. (2006). Airway obstruction due to metastatic renal cell carcinoma of the tongue. Oral Surgery, Oral Medicine, Oral Pathology. *Oral Radiology, and Endodontics, 101*(3):e76-e78.

Venuta, F., Rendina, E. A., & De Giacomo, T., et al. (2002). Nd:YAG laser reduction of lung cancer invading the airway as a bridge to surgery and palliative care. *Annals of Thoracic Surgery, 74*(4):995-998.

Wickham, R. (2002). Dyspnea: Recognizing and managing an invisible problem. *Oncology Nursing Forum,* Online. *29*(6):925-934.

END-OF-LIFE CARE

CYNTHIA BROWN • KATHLEEN MURPHY-ENDE

PATHOPHYSIOLOGICAL MECHANISMS

The dying process is a complex physiologic response to end-stage illness. It is characterized by symptoms that require intensive interventions to ensure comfort for the patient and a sense of well-being for the caregiver. Death can happen suddenly, but in malignant conditions, the dying process often begins several months before death occurs. Symptoms such as decreased activity, anorexia, pain, drowsiness, anxiety, depression, shortness of breath, constipation, and weakness may occur simultaneously (Potter et al., 2003; Bruera & Neumann, 1999). As death nears, signs and symptoms include fever, purple-blue discoloration and coolness of the distal extremities, anorexia, dysphagia, constipation, mental status changes, irregular breathing patterns, congestion, cough, inability to clear secretions, a decrease in urine output, and incontinence.

Fever is a result of a rise in the body's set-point temperature, which is regulated by the preoptic region of the anterior hypothalamus. The set point can be raised by a number of factors, including the release of pyrogens produced by infectious agents or the immune system, tumor infiltration of the thermoregulatory area of the brain, obstructive tumors of the gastrointestinal (GI) or genitourinary (GU) tract, adrenal carcinomas, necrotic tumors, leukemia, multiple myeloma, Ewing's sarcoma, lymphoma, and inflammatory processes. Antipyretics (e.g., acetaminophen) can bring down the set point to a lower or normal body temperature (Rhiner & Slatkin, 2001).

Cardiac output decreases, causing mottling and coolness of the extremities, tachycardia, and hypotension. Renal failure occurs when the diminishing cardiac output reduces the circulation through the kidneys, resulting in decreased urine output (Matzo, 2001).

Changes in the GI system begin with changes in taste and a loss of appetite. Liver involvement, ascites, and tumor obstruction cause nausea and vomiting. Immobility, a decreased intake of fiber and fluids, decreased colonic peristalsis, and tumor compression result in constipation or obstruction.

Neurologic changes range from mild confusion to delirium or severe agitation. Underlying causes include the accumulation of toxins from renal or liver failure, hepatic encephalopathy, acidosis, metabolic and electrolyte imbalances, medication effects, hypoxia, sleep deprivation, sepsis, and even bowel obstruction. Patients may acknowledge people or spirits in the room that are apparent to no one else, or they may talk to or about those who have already died. This is a phenomenon of nearing death awareness that many nurses have observed and documented, and it is not necessarily confusion or delirium. The level of consciousness may decline to an unresponsive state.

Pulmonary changes include inability to clear secretions from the throat, periods of apnea that become longer and, in the final stages, breathing with mandibular movement during the last few hours. These changes arise from decreased blood perfusion to the brainstem, which slows the impulses from the respiratory centers in the brain (Brasher, 2002).

Decreased urine output may occur as a result of dehydration or renal failure. Incontinence may occur as sphincter control is lost or because the patient is unable to communicate personal needs.

EPIDEMIOLOGY AND ETIOLOGY

In 2005 there were 578,280 cancer deaths in the United States (American Cancer Society, 2005). A recent study found that the mortality rate among patients with cancer admitted to the ICU is 45.7% (Thiery et al., 2005), and the mortality rate for patients with cancer who are mechanically ventilated is 60% to 70% (Azoulay et al., 2001). Patients who undergo bone marrow transplantation and who require mechanical ventilation in an ICU have an 80% mortality rate (Bach et al., 2001). Initiation of the do not resuscitate (DNR) order served as a decision point in limiting treatment, such as withholding or withdrawing life-supporting interventions; this resulted in the death or discharge of 98% of ICU patients with cancer (Smedira et al., 1990).

RISK PROFILE

Death in the ICU

Lack of or disregard for an advance directive. The SUPPORT (1995) study involved 960 people who had requested no resuscitation. The study found that the DNR order was implemented for only half of these patients, and one third of the patients died while hospitalized.

Allogeneic bone marrow transplantation (BMT) with relapsed or recurrent cancer and poor performance status as a result of the cancer or the cancer treatment side effects (Groeger et al., 1998) and readmission soon after BMT (Karamlou et al., 2003).

Lack of clarification of end-of-life goals (Field & Cassell, 1997).

Poor functional status, high tumor burden, and presence of co-morbidities (Karamlou et al., 2003).

Patients with disseminated intravascular coagulation and those requiring vasopressors are more likely to die. Prolonged mechanical ventilation and ventilation for longer than 24 hours after admission increases the risk of death (Groeger et al., 1999). Mechanical ventilation with multiorgan failure also is a poor prognostic indicator (Bach et al., 2001).

PROGNOSIS

The prognosis for patients with advanced cancer is based on syndrome manifestations, especially physical dependence, anorexia-cachexia, and lymphopenia (Glare & Christakis, 2004). Clinical variables predictive of survival include performance status, anorexia, cognitive failure, dyspnea, dry mouth, weight loss, and dysphagia (Vigano et al., 2000). Prognostication by the physician or nurse practitioner is helpful in providing the patient and family with information so that they can set goals and priorities, as well as develop coping mechanisms for dealing with loss and grief. Prognostic guidelines may provide the impetus for decision making; may open up communication among the patient, the family, and health care providers; and may establish the need for referrals to end of life resources (Glare & Christakis, 2004). Cultural, sociologic, religious, and spiritual variables affect the patient's and family's willingness to discuss the prognosis, as well as the nurse's comfort level in predicting death. These factors influence the type of information patients and families are willing to accept or believe, and also what the nurse is willing to discuss with them.

PROFESSIONAL ASSESSMENT CRITERIA (PAC)

1. Comprehensive nursing assessment includes evaluating the physical, psychological, spiritual, emotional, and social elements of the patient and family.
2. The patient's and family's goals of care must be determined.
3. Diagnostic testing is obtained if the information is needed to help with symptom management or the prognosis.

NURSING CARE AND TREATMENT

1. **Provide guidance and counseling in the decision-making process.** The legal basis for decision making includes knowledge of the provisions of the Patient Self-Determination Act (PSDA), which went into effect in December, 1991. This federal law requires all facilities that receive either Medicare or Medicaid funding to inform the patient that the person has the right to accept or refuse any treatment or medical care. Also, the facility is required to recognize advance directives. A health care proxy (power of attorney for health care) may be appointed to substitute judgment in the event the patient is unable to express his or her wishes about health care decisions or if the patient lacks decision-making capacity. Naming a power of attorney for health care decisions allows for decision making under changing circumstances. A *living will* is a form of advance directive that states the patient's wishes; it is a legal document, but it does not appoint a power of attorney for health care. Most living wills are requests that curatively oriented treatments not be initiated or, if initiated, are stopped once the person is considered to have a terminal condition or to be in a persistent vegetative state (Project Grace, 2006; AHRQ, 2001). Living wills may also call for measures to prolong life. The accepted format for advance-directive documents varies from state to state. If a health care proxy has not been appointed, some states give the next of kin the authority to make decisions. The PSDA is legally grounded in the right to privacy and the right of a competent person to make decisions about treatments. The concept of *autonomy* is the underpinning of this law, which reflects the dominant value system of the United States. However, autonomy may not be as valued in other cultures (Douglas, 2001). Advanced practice oncology nurses follow the ethical code as interpreted by the American Nurses Association (2001), which regards autonomy as an important element of patient care.
2. **Provide aggressive pain management (see Chapter 36).**
3. **Manage nausea and vomiting.** These symptoms may be caused by medications, abdominal or brain tumors, anxiety, gastritis, bowel obstruction, constipation, hypercalcemia, hypokalemia, hypernatremia or hyponatremia, dehydration, uremia, or infection. Treat the underlying cause if known; for example, stop using irritating medications or *switch* to a less irritating form. Use dexamethasone for increased intracranial pressure caused by brain tumors, benzodiazepines for anxiety, and H_2 blockers for gastritis. If the etiology is not known, prochlorperazine can be started at a dosage of 25 mg given rectally every 12 hours. Nonpharmacologic interventions include eliminating offending foods and odors and alterations in the diet until symptoms resolve (Murphy-Ende, 2006a).

4. **Manage dysphagia**. Difficulty swallowing may be caused by candidiasis, infection, compression of the esophagus by tumor, esophageal erosion, brain metastasis, or proximal muscle weakness. Candidiasis infections should be treated with antifungal medications (e.g., nystatin). Radiation treatment may be used to shrink tumors, and steroids may be given to reduce swelling. Soft foods or liquids may be more tolerable; however, if the patient is not hungry, forcing the issue of eating may cause distress. Tube feeding may or may not be indicated, depending on the individual patient's prognosis and goals of care.

5. **Manage xerostomia**. Thirst is the conscious desire for water, which may be accompanied by dry lips, dry mouth, and polydipsia. However, thirst is not a reflection of fluid status (Murphy-Ende, 2006b). Anticholinergic drugs, the effects of radiation, and oral tumors may create a dry mouth. Treatment should be directed at the underlying cause of thirst; however, if thirst is due to side effects of pain medications, the medications need to be continued. Liquids can be given as ice chips, through the end of a straw, or with an eye dropper or a small syringe. Oral care with a moist swab should be provided frequently, and family members can be taught to perform this task. If oral candidiasis is present, treatment with nystatin oral solution (as either a swish-and-swallow or a troche) may provide relief. Hard candy or gum (preferably sugar free) can be helpful. Pilocarpine may be used when the salivary glands are no longer functioning, as in the case of radiation damage (Murphy-Ende, 2006c).

6. **Anticipate and manage constipation**. Constipation is a predictable side effect of opioids, dehydration, and immobility, and it must be managed aggressively. When opioids are started, a stimulant (e.g., senna) should be started along with a stool softener (e.g., docusate sodium). The dose of senna and bisacodyl is titrated to produce a comfortable bowel movement at least every 3 days. Milk of Magnesia (30 mL) may be added if no bowel movement occurs within 72 hours. A bisacodyl suppository may be administered daily as needed. Enemas may also be helpful but can be uncomfortable for the patient. If the patient is impacted, use an oil-retention enema and allow it to be absorbed before disimpaction.

7. **Manage diarrhea**. Diarrhea may lead to dehydration and electrolyte imbalance and may compromise the integrity of the skin, causing pain, excoriation, and fungal growth. Before administering an antidiarrheal agent, rule out impaction and infectious diarrhea. For noninfectious diarrhea, administer loperamide (Imodium) 2 mg tab (liquid, 1 mg/5 mL) by mouth. The dose is 4 mg after the initial acute episode of diarrhea, then 2 mg after each unformed stool, up to a maximum of 16 mg/day. If loperamide is ineffective, start diphenoxylate hydrochloride with atropine sulfate (Lomotil); the initial dose is 15-20 mg/day by mouth in three or four divided doses, then 5-15 mg/day in two or three divided doses (Hodgson & Kizior, 2007). Skin care includes washing after each episode, followed by application of a petroleum-based, zinc oxide–based, or dimethicone-based ointment.

8. **Manage dyspnea**. Dyspnea is the uncomfortable awareness of breathlessness, which can be minimized with pharmacologic and nonpharmacologic interventions. Treating the underlying etiology, when possible, is the first line of treatment. Oxygen, blood transfusions, radiation or chemotherapy, and thoracentesis may be indicated if these interventions will treat the underlying problem rapidly enough. Nonpharmacologic treatments include breathing techniques used for COPD, fans, an open door or window, cool room temperature, and positioning the patient upright, with frequent repositioning as tolerated. Explain the etiology and reassure the patient that treatment to alleviate breathlessness is a priority. Medications to consider include morphine sulfate, bronchodilators, corticosteroids, anxiolytics, diuretics, and anticholinergics. Fluid overload or edema may contribute to dyspnea and must be monitored and

treated. Airway congestion, referred to as the "death rattle," is emotionally disturbing for the family. The congestion may be loud, requiring support and education of the family to emphasize that the patient is not "drowning." Atropine drops, tabs, or patches may be used to dry secretions and minimize audible breathing, and gentle oral suctioning (not deep suctioning) can be done to remove excess secretions (Dudgeon, 2001). (See Chapter 12).

9. **Manage cough.** The cough may be dry or productive, and the patient may or may not be able to expectorate the sputum. Patients nearing the end of life may have difficulty clearing the airway because of weakness. Identifying and treating the cause of the cough, when possible, is helpful. For infections, antibiotics should be considered. Antitussives (e.g., codeine and other opioids) help suppress the cough. Expectorants help bring up secretions. Anticholinergics (e.g., atropine) are used to dry secretions. Diuretics are used if heart failure is contributing to the symptoms of cough. Nonpharmacologic approaches include humidifying air/oxygen, suctioning, repositioning, limiting talking, and using a word board if talking initiates coughing spells.

10. **Manage pruritus and rash.** These conditions can have either an endogenous or an exogenous etiology. Endogenous causes (e.g., malignancy, endocrine abnormalities, dermatitis, infection, renal failure, and hepatic dysfunction) should be identified and treated if possible. Medication-induced pruritus should be assessed and the medications discontinued. In patients with advanced cancer, opioids may be a causative factor, therefore opioids should be rotated or an antihistamine (e.g., diphenhydramine) should be added. Steroids can be used orally, parenterally, or topically to manage pruritus (Rhiner & Slatkin, 2001). Dry skin can be treated with mild soap and lotions that contain oil or aloe. Cool compresses over the affected sites may offer temporary relief. Rashes should be noted, documented, diagnosed, and treated. Treatment of rash and pruritus is directed at providing symptomatic relief and eliminating causative factors. Follow-up evaluation is necessary to evaluate the effectiveness of treatment and continued symptom management (Murphy-Ende, 2006d).

11. **Manage fever.** Consistency in either treating or not treating fever is important so that the patient's set-point temperature is not rising and falling, causing chills and shaking. Acetaminophen can be used either orally or rectally. NSAIDs can also be used either solely or alternately with the acetaminophen. Nonpharmacologic measures include using a cool cloth or tepid bath and light clothing or covers. It is important for families to understand that the elevated temperature may be a natural part of the dying process and that it is not necessarily caused by an infection.

12. **Manage delirium.** Delirium is an acute confusional state. The etiology may be brain involvement, paraneoplastic syndrome, encephalopathy (metabolic, anoxic, or septic), electrolyte imbalance, or toxic metabolites of drugs. When the etiology of acute delirium can be determined, the underlying cause is treated. Delirium of unknown cause can be treated with haloperidol. Diphenhydramine can be used to prevent extrapyramidal reactions to haloperidol and to provide sedation. Treatment focuses on symptom control, family teaching, and support (NCCN, 2005). (For detailed information on delirium, see Chapter 7.)

13. **Manage agitation.** Agitation can lead to injury of the patient or health care worker. Therefore a quiet environment must be created, and the patient must be positioned within full view of the staff. All invasive lines, catheters, and devices should be triaged and removed if possible to prevent harm to the patient if self-removal is an issue. Dying patients should not be restrained; no lines or medical devices are important enough at this stage to warrant protection by restraining the patient. Medications can be helpful (e.g., haloperidol 5-10 mg given PO, SQ, IV, or IM and repeated after 30 minutes). A benzodiazepine (e.g., Ativan 1-2 mg) can be given for added effect.

A sitter should be requested to protect the patient from self-harm (Wrede-Seaman, 1999). (For detailed information, see Chapter 7.)

14. **Manage confusion**. Confusion is common in the elderly, especially in a setting other than their usual environment. Other causes include drugs, impaction, a full bladder, pain, brain metastasis, cerebrovascular accident, metabolic imbalances, hypoglycemia, infection, withdrawal from alcohol or benzodiazepines, fear, and anxiety. Treat the underlying cause when possible. Reorient the patient and provide a calm, quiet environment that is well-lit during the day. Maintain continuity of caregivers and routine (see Chapter 7).

15. **Manage anxiety and depression**. Determine whether the patient has a past history of anxiety or depression, and if so, how it was treated. Other issues that may contribute to signs and symptoms of anxiety and depression include fear of dying, hypoxia, dyspnea, and psychological distress, which is closely related to spiritual distress and depression. Managing symptoms such as dyspnea can reduce anxiety. (For detailed information, see Chapter 8.)

16. **Manage spiritual distress**. The spiritual needs of the patient are incorporated into nursing care as a way to assist the dying person and family in finding meaning and resolution through exploration of life experiences or inner connection to a higher reality through a spiritual belief system. Taking time to actively listen to the patient's interpretation of life's purpose, struggles, fears, hopes, and relationships can help the individual find meaning in his or her death. Facilitating a life review through pictures or stories is one way to help the dying person discover meaning. Reconciliation of relationships, forgiveness of self and others, and completion of tasks become part of the closure of life. The care team should include nondenominational clergy, who can address spiritual issues and help the dying person access spiritual care from the community.

17. **Provide the patient and family with psychological support and counseling**. The nurse's interpersonal skills, clinical knowledge, and comfort with death will facilitate family and patient discussions about end of life choices (AHRQ, 2001). Educate the patient and family about the end of life process, such as lack of appetite, fatigue, respiratory congestion, and mental status changes, and provide anticipatory guidance on the symptoms of organ failure. Families may find the physical changes in the patient very difficult to accept, therefore the teaching may need to be repeated before the family begins to accept these changes. An important task in the process of acceptance is for family members to tell their story several times and to different people. Model for the family the care of the dying by speaking to the patient with the assumption that the patient can hear at all times. Maintain the patient's "voice" and autonomy in the dying process by eliciting the patient's values and preferences and advocating for the patient. The patient may be too weak to do this and needs the advocacy skills of the nurse (Smith et al., 2002). The assessment of end of life goals is a dynamic process that should be revisited as the patient's condition changes. It is important to emphasize to the family and patient that withdrawal of technology does not mean withdrawal of care. When patients experience nearing death awareness, the nurse's role is to provide education and support to the family and to help decipher the metaphors the dying person is communicating (Callanan & Kelley, 1992).

EVIDENCE-BASED PRACTICE UPDATES

1. Despite the media focus on living wills and end of life choices, the Pew Research Group (2006) noted that although 95% of the participants in their study knew about living wills, only 29% actually had a living will that stated their end of life preferences.

2. A qualitative study that assessed the perceptions of bereaved family members about the end-of-life care their deceased relatives received found a positive correlation between effective communication with nurses, physicians, and multidisciplinary health care providers about end of life and satisfaction with the care the relative received (Royak-Schaler et al., 2006).

3. In a study of adult critical care admissions to a large tertiary care center over an 8-month period, 334 deaths were recorded from 4882 CCU admissions (a mortality rate of 6.8%). The investigators found that at the time of death in the CCU, life support had been withdrawn in 42% of patients; 39% received full support; 8% were declared brain dead; and 37% had experienced unsuccessful attempts at resuscitation. When support was withdrawn, 57% died in less than 1 hour; 42% died within 1 to 24 hours; and 1% died after 24 hours (Lindgren et al., 2006). The investigators concluded that knowledge of the patient's wishes and documentation of those wishes in the form of an advance directive could prevent transfers to the CCU or, once the patient was in the CCU, could facilitate the direction of care to avoid unwanted medical interventions. Therefore early discussion of the patient's wishes is an important role of the health care team, and most important, of the nurse practitioner.

4. An investigation into how patients process their values and make decisions through story telling confirmed the importance of listening as a means to help patients become partners in their own health care. Active listening allows the health care provider to support the patient in decision making (Young & Rodriguez, 2006).

5. In an analysis of 58 studies, Gomes and Higginson (2006) found that the factors that predicted the likelihood of death occurring at home included the availability of regional health care services able to support a home death, the ability of families to care for a patient, and the patient's personal preference to die at home.

TEACHING AND EDUCATION

1. Dying is a multidimensional process. It encompasses physical symptoms; relationships with oneself, others, and God; hope; and a sense of independence and meaning in the face of illness (McMillan & Weitzner, 1998). The physical, social, emotional, and spiritual domains influence each other.

2. Tests and procedures are limited to those that will provide information that can be used to plan comfort measures. The focus of care is on comfort, and testing may be uncomfortable or unnecessary.

3. The patient may experience nearing death awareness, as described by Callanan and Kelley (1992). This is a phenomenon in which the patient begins speaking to people who have died and also speaks metaphorically of taking a trip or going somewhere. During this time the patient may meticulously pick at the air or at the sheets with a pincer reflex.

4. Consider hospice services. Hospices provide bereavement services to survivors regardless of whether the deceased was admitted into hospice services. Hospices also are helpful for educating the patient and family before the patient is admitted into hospice. This allows the patient and family to make informed decisions about the services they do and do not want.

5. **Web sites for information:**
   - National Hospice and Palliative Care Organization (provides information regarding end of life research and patient information regarding hospice care): www.nhpco.org
   - American Academy of Hospice and Palliative Medicine (provides conferences and tools to assist health care team members in providing end of life care): http://www.aahpm.org/resources/

- American Cancer Society (provides the results of cancer research, statistics, and educational resources for patients, caregivers, and health care providers): http://www.cancer.org
- Center to Advance Palliative Care: http://www.capc.org
- Hospice and Palliative Nurses Association (provides support to hospice and palliative care nurses through educational opportunities and nursing research): http://www.hpna.org
- End of Life/Palliative Education Resource Center (EPERC) (provides educational resources for end of life care): http://www.eperc.mcw.edu
- Growthhouse (an information clearinghouse for end of life care): http://www.growthhouse.org
- Epidemiology of Dying and End of Life Experience: http://www.edeledata.org
- Project Grace (provides a glossary of terms related to end of life decision making, as well as guidelines and a template for advance directives): http://www.pgrace.org
- From Aging with Dignity (provides practical information, advice, and the legal tools needed to construct a very detailed advance directive): http://www.fivewishes.org

NURSING DIAGNOSES

1. **Decisional conflict** related to uncertainty about choices and delayed decision making (e.g., do not resuscitate orders, withdrawing or starting mechanical ventilation, dialysis, and artificial nutrition and hydration)
2. **Spiritual distress** related to fear of death, grief, and conflict in relationship with God (however the person defines God), belief system, and others
3. **Hopelessness** related to terminal illness and lack of time to complete life tasks
4. **Chronic pain** related to patient/family misconceptions about the use of pain medications and professional/system obstacles to pain management
5. **Grieving** related to terminal illness

EVALUATION AND DESIRED OUTCOMES

1. The patient and family will be able to verbalize their values, choose among different options while noting how each choice reflects the family's and the individual's value system, and make a decision that they believe to be the best one possible, even when none of the available choices can be considered good.
2. The patient will be able to express spiritual beliefs and rituals, accessing spiritual resources.
3. The patient will resolve outstanding gaps in communication and resolve conflicts or issues with others.
4. The patient will reframe goals and identify specific activities that can be accomplished in the time remaining. Hope may be focused on time with family, a comfortable death, and hopes that are in the immediate future. The hope for life after death may also be verbalized (Herth, 1993).
5. The patient will state that his or her pain is at or below an acceptable level, as established by the patient. If the patient is unable to communicate, minimal or no nonverbal indicators of pain will be seen, and family caregivers will indicate that comfort has been obtained.
6. The patient will express his or her grief to the clinician and significant others and discuss a future in which the patient is no longer alive.

DISCHARGE PLANNING AND FOLLOW-UP CARE

- Arrange for hospice services (hospice inpatient unit or hospital-based, freestanding, or home hospice care). Hospice services are provided through an interdisciplinary team consisting of a physician, nurse, home health aide, social worker, and chaplain, who work to support the end of life goals of the patient and family.
- Provide information on caregiver support, respite care, and resources and education on care giving roles and issues.
- Arrange for medical equipment (e.g., hospital bed, oxygen, commode, shower chair, and wheelchair).
- Arrange for medications for symptom management. Hospice may prearrange delivery; if not, medications for symptom management should be in the home before the patient arrives. Provide a complete list of medications, their purpose, dosage, route, frequency, and side effects.
- Provide a list of people to contact and things to do near or after the patient's death.
- Send a follow-up letter or make a phone call to the family after the patient's death. Provide a referral to after-death bereavement counseling services as appropriate.

REVIEW QUESTIONS

QUESTIONS

1. Mr. Long is in the ICU with his family around him. He has no less than five family members around his bed. For a week the ICU staff has instructed the family to hold Mr. Long's arms and legs down. He is also restrained to protect the respiratory trumpet in his right nostril and the feeding tube in his left nostril. The family has found Mr. Long's living will, which states that he does not want a feeding tube. Although the living will was brought in 2 days ago and the physician has seen the document, the feeding tube has not been removed. The family has requested that the hospital administration intervene on behalf of Mr. Long. The legal precedence that supports Mr. Long's living will is:
   1. The Patient Self-Determination Act (PSDA)
   2. Hospital policy
   3. There is no legal precedence; the patient does not have any choices.
   4. Both a and b

2. Hospice home care is planned for Mr. Long, and his tube feeding is discontinued. The palliative care nurse practitioner is planning for Mr. Long to arrive home tonight. Mr. Long is still restrained and continues to have his limbs held down by his family members at his bedside. The nurse practitioner notes that Mr. Long is moaning and furrowing his eyebrows as he attempts to pull his arms up. The NP orders the following medications to be available before the patient arrives home:
   1. Liquid morphine for pain and lorazepam for agitation
   2. A bed equipped with similar restraints
   3. Continuous care to monitor the patient in the hospital
   4. Both a and c

3. Mr. Long arrives home, and his hospice nurse is there to admit him to the program. Upon his arrival in the home, she begins to medicate him for pain and anxiety. As the paramedics transfer the patient to the hospice bed, they unfasten his restraints and prepare to fasten them to his hospice bed. The hospice nurse:
   1. Does not stop the paramedics; the patient is dying and needs to be protected from hurting himself
   2. Stops the paramedics and unfastens the restraints from the patient's wrists and ankles, telling

the paramedics that appropriate management of the patient's symptoms will enable the patient to be free of restraints

3. Asks the family whether they would like the patient restrained

4. Directs the paramedics to return this out-of-control patient to the emergency department

4. **Mr. Long is medicated appropriately for pain and anxiety. He begins to breathe easier and relax. When he sees his family around his bed, he begins to raise his arms. The family reacts by holding down his arms, as they were instructed to do in the hospital. The hospice nurse:**

1. Assists the family while she ties the restraints to the patient

2. Asks the family to allow the patient to move freely and assists the patient

3. Instructs the family to have more family members around the bed if they do not want the patient restrained

4. Administers haloperidol 5 mg orally to treat delirium

5. **Finally, after a week of being confined to bed, Mr. Long is able sit up and hugs each person around his bed. He then looks up and says, "Hello, George!" The family knows that Mr. Long's brother, George, died years ago. The family looks to the hospice nurse for guidance. The hospice nurse:**

1. Administers haloperidol 0.5 mg orally

2. Asks the family whether Mr. Long has a history of psychotic episodes

3. Teaches the family that this is a normal event in the dying process, called nearing death awareness, and that it is considered a peaceful occurrence for the patient. If the patient becomes agitated or disturbed by these events, they will be reassessed.

4. Tells the family that it won't be long now; George is an angel who has come to take Mr. Long away

6. **At the end of life, which of the following is most important:**

1. Monitoring a daily serum chemistry

2. Monitoring vital signs

3. Maintaining pain control

4. Ensuring that the patient is eating

7. **Mr. Long states that he has lost all his sense of hope. A reframing statement would be:**

1. "There is no hope for cure."

2. "The hopes you had at one time may not be possible. Can you think of anything you are hoping for now?"

3. "Mr. Long, I promise we will keep you comfortable and out of pain."

4. "Are you in pain?"

8. **The nursing assistant reports that Mrs. Jones has been upset all day because she believes that her cancer has advanced and her doctor has not been honest with her about her prognosis. If the doctor has not been truthful, this is a violation of the moral principle of:**

1. Justice

2. Confidentiality

3. Veracity

4. Her living will

9. **An important skill that helps the nurse care for the dying patient and family is:**

1. The ability to talk about death frequently with the patient

2. Listening to the patient talk about his thoughts about his death

3. Acting as if death will not occur and changing the topic to avoid distress

4. Reassuring the patient and family that pain can always be well controlled

10. **Which of the following statements is false:**

1. Pruritus can be a side effect of an opioid, and it usually subsides after a few days.

2. Dyspnea can be treated with atropine.

3. Nausea is a common symptom at the end of life and should be treated with calcium supplements.

4. The nurse's skills as an advocate help maintain the "voice" of the patient.

ANSWERS

1. *Answer: 1*
   Rationale: The PSDA is a federal law that requires institutions to notify patients about the availability of formal advance directives, in which the patient can direct his or her care, before any event that may leave the patient unable to make those wishes known.

2. *Answer: 1*
   Rationale: The patient is expressing nonverbal signs of pain by moaning and furrowing his eyebrows. His pain will be managed with opioids, and his anxiety and agitation will be treated with benzodiazepines and physical and psychological interventions.

3. *Answer: 2*
   Rationale: Restraining a hospice patient is not necessary. Symptoms should be managed first with medication and attention to all the patient's needs, physical, social, emotional, and spiritual.

4. *Answer: 2*
   Rationale: The patient is in the home setting and should be allowed to enjoy moving freely, as long as he is not showing signs of aggression or of endangering himself or others. An initial dose of haloperidol is 0.5 mg (up to 5 mg) three times a day. In the elderly, it is best to start with a lower dose.

5. *Answer: 3*
   Rationale: People who are dying may note that family members who have already died are in the room speaking with them. This is an uncommon phenomenon called *nearing death awareness*, and it is a pleasant event for the patient that requires no intervention except family education and support.

6. *Answer: 3*
   Rationale: Comfort is the patient's most important need at this time. Monitoring of vital signs and laboratory tests are not useful unless they will alter the plan of care.

7. *Answer: 2*
   Rationale: This answer reframes the statement and helps Mr. Long consider other aspects of his life that are important to him, as well as events that he realistically may be able to anticipate. Although assessing for pain and symptoms is important, talking about them now distracts from the topic of hope.

8. *Answer: 3*
   Veracity is the moral principle of truth telling, and it is a component of informed consent.

9. *Answer: 2*
   Rationale: Being comfortable with the subject of death means that the nurse has explored his or her experiences and feelings about death and is prepared to help the patient and family through the experience of death and dying by active listening. The topic of death need not be brought up frequently, and this can even be offensive to the patient, who knows that he or she is dying. Most of the time pain is well controlled, but in some situations it cannot be controlled completely.

10. *Answer: 3*
    Rationale: Answer 3 is false, because nausea is sometimes caused by hypercalcemia and can be treated successfully by treating the underlying cause and using the appropriate antiemetic.

REFERENCES

Agency for Healthcare Research and Quality (AHRQ). (2001). Making health care safer: A critical analysis of patient safety practices. (Publication No. 01-E058). Retrieved May 20, 2006, from http://www.ahrq.gov/clinic/ptsafety/index.html#toc.

American Cancer Society (2005). Estimated cancer deaths for selected cancer sites by state, 2005. Retrieved May 29, 2006, from http://www.cancer.org/downloads/stt/Estimated_Cancer_Deaths_for_Selected_Cancer_Sites_by_State,_US,_2005.pdf.

American Nurses Association (2001). *Code of ethics for nurses with interpretive statements*. Washington, D.C: American Nurses Association.

Azoulay, E., Alberti, A., & Bornstain, C., et al. (2001). Improved survival in cancer patients requiring mechanical ventilatory support: Impact of noninvasive mechanical ventilatory support. *Critical Care Medicine, 3*:519-525.

Bach, P. B., Schrag, D., & Nierman, D. M., et al. (2001). Identification of poor prognostic features among patients requiring mechanical ventilation after hematopoietic stem cell transplant. *Blood, 98*:3234-3240.

Brasher, V. L. (2002). Alterations of pulmonary function. In K. L. McCance, & S. E. Huether (Eds.), *Pathophysiology: The biologic basis for disease in adults and children* (pp. 1105-1145). St. Louis: Mosby.

Bruera, E., & Neumann, C. M. (1999). Respective limits of palliative care and oncology in the supportive care of cancer patients. *Support Care Cancer, 7*:321-327.

Callanan, M., & Kelley, P. (1992). *Final gifts*. New York: Bantam.

Douglas, M. R. (2001). Ethics and nursing practice. In N. Brent, (Ed.), *Nurses and the law: A guide to principles and applications*. (2nd ed.). (pp. 29-42). Philadelphia: WB Saunders.

Dudgeon, D. (2001). Dyspnea, death rattle and cough. In B. R. Ferrel, & N. Coyle (Eds.), *Textbook of palliative nursing* (pp. 245-261). New York: Oxford University Press.

Field, M. J., & Cassel, C. K. (1997). *Approaching death: Improving care at the end of life*. Washington, D. C.: National Academy Press.

Glare, P., & Christakis, N. (2004). Predicting survival in patients with advanced disease. In D. Doyle, G. Hanks, N. Cherny, & K. Calman (Eds.), *Oxford textbook of palliative care (pp.29-42)*(3rd ed.). New York: Oxford University Press.

Gomes, B., & Higginson, I. J. (2006). Factors influencing death at home in terminally ill patients with cancer: Systemic review. *British Medical Journal, 332*:515-521.

Groeger, J. S., Lemeshow, S., & Price, K., et al. (1998). Multicenter outcome study of cancer patients admitted to the intensive care unit: A probability of mortality model. *Journal of Clinical Oncology, 16*:761-770.

Groeger, J. S., White, P., & Nierman, D. M., et al. (1999). Outcome for cancer patients requiring mechanical ventilation. *Journal of Clinical Oncology, 17*:991-997.

Herth, K. (1993). Hope in older adults in community and institutional settings. *Issues in Mental Health Nursing, 14*:139-156.

Hodgson, B., & Kizior, R. (2007). *Nursing drug handbook*. St Louis: W. B. Saunders.

Karamlou, K., Nichols, D. J., & Nichols, C. R. (2003). Intensive care unit outcomes in elderly cancer patients. *Critical Care Clinician, 19*:657-675.

Lindgren, V. A., Barnett, S. D., & Bloom, R. I. (2006). Who is dying in our critical care units?. *Journal of Nursing Care Quality, 21*:78-85.

Matzo, M. L. (2001). Peri-death nursing care. In M. L. Matzo, & D. W. Sherman (Eds.), *Palliative care nursing: Quality care to the end of life* (pp. 487-511). New York: Springer Publishing.

McMillan, S. C., & Weitzner, M. (1998). Quality of life in cancer patients. *Cancer Practice, 6*:282-288.

Murphy-Ende, K. (2006a). Nausea and vomiting. In D. Camp-Sorrel, & R. Hawkins (Eds.), *Clinical manual for the oncology advanced practice nurse* (pp. 465-471). Pittsburgh: Oncology Nursing Society.

Murphy-Ende, K. (2006b). Dynamics of fluids and electrolytes. In C. Chernecky, D. Macklin, & K. Murphy-Ende (Eds.), *Fluid and electrolytes* (pp. 8-57). Philadelphia: W. B. Saunders.

Murphy-Ende, K. (2006c). Thirst. In D. Camp-Sorrell, & R. Hawkins (Eds.), *Clinical manual for the oncology advanced practice nurse* (pp. 997-1001). Pittsburgh: Oncology Nursing Society.

Murphy-Ende, K. (2006d). Rash. In D. Camp-Sorrell, & R. Hawkins (Eds.), *Clinical manual for the oncology advanced practice nurse* (pp. 95-103). Pittsburgh: Oncology Nursing Society.

National Comprehensive Cancer Network (NCCN) (2005). Palliative care. In *Clinical practice guidelines in oncology*. Retrieved June 24, 2006, from http://www.nccn.org/professionals/physician_gls/default.asp.

Potter, J., Hami, F., & Bryan, T., et al. (2003). Symptoms in 400 patients referred to palliative care services: Prevalence and patterns. *Palliative Medicine, 17*:310-314.

Project Grace. (2006). Glossary of terms. Retrieved May 20, 2006, from http://www.pgrace.org/glossary.htm.

Research Group (2006). Strong public support for the right to die: More Americans discussing—and planning—end-of-life treatment. Retrieved May 20, 2006, from http://people-press.org/reports/pdf/266.pdf.

Rhiner, M., & Slatkin, N. E. (2001). Pruritus, fever, and sweats. In B. R. Ferrel, & N. Coyle (Eds.), *Textbook of palliative nursing* (pp. 245-261). New York: Oxford University Press.

Royak-Schaler, R., Gadalla, S. M., & Lemkaw, J. P., et al. (2006). Family perspectives on communication with health care providers during end-of-life care. *Oncology Nursing Forum, 33*(4):753-760.

Smedira, N. J., Evans, B. H., & Grais, L. S., et al. (1990). Withholding and withdrawal of life support from the critically ill. *New England Journal of Medicine, 5:*309-315.

Smith, N. L., Kotthoff-Burrell, E., & Post, L. F. (2002). Protecting the patient's voice on the team. In M. D. Mezey, C. K. Cassel, & M. M. Bottrell (Eds.), *Ethical patient care: A casebook for geriatric health care teams.* (pp. 83-101). Baltimore: The Johns Hopkins University Press.

SUPPORT Principal Investigators. (1995). A controlled trial to improve care for seriously ill hospitalized patients: the Study to Understand Prognoses and Preferences for Outcomes and Risks of Treatments (SUPPORT). *Journal of the American Medical Association, 274:*1591-1598.

Thiery, G., Azoulay, E., & Darmon, M., et al. (2005). Outcome of cancer patients considered for intensive care unit admission: A hospital-wide prospective study. *Journal of Clinical Oncology, 23:*4406-4413.

Vigano, A., Bruera, E., & Jhangri, G. S., et al. (2000). Clinical survival predictors in patients with advanced cancer. *Archives of Internal Medicine, 160:*861-868.

Wrede-Seaman, L. (1999). *Symptom management handbook: A handbook for palliative care* (pp. 14-19). Yakima, WA:Intellicard.

Young, A. J., & Rodriguez, K. L. (2006). The role of narrative in discussing end-of-life care: Eliciting values and goals from text, context, and subtext. *Health Communication, 19:*49-59.

ESOPHAGEAL VARICES

LORI ANN BROWN

PATHOPHYSIOLOGICAL MECHANISMS

Esophageal varices are dilated blood vessels in the wall of the esophagus; they are often described as hemorrhoids of the esophagus. Varices are caused by liver disease and can lead to serious complications, including death.

Portal hypertension is the primary cause of esophageal varices. Blood flow through the liver is diminished, which increases blood flow through the microscopic blood vessels in the esophageal wall. As the blood flow increases, the blood vessels begin to dilate. This dilation can be profound.

The blood vessels continue to dilate until they become large enough to rupture. Rupture of esophageal varices rapidly becomes an emergency situation. The mortality rate associated with rupture is high. Treatment of the esophageal varices is first directed toward immediately controlling the bleeding, then toward long-term medical therapy. Immediate control of the bleeding usually is accomplished endoscopically. The goal of medical management and long-term therapy is to reduce the risk of bleeding.

Patients with cirrhosis have a disorganization of hepatic tissues that is caused by fibrosis and nodular regeneration. The changes in liver structure lead to an increase in the portal venous pressure (i.e., portal hypertension) (Chambers, 2001). New vascular channels may develop and form shunts. As a result, venous blood in the splanchnic system may be diverted from the liver to the systemic circulation through the development of connections to neighboring low-pressure veins. These connections are known as *collateral circulation* (Chambers, 2001).

The normal portal venous pressure is 2 to 6 mm Hg. Obstruction of the portal venous system leads to increased portal pressure. An elevated portal venous pressure distends the veins proximal to the site of the blockage. This distention increases the capillary pressure in organs drained by the obstructed veins. As the pressure in these veins increases, they become distended with blood, the vessels enlarge, and varices develop. For varices to form, the portal venous pressure must exceed 10 mm Hg (Chambers, 2001).

Rupture of esophageal varices, which is often painless, results in hemorrhage with hematemesis and/or bloody stools. Rupture is caused by a combination of elevated portal venous pressure and erosion of varices by gastric acid.

EPIDEMIOLOGY AND ETIOLOGY

Research data on the outcome in patients with hemorrhagic esophageal varices are grim; a large percentage of these patients either die or suffer from rebleeding. However, according to the Hospital Discharge Register and the Causes of Death Register (Stokkeland et al., 2006), patient outcomes over the past 35 years have improved. The 5-year survival rate in men younger than 50 years of age has increased from 31% to 49%. The mortality rate for esophageal variceal bleeding, on the first event, is 40% to 70%. Huether (2002) found that, "Mortality from ruptured esophageal varices in general ranges from 30% to 60%."

Mortality is related to a number of factors, including liver failure, sepsis, exsanguination, and cerebral edema.

Research has shown that a combination of better treatment regimens and prophylactic treatment options has improved the mortality rate in esophageal variceal hemorrhage. (Herrine, 2005). According to Wu and Chan (2005), both the rebleeding and mortality rates of variceal hemorrhage have been reduced significantly as a result of advances in endoscopic therapy and the use of vasoactive agents. These researchers also credit the use of antibiotic prophylaxis and portasystemic shunts for the decline in the mortality rate (Wu & Chan, 2005).

Not only are esophageal varices associated with a high mortality rate, they also are associated with high health care costs. Both beta blockers and endoscopic procedures have proven to be effective treatment methods, but early detection is still crucial to reducing the risk of hemorrhage, morbidity, and mortality (Suzuki et al., 2005).

Esophageal varices are associated with a higher mortality rate than any other symptom of portal hypertension, and cirrhosis is the most common cause of portal hypertension, accounting for 84% of all cases (Oura et al., 1994).

RISK PROFILE

The populations at greatest risk for the development of esophageal varices are individuals who tend to have a history of chronic cirrhosis, liver cancer, or metastasis. Determinants of the risk of developing esophageal varices include:

- Alcohol-induced cirrhosis
- Hepatocellular carcinoma or cancer metastatic to the liver
- Portal venous pressure greater than 10 mm Hg
- Liver failure
- Liver-associated ascites
- Aortopexy (superior vena cava syndrome) in children
- Use of protease inhibitors
- Ovarian cancer
- Esophageal cancer
- Cholangiocarcinoma, Klatskin's tumors
- History of esophageal varices or previous bleed (Sidhu & Wilbur, 2005)
- Increased portal pressure with longitudinal red streaks or spots or diffuse erythema seen during endoscopy (Sidhu & Wilbur, 2005)
- Larger varices pose a greater risk of hemorrhage (Sidhu & Wilbur, 2005).
- Laboratory abnormalities include increased bilirubin and elevated liver function tests.
- Patients at risk for rebleeding of an esophageal varix include:
  - Those with a history of alcoholism
  - The elderly and patients who suffered shock episodes during the initial hemorrhage
  - Patients with multiple co-morbidities, especially liver cancer and cirrhosis
  - Patients with a bleeding coagulopathy

PROGNOSIS

If esophageal varices are left untreated, the prognosis is poor, and death could occur by profound hemorrhage or airway obstruction. Esophageal variceal bleeding can resolve spontaneously, but early treatment and close monitoring are indicated.

After the initial bleeding episode, the patient is at a risk for rebleeding. Huether (2002) found that "Recurrent bleeding indicates a poor prognosis; most patients die within one year."

PROFESSIONAL ASSESSMENT CRITERIA (PAC)

1. **Hematemesis**: Vomiting of either bright red or coffee ground-like blood.
2. **Signs and symptoms of hemorrhage**: Hypotension, tachycardia, dizziness, dyspnea, tachypnea, restlessness, anxiety, decreased level of consciousness, decreased urine output, and cool, clammy skin.
3. **Signs and symptoms of shock**: Hypotension, decreased cardiac output, bradycardia.
4. **Signs and symptoms of liver failure:** Jaundice, ascites, splenomegaly, venous hums, weakness, malaise, anorexia, nausea and vomiting, weight loss, abdominal pain, edema, dark urine, encephalopathy.
5. The **Child-Pugh classification** (sometimes called the *Child-Turcotte-Pugh Score*) is used to assess chronic liver cirrhosis, to determine the prognosis and treatment options, and to evaluate the patient for liver transplantation. The score uses five clinical measures of liver disease. Each measure is assigned 1 to 3 points, with 3 representing the severest condition (Table 14-1).

NURSING CARE AND TREATMENT

The treatment of esophageal varices is a collaborative effort that includes nursing assessment and interventions, pharmacologic therapy, and interventional procedures or surgery. Once esophageal varices rupture and begin to hemorrhage, medical treatment becomes an emergent situation requiring immediate care.

1. Rupture of esophageal varices requires the following interventions:
   - Maintain an open airway, position the patient to enhance breathing and expulsion of hematemesis, and suction excess secretions and blood.
   - Assess the rate and volume of bleeding. Assess blood pressure and pulse with the patient in the supine position and in the sitting position.
   - Insert an IV access and administer fluids and blood products, rapid infusion of 5% dextrose, and a colloid solution until blood pressure is restored and urine output is adequate.
   - Obtain a blood specimen for hemoglobin, hematocrit, PT, PTT, platelets, type and cross-match, electrolytes, and renal and liver function tests.

Table 14-1	CHILD-PUGH CLASSIFICATION OF LIVER DISEASE		
Parameter	**1 Point**	**2 Points**	**3 Points**
Bilirubin (total)	<34 mcgmol/L (<2 mg/dL)	34-50 mcgmol/L (2-3 mg/dL)	>50 mcgmol/L (>3 mg/dL)
Serum albumin	>35 mg/L	28-35 mg/L	<28 mg/L
INR	<1.7	1.71-2.20	> 2.20
Ascites	None	Suppressed with medication	Refractory
Hepatic encephalopathy	None	Grade I or II (or suppressed with medication)	Grade III or IV (or refractory)
Prognosis for Liver Disease Based on the Total Score			
Points	*Class*	*Life Expectancy*	*Perioperative Mortality*
5-6	A	15-20 months	10%
7-9	B	Candidate for transplantation	30%
10-15	C	1-3 months	82%

Modified from Pugh, R. N., Murrray-Lyon, I. M., & Dawson, J. L., et al. (1973). Transection of the oesophagus for bleeding oesophageal varices. *British Journal of Surgery, 60*(8), 646-649.

- Correct clotting factor deficiencies with fresh frozen plasma, fresh blood, and vitamin K_1.
- Insert a nasogastric tube to assess the severity of bleeding and to lavage gastric contents before endoscopy.
- Prepare for pharmacologic therapy (octreotide or somatostatin) and endoscopy as soon as the patient has been resuscitated. The aim is to establish the cause and to control the bleeding.

2. In nonemergency situations, determine whether the patient is hemodynamically stable or unstable.
3. Assess for coughing and choking and maintain the airway.
4. Infuse IV fluid replacement with isotonic fluids (avoid lactate solutions) and monitor response to fluid replacement.
5. Replace clotting factors.
6. Prepare for possible procedures such as endoscopic variceal sclerotherapy.
7. Assess for signs of slow bleeding and anemia.
8. Hallmark signs and symptoms of bleeding include coughing or choking; cool, dusky skin; and altered mentation.
9. Monitor vital signs for rapid pulse, high blood pressure initially (due to vasoconstrictive compensatory response, then may become low), tachypnea, low central venous pressure, low pulmonary artery pressure, low to normal temperature.
10. Assess for other co-morbidities and medical history.
11. Significant laboratory values:
    - Low hemoglobin and hematocrit
    - Elevated INR (prolonged PT)
    - Decreased platelets
    - Elevated WBC
    - Hyperkalemia
    - Hypernatremia
    - Elevated BUN and creatinine
    - Elevated ammonia
    - Elevated lactate
    - Elevated liver function tests (high alanine aminotransferase [ALT], high aspartate aminotransferase [AST])
    - ABGs (metabolic acidosis)
    - Occult blood in stool
    - High urine specific gravity
12. Pharmacologic therapy:
    - Patients with esophageal varices and no prior history of variceal hemorrhage should be treated with nonselective beta-adrenergic blockers (e.g., propranolol, nadolol, timolol), provided that the use of beta blockers is not contraindicated. Garcia-Tsao (2006) found that, "Therapy with nonselective beta blockers is the gold standard in the prevention of first variceal hemorrhage in patients with medium to large varices and has been compared to endoscopic variceal ligation in several randomized trials." Beta blocker therapy has proven to reduce the risk of first bleeding in patients with evidence of varices and recurrent bleeding and mortality in patients with a history of previous variceal hemorrhage. Beta blockers lower portal hypertension by reducing cardiac output, which leads to splanchnic vasoconstriction and a reduction in portal pressures. Beta blockers reduce the risk of recurrent bleeding by 34% and mortality by 26% (Wilbur & Sidhu, 2005).
    - Vasopressin (Pitressin) is a synthetic antidiuretic hormone. It causes vasoconstriction of the splanchnic arteriolar bed, which reduces portal pressure. Reducing portal

pressure and hepatic blood flow decreases bleeding. Vasopressin can have many harmful side effects, specifically cardiac side effects. Vasoconstriction of the coronary arteries can cause chest pain and dysrhythmias. Patients treated with vasopressin must be on continuous ECG monitoring. The dosing of vasopressin ranges from 0.2 to 0.9 units/minute IV.

- Octreotide (Sandostatin), another medication used in the treatment of bleeding esophageal varices, is a long-acting somatostatin. Like vasopressin, octreotide causes splanchnic vasoconstriction. However, it causes selective vasoconstriction, therefore the cardiac side effects are not evident. The dosing of octreotide is an initial IV bolus of 50 mcg, then 50 mcg/hr for up to 5 days.

13. Endoscopic therapy: A sclerosing agent is injected into the bleeding varix and also into the tissue surrounding it. Endoscopic sclerotherapy is successful in controlling acute esophageal variceal bleeding in up to 90% of patients. Control should be obtained with one or two sessions. Patients who continue to bleed after two sessions should be considered for alternative methods to control the bleeding. The American Society for Gastrointestinal Endoscopy (ASGE) (2005). Found that, "Complications of sclerotherapy may be life-threatening (mortality rate, 0% to 11%). These include injection-induced bleeding, postinjection ulceration with delayed bleeding (2% to 13%), esophageal perforation (0% to 6%), and sepsis (0% to 7%). Other possible complications include chest pain (25% to 50%), fever (20% to 40%), esophageal ulcers (30% to 78%), pleural effusion (16% to 48%), esophageal stricture (3% to 59%), and dysphagia not due to stricture (4%)."

14. *Endoscopic variceal ligation (banding)*: This procedure is based on the widely used technique of rubber-band ligation of hemorrhoids. Up to 10 bands can be applied to the varix. The esophageal mucosa and the submucosa containing varices are bound, causing subsequent strangulation, sloughing, and eventual fibrosis, resulting in obliteration of the varices.

15. *Surgical/procedural therapy*: Approximately 5% to 10% of patients with esophageal variceal hemorrhage have conditions that cannot be controlled by endoscopic and/or pharmacologic treatment. Balloon tamponade (e.g., Minnesota tube, Sengstaken-Blakemore tube, Linton-Nachlas tube) may be used as a temporary option to manage these cases. Definitive salvage options may include the following:

- Portosystemic shunt
- Liver transplantation (the treatment of choice in patients with advanced liver disease)
- Percutaneous transhepatic embolization (PTE) of gastroesophageal varices: This procedure involves catheterization of the gastric collaterals that supply blood to varices via the transhepatic route. Generally, this procedure is less effective than endoscopic sclerotherapy for treatment of variceal hemorrhage and is much less effective than medical and surgical options. Therefore it should be reserved for situations in which acute variceal bleeding is not controlled by pharmaceutical treatment, endoscopic sclerotherapy, or endoscopic variceal ligation, and surgical management is contraindicated.
- Transjugular intrahepatic portosystemic shunts (TIPS): This technique is an effective salvage procedure for stopping acute variceal hemorrhage after failure of medical and endoscopic treatment. A stent is placed between the hepatic and portal veins, creating a portosystemic shunt in the liver. The shunt reduces portal hypertension, which in turn reduces bleeding. However, the TIPS procedure is associated with a number of complications. Chambers (2001) found that, "There is a high rate (50%) of reocclusion within one year." An even greater risk is that the patient may experience hepatic encephalopathy and ultimately die. Catalano and colleagues (2005) found that, "Encephalopathy occurs in 13% to 47% of patients." According to Wu

and Chan (2005), "The TIPS procedure should only be used as a rescue therapy once all other treatment options have failed."

- Balloon tamponade: In this procedure, a Sengstaken-Blakemore tube is inserted and the patient must be monitored in an ICU setting. The tube has three lumens: one for gastric aspiration, one for inflation of the esophageal balloon, and one for inflation of the gastric balloon. Inflation of the balloon ports puts pressure on the vessels serving the varices. This pressure reduces blood flow, stopping the variceal bleeding. The nurse or physician must insert the tip of the balloon into the stomach, then inflate it and clamp it. Next, the tube is withdrawn until resistance is met, so that pressure is applied at the gastroesophageal junction. A proper amount of traction must be applied to sustain enough pressure on the bleeding vessel. If bleeding does not stop when the gastric balloon is inflated, the esophageal balloon must be inflated next. Normal inflation pressure is 20 to 45 mm Hg. In maintenance of the Sengstaken-Blakemore tube, airway protection is essential, and IV sedation may be necessary to relieve anxiety and discomfort. Hemostats and scissors must be kept at the bedside at all times in case the airway becomes compromised and the tube needs to be severed immediately. Specific care of the Sengstaken-Blakemore tube involves the following:
- Secure the airway with an endotracheal tube.
- Monitor vital signs.
- Obtain IV access, preferably a central line.
- Obtain laboratory tests: hemoglobin, hematocrit, PT, PTT, INR, platelets, white blood cells, liver function tests, potassium, sodium, type and cross-match, and ABGs.
- Connect nasogastric tube to continuous suction.
- Keep patient NPO because the person is at high risk for aspiration.
- Correct coagulopathies with transfusion of FFP.
- Transfuse packed red blood cells as determined by hemoglobin values.
- Administer medications as prescribed.
- Prepare for endoscopy.

EVIDENCE-BASED PRACTICE UPDATES

1. Beta-blocker therapy has proven to reduce the risk of initial bleeding in patients with esophageal varices, as well as recurrent bleeding episodes in patients with a history of esophageal variceal hemorrhage (Sidhu & Wilbur, 2005).
2. Studies have shown that band ligation has replaced sclerotherapy as the first-line endoscopic treatment for esophageal varices (Wu & Chan, 2005).
3. Morbidity and mortality are significantly reduced in patients who undergo aggressive pre-endoscopic resuscitation. Optimal resuscitation before endoscopy and proper pharmacologic management after endoscopy seem to be as crucial to the management of patients with upper GI bleeding as meticulous hemostatic techniques during the procedure (Wassef, 2004). The same study found a reduction in postprocedural MI with aggressive pre-endoscopic resuscitation.
4. Morbidity and mortality are significantly reduced in patients with esophageal variceal hemorrhage who undergo aggressive pre-endoscopic resuscitation (Wassef, 2004).
5. Band ligation of esophageal varices is associated with a higher incidence of fundal varices and worsening portal hypertensive gastropathy compared to sclerotherapy (Sarwar et al., 2006).
6. The TIPS procedure is recommended only when the patient's condition fails to respond to pharmacologic and endoscopic therapy (Garcia-Tsao, 2006).
7. Endoscopic screening is recommended for patients diagnosed with cirrhosis (Suzuki et al., 2005).

TEACHING AND EDUCATION

1. Discuss the plan of care and treatment options with the patient and family. Explain the rationale for frequent monitoring of signs and symptoms, vital signs, and laboratory and diagnostic tests.
2. Educate the patient about his or her prescribed medications (i.e., name, purpose, dosage, frequency, route, and side effects). Teach the patient to schedule medications, and emphasize the importance of taking them as prescribed. Warn the patient not to discontinue beta blockers abruptly without first contacting the physician or nurse practitioner. During vasopressin infusion, instruct the patient or family to notify the nurse if the patient has any chest pain.
3. Obtain informed consent regarding the risks and benefits of the various interventions and procedures. Explain the procedures and the nursing care involved and encourage and answer questions.
4. Explain the rationale for administration of blood products.

NURSING DIAGNOSES

1. **Deficient fluid volume** related to hemorrhage
2. **Ineffective tissue perfusion**, cardiopulmonary, related to decreased circulating blood volume
3. **Impaired gas exchange** related to loss of oxygen-carrying capacity
4. **Risk for aspiration** of blood related to vomiting of gastric contents
5. **Deficient knowledge** related to disease process and therapeutic interventions

EVALUATION AND DESIRED OUTCOMES

1. Bleeding will be resolved or controlled.
2. Airway will be open.
3. Lung sounds will be clear, and ventilatory support will be discontinued.
4. Systolic blood pressure will return to normal.
5. Hematocrit will be within normal limits within 24 hours of last transfusion.
6. Laboratory values will be within normal limits.
7. Intake and output will be balanced, with a urine output of 30 mL/hr or greater.
8. Bowel function will return to normal.
9. The patient and family will verbalize the care plan and the treatment options.

DISCHARGE PLANNING AND FOLLOW-UP CARE

- Educate the patient about his or her medications (purpose, name, dosage, route, frequency, and side effects).
- Teach the patient how to identify signs and symptoms of esophageal bleeding.
- Educate the patient in the assessment of his or her alcohol use. Provide basic counseling and education, referral to an alcohol and drug abuse counselor, and Alcoholics Anonymous meeting locations. Assist the patient to identify support persons.
- Stress the importance of keeping and obtaining follow-up medical and counseling appointments and procedures.
- Explain when to notify the physician or nurse practitioner: any episode of vomiting blood and signs of liver failure (jaundice, pruritus, change in mentation).

REVIEW QUESTIONS

QUESTIONS

1. **The first priority in the management of acute GI bleeding is to:**
   1. Hemodynamically stabilize the patient
   2. Diagnose the cause of the bleed
   3. Prepare for emergency sclerotherapy
   4. Administer IV vasopressin

2. **A therapy specifically for patients with variceal upper GI bleeding is:**
   1. Chemotherapy
   2. Insertion of a Swan Ganz catheter
   3. Radiation
   4. Sclerotherapy

3. **Octreotide:**
   1. Is also known as dexamethasone
   2. Carries a risk of cardiac side effects
   3. Causes splanchnic vasoconstriction, which reduces variceal bleeding
   4. Is administered PO

4. **The nurse must monitor the patient with bleeding esophageal varices for signs and symptoms of:**
   1. Shock
   2. Fever
   3. Deep vein thrombosis
   4. Seizures

5. **Esophageal varices begin to bleed when _____ hypertension occurs:**
   1. Malignant
   2. Portal
   3. Pulmonary
   4. Idiopathic

6. **If esophageal varices are not treated, the patient faces a high risk of:**
   1. Myocardial infarction
   2. Death
   3. AIDS
   4. Stroke

7. **A/an _____ tube may be inserted to tamponade bleeding varices:**
   1. Endotracheal tube
   2. Sengstaken-Blakemore tube
   3. Nasogastric tube
   4. PEG tube

8. **A primary nursing intervention in the management of patients with bleeding esophageal varices is:**
   1. Pain control
   2. Ensuring IV access
   3. Airway management
   4. Administration of vasopressin

9. **The medications used to prevent bleeding in patients with esophageal varices are:**
   1. Calcium channel blockers
   2. Antihistamines
   3. Beta blockers
   4. Steroids

10. **The patient population at greatest risk for esophageal varices is:**
    1. Children
    2. Patients with cirrhosis
    3. Females
    4. Patients with diabetes

ANSWERS

1. *Answer: 1*
   Rationale: Controlling the bleeding and maintaining hemodynamic status is the first priority.

2. *Answer: 4*
   Rationale: Sclerotherapy is the only option listed that is specific to the treatment of esophageal variceal hemorrhage.

3. *Answer: 3*
   Rationale: Octreotide is administered IV and reduces bleeding by causing vasoconstriction.

4. *Answer: 1*
   Rationale: With esophageal varices, the patient is at risk of hemorrhage and multiple organ failure.

5. *Answer: 2*
   Rationale: Increasing portal venous pressures causes the varix to rupture and hemorrhage.

6. *Answer: 2*
   Rationale: Hemorrhagic shock may lead to death if esophageal varices go untreated.

7. *Answer: 2*
Rationale: The Sengstaken-Blakemore tube provides compression at the site of the varices.

8. *Answer: 3*
Rationale: Maintaining an open airway and preventing aspiration are critical in patients with bleeding esophageal varies. Pain control is always important and should be assessed, but esophageal bleeding usually is not painful.

9. *Answer: 3*
Rationale: Beta blockers reduce cardiac output, which reduces portal blood flow, leading to decreased bleeding.

10. *Answer: 2*
Rationale: Chronic cirrhotic liver disease is the primary risk factor for esophageal varices.

REFERENCES

Catalano, G., Urbani, L., & DeSimone, P., et al. (2005). Expanding indications for TIPSS: Portal decompression before elective oncologic gastric surgery in cirrhotic patients. *Journal of Clinical Gastroenterology, 39*:921-923.

Chambers, J. E. (2001). Gastrointestinal alterations. In Sole, M. L., Lamborn, M., & Harts Lorn, J. (Eds.), *Introduction to critical care nursing.* (3rd ed.). (pp. 459-508). Philadelphia: W.B. Saunders.

Day, M. W. (2005). Esophagogastric tamponade tube. In K. K. Calson, & D. J. Wiegand (Eds.), *AACN procedure manual for critical care.* (5th ed.). (pp. 861-869). Philadelphia: W.B. Saunders.

Doctorslounge. (2006). Child-Pugh Score. Retrieved July, 9, 2006, from http://www.doctorslounge.net/clinlounge/scores/child.html.

Garcia-Tsao, G. (2006). Portal hypertension. *Current Opinion in Gastroenterology, 22*(3):254-262.

Giannini, E. G., Botta, F., & Borro, P., et al. (2005). Application of platelet count/spleen diameter ratio to rule out the presence of esophageal varices in patients with cirrhosis: A validation study based on follow-up. *Digestive and Liver Disease, 37*(10):779-785.

Grace, N. D. (1997). Diagnosis and treatment of gastrointestinal bleeding secondary to portal hypertension. American College of Gastroenterology practice parameters committee, *American College of Gastroenterology, 7*:1081-1091.

Herrine, S. K. (2005). Advances in the treatment of complications of cirrhosis and portal hypertension-variceal bleeding. Retrieved September 15, 2006, from http://www.medscape.com/viewarticle/518704.

Huether, S. E. (2002). Alterations of digestive function. In K. McCance, & S. E. Huether (Eds.), *Pathophysiology: The biologic basis for disease in adults and children.* (4th ed.). (pp. 1261-1313). St. Louis: Mosby.

Mukherjee, S., & Sorrell, M. F. (2005a). Beta blockers to prevent esophageal varices: An unfulfilled promise. *New England Journal of Medicine, 353*(21):2288-2290.

Olsen, S., Arteaga, T., & Brown, R. S. (2005). Is variceal banding more effective than beta blockade in primary prophylaxis for variceal hemorrhage? *Evidence-Based Gastroenterology, 6*(3):73-76.

Oura, S., Kojima, K., & Fukasawa, M., et al. (1994). Etiology and management of esophageal varices. *Nippon Rinsho, 52*:80-84.

Sarwar, S., Khan, A. A., & Alam, A., et al. (2006). Effect of band ligation on portal hypertensive gastropathy and development of fundal varices. *Journal of Ayub Medical College, 18*(1):32-35.

Siduh, K., & Wilbur, K. (2005). Beta blocker prophylaxis for patients with variceal hemorrhage. *Journal of Clinical Gastroenterology, 39*:435-440.

Spratto, G. R., & Woods, A. L. (2003). *PDR nurse's drug handbook 2004.* New York: Thomson.

Stokkeland, K., Brandt, L., Ekbom, A., & Hultcrantz, R. (2006). Improved prognosis for patients hospitalized with esophageal varicies in Sweden 1969-2002. *Hepatology, 43*:500-505.

Suzuki, A., Mendes, F., & Lindor, K. (2005). Diagnostic model of esophageal varices in alcoholic liver disease. *European Journal of Gastroenterology and Hepatology, 17*:307-309.

The American Society for Gastrointestinal Endoscopy (ASGE). (2006). *Role of endoscopic sclerotherapy.* Retrieved April 19, 2006, from http://www.sages.org/sg_asgepub1019.html.

Wassef, W. (2004). Upper gastrointestinal bleeding. *Current Opinion in Gastroenterology, 20*(6):546-556.

Williams, B. J., Mulvihill, D. M., & Pettus, B. F., et al. (2006). Pediatric superior vena cava syndrome: Assessment at low radiation dose 64, slice CT angiography. *Journal of Thoracic Imaging, 21*(1):71-72.

Wu, J. C., & Chan, F. K. (2005). Esophageal bleeding disorders. *Current Opinion in Gastroenterology, 21*:485-489.

ETHICS IN ADULT ONCOLOGY AND CRITICAL CARE NURSING

MARLENE M. ROSENKOETTER

THE DISCIPLINE OF ETHICS

Ethics is sometimes referred to as moral philosophy. It includes the study and decisions involved in determining "right" and "wrong" behavior. Ethics is concerned with "the study of social morality and philosophical reflection on its norms and practices" (Burkhardt & Nathaniel, 2002).

The three main areas of ethics are metaethics, normative ethics, and applied ethics. *Metaethics* asks questions about the nature of goodness or badness, rather than what is actually good or bad, right or wrong, behavior (Moral Philosophsophy.info, 2005). It focuses on universal truths, where our ethical principles originate, as well as on what these truths mean, and our reasoning. It considers whether there are things that are good or bad independent of us, or whether they are something that we have actually invented. *Normative ethics* is more about how we should live our lives, good habits that we should adopt, and the consequences of our actions on others. Two types of normative ethics are *virtue ethics* and *deontology*. *Virtues* are considered traits or acts that are good to have, in contrast to *vices*, which are not. Deontology suggests that certain things are right or wrong, regardless of their consequences. *Applied ethics* is the practical side of ethics, or the use of ethical principles to determine what is right or wrong for us to do. Applied ethics focuses on the issues and dilemmas that we face, such as abortion, assisted suicide, do not resuscitate, and the right to die.

So where do we get our own *personal* ethical beliefs? They begin in our formative years with the teachings of parents, relatives, and friends. They are influenced by the religious beliefs that we adopt and hold to be true, by the cultures of which we are a part, and by the education we receive. At the point of entry into nursing, each of us was taught what behaviors were appropriate and expected of us, as well as standards and practices that were considered "professional." These were intertwined to form a belief system that we use to make ethical decisions. Understanding our own values, acknowledging those values, and understanding where they came from is essential for sound ethical decision making in clinical practice. In order to understand the ethical beliefs and the decisions of patients and families, it is equally important to understand *their* backgrounds, *their* cultures (Jecker, 1997), *their* religions, and *their* social norms. Without such an understanding, the needs of the patient and family and the interventions by nurses and other health professionals may be in conflict. Consider for a moment how you would approach each patient differently if one is Native American, one is Jewish, or one is Islamic, or one was born in the Far East or South America. The backgrounds of these patients may well be different from yours and are certainly different from one another.

Patients and their families cannot be viewed in isolation, and they cannot be approached solely from the perspective of your personal beliefs. They have the right to receive and participate in health care from their own perspectives and their own systems.

PRINCIPLES OF ETHICS

"Ethical principles are basic and obvious moral truths that guide deliberation and action" (Burkhardt & Nathaniel, 2002). The eight ethical principles considered here are autonomy, beneficence, nonmaleficence, justice, confidentiality, veracity, fidelity, and privacy.

Autonomy is the quality or state of being self-governing and of having moral independence and self-determination. The patient has a right to make his or her own decisions, assuming the capacity and the ability to do so. This principle is one that frequently causes serious ethical dilemmas in the critical care setting. The patient may be greatly incapacitated, on a ventilator, heavily sedated, and unaware of his or her surroundings or condition. At this point, other people necessarily step in and make decisions that include life and death situations. This places additional moral, emotional, and cognitive demands on the family surrogate (Meeker & Jezewski, 2005). In 2005 the American Association of Critical-Care Nurses (AACN) issued a public policy statement on the role of the critical care nurse as a patient advocate (AACN, 2005). This includes respect and support the patient (or surrogate) in autonomous, informed decision making and to intercede for patients who cannot speak for themselves in situations involving immediate action.

Beneficence is the quality or state of being *beneficent* (i.e., doing what is good). *Nonmaleficence* is the counterpart term (i.e., not doing harm). Physicians, nurses, specialty therapists, and clergy are assumed to be beneficent and not to want to intentionally do harm to a patient. The questions, however, are: What is good? What is harm? When does a medical intervention cease to be doing good for a patient and does harm? Such deliberations often stem from or involve ethical dilemmas. For whom is the decision good? To whom will it cause harm? If a patient *could* receive an experimental drug that *might* reverse a condition, will it cause harm, and, if it will cause harm, will the harm be exceeded by the good the drug could do? What if the patient prefers to use alternative therapies that are not within the mainstream of medical practice? The terms *alternative* and *complementary* are used to refer to nontraditional methods of diagnosing, preventing, or treating a particular disorder. Many cancer patients, for example, may find that these approaches relieve their symptoms or side effects, ease their pain and suffering, and generally enhance their lives during the course of their treatment (ACS, 2006).The patient has the autonomous right to use such therapies. The American Holistic Nurses Association suggests that nurses draw upon and use both conventional and complementary and alternative (CAM) modalities and that both are within the scope of nursing practice (AHNA, 2004). Therefore the use of such approaches not only is within the rights of the patient, it also is appropriate in nursing practice. Ethical questions arise when the patient chooses to use such treatments in lieu of traditional medicine and the nurse is asked to participate in their administration. This can pose a conflict between the patient's right to autonomous decision making and the nurse's observance of the principles of beneficence and nonmaleficence.

Experimental procedures can create similar issues. The Oncology Nursing Society has taken a position on cancer clinical trials, indicating that, "Every person diagnosed with cancer must have the right to participate in a clinical trail if medically indicated" (ONS, 2004a). Clinical trials, of course, must follow agency policies regarding informed consent, and patients must be advised of their rights as human subjects, including the risks and benefits of experimental drugs and devices.

The obligation to do good and the obligation not to do harm clearly arise in the issue of assisted suicide, namely, "Any act that entails making a means of suicide available to a patient with knowledge of the patient's intention" (ONS, 2004b). The ONS statement affirms that any requests for assisted suicide should include an open discussion of the request, but nurses are to uphold the ethical code and standards of the profession and may refuse to participate in any state where assisted suicide is legal. The American Nurses

Association's position statement on assisted suicide reads, "Nursing has a social contract with society that is based on trust and therefore patients must be able to trust that nurses will not actively take human life" and, "Nurse participation in assisted suicide is incongruent with the accepted norms and fundamental attributes of the profession" (ANA, 1994a). Nurses continue to be confronted and struggle with the complex moral and professional issues related to assisted suicide (Scanlon & Rushton, 1996). With regard to active euthanasia, the ANA states, "The nurse should not participate in active euthanasia because such an act is in direct violation of the *Code for Nurses with Interpretive Statements*" (ANA, 1994b, 2001). This has recently been made even more clear in the case of two nurses and a physician charged with intentionally ending the lives of patients in the aftermath of Hurricane Katrina (NPR, 2006).

The ethical principle of *justice* implies that the nurse will be fair and impartial while conforming to truth and reason in decision making. This principle is a key point where issues of ethics and human rights intersect (ANA, 1991a). The principle of justice is particularly important in the use and distribution of critical care resources and services. Does everyone have an equal right to receive the same level and quality of health care? Who should be the recipient of a heart or a lung available for transplant? All these decisions involve not only the high-quality health care available in the United States but also the cost of health care. In 1960, U.S. health care expenditures accounted for about 5% of the gross domestic product (GDP); in 2000, that figure had grown to more than 13% (AHRQ, 2002). This is a higher percentage than in any other country in the world. Health spending in the United States topped $1.8 trillion in 2004, accounting for about 17.3% of the GDP (Fleck, 2006). The health care share of the GDP is expected to increase from 15.3% in 2003 to 18.7% by 2014 (Heffler et al., 2005).

Technology has forever changed the health care landscape. Surgical techniques, vascular access, computerization of complex procedures, genome research, and a variety of medical advances have made interventions possible that previously were not only unavailable but completely unknown. Concerns are heightened when we consider the cost of these interventions, their appropriate use, and the consequences of their use. In the greater health care system, ongoing concern focuses on the availability and distribution of health care dollars, including care for individuals who have limited or no insurance. According to the ANA position statement on ethics and human rights, "Human beings deserve respect as ends in themselves, and therefore, deserve nursing services that are equitable in terms of accessibility, availability, affordability and quality" (ANA, 1991a). In a society in which sophisticated and advanced health care is available, ethical dilemmas will continue to emerge concerning who should be the recipients of available resources.

Confidentiality is the concept of nondisclosure of information that is private, personal, or when disclosure could be harmful to another person. As of 2003, the Health Insurance Portability and Accountability Act of 1996 (HIPAA) protects any information that identifies an individual and that is not an educational or employment record. Patients have the right to see, copy, and supplement their medical records, and hospitals must have safeguards in place to protect identifying information (Health Privacy Project, 2000). Nurses in oncology and critical care settings are equally responsible under federal law for protecting the privacy and confidentiality of all information pertaining to patients. This means that nurses are forbidden to discuss patients in places such as the lobby, elevators, and cafeterias, as was customary in previous years. This can be very difficult in critical care settings, where the proximity of one patient to another easily lends itself to a violation of the standards. Nevertheless, all precautions must be taken to safeguard the confidentiality of the patient. Privacy and confidentiality have come to the forefront with the developments in technology, such as facsimile machines and wireless computer networks, which have changed the delivery of health care (ANA, 2005). The use of technology creates the potential for unintentional breaches of confidentiality in the transmission of health care information.

Closely related to confidentiality are the principles of veracity, fidelity, and privacy. *Veracity* refers to truth telling, which has many ramifications in the critical care setting. Nurses are quite passionate about patients' rights, and, in an absence of truth, nurses find themselves in unethical situations (Turkoski, 2001). Martin (1993) examined the issue of veracity with regard to the four tenets of autonomy, justice, beneficence, and nonmalefi-cence. She concluded that lying to patients has no moral justification. Yet, when a patient asks, "Am I going to die?" "Do I have cancer?" "Is my son dead?" do you always answer truthfully? How do you make the decision on what to say? Do you tell the patient what the family does not know, or what the family has requested that the patient not be told, even though, at the same time, you feel that the patient has the right to know? Each situation is unique, and decision making is complicated by the beliefs of the patient, the family, the physician, and even society (Blake, 1996).

Fidelity means promise keeping in an ethical context. It is the virtue of faithfulness; being true to our commitments and obligations to others. These commitments relate to the obligations that are implicit in a trusting relationship, including confidentiality and keep-ing promises. If the family is promised that the patient will not have pain or suffer at the end of his or her life, then the nurse has the responsibility to keep this promise. Nurses "must use effective doses of medications prescribed for symptom control and nurses have a moral obligation to advocate on behalf of the patient when prescribed medication is insufficiently managing pain and other distressing symptoms" (ANA, 2003a). The principle of fidelity is closely related to the principle of autonomy. Failure to keep promises made to others denies them the opportunity to exercise their freedom of choice in the relationship, which limits their autonomy.

Each patient and family has the right to autonomous decision making and respect for their *privacy*. Allowing them time alone to discuss issues, freeing them from unauthor-ized intrusion, and providing informed consent are assumed. With the advent of compu-terized documentation and records, scheduling, reporting of diagnostics, and certainly communications between the patient and other health care professionals, the potential for technologic intrusion into privacy emerged. HIPAA has changed all of that and has directed that patients and families be assured of their privacy. As mentioned, however, in a close physical environment such as a critical care unit, invasion of that privacy can easily occur. The nurse is responsible for protecting privacy and making every attempt to maintain it.

CODES OF ETHICS

Virtually every discipline and every field of endeavor now has a code of ethics. Psychology, social work, and criminal justice, as well as newspapers, businesses, manufacturing com-panies, and real estate agencies, all have codes of ethics, but none could be more basic or more critical than the codes of ethics that affect the lives of patients and their families. Two codes of ethics are essential for nurses: the ANA Code of Ethics for Nurses with Interpretative Statements (ANA, 2001) and the International Council of Nurses (ICN) Code of Ethics for Nurses (ICN, 2000). These two documents set forth the ethical standards that nurses are expected to follow and against which their behaviors can be evaluated, including in a court of law. In fact, in 1994 the ANA published a position statement that stated the ANA believes the nine Provisions of the Code are nonnegotiable and every nurse has an obligation to abide by them (ANA, 1994b). Every nurse is responsible for reading, understanding, and keeping readily available copies of the ANA and ICN codes, which can be consulted when difficult situations and ethical dilemmas arise. These documents can be the focus of dialog and reflection, as well as a source of understanding, support, and direction in ethically complex situations.

ADVANCE DIRECTIVES

The Patient Self-Determination Act, which took effect in 1991, applies to all health care institutions and providers (*Federal Register, 2003*). It requires that all individuals receiving medical care be provided with written information about their rights, including the right to accept or refuse treatment (Kyba, 2002) and the right to have advance directives. They must be made aware of their right to make decisions upon admission (ANA, 1991b). Nurses are responsible for ensuring that the patient is made aware of these rights, unless the patient is incapable of understanding the information or of making a decision, in which case the information goes to the family.

The term *advance directive* refers to the living will and the health care power of attorney. These give instructions about future medical care if the person is unable to participate in medical decisions because of serious illness or incapacity (NHPCO, n. d.). A *living will* is a written document in which a patient's wishes about medical treatment are described so that if the person becomes unable to communicate those wishes, others will do so on his or her behalf. The *health care power of attorney* is a legal document in which the individual appoints a specific person to make decisions about his or her health care in the event the person becomes unable to make decisions or to communicate personal wishes. An important point is that the states regulate the use of advance directives differently. If the person is hospitalized in a state different from the one in which the papers were signed, their use could be different from that originally anticipated by the patient and family. Nurses need to be aware of hospital policies and state regulations covering advance directives, including do not resuscitate orders (ANA, 2003b). They also need to be in a position to discuss these issues with the patient and the family members responsible for invoking the patient's wishes. Nurses need to keep in mind that the patient can change these directives at any time, and those changes need to be shared with the family. (See Chapter 13 on end of life care.)

ETHICAL DILEMMAS AND MORAL DISTRESS

The AACN's position statement on moral distress states that it occurs when, "You know the ethically appropriate action to take, but are unable to act upon it" and/or "You act in a manner contrary to your personal and professional values, which undermines your integrity and authenticity" (AACN, 2006). The AACN further indicated that in one study nearly 50% of nurses had acted against their consciences in providing care to their terminally ill patients. Moral distress is a serious issue among oncology and critical care nurses (Elpern et al., 2005).

A number of complex and complicated issues contribute to moral distress in the oncology and critical care environments. For example, when no viable medical interventions are left to treat the patient, the decision may be made to withhold further treatments or to discontinue those in place. Either decision can be difficult and extremely traumatic for the families of patients and for the staff (van Rooyen et al., 2005) and can create ethical concerns for nurses. Moreover, a study of 1000 internists found that a large percentage of these physicians would be unwilling to comply with some of patients' wishes to withhold or withdraw life-sustaining treatment (Farber et al., 2006). This complicates matters even more. Ethics committees are frequently consulted in these situations to provide assistance with decision making and to assist family members, as well as staff members, with their feelings and concerns. One problem is that intentionally withholding life-prolonging treatment may be equated with intentionally causing death and even involve self-deception (Sayers & Perera, 2002). In 1992 the ANA issued a position statement on foregoing nutrition and hydration, a statement that can be very helpful to all nurses. The document states that, "The decision to withhold artificial nutrition and hydration should be made by the patient or surrogate with the health care team." This should be distinguished from withholding the provision of food and water. The Robert Wood Johnson Foundation suggests that, "Artificial nutrition and hydration is a medical treatment that may be refused [by] any patient who has the ability to make decisions" (RWJF, 2006). In recent years, the inclusion of do not resuscitate orders (ANA, 2003) and artificial nutrition and hydration treatments have become more important in advanced care planning (Gillick, 2006).

A basic consideration in these decisions is the issue of *medical futility*. By definition, *futility* means being ineffective or serving no useful purpose. Such decisions must include the beliefs and values of the patient, family, physician, nurses, and other members of the health care team. Pellegrino (2005) suggests that the definition of futility should weigh these factors: effectiveness, benefits, and burdens. *Effectiveness* means determining whether an intervention would alter the course of a disease or symptom; this is a decision most often made by the physician. *Benefits* involve the patient, the family, or both and focus on whether the treatment would be worthwhile for the patient. *Burdens* include the potential physical, financial, and emotional consequences. Although the nurse's role in determining medical futility varies considerably from one setting to another, nurses can play an important role by assisting families to understand the issues and actively participate in the decision-making process (Heland, 2006). A fundamental point is that easing death can be a fulfilling contribution and can reduce the suffering and enrich the lives of both patients and families (Reynolds et al., 2005). Yet, "mercy killings" are not an acceptable practice, regardless of the circumstances.

ETHICAL DECISION MAKING

Having a framework for ethical decision making provides the nurse with a foundation not only for dialog but for the process of resolution. While there are variations in frameworks, they essentially include the following questions.

1. Is an ethical dilemma emerging or has one emerged?
2. Who are the parties involved who need to discuss the potential or existing dilemma?
3. What is the relevant information?
   - What is the medical information?
   - What are the facts? What is *not* known?
   - What information is in the medical record?
   - What does the patient tell me (if able)?
   - What do family members or friends tell me?
   - What is the prognosis?
   - What are the sociocultural and religious factors involved?
   - What are *currently* the probable outcomes?
4. Who is capable of making decisions?
   - What is the capacity of the patient for making decisions?
   - If the patient is not capable of resolving ethical dilemmas, who is?
   - What surrogate is capable and available to make decisions?
5. What are the ethical dilemmas?
   - What ethical principles are involved?
   - What is the nature of each dilemma?
   - On what do the parties involved agree?
   - On what do the parties involved disagree?
   - What issues or factors are important to each party involved?
   - Is an ethics consult or ethics committee desired by any involved party?
   - Have all of the involved parties met to discuss the dilemmas?

6. What are the legal and moral issues?
   - Are advance directives needed or available?
   - If the patient is not capable of making the decision, who is legally capable?
   - What is the projected cost to all parties involved?
   - What is the appropriate distribution of resources in the situation?
7. What are the options?
   - What parties endorse which options?
   - What are the consequences of each option?
8. What are the projected outcomes?
   - What outcomes are desired?
   - What outcomes may be possible?
   - What are the risks and benefits to the patient and other involved parties?
   - What outcomes are acceptable and unacceptable to each of the parties involved?
   - Who will be affected by the outcomes?
   - Where is there agreement?
9. What are the "final" decisions?
10. What are the outcomes of any decisions?
    - How do the parties involved feel about the outcomes?
    - What are the consequences of the outcomes for the patient and involved parties?
11. What have I learned from this process or the decisions?
12. What would I do differently in the future?

HOSPITAL ETHICS COMMITTEES (HECS)

Ethical dilemmas are common in health care settings. They have increased dramatically over the past few decades with the explosion in technology, greater access to sophisticated health care in secondary and tertiary facilities, the development of newer and often expensive medical interventions, and the demands of our society for equal access to equal care by everyone. Hospitals now are required to have some type of committee or process in place to deal with health care dilemmas. The main impetus for this arose from the decision of the New Jersey Supreme Court in the Karen Quinlan case. The court indicated that ethics committees, rather than courts, should be the focus of decisions involving the withdrawal of life support systems (O'Rourke, 1983). In 1987 Maryland became the first state to enact legislation requiring every hospital in the state to have an ethics committee (MHECN, 2005).

A hospital ethics committee (HEC) can have a variety of different functions and compositions of members. It frequently includes clergy, clinical ethicists, nurses, physicians, and social workers (Fowler, 1990, 1986; Fowler & Levine-Ariff, 1987). A study of religious-affiliated hospitals found that members might also include administrators, community representatives, attorneys, and patient advocates (Higgins & Lemke, 1995). The roles and functions of the committee and the frequency of meetings can vary widely. The important point is that nurses, patients, and family members must understand how to contact the committee and how to request an ethics consult. Ethics committees do not make decisions; rather, they help others make their own decisions. Ethics committees are able to collect relevant medical information and sort through it. One of their first responsibilities is to identify who the decision makers will be and the role of the patient in the decision-making process. If the patient is unable to make a decision, who is the most responsible party? Do advance directives exist, and, if so, what are they? Another role is to get the various parties together to discuss their ideas, dilemmas, and concerns. Are there any legal issues involved? Everyone can then consider any recommendations the committee wants to make (Freer, 1997), as well as their own, and move toward a meaningful resolution.

SUMMARY

Advances in technology and medicine have heightened the focus on ethical decision making for oncology and critical care nurses. Dilemmas are common in clinical practice. Nurses have a major role in resolving existing dilemmas while assisting patients and families with their decisions. They serve as resources for values clarification, explaining legal issues, interpreting the ANA and ICN codes, and educating interdisciplinary team members on the ethical decision-making process.

REVIEW QUESTIONS

QUESTIONS

1. **Deontology is the study of ethics that:**
   1. Suggests what is right and wrong, regardless of the consequences
   2. Establishes principles that a person can use to determine what is right and wrong
   3. Examines traits that a person should and should not have
   4. Asks questions about the nature of goodness

2. **Our personal ethical beliefs are derived from:**
   1. Our religious beliefs
   2. Our culture
   3. Our parents and families
   4. All of the above

3. **In reporting a medication error, you are applying which principles?**
   1. Beneficence and justice
   2. Nonmaleficence and veracity
   3. Autonomy and fidelity
   4. Confidentiality and justice

4. **Use of the ANA Code of Ethics is:**
   1. Legally required
   2. Decided by the hospital administrator
   3. A source of concern for nurses
   4. Nonnegotiable in practice

5. **The Patient Self-Determination Act of 2003:**
   1. Applies to all health care institutions and health care providers
   2. Was developed to protect patients involved in clinical drug trials
   3. States that patients are responsible for following their medical regimen
   4. Applies only to care prescribed by physicians and does not concern nurses

6. **Which of the following statements is accurate regarding advance directives (more than one answer may apply):**
   1. They can be changed at any time by the patient.
   2. They are written documents determined by family members.
   3. Their use and interpretation is the same from state to state.
   4. They are legally binding documents.

7. **Nurse participation in assisted suicide and euthanasia:**
   1. Is not within the acceptable ethical standards and practice of nursing
   2. Is permitted in all states when the death is attended by a qualified physician
   3. Can be carried out with the written consent of family members
   4. Requires advanced practice certification

8. **The first step in resolving any ethical dilemma is to:**
   1. Talk with the patient to determine the issues
   2. Find out what the legal and moral issues are
   3. Get the medical facts and all related information
   4. Assess the options for resolution of the dilemma

9. **The primary purpose of an ethics committee is to:**
   1. Determine what should be done to resolve the dilemma

2. Coordinate the efforts of the health care team
3. Determine the legal implications for the hospital
4. Assist the patient, the family, or both with making their own decisions

10. **The role (or roles) of the nurse in any ethical dilemma is:**
    1. To assist family members and the patient, if appropriate, to solve their dilemmas
    2. To tell the family members the decision that the nurse believes is best
    3. To report research to families in order to influence their final decisions
    4. To screen patients and families from interventions by ethics committees

ANSWERS

1. **Answer: 1**
   Rationale: Deontology suggests that certain things are right or wrong, regardless of their consequences.

2. **Answer: 4**
   Rationale: Our ethical beliefs come from many sources throughout our lives and are influenced directly by the systems and societies in which we live.

3. **Answer: 2**
   Rationale: The two applicable principles in this case are not to do harm and truth telling.

4. **Answer: 4**
   Rationale: Use of the code is nonnegotiable in nursing practice.

5. **Answer: 1**
   Rationale: This law applies to all health care programs, providers, and agencies.

6. **Answer: 1**
   Rationale: Patients have a right to change advance directives. Advance directives interpretation vary from state to state.

7. **Answer: 1**
   Rationale: Assisted suicide and euthanasia are violations of the Code of Ethics for Nurses.

8. **Answer: 3**
   Rationale: The first step is to get the facts on medical information, the prognosis, and the various sociocultural, religious, and related elements.

9. **Answer: 4**
   Rationale: The ethics committee serves in a consulting role to help other people make their own decisions.

10. **Answer: 1**
    Rationale: The nurse provides support to allow patients and families to make their own decisions.

WEB SITE RESOURCES FOR INFORMATION ON ETHICS ISSUES

AMA Institute for Ethics
- http://www.ama-assn.org/ama/pub/category/2558.html

American Association of Critical-Care Nurses
- http://www.aacn.org/AACN/aacnhome.nsf/vwdoc/AboutAACN

Classic Texts in Ethics
- http://ethics.acusd.edu/books.html

Codes of Ethics in Health Care
- http://ethics.iit.edu/codes/health.html

Ethics Resource Center
- http://www.ethics.org/

Kennedy Institute of Ethics
- http://kennedyinstitute.georgetown.edu/index.htm

National Institute of Ethics
- http://www.ethicsinstitute.com/

Normative Ethics and Principles
- http://www.stedwards.edu/ursery/norm.htm

WEB SITE RESOURCES FOR INFORMATION ON ETHICS ISSUES–cont'd

NYSNA Position Statement: Role of the Registered Professional Nurse in Ethical Decision-Making
- http://www.nysna.org/programs/nai/practice/positions/position6.htm

Online Guide to Ethics and Moral Philosophy
- http://caae.phil.cmu.edu/Cavalier/80130/

Religious Beliefs Affecting Health Care Resource
- http://www.healthsystem.virginia.edu/internet/chaplaincy/rbpahc.cfm

The Philosophy of Ethics
- http://www.philosophyarchive.com/concept.php?philosophy=Ethics

The Hasting Center
- http://www.thehastingscenter.org/

The Kenan Institute for Ethics
- http://kenan.ethics.duke.edu

World Cultures at Yahoo
- http://dir.yahoo.com/Society_and_Culture/Cultures_and_Groups/Cultures/

World Cultures
- http://www.wsu.edu:8080/~dee/WORLD.HTM

World Religions Online Guide
- http://www.world-religions.info/

Wikipedia Online Encyclopedia
- http://en.wikipedia.org/wiki/Ethics

From Schroeter, K., & Gaylor, G. (2006). Ethical considerations in organ donation for critical care nurses. Retrieved July 6, 2006, from http://jeffline.tju.edu/Education/dl/health_policy/syllabus/popup_ccnurse.html

REFERENCES

AACN. (2006). Position statement: Moral distress. Retrieved July 9, 2006, from http://www.aacn.org/AACN/pubpolcy.nsf/Files/MDPS/$file/Moral%20Distress%20_1_7.8.06.pdf.

AACN. (2005). Public policy: Role of the critical care nurse. Retrieved April 24, 2006, from http://www.aacn.org.

American Cancer Society (ACS). (2006). Complementary and alternative therapies. Retrieved July 9, 2006, from http://www.cancer.org/docroot/ETO/ETO_5.asp?sitearea=ETO.

American Holistic Nurses Association (AHNA). (2004). Position on the role of nurses in the practice of complementary and alternative therapies. Retrieved February 8, 2006. from http://www.ahna.org/about/statements.html.

AHRQ. (2002). Fact sheet: Health care costs. Retrieved July 7, 2006, from http://www.ahrq.gov/news/costsfact.htm.

ANA. (2005). Position statements: Privacy and confidentiality. Retrieved April 24, 2006, from http://nursingworld.org/readroom/position/ethics/etprivcy.htm.

ANA. (2003a). Position statement: Pain management and control of distressing symptoms in dying patients. Retrieved July 8, 2006, from http://www.nursingworld.org/readroom/position/ethics/etpain.htm.

ANA. (2003b). Position statement: Nursing care and do-not-resuscitate (DNR) decisions. Retrieved July 9, 2006, from http://www.nursingworld.org/readroom/position/ethics/etdnr.htm.

ANA. (2001). *Code of ethics for nurses with interpretive statements.* Silver Spring, MD: ANA.

ANA. (1994a). Position statement: Assisted suicide. Retrieved July 9, 2006, from http://www.nursingworld.org/readroom/position/ethics/etsuic.htm.

ANA. (1994b). *Position statement: The nonnegotiable nature of the ANA Code for Nurses with Interpretive Statements.* Washington, DC: ANA.

ANA. (1992). *Position statement: Foregoing nutrition and hydration.* Washington, DC: ANA.

ANA. (1991a). Ethics and human rights position statements: Ethics and human rights. Retrieved April 24, 2006, from http://nursingworld.org/readroom/position/ethics/prtetethr.htm.

ANA. (1991b). *Position statement: Nursing and the Patient Self-Determination Act.* Washington, DC: ANA.

Blake, C. (1996). *Nurses' reflections on ethical decision-making.* Fordham University (EdD, Dissertation).

Burkhardt, M., & Nathaniel, A. (2002). *Ethics and issues in contemporary nursing.* (2nd ed.). Clifton Park, NY: Delmar, Thomson Learning.

Elpern, E., Covert, B., & Kleinpell, R. (2005). Moral distress of staff nurses in a medical intensive care unit. *American Journal of Critical Care, 14*(6):523-530.

Farber, N., Simpson, P., & Salam, T., et al. (2006). Physicians' decisions to withhold and withdraw life-sustaining treatment. *Archives of Internal Medicine, 166*(5):560-564.

Federal Register. (2003). Health insurance reform: Security standards. Retrieved May 18, 2007 from http://aspe.hhs.gov/admnsimp/.

Fleck, L. (2006). The costs of caring: Who pays? Who profits? Who panders?. *Hastings Center Report, 36*(3):13-17.

Fowler, M. (1990). Reflections on ethics consultation in critical care. *Nursing Clinics of North America, 2*(3):431-435.

Fowler, M., & Levine-Ariff, J. (Eds.), (1987). *Ethics at the bedside: A source book for the critical care nurse.* Philadelphia: J. B. Lippincott.

Fowler, M. (1986). The role of the clinical ethicist. *Heart & Lung, 15*(3):318-319.

Freer, J. (1997). Ethics Committee core curriculum: How to perform an ethics consult. UB Center for Clinical Ethics and Humanities in Health Care. Retrieved May 18, 2006, from http://wings.buffalo.edu/faculty/research/bioethics/man-case.html.

GDP. (2006). Fact sheet: Health care costs—background. Retrieved July 7, 2006, from http://www.ahrq.gov/news/costsfact.htm. no date

Gillick, M. (2006). The use of advance care planning to guide decisions about artificial nutrition and hydration. *Nutrition in Clinical Practice, 21*(2):126-133.

Health Privacy Project. (2000). Health privacy: Know your rights. Retrieved May 23, 2006, from http://www.healthprivacy.org.

Heffler, S., Smith, S., & Keehan, S., et al. (2005). Trends: U. S. health spending projections for 2004–2014. *Health Affairs, 23:*W5-W74.

Heland, M. (2006). Fruitful or futile: Intensive care nurses' experiences and perceptions of medical futility. *Australian Critical Care, 19*(1):25-31.

Higgins, R., & Lemke, S. (1995). Ethics committees in Southern Baptist–related hospitals: Survey results and analysis. Paper presented at the American Academy of Religion, Dallas, Texas, 1995. Retrieved May 18, 2006, from http://www.nobts.edu/Faculty/ItoR/LemkeSW/Personal/ecsurvey.html. Author only provided a year presented

HIPAA. (2006). Title II, the Health Insurance Portability and Accountability Act of 1996. Retrieved 5/23/2006 from http://www.hipaa.org.

ICN. (2000). *The ICN code of ethics for nurses.* Geneva: ICN.

Jecker, N. (1997). Principles and methods of ethical decision making in critical care nursing. *Critical Care Nursing Clinics of North America, 9*(1):29-33.

Kyba, F. (2002). Legal and ethical issues in end-of-life care. *Critical Care Nursing Clinics of North America, 14*(2):141-155.

Martin, J. (1993). Lying to patients: Can it ever be justified. *Nursing Standard, 7*(18):29-31.

Meeker, M., & Jezewski, M. (2005). Family decision making at end of life. *Palliative & Supportive Care, 3*(2):131-142.

MHECN. (2005). The Maryland Healthcare Ethics Committee Network. University of Maryland School of Law. Retrieved May 18, 2006, from That's it. http://www.law.umaryland.edu/specialty/mhecn/index.asp.

Moral Philosophy.info. (2005). Metaethics. Retrieved May 2, 2006, from http://www.moralphilosophy.info/html.

National Hospice and Palliative Care Organization (NHPCO). (n. d.). Glossary of terms about end-of-life decision-making: Caring connections. Retrieved May 24, 2006, from http://www.caringinfo.org.

NPR. (2006). Doctors, nurses charged in post-Katrina deaths. National Public Radio, July 18, 2006. Retrieved July 25, 2006, from http://www.npr.org/documents/2006/jul/nolacharges.pdf.

ONS. (2004a). *Position statement: Cancer research and cancer clinical trials.* Pittsburgh: Oncology Nursing Society.

ONS. (2004b). Oncology Nursing Society position on the nurse's response to the patient requesting assisted suicide. Retrieved July 8, 2006, from http://www.ons.org/publications/positions/AssistedSuicide.shtml.

O'Rourke, K. (1983). Ethics committees in hospitals. Retrieved May 18, 2006, from http://www.op.org/domcentral/study/kor/83050409.htm.

Pellegrino, E. (2005). Decisions at the end of life: The abuse of the concept of futility. *Practical Bioethics,* *1*(3):3-6.

Reynolds, S., Cooper, A., & McKneally, M. (2005). Withdrawing life-sustaining treatment: Ethical considerations. *Thoracic Surgery Clinics, 15*(4):469-480.

Robert Wood Johnson Foundation (RWJF). (2006). *When patients cannot eat or drink: Understanding artificial nutrition and hydration.* Princeton, NJ: Robert Wood Johnson Foundation.

Scanlon, C., & Rushton, C. (1996). Assisted suicide: Clinical realities and ethical challenges. *American Journal of Critical Care, 5*(6):397-403.

Sayers, G., & Perera, S. (2002). Withholding life prolonging treatment, and self deception. *Journal of Medical Ethics, 28*(6):347-352.

Turkoski, B. (2001). Ethics in the absence of truth. *Home Healthcare Nurse, 19*(4):218-222.

van Rooyen, D., Elfick, M., & Strumpher, J. (2005). Registered nurses' experiences of the withdrawal of treatment from the critically ill patient in an intensive care unit. *South African Journal of Nursing, 28*(1):42-51.

FEVER

ANGELA L. DANIEL

PATHOPHYSIOLOGICAL MECHANISMS

The human body uses a complex interaction of systems to maintain homeostasis. As a component of homeostasis, the body maintains a temperature between 36.1° C (97° F) and 37.4° C (99.3° F), with cyclic fluctuations throughout the day. Variations above or below these "normal" parameters can be a signal of disease. For the patient with cancer, fever may be defined as one temperature reading greater than 38.3° C (101° F) or three readings, 1 hour or more apart, greater than 38° C (100.4 °F) within 24 hours (Dalal & Zhukovsky, 2006). It is imperative to recognize that for the patient with cancer, especially the patient with neutropenia, fever may be the initial and only indicator of a change in status and a need for immediate intervention.

Elevation of the core body temperature has long been recognized as a symptom of the onset of disease. However, an elevated temperature is a single component of a larger and more complex physiologic response to disease called the *febrile response* (Fig. 16.1). During the febrile response, a complex interaction of immunologic, endocrine, behavioral, neural, and cytokine-mediated processes occurs to alter the body's temperature (Mackowiak, 2006). These systems are coordinated by the hypothalamus to maintain a homeostatic core body temperature.

The hypothalamus is considered the thermostat for the body, and it is an integral component of the febrile response. The body normally maintains temperature through the balanced production and dissipation of heat. However, external factors, such as an increased external temperature or the introduction of endogenous or exogenous pyrogens, can cause regulatory malfunction in the hypothalamus, resulting in a hyperthermic state. During this hyperthermic state, or fever, a new hypothalamic set point is initiated for the body's core temperature.

Fever has three routinely accepted phases: chill, fever, and flush. During the initial chill phase, the sympathetic nervous system is activated and vasoconstriction occurs in the cutaneous blood vessels. Shivering may begin to generate heat through muscle activation. Sweat production is inhibited and neurotransmitters are secreted, leading to increases in cell metabolism, heat production, and body temperature (Dalal & Zhukovsky, 2006). During this initial phase, the individual may perceive himself or herself to be cold and may try to get warm, perhaps by using blankets or putting on extra clothing. These behavioral actions contribute to heat conservation and raise the body's core temperature to the new set point. However, in a patient with cancer, the immune system may be blunted to such an extent that the person is unable to mount even the first sign of infection or a mild febrile response. In addition, patients with cancer are subject to polypharmacy; antipyretics may be given before a blood transfusion, and corticosteroids may be used to reduce inflammation. All these factors may diminish the body's ability to recognize a pyrogen and release the appropriate mediators to initiate a febrile response.

Once the new hyperthermic set point is reached, heat production is balanced by heat loss, and the body maintains this temperature through negative feedback mechanisms. Heat-sensitive receptors in the hypothalamus and throughout the body recognize the

Febrile Response

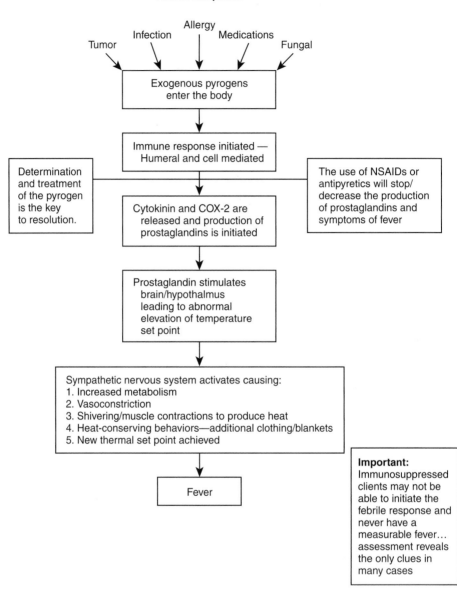

Fig. 16.1 • The febrile response.

elevated temperature and reduce the stimulation of the sympathetic nervous system, thereby maintaining the newly elevated body temperature. This is the second, or fever, phase.

In the final phase of fever, the flush phase, the hypothalamus recognizes resolution of the cause of the elevated temperature and returns to the routine body temperature. Once the pyrogens and toxins have been controlled or antipyretic therapy has been initiated, the hypothalamus initiates a reverse cycle in which the sympathetic nervous system is inhibited.

This causes cutaneous vasodilation, diaphoresis, and a decrease in cell metabolism. These mechanisms promote heat loss and the body's return to the new, lower set point.

Cytokine Mediators

When exogenous pyrogens enter a host, an inflammatory response is initiated. Macrophages and phagocytic cells recognize an invader, and proinflammatory cytokinines are produced and released into the circulation, stimulating the production of prostaglandins. The cytokinines include interleukins 1B (IL-1B), 6 (IL-6), interferon, and tumor necrosis factor (TNF). In addition to producing prostaglandins, these cytokinin mediators are thought to stimulate central production of the inducible enzyme cyclooxygenase-2 (COX-2) (Dalal & Zhukovsky, 2006). Current research suggests that it is this prostaglandin production that activates the thermoregulatory aspects of the hypothalamus and begins the febrile response and fever. Another factor is that a person loses about 1% of the body's immune function each year after age 30; therefore a person who is 80 years old has about 50% of his or her original immunity, which leads to lower regulation levels.

EPIDEMIOLOGY AND ETIOLOGY

Patients with cancer are a subgroup of patients who may be both immunocompromised and physically debilitated (Smeltzer & Barel, 2004). Consequently, recognizing and diagnosing the cause of fever in a patient with cancer often is a difficult and time-consuming endeavor. In these patients, the signs and symptoms that signal a change in their condition may be subtle and difficult to differentiate. It is imperative that clinicians be alert for and recognize subtle signs and symptoms and that they evaluate each as the potential initiator of fever.

Typically, fever in the oncology patient is caused by infection, the tumor itself (paraneoplastic fever), medications, blood product transfusions, and graft versus host disease. Other, less frequent causes include narcotic drug withdrawal (specifically benzodiazepines), neuroleptic malignant syndrome, and obstruction of a viscus organ (e.g., bowel or bladder). In addition, co-morbid conditions should be evaluated as a cause of fever. Cerebrovascular accidents, thrombosis, and connective tissue disorders may also induce a hyperthermic state.

Infection

Infection is one of the most common causes of fever in patients with cancer, and it is associated with high rates of morbidity and mortality. Without rapid intervention and treatment (i.e., within 48 hours), the mortality rate among patients with cancer who have a fever caused by infection can be as high as 70%. The severity of infection is inversely proportional to the number of circulating neutrophils; therefore patients who are neutropenic are at a much higher risk for more frequent and severe infections than patients who are not immunocompromised. In patients with neutropenia (defined by an absolute neutrophil count [ANC] of less than 500 cells/mm^3), fever should be considered an absolute emergency and intervention begun immediately. An additional factor in predicting outcomes is the nadir of the neutropenic causative agent and the nadir of the neutropenia itself. An antineoplastic agent with a short nadir leads to rapid depletion of neutrophils and puts the patient at much higher risk of infection, sepsis, and death. One area that requires continued research in oncology is the relationship between chemotherapeutic agent nadirs and patients' risk for neutropenia. Certain chemotherapeutic regimens (Crawford et al., 2005) correlate with a higher risk of neutropenia (Table 16-1). Research seems to support the prophylactic use of colony-stimulating factors in these high-risk patients (Rolston, 2004).

Neutropenic patients are at the highest risk for infection (Baden & Rubin, 2002). The organisms that cause the infections are related to the geographic and site-specific origin of

Table 16-1	CHEMOTHERAPEUTIC AGENTS CORRELATED WITH A HIGHER RISK OF NEUTROPENIA	
Type of Cancer	**Treatment**
Breast cancer	Doxorubicin, cyclophosphamide, docetaxel (ACT)
	Doxorubicin, paclitaxel (AT)
	Docetaxel, doxorubicin, cyclophosphamide (TAC)
Non-Hodgkin's lymphoma	Vincristine, doxorubicin, prednisone, etoposide, bleomycin, cyclophosphamide (VAPEC-B)
	Dexamethasone, cisplatin, cytarabine (DHAP)
	Etoposide, methylprednisolone, cisplatin, cytarabine (ESHAP)
Ovarian cancer	Topotecan
	Paclitaxel
	Docetaxel
Testicular cancer	Vinblastine, ifosfamide, cisplatin (VIP)
Non-small cell lung cancer	Cyclophosphamide, doxorubicin, etoposide (CAE)
	Topotecan
	Topotecan, paclitaxel (Top T)

Data from Crawford, J., Althaus, B., Armitage, J., et al. (2005). The NCCN 2005 myeloid growth factors clinical practice guidelines in oncology. *Journal National Cancer Network, 3*(4):540–555.

the infection. The most common sites of infection in patients with cancer are the pharynx, lower esophagus, lung, perineum, anus, eye, skin, periodontium, vascular catheter access sites, and tissue around the nails (Urabe, 2004). Some common organisms have been associated with specific sites (Table 16-2) (Hughes et al., 2002). The clinician should pay close attention to these sites and inspect and evaluate any redness, tenderness, drainage, or abnormal conditions. As mentioned, in oncology patients the body's ability to mount an effective immune response may be significantly blunted, and subtle abnormalities may be the only signal of infection.

A significant proportion of the fever-causing infections in patients with cancer now are gram positive in nature. The main culprits are staphylococci (*S. aureus* and *S. epidermidis*), streptococci (e.g., *S. pneumoniae*, a common cause of pneumococcal pneumonia), enterococci, and strep A and B. These organisms must be treated; however, immediate initiation of a glycopeptide antimicrobial (vancomycin) is not necessarily required unless the patient's symptoms are consistent with sepsis or an exact pathogen has been identified.

Gram-negative organisms are a less likely pathogen in patients with cancer. However, gram-negative bacilli and cocci are potentially the most deadly and therefore require

Table 16-2	COMMON SITES, CAUSES, AND SYMPTOMS OF INFECTION	
Site	**Cause**	**Symptoms**
Cutaneous	*S. aureus, streptococci*	Cellulitis, abscesses, folliculitis
Pulmonary	*S. aureus, P. aeruginosa*	Adventitious breath sounds, cough,
	H. influenzae, S. pneumoniae	fever, dyspnea
Sepsis	*S. aureus, P. aeruginosa,*	Hypotension, tachycardia,
	Enterobacter spp.	decreased mentation,
		nausea/vomiting
UTI	*E. coli*	Urgency and frequency in voiding
Insertion sites/catheters	*S. aureus*/coagulase negative Staphylococci, *P. aeruginosa*	Redness at site and sepsis symptoms

Data from Hughes, W., Armstrong, D., & Bodye., G., et al. (2002). 2002 Guidelines for the use of antimicrobial agents in neutropenic patients with cancer. *Clinical Infectious Diseases, 34*(6):730–751.

immediate treatment to prevent sepsis and progression. Because gram-negative organisms can be isolated from multiple sites in a patient with cancer, the sites of origin (e.g., urinary tract, pulmonary and gastrointestinal tracts) must be evaluated extensively for potential infection-causing organisms. Gram-negative organisms (e.g., *Escherichia coli* and *Klebsiella* and *Pseudomonas* spp.) require immediate, broad-spectrum antimicrobial coverage because of the potentially rapid and overwhelming effects of sepsis in a patient with cancer. Even though gram-positive organisms are seen more often in these patients, progression of gram-negative infections is associated with a higher mortality rate (Klastersky, 2004).

Fungal Infections

During the initial neutropenic episode, bacterial infections are most prevalent. However, as the host remains neutropenic, the risk for fungal infections increases. Fungal infections in a patient with cancer can be either a primary cause of illness or a secondary opportunistic infection that occurs in a patient being treated with antimicrobials. By far the most common cause of fungal infections is *Candida albicans,* and *Aspergillus* organisms are a distant second (Wingard, 2004). In a patient with fever, especially a neutropenic patient, fungal infection is often seen when the patient is not responding to broad-spectrum anti-microbial therapy. The clinical manifestations of both *Candida* and *Aspergillus* infections have a high likelihood of fever associated with infection (Wingard, 2004) and may mimic symptoms of a bacterial infection.

A continuing challenge for health care providers is how to rapidly identify patients experiencing fever who are potentially neutropenic and in need of antifungal therapy. In the past, empiric antifungal therapy usually consisted of deoxycholate (amphotericin B [Amp B]). However, this antifungal medication has been associated with serious toxicities, including nephrotoxicity, phlebitis at the infusion site, and anemia. Although amphotericin B is still used, newer antifungals have emerged. Among these are the "azoles" (e.g., fluconazole, itraconazole, ketoconazole, and voriconazole), which have been shown to have fewer toxicities (Wingard, 2004). However, as with any medication regimen, the patient's response to treatment must be monitored continuously and adjusted as necessary.

Paraneoplastic Fever

Fever is a common associated illness with some cancers and may parallel the progression of the tumor or cancer. Paraneoplastic fevers are most often associated with Hodgkin's lymphoma. However, several other types of cancer are coming to be associated with paraneoplastic fever. Cancers such as acute leukemia, lymphoma, renal cell carcinoma, bone sarcoma, adrenal carcinoma, and pheochromocytoma are associated with paraneoplastic fever. Cancers involving solid tumors (e.g., breast, lung, and colon cancers) are not normally associated with this type of fever (Dalal & Zhukovsky, 2006). The definitive treatment for paraneoplastic fever is treatment of the underlying malignancy. In the absence of effective antineoplastic therapy, treatment with nonsteroidal antiinflammatory drugs (NSAIDs) is the treatment of choice. A common choice of NSAID for this type of fever is naproxen (Naprosyn), and response to initiation of this therapy has been used to diagnose tumor-associated fevers. However, chronic use of NSAIDs may cause bleeding problems, therefore the patient needs continued follow-up and teaching regarding the signs and symptoms of undesired bleeding, such as black, tarry stools, excessive bruising, and worsening or abnormal fatigue. These symptoms should be reported to the caregiver immediately.

Medication-Related Fever

The diagnosis of medication-induced fever in an oncology patient is often a diagnosis of exclusion, except for specific medications (Box 16-1). These include biologic modifiers (interferon, TNF), bleomycin, and amphotericin B. These drugs routinely cause fevers, and the patient may need to be treated prophylactically before initiation of therapy. Premedication with NSAIDs, acetaminophen, or corticosteroids may lessen the fever. In most cases, a fever related to medication administration resolves once the drug therapy is stopped. Other medications that may cause fever are antibiotics, cardiac medications, antiseizure medications, cytotoxics, and growth factors. In a review study, antibiotic therapy accounted for approximately 31% of drug-related fevers (Dalal & Zhukovsky, 2006). However, patients with cancer are not exempt from cardiovascular disease, diabetes, seizures, and infection, therefore the medications used to treat these conditions should routinely be evaluated in cases of suspected medication-induced fever.

Blood Product–Related Fever

Patients with cancer often are treated with antineoplastic medications aimed at killing the rapidly multiplying cancer cells. Because these therapies may also deplete the patient's blood counts, multiple transfusions of blood products may be required. Fever in response to transfusions is not uncommon in oncology patients. The febrile response is thought to be a result of antibody production by the body as a defense against antigens on the donors' cells and the resulting inflammatory response. The more transfusions a patient receives, the greater the likelihood of a febrile reaction. Treatment of this type of fever includes premedication with acetaminophen and diphenhydramine. In addition, use of blood products that have been irradiated and depleted of leukocytes can minimize these reactions.

BOX 16-1	MEDICATIONS THAT MAY CAUSE FEVER

5-Flucytosine (Ancobon)
Acycloguanosine (Acyclovir)
Allopurinol (Zyloprim)
Deoxycholate (Amphotericin B)
Bleomycin
Captopril (Capoten)
Cimetidine (Tagamet)
Clofibrate (Clofarabine)
Erythromycin (Ery-tab, Eryc, EES)
Fluconazole (Diflucan)
Heparin sodium
Hydralazine (Apresoline)
Hydrochlorothiazide (HCTZ)
Immunoglobulins (Carimune, Gamunex, Gammagard, BayGam, Flebogamma, RhoGAM, Panglobulin, Polygamy)
Interferons (Avonex, Alferon, Intron, Roferon, Infergen, Rebetron, Rebif, Betaseron, Actimmune)
Isoniazid (INH)
Meperidine (Demerol)
Methotrexate (MTX)
Methyldopa (Aldomet)
Nifedipine (Procardia)
Nitrofurantoin (Marcobid, Macrodantin)
Penicillin's (Bicillin, Amoxil, Augmentin, Unasyn, Zosyn, Timentin)
Phenytoin (Dilantin)
Procainamide (Procanbid)
Vaccines (Attenuvax, Comvax, Harvix, Meruvax, M-M-R II, Pneumovax, Prevnar, rabies vaccine, Varivax)

RISK PROFILE

The risk of negative outcomes associated with fever in a patient with cancer directly correlates with the patient's immune status and exposure to infective agents. As discussed previously, a patient with protracted neutropenia or one who is prescribed an antineoplastic agent with a longer nadir has a greater potential for infection and thus the potential for fever. Patients with cancer who are more at risk for infection and fever can be divided into three categories based on (1) the local epidemiology, with the highest risk seen in hospitalized patients; (2) the type of cancer for which the patient is undergoing treatment, with the highest risk seen in patients with leukemia, lymphoma, brain tumors, or sarcoma; and (3) the patient's condition at the time of infection, with the highest risk seen in patients who are physically debilitated or at the lowest point in the nadir.

To use the local epidemiology as part of the evaluation and treatment of a patient with fever, the patient's local environment must be assessed. More precisely, this is the environment in which the patient was exposed to the causative agent or became ill. Such areas include the health care environment and the community environment. The two environments have similar patterns, but their circumstances may dictate different courses of treatment. For example, with nosocomial infections, antibiotics may prove less efficacious, and multiple protocols may be initiated because the organisms may have developed resistance to routine antibiotics. Community-acquired infections may involve more virulent toxins, but they may respond to treatment more quickly. Education of the patient at higher risk for community-acquired infections should center around hygiene (e.g., hand washing), good housekeeping skills, and the need to change furnace and air conditioning filters every month or as specified by the appliance's manufacturer.

Risk for Nosocomial Infections

- Severe, ongoing illness, such as diabetes, cardiovascular disease, renal disease, and respiratory disease (e.g., COPD, asthma)
- Previous treatment with antimicrobial agents
- Immunosuppression
- Invasive procedures, such as insertion of a central IV line or a Foley catheter
- Advanced age (over 60 years old)
- Repeated contact with any health care system

Risk for Community-Acquired Infection

- Severe, ongoing illness, such as COPD, asthma, diabetes, cardiovascular disease, and renal disease
- Immunosuppression
- Crowded living environment or exposure to crowds in malls or shopping areas
- Exposure to child care and children
- Poor hygiene, especially around tubes and skin folds
- International travel or exposure to individuals returning from travel
- Recent vaccination with live vaccines

Risk Associated with Cancer Type

The type of cancer is an additional factor for fever. Patients at higher risk for fever related to the malignancy are those with:

- Malignancy that affects the humeral immune system (e.g., Hodgkin disease and non-Hodgkin lymphoma)

- Tumors that produce antigens, which elicit an immune response (e.g., renal cell carcinoma, pheochromocytoma)
- Brain tumors that affect the thermoregulatory center of the brain
- Metastatic disease to the liver from a primary site, such as the breast, bone, or colon
- Malignancies that affect the blood, such as leukemia (ALL, ALM, hairy cell, CLL, CLM) and essential thrombocytopenia

The cause of fever cannot be differentiated based on the tumor type. However, the practitioner who knows that some patients are at higher risk for fever from sources other than infection can make more precise assessments and evaluations.

Risk Associated with the Patient's Condition

Patients at higher risk for fever from infection have some common traits, including the following:

- Immunosuppression resulting from bone marrow suppression caused by chemotherapy or radiation therapy
- Neutropenia (ANC less than 500 mm^3)
- Impaired phagocyte function or other deficits in the immune response
- Alteration in the external physical defense barriers (e.g., skin integrity, mucosa, presence of a surgical incision)
- Splenic dysfunction
- Impairment of T-lymphocyte and phagocyte function as a result of irradiation or radiotherapy
- Dehydration, in which hypernatremia or a loss of fluid affects the hypothalamus and temperature regulation

PROGNOSIS

The prognosis for febrile patients with cancer is directly correlated with the patient's condition and the length of time to initiation of treatment. Patients with cancer often are febrile at home and do not turn to the health care system immediately. Clinical practitioners recognize that prompt intervention and treatment of the patient with cancer is imperative and that initiation of antimicrobial therapy in the febrile neutropenic patient reduces mortality and morbidity in these patients (Nirenberg et al., 2004). As response times have improved, and health care providers increasingly have recognized the emergent nature of fever in a patient with cancer, mortality rates have declined; fewer than 10% of febrile neutropenic patients succumb to the infection after initiation of prompt treatment (Nirenberg et al., 2004). Key points of the treatment strategy for patients with cancer are (1) determining the accurate course of treatment in the febrile patient and (2) beginning antimicrobial therapy within 12 to 24 hours of the onset of fever in neutropenic patients. Because mortality rates from fever can run as high as 75% in neutropenic patients, a fever that goes untreated for 48 hours after onset is an absolute emergency and should be treated as such.

PROFESSIONAL ASSESSMENT CRITERIA (PAC)

Rapid, focused assessment of the febrile patient is an essential part of treatment. Advanced practice nurses should perform a thorough examination to determine a focal cause of the fever, including obtaining subjective and objective data.

Subjective Data

1. Presenting symptoms: onset, exacerbating factors, controlling factors, associated symptoms
2. Length of treatment for and diagnosis of cancer
3. Nature and duration of antineoplastic therapy
4. Previous infections and treatment with antibiotics
5. History of fevers associated with disease or tumor
6. Previous medical procedures and recent injections or venipunctures
7. Allergies and drug reactions
8. Last hospitalization or exposure to crowds
9. History of travel or exposure to insects or animals

Objective Data

1. Physical examination (initially and daily)
   - Vital signs: tachycardia, hypotension, fever
   - General appearance: pale, flushed, lethargic
   - Neurologic examination for deficits or changes
   - Integumentary evaluation for rashes, lesions, redness, or otherwise abnormal areas
   - Oral examination for mucosal integrity or lesions
   - Sinus palpation for tenderness or drainage
   - Palpation of lymph nodes for size and tenderness
   - Pulmonary evaluation for adventitious or decreased breath sounds
   - Cardiac evaluation for S1/S2, murmurs, rate, rhythm, presence of rub
   - Abdomen for bowel sounds, masses, tenderness, or rebound
   - CVA tenderness posteriorly
   - Urogenital and perirectal examination for skin integrity and lesions or tenderness
2. Blood culture ×2 for bacteria and fungi
   - Blood culture from each catheter lumen or port (if placed); one peripheral blood culture
3. CBC with differential, ANC, electrolytes, liver and renal function studies
4. Chest x-ray film if symptoms are present or in any case of suspicion
5. Sputum and wound cultures
6. Urinalysis and culture

   NOTE: *Cultures should be collected immediately, before antibiotic therapy is initiated. Do NOT wait for results of cultures before initiating antimicrobial therapy.*

   Assessment, evaluation, and consideration of even the slightest abnormal finding could lead to diagnosis in patients who are immunocompromised. These patients often are unable to mount a full-scale immune response, therefore they may not show the signs and symptoms expected in an uncompromised patient.

NURSING CARE AND TREATMENT

In the patient with cancer, the hallmark of effective treatment is rapid assessment and differentiation of potential causes of fever. The most effective treatment for fever is treatment of the underlying causative agent. In the neutropenic patient, the causative agent most likely is infectious. In neutropenic and immunosuppressed patients, prompt empiric initiation of broad-spectrum antimicrobial therapy is recognized as an essential component of effective therapy (Box 16-2) (Baltic et al, 2002).

In addition, treatment for fever in a patient with cancer, especially one who does not respond to antimicrobial therapy, should include evaluation for fungal infection. Fungal infections may present similarly to bacterial infections, but they do not respond to antimicrobial therapy. In such cases, initiation of an antifungal drug, such as intravenous deoxycholate (amphotericin B) or fluconazole (Nizoral), is the treatment of choice.

Antipyretics

The use of antipyretics cannot be overlooked in the treatment of fever in patients with cancer. Fever may enhance the body's defense mechanisms, and although antipyretics may suppress the fever and its uncomfortable side effects, the causative agent remains, and evaluation should continue. Antipyretic medications do not treat the cause of the fever; they may relieve symptoms and assist the body in recovering or recuperating from the increased metabolic demands initiated by a fever. Each degree of elevation in temperature results in a 7% increase in the metabolic rate and increased demands on the heart (Ezzone, 2000).

BOX 16-2   **GUIDELINES FOR INITIATING ANTIMICROBIAL THERAPY IN THE NEUTROPENIC OR IMMUNOSUPPRESSED PATIENT**

Regimen 1
Treatment with oral antibiotics in low-risk patients who:
- Show no neurologic or mental changes.
- Show no absolute focus of bacterial infection, or signs or symptoms of systemic infection.
- Have a suspected length and resolution of neutropenia within 7 to 10 days.
- Have a malignancy in remission.
- Have a negative chest x-ray film (CXR)
- Do not have an intravenous catheter site infection.
Medications: Quinolone-based combinations, such as ciprofloxacin plus amoxicillin-clavulanate.

Regimen 2
Treatment with a single antimicrobial agent given intravenously:
- Considered as effective as multidrug therapy in uncomplicated episodes of febrile neutropenia.
- Requires close monitoring for adverse reactions, drug resistance, and secondary infections.
Medications: A third- or fourth-generation cephalosporin, such as ceftazidime (Fortaz) or cefepime (Maxipime), or a carbapenem (imipenem-cilastatin or meropenem).

Regimen 3
Treatment using a multidrug approach without a glycopeptide (vancomycin):
- Has potential synergistic action against gram-negative organisms, and little drug resistance is generated during therapy.
- Disadvantages include lack of efficacy against gram-positive organisms.
- Assess closely for nephrotoxicity with use of aminoglycosides.
Medications: An aminoglycoside (gentamicin, tobramycin, or amikacin) with an antipseudomonal carboxypenicillin or ureidopenicillin (ticarcillin-clavulanic acid or piperacillin). A second combination may include an aminoglycoside with ceftazidime.

Regimen 4
Treatment using a multidrug approach with a glycopeptide (vancomycin):
- Limited use related to emerging vancomycin-resistant gram-positive organisms.
- Vancomycin should be used in cases involving:
1 Clinically suspected, serious catheter-related infections.
2 Known colonization with penicillin- and cephalosporin-resistance pneumococci or methicillin-resistant *S. aureus* (MRSA).
3 Positive blood culture for gram-positive bacteria.
4 Hypotension or signs of shock (Hughes et al., 2002).
Medications: Medications as listed previously in regimens 1-3, with the addition of vancomycin.

Data from Hughes, W., Armstrong, D., & Bodye., G., et al. (2002). 2002 Guidelines for the use of antimicrobial agents in neutropenic patients with cancer. *Clinical Infectious Disease, 34*(6):730-751.

An elevated temperature is also associated with increased oxygen and nutritional demands. These additional demands are especially significant in debilitated patients with cancer, who can least compensate for the extra demands. Emphasis must be placed on monitoring of fluid and electrolyte status and correcting imbalances and on maintaining cardiac output and homeostasis. In the past it was thought that substantial cardiac stress occurred when the body temperature exceeded 42° C (107.6° F). However, recent research (Robins et al, 2006) has documented that cardiac stress is maximal at temperatures of 39.5° C (103.1° F) to 40° C (104° F). Therefore practitioners should be concerned about the cardiac status of their patients long before temperatures reach 42° C (107.6° F) (Robins et al., 2006).

Acetaminophen and NSAIDS are widely prescribed antipyretics. These medications work by lowering the hypothalamic set point and inhibiting COX production. Salicylates may also be used and have similar results; however, they must be used with extreme caution in patients at risk for thrombocytopenia because of aspirin's effect on platelets. Salicylates should not be the first choice for treatment of patients with gastric ulcers or hepatic or renal disease, patients with clotting disorders, or patients taking anticoagulants. The effects of COX-2 inhibitors (e.g., Celebrex) are similar to those of NSAIDs; however, their side effects are under scrutiny, and these drugs are rarely used as antipyretics.

Fluid Replacement

Fever increases the metabolic demands on the body, and fluid depletion and dehydration may become significant issues. In addition, dehydration may be a cause of fever. Patients with fever should be encouraged to increase their intake of water or juices. In hospitalized patients, intravenous fluid replacement should be initiated for maintenance to prevent dehydration and maintain kidney function.

Comfort Measures

The evaluation and treatment of fever should be prioritized such that the most serious or life-threatening causes are evaluated first. Even so, a patient with fever experiences discomfort from an alteration in body temperature, chills, diaphoresis, joint pain with stiffness, and fatigue. These by themselves may not be life-threatening, but they are symptoms that may significantly alter the patient's quality of life, and comfort measures should be implemented. Comfort measures include light clothing, tepid baths, replacing wet clothing and blankets when necessary, adjusting the ambient temperature in the patient's room for comfort, and preventing drafts (NCI, 2006). Additional measures include applying lubricants to the lips and providing ice chips to keep buccal membranes moist, as well as maintaining an environment conducive to rest.

EVIDENCE-BASED PRACTICE UPDATES

1. Febrile neutropenia (ANC less than 500 mm^3) represents an absolute emergency; initiation of empiric antimicrobial therapy is recommended within 48 hours of the onset of fever (Kanamaru & Tatsumi, 2004).
2. Discontinuation of empiric antimicrobial therapy is directly correlated with the neutrophil count. If the ANC is greater than 500 mm^3 for 2 days and the patient is afebrile for longer than 48 hours without an identified pathogen, discontinuation of therapy may be considered (Hughes et al., 2002).
3. Gram-positive organisms account for 60% to 70% of infections in patients with cancer. However, 15% to 20% of infections in patients with cancer are polymicrobial, and a high percentage have a gram-negative component (Rolston, 2004).

TEACHING AND EDUCATION

Fever: Report temperatures greater than 38.3° C (101° F) to health care provider.

Antipyretics: Take the appropriate dose of these drugs: ibuprofen 400 mg q6-8hr, acetaminophen to a maximum of 4 g/day.

Nutrition: Eat frequent, small, high-calorie meals.

Fluids: Increase fluid intake to 2 to 3 L/day to maintain hydration.

Fatigue: Get adequate rest and short periods of exercise to compensate for fatigue.

Medications: Take all medications as prescribed until the course is completed or the health care provider instructs you to discontinue them.

Signs and symptoms of infection and sepsis: Be alert to small changes in your body that may signal the development of infection and sepsis.

Web sites for information:
- National Cancer Institute: www.cancer.gov
- Alliance of Breast Cancer Organizations: www.nabco.org
- National Ovarian Cancer Coalition: www.ovarian.org
- Alliance for Lung Cancer Support, Advocacy and Education: www.alcase.org
- Medline Plus: http://medlineplus.gov
- Quackwatch: www.quackwatch.org

NURSING DIAGNOSES

While treating the patient and using a focused diagnostic process, nurses have the tools to assist patients beyond the provisions of the strict medical model. Nursing diagnoses allow care to be structured more specifically for each patient. In addition to the patient's needs, they take into account his or her support system and family, enabling the nurse to educate the patient and family about the disease process.

1. **Ineffective thermoregulation** related to infection, transfusion of blood and blood products, tumor, dehydration, and medication administration, as manifested by a temperature greater than 38.3° C (101° F) or three temperatures at least 1 hour apart within a 24-hour period greater than 38° C (100.4° F)
2. **Risk for infection** related to myelosuppression/neutropenia, altered cell-mediated or humeral immune response, exposure to exogenous pathogenic organisms, altered skin integrity, and insertion and maintenance of invasive lines
3. **Imbalanced nutrition: less than body requirements** related to metabolic demands greater than intake, anorexia, cachexia, and malabsorption, as manifested by a decrease in weight of 10% during treatment or the acute episode
4. **Risk for deficient fluid volume** related to decreased PO intake, increased insensible loss during fever, and increased metabolic requirements during fever
5. **Deficient knowledge** related to disease and its progression, assessing signs and symptoms of fever, assessing signs and symptoms of infection, need for rapid assessment and intervention for fever and febrile response, and family involvement in delivery of care in home setting

EVALUATION AND DESIRED OUTCOMES

1. The patient will verbalize and demonstrate two techniques for monitoring his or her temperature.
2. The patient will have no signs or symptoms of infection.
3. The patient will maintain the current body weight and nutritional status.
4. CBC/electrolytes/CXR or other diagnostic tests for infection will improve or be within normal limits.
5. The patient's temperature will be within normal limits: 36.1° C (97° F) to 37.4° C (99.3° F).

DISCHARGE PLANNING AND FOLLOW-UP CARE

- Educate the patient and family about the signs and symptoms of infection in neutropenia.
- Discuss various factors with the family and caregivers to formulate a discharge plan:
  - The patient's current health status
  - Expectations for the course of therapy
  - Expected outcomes
  - Potential complications
  - Potential adverse reactions or effects of therapy
  - Actions to initiate if perceived problems occur
- Discuss symptomatic support of the patient (e.g., oxygen, a feeding tube, pain medication).
- Educate the patient about techniques to avoid exposure to toxic or infectious agents (e.g., avoiding crowds, avoiding children or other people who are or are likely to be ill)
- Teach and have the patient verbalize a protocol for contacting the health care provider if fever or signs of infection are discovered.
- Follow-up with a health care provider should occur within 1 week of discharge from the hospital if the patient is asymptomatic and no other difficulties are noted. However, patient education regarding abnormal signs and symptoms should reinforce the need to contact the health care provider immediately if problems appear. The patient must call the health care provider for each new febrile episode, and ongoing discussion should focus on ways to avoid contact with toxins or infectious agents.

REVIEW QUESTIONS

QUESTIONS

1. The nurse is developing a plan of care for a neutropenic patient being discharged after admission for nausea and vomiting with stomatitis. The nurse recognizes the need for further teaching when the patient states:
   1. "I will need to avoid citrus juices and fruits until I heal."
   2. "I will need to come back to the physician's office next week for a follow-up visit."
   3. "I will need to wash my hands frequently to avoid getting sick."
   4. "I will need to stand 3 to 5 feet away from someone who is coughing."

2. A patient who is receiving chemotherapy for prostate cancer develops myelosuppression. The teaching plan for this patient would include:
   1. Increasing his intake of fresh fruits and vegetables
   2. Treating a sore throat with over-the-counter lozenges

3. Permission to receive a live/attenuated flu vaccine within 5 to 7 days of discharge
4. Washing his hands frequently and avoiding crowds to reduce the potential for infection

3. After a patient receives chemotherapy for breast cancer, her platelet count falls to 98,000/mcL. The term the nurse should use to describe this low platelet count is:
   1. Neutropenia
   2. Leukopenia
   3. Anemia
   4. Thrombocytopenia

4. A patient diagnosed with renal carcinoma is admitted to the emergency department with a temperature of 38.3° C (101° F). The patient's vital signs are as follows: P-116, R-24, BP-106/62, SaO$_2$-92% on room air. The patient's family states that the patient is just not acting like herself. Your immediate nursing action would be to:
   1. Complete a thorough subjective and objective assessment
   2. Initiate antimicrobial therapy immediately upon arrival to the room
   3. Initiate oxygen at 2 L and an IV of NS at 125 mL/hr
   4. Draw three sets of blood cultures and begin narrow-spectrum antimicrobial therapy focused on gram-negative organisms

5. A patient contacts the health care provider with a complaint of fever for the past 24 hours of 37.9° C (100.3° F). The patient is 12 days post chemotherapy, with a nadir of 5 days. He denies having a cough, urinary symptoms, or fatigue. The patient has a prior medical history of seizures treated with Dilantin and supraventricular tachycardia (SVT) after an MI that is controlled with a beta blocker. There is a high index of suspicion that this patient's fever may be caused by:
   1. Infection
   2. Paraneoplastic factors
   3. Medications
   4. Blood transfusions

6. A patient presents with complaints of a fever, which is measured orally as 38.4° C (101.2° F). His lab work is as follows: WBCs, 1200 mcL RBC, 3.2 mil/mcL; platelets, 32,000/mcL. He has NS infusing at 125 mL/hr for hydration. He is dressed in multiple layers of clothing and has three blankets. He requests medication for his fever. You recognize that the best drug choice for this patient is:
   1. Naprosyn
   2. Ibuprofen
   3. Aspirin
   4. Acetaminophen

7. A patient was admitted to the unit 7 days ago with a fever of 38.3° C (101° F). He is 10 days post chemotherapy, with a nadir of 10 days. He is being treated with a broad-spectrum antibiotic but remains febrile after 7 days. His symptoms are essentially unchanged. As this patient's health care provider, you suspect an infection caused by:
   1. A gram-positive organism
   2. A gram-negative organism
   3. A methicillin-resistant gram-negative organism
   4. Pathogenic fungi

8. The nursing diagnosis that would best apply to the patient being discharged from the hospital with stomatitis would be:
   1. Imbalanced nutrition: less than body requirements
   2. Risk for infection
   3. Impaired skin integrity
   4. Risk for imbalanced fluid volume

9. Which of the following statements about COX-2 inhibitors is correct:
   1. COX-2 inhibitors show greater analgesic activity than traditional NSAIDs with less gastric upset.
   2. COX-2 inhibitors do not affect the kidneys.
   3. COX-2 inhibitors show antiinflammatory activity similar to that of the traditional NSAIDs.
   4. COX-2 inhibitors are cardioprotective.

10. **A patient is discharged home, although he is still at high risk for infection. Patient teaching for this individual would include:**
    1. The health care practitioner should be notified within 48 hours if fever presents.
    2. The patient should take his temperature every 4 hours while he is at high risk for infection, and he should call the practitioner if his temperature is 38° C (101° F) or higher.
    3. Tachycardia is a reliable sign of impending infection in conjunction with a fever.
    4. The patient should take his temperature by the axillary method once an hour while he is at high risk for infection, and he should notify the practitioner if his temperature is higher than 37.9° C (100.1° F).

ANSWERS

1. **Answer: 4**
    Rationale: The patient should avoid crowds and people who are ill. A short distance, such as 3 to 5 feet, is not effective in reducing exposure to airborne viruses and bacteria, which can be transmitted through sneezes or coughs.

2. **Answer: 4**
    Rationale: Washing the hands is the first-line and best defense against infection. Chemotherapy affects all types of cells, and the patient should not be vaccinated or eat fruits and fresh vegetables until the myelosuppression has resolved.

3. **Answer: 4**
    Rationale: Thrombocytopenia is the correct term for a lower than normal platelet count.

4. **Answer: 1**
    Rationale: Although antimicrobials are a high priority, a thorough history and physical examination will direct the practitioner in prescribing antimicrobials and supportive treatment.

5. **Answer: 3**
    Rationale: This patient has a low risk for neutropenia. He is experiencing a low-grade fever and is undergoing polypharmacy for his co-morbidities. The seizure and cardiac medications may cause fever. The patient has no other symptoms suggestive of an infectious cause. However, infection needs to be ruled out before a diagnosis of medication-induced fever can be made.

6. **Answer: 4**
    Rationale: This patient has a low platelet count, and all the medications listed, except acetaminophen, affect platelets and clotting. Acetaminophen is the best choice of antipyretic for this patient.

7. **Answer: 4**
    Rationale: This patient is being treated empirically for infection but has shown no response. Fungal infections often present similarly to bacterial infections, but they do not respond to antimicrobial therapy. Fungal infection should also be suspected in patients who may be neutropenic for longer periods of time because of treatment with antineoplastic agents.

8. **Answer: 3**
    Rationale: Although the patient is at risk for fluid imbalance and nutritional imbalance, the impaired skin integrity presents a higher level of risk in this patient's care and is the higher level nursing diagnosis.

9. **Answer: 3**
    Rationale: COX-2 inhibitors are GI protective, not cardioprotective. They function similarly to other NSAIDs, but their side effects are under scrutiny.

10. **Answer: 2**
    Rationale: Patients at high risk for infection should monitor their temperature frequently; however, every hour is a bit excessive. Tachycardia is not a reliable sign of infection and may be a symptom of many conditions. The patient should take his temperature every 4 hours, and he should call the practitioner if his temperature is 38° C (101° F) or higher.

REFERENCES

Baden, L., & Rubin, R. (2002). Fever, neutropenia, and the second law of thermodynamics. *Annals of Internal Medicine, 137*(2):123-124.

Baltic, T., Scholsser, E., & Bedell, M. (2002). Neutropenic fever: One institution's quality improvement project to decrease time from patient arrival to initiation of antibiotic therapy. *Clinical Journal of Oncology Nursing, 6*(6):337-340.

Crawford, J., Althaus, B., & Armitage, J. (2005). The NCCN 2005 Myeloid growth factors clinical practice guidelines in oncology. *Journal of the National Comprehensive Cancer Network: JNCCN, 3*(4):540-555.

Dalal, S., & Zhukovsky, D. (2006). Pathophysiology and management of fever. *Journal of Supportive Oncology, 4*(1):9-16.

Ezzone, S. (2000). Fever. In D. Camp-Sorrell, & R. Hawkins (Eds.), *Clinical manual for the oncology advance nurse practitioner* (pp. 813-824). Pittsburgh: PA: Oncology Nursing Society.

Hughes, W., Armstrong, D., & Bodey, G., et al. (2002). 2002 Guidelines for the use of antimicrobial agents in neutropenic patients with cancer. *Clinical Infectious Diseases, 34*(6):730-751.

Kanamaru, A., & Tatsumi, Y. (2004). Microbiological data for patients with febrile neutropenia. *Clinical Infectious Diseases, 39*(Suppl 1):7-10.

Klastersky, J. (2004). Management of fever in neutropenic patients with different risks of complications. *Clinical Infectious Diseases, 39*(Suppl 1):32-37.

Mackowiak, P. (2006). Pathophysiology and management of fever: We know less than we should. *Journal of Supportive Oncology, 4*(1):21-22.

National Cancer Institute (NCI). (2006). *Fever, sweat, and hot flashes.* Retrieved April 11, 2006, from http://www.cancer.gov/cancertopics/pdq/supportivecare/fever/healthprofessional.

Nirenberg, A., Mulhearn, L., & Lin, S., et al. (2004). Emergency department waiting times for patients with cancer with febrile neutropenia: A pilot study. *Oncology Nursing Forum, 31*(4):711-715.

Robins, H., Brandt, K., & Longo, W. (2006). Pathophysiology and management of fever revisited. *Journal of Supportive Oncology, 4*(6):265-266.

Rolston, K. (2004). The Infectious Diseases Society of America 2002 guidelines for the use of antimicrobial agents in patients with cancer and neutropenia: Salient features and comments. *Clinical Infectious Diseases, 39*(Suppl 1):44-48.

Smeltzer, S., & Bare, B. (2004). *Oncology: Nursing management in cancer care* (pp. 315-368). Philadelphia: Lippincott Williams & Wilkins.

Urabe, A. (2004). Clinical features of the neutropenic host: Definitions and initial evaluation. *Clinical Infectious Diseases, 39*(1),s53-s55.

Wingard, J. (2004). Empirical antifungal therapy in treating febrile neutropenic patients. *Clinical Infectious Diseases, 39*(1),s38-s43.

Gastrointestinal Obstruction: Biliary, Gastric, and Bowel Obstructions

KATHLEEN MURPHY-ENDE

This chapter covers three types of gastrointestinal obstructive problems: biliary obstruction, gastric obstruction, and bowel obstruction. Obstructive disorders of the biliary and gastrointestinal tract are common complications in patients with advanced gastrointestinal, abdominal, pelvic, and hepatobiliary malignancies. Patients with an obstructive process are acutely ill and require intensive nursing care directed at symptom control.

BILIARY OBSTRUCTION

PATHOPHYSIOLOGICAL MECHANISMS

Obstruction of the biliary tract occurs when the hepatic or extrahepatic biliary ducts are occluded, causing a decrease in or obstructed flow of bile. Obstruction of the biliary tree may be caused by malignant or nonmalignant conditions.

Bile, which is produced by the hepatocytes, contains bile salts, water, cholesterol, electrolytes, and bilirubin. Bilirubin is the end product of heme degradation. The main function of bile is to emulsify fats. Half of the bile produced moves from the liver into the duodenum though a system of ducts, which ultimately drains into the common bile duct (CBD). The CBD passes through the head of the pancreas for about 2 centimeters before passing through the ampulla of Vater into the duodenum. In the liver, the bile is collected into the small bile canaliculi, which are small ducts surrounding the hepatocytes. The canaliculi empty into progressively larger ducts into the hepatic and common bile duct. Bile then is delivered to the gallbladder for concentration and storage or directly into the intestine (Corwin, 2000). About 50% of bile is stored in the gallbladder; after a person eats, it is released into the cystic duct, which joins the hepatic ducts from the liver to form the common bile duct.

Any occlusion of bile flow through the bile ducts may lead to obstructive jaundice. Biliary obstruction may arise from intrinsic occlusion or extrinsic compression. *Jaundice* is an excess of bilirubin in the blood; it is referred to as *icterus* when it is visible in the sclera or the skin. Obstruction of the bile canaliculi caused by a hepatic tumor, inflammation, or calculi causes intrahepatic jaundice. Because obstruction at this level reduces the flow of conjugated bilirubin into the bile duct, the amount of conjugated bilirubin absorbed into the blood increases. Posthepatic obstructive jaundice occurs when the bile flow is blocked at the level of the extrahepatic bile ducts by a tumor, porta hepatis lymphadenopathy, or gallstones. The liver is able to conjugate bilirubin, but the bilirubin is unable to reach the small intestine; therefore it enters the bloodstream, where most of it is excreted by the kidneys into the urine. If the obstruction persists, the bile canaliculi become congested and rupture, spilling bile into the lymph and bloodstream. Bilirubin binds to elastic tissue, causing the characteristic color changes of yellow skin and sclera.

EPIDEMIOLOGY AND ETIOLOGY

In the United States the incidence of biliary obstruction is approximately 5 per 1000 people. Biliary obstruction in patients with cancer may arise from mechanical causes, such as a primary or metastatic tumor, and it may be either intrahepatic or extrahepatic. Nonmalignant causes of biliary obstruction include gallstones, hepatic artery thrombosis, sclerosing cholangitis, iatrogenic conditions, pancreatitis, and biliary stricture secondary to previous surgery or hepatic intraarterial chemotherapy. Gallstones, the most common cause of biliary obstruction, have a higher incidence in females, individuals of Hispanic and Northern European origin, and prima women (Bonheur et al., 2006). Infectious causes of obstruction include HIV and oriental and parasitic cholangitis. Other, less common causes are Caroli's disease, Mirizzi's syndrome, and retroperitoneal fibrosis.

RISK PROFILE

- Patients with advanced malignancy in or near the biliary ducts are at risk for developing obstruction from tumor invasion.
- Malignant causes include cancer of the pancreas, ampullary carcinoma, and cholangiocarcinoma (Kichian & Bain, 2004). Metastatic lymphoma and melanoma have also been identified as causes of extrahepatic biliary obstruction (Stellato, 1987).
- Hepatic intraarterial chemotherapy with 5-fluoropyrimidines may cause obstructive jaundice by causing bile duct strictures (Shea et al., 1986).
- Enlarged lymph nodes at the porta hepatis may present a risk of obstruction.
- Nonmalignant causes include gallstones, chronic pancreatitis, and biliary stricture.

PROGNOSIS

Patients with biliary obstruction arising from pancreatic cancer, cholangiocarcinoma, and metastatic disease are at risk of developing ascending cholangitis. Surgical bypass or stenting, if done early in the disease process, may prolong life and improve symptoms. Unfortunately, these procedures may not always be possible in advanced disease, in which case life expectancy is limited. The mortality and morbidity of biliary obstruction depend on the cause of the obstruction. The duration of palliation by stenting depends on the disease and the type of stent used. (Earnshaw et al., 1992). Patients with biliary obstruction are gravely ill because of the obstruction and infection; however, treatment with antibiotics and GI procedures may dramatically improve their physical condition and symptoms.

PROFESSIONAL ASSESSMENT CRITERIA (PAC)

1. A **complete history and physical examination** are important in the evaluation and treatment of biliary obstruction. The following information should be obtained:

- Cancer history and treatment, including surgery, hepatic artery chemotherapy, and radiation
- Surgical history
- Medical history of gallstones, biliary colic, liver disease, pancreatitis, and risk factors for or a history of hepatitis
- Current medications and past use of hepatotoxic agents, drug use, and alcohol
- Review of systems, with attention to symptoms of pain in the right upper quadrant, anorexia, dyspepsia, nausea, weight loss, low-grade fever, fatigue, diarrhea, and symptoms of jaundice. The most obvious signs and symptoms of biliary obstruction, which are caused by jaundice, include pruritus, darkening or yellow skin, dark/frothy urine, pale or clay-colored stools, and bruising.

2. The **physical exam** may reveal weight loss or a low-grade temperature. The skin should be examined for jaundice, which in fair-skinned patients is most noticeable on the face, trunk, and sclerae, and in dark-skinned patients on the sclerae, conjunctivae, and hard palate. Examining the skin in natural sunlight is superior to examination in indoor light because jaundice may not be detectable in artificial lighting. Scratch marks and bruising are other noteworthy findings. In cirrhosis, purpuric spots, vascular angiomas, and palmar erythema may be present. Ecchymoses may be seen in obstructive or hepatocellular disease. The physical findings on the abdominal exam will vary, depending on the etiology of the obstruction. Dilated periumbilical veins indicate portal collateral circulation and cirrhosis. Ascites may be present in metastatic disease or cirrhosis. A right upper quadrant mass, hepatomegaly with a bruit, or splenomegaly may be present. The gallbladder may be palpable with obstruction of the common bile duct. The practitioner should also palpate for lymphadenopathy.

3. **Laboratory diagnostics**: The purpose of obtaining laboratory data is to distinguish between obstructive and nonobstructive (intrahepatic cholestasis) jaundice. A complete blood count (CBC) is done to check for anemia and hemolysis. A positive direct Coombs' test is seen in hemolytic anemia. The total and direct bilirubin levels are elevated with obstruction. An increased indirect (free or unconjugated) bilirubin is seen in nonobstructive jaundice, such as autoimmune hemolysis, cirrhosis, and viral and drug-induced hepatitis. Liver function tests are useful, but it is important to realize that results will vary, depending on the extent of the obstruction or disease. Increased aspartate transaminase (AST) or alanine transaminase (ALT) with an increased bilirubin level indicates hepatocellular disease or injury. A normal or mildly elevated AST with an elevated bilirubin is seen in intrahepatic cholestasis and biliary obstruction. Elevated alkaline phosphatase and ALT levels three times the normal indicate obstruction or prolonged cholestasis. A decreased albumin may be seen in hepatocellular disease. The urine often is positive for bilirubin. The prothrombin time may be prolonged with cholestasis, obstruction, or hepatocellular injury. Lipase and amylase are elevated with pancreatitis. Hepatitis titers should be ordered if viral hepatitis is suspected.

4. **Imaging studies**: Radiographic studies frequently are performed to determine the etiology of the obstruction. Evaluation of the liver by ultrasound is done to differentiate between obstructive and nonobstructive jaundice, and it may also detect cirrhosis, hepatic abscess, cysts, hematoma, and tumors. This noninvasive procedure is helpful for viewing the intrahepatic duct structure and areas of the gallbladder (Bonheur et al., 2006). However, visualization may be poor as a result of obesity or overlying bowel gas. CT scanning with intravenous contrast may be necessary if the ultrasound exam is inconclusive. CT scans allow assessment of the liver's size and structure, as well as abnormalities, but they are more expensive. Scintiscans, which are rarely used in clinical practice, have been used to distinguish between hepatocellular dysfunction and extrahepatic obstruction. However, they are not used as initial imaging; rather, they tend to be

reserved for demonstrating a bile leak or evaluating stent placement (Drane, 1991). Percutaneous transhepatic cholangiography, which is used only when a percutaneous drain is placed, may help in the study of the anatomic details. Although rare, side effects of bleeding, biliary leakage, and sepsis can occur after this procedure. Endoscopic retrograde cholangiopancreatography (ERCP) is useful for patients who have pancreatic disease, because a view of the pancreatic ducts can also be obtained (Bonheur et al., 2006). Magnetic resonance cholangiopancreatography, when available, may be useful and reduces the need for invasive cholangiography (Lillemoe, 1999).

NURSING CARE AND TREATMENT

1. Palliation may be approached by biliary surgical bypass, stenting, and external drainage, and palliative approaches occasionally may be combined with chemotherapy and radiation. Malignant biliary obstruction may be treated by several different procedures, depending on the location and degree of obstruction and the patient's medical status and prognosis. Nursing care varies according to the type of procedure used, therefore nurses who care for these patients should be familiar with the following procedures:
   - Biliary bypass surgical procedures are performed to provide palliation in unresectable or recurrent tumors.
   - Preoperative biliary drainage in patients undergoing pancreatic surgery for malignancy is commonly performed but is associated with an increased incidence of infection and pancreatic fistulae (Lillemoe, 1999).
   - Choledochojejunostomy or hepaticojejunostomy can be done to relieve jaundice caused by extrahepatic obstruction.
   - A Roux-en-Y choledochojejunostomy can be done to treat obstruction of the common bile duct near the cystic duct junction. This procedure involves taking a loop of the jejunum and anastomosing it to the common or left hepatic duct.
   - Insertion of external biliary drains has been used to relieve obstruction preoperatively and for inoperable tumors. External drains require more nursing care, including flushing, dressing changes, and skin care; tubes may need to be changed every few months to prevent occlusion.
   - Insertion of internal biliary stents, endoscopically or percutaneously, has become accepted practice for palliative management. Endoscopic retrograde cholangiopancreatography (ERCP) of malignant obstructive jaundice. Stents may be plastic or metal. However, percutaneous transhepatic stent placement is associated with a high risk of sepsis, biliary leakage, and hemorrhage (Joseph et al., 1986). Currently, internal expandable stents are acceptable for use in patients with a very limited life span (Lee et al., 1997).
2. **Administration of antibiotics**: Cephalosporins covering both gram-negative and gram-positive bacteria are commonly used.
3. **The preprocedural workup** includes review of the procedure and obtaining informed consent. Check laboratory results for coagulation parameters, prothrombin time, activated partial thromboplastin time, hematocrit, white blood count, platelet count, and liver function tests.
4. The period immediately after stent or drain placement requires close monitoring of the site and tube for signs of wound infection and tube patency. Temperature is monitored for infection. Assess for complications such as sepsis, peritonitis, hemorrhage, and pneumothorax. A sterile dressing change should be done every day for the first 5 days, then every 2 to 3 days. The nurse should monitor laboratory results, checking for electrolyte and bicarbonate imbalances. The bilirubin level should return to normal within 10 days after the procedure.

5. Care of external biliary drains or percutaneous transhepatic biliary stents should include teaching the patient and family about the skin, dressing, and catheter care. The drain is flushed every 8 to 24 hours with 10 to 20 mL of normal saline to keep the lines patent. The skin and exit site should be checked twice a day for signs of skin breakdown or infection. The skin around the drain should be washed daily, or more often if drainage occurs, and a clean dressing should be applied. The patient or family should be taught basic drain care and how to check for and report signs of infection, such as persistent pain, fever, or chills. Signs of stent occlusion or dislocation, such as recurrent jaundice or pruritus, should be reported immediately.

6. Pruritus is a frequent symptom in malignant biliary obstruction. The accumulation of bile salts in the skin is presumed to be the causative mechanism for pruritus, but other mediators that may contribute are histamine, kallikreins, prostaglandins, substance P, and endogenous opioids (Khandelwal & Malet, 1994). Pruritus associated with biliary obstruction can range from mild to severe. Several medications are used to manage the condition, with varying efficacy:

   • Cholestyramine 4-6 g PO 30 minutes before meals to absorb bile acids. Side effects include fat malabsorption, possible altered absorption of other medications, and constipation.
   • Antihistamines, such as hydroxyzine 25-50 mg PO TID. Major side effects are drowsiness, dizziness, and dry mouth. The sedative effect may be helpful for aiding sleeping
   • Phenothiazines, such as prochlorperazine 10 mg PO q8h. Side effects include sedation, akathisia, extrapyramidal reactions, dry mouth, and orthostatic hypotension.
   • H_2-receptor blockers, such as ranitidine 150 mg PO BID, can be added to any of the previously listed medications if symptoms persist. Side effects include dizziness, headache, and diarrhea.
   • 5-HT3 antagonists, such as ondansetron, have been used for cholestatic pruritus (Radere et al., 1994). Side effects may include headache, dizziness, and myalgias.
   • Topical steroid creams, such as triamcinolone 0.1% ointment/cream BID. Steroid creams should never be used long term.
   • Creams compounded with antidepressants, such as doxepin, may also be tried. They are thought to inhibit H_1 and H_2 receptors, thus reducing pruritus.
   • Cream mixture of local anesthetics lidocaine and prilocaine (EMLA) BID to affected areas.
   • Skin care includes bathing using mild soap and oil or lotion without alcohol. Moisturizing agents such as Aveeno, Aquaphor, and Neutrogena Sesame Oil are helpful for dry skin. Provide assistance with frequent turning and repositioning. Keep the patient's nails trimmed short and filed to reduce trauma from scratching. Avoid hot baths. Cool compresses may be applied to the skin during episodes of acute pruritus. Cool, dry temperatures may reduce sweating and pruritus.

7. Pain may or may not be present with obstruction, depending on the etiology of the obstruction. The patient with pancreatic cancer may have a significant amount of pain, requiring pain assessment with around-the-clock or long-acting opioids. Perform a detailed pain assessment, and teach the patient to keep a diary of pain intensity, as well as the use of analgesics, and their effectiveness. Ongoing pain assessment and evaluation are required.

8. Nausea and anorexia can lead to altered nutrition. The impact of low-grade nausea on nutrition and quality of life should not be underestimated. Nausea should be assessed regularly and controlled with antiemetics including:

   • Phenothiazines, such as prochlorperazine 10 mg PO q6h or 10 mg IV or IM q4h. Side effects include sedation, akathisia, extrapyramidal reactions, dry mouth, and orthostatic hypotension.
   • Benzodiazepines, such as lorazepam 0.5-1 mg PO q4-6h or IV q4h. Side effects include sedation, anterograde amnesia, dizziness, and disorientation.

- Serotonin antagonists, such as dolasetron or Anzemet, may be helpful, but unfortunately many insurance companies cover the cost of these agents only for chemotherapy-induced nausea. Side effects include headache and dizziness. The nurse should regularly evaluate the effectiveness of the medications.
- Nonpharmacologic approaches for low-grade nausea include relaxation, hypnosis, imagery, diversion, and dietary modification.
9. **Nutrition**: Anorexia and altered taste occur with elevated bilirubin and liver function tests. Nutritional supplements and small, frequent, high-calorie, high-protein snacks are better tolerated than large meals. The patient should avoid drinking liquids close to snack time to avoid feeling full. For some patients, cold food may be more appealing than warm food with aromas. It is important to teach the family to offer snacks without pushing food. Enteral or parenteral supplements may be appropriate to consider as an early intervention in patients with a good prognosis or in malnourished patients with stable disease. Appetite stimulants may be helpful, such as megestrol acetate 400-800 mg PO daily or 80 mg PO 4 times a day. Side effects may include rash and fluid retention. Sensitive patient and family education for the terminally ill should include the anticipation of continual weight loss as an expected symptom.
10. Patients in the terminal phase should be treated and kept comfortable with palliative nursing care. Consultation with the palliative care nurse practitioner is helpful for developing a plan of care, reviewing and suggesting medications, and providing patient and family education and support.

EVIDENCE-BASED PRACTICE UPDATES

1. For patients with unresectable pancreatic tumors, a randomized trial has demonstrated a reduced hospital stay and similar morbidity and mortality with endoscopic stent placement compared to surgical bypass (Anderson et al., 1989).
2. Endoscopic stent placement has increased recurrent jaundice caused by an occluded or dislodged stent, and cholangitis occurs in 13% to 60% of patients (Frakes et al., 1993).
3. Quality of life is improved in patients with biliary obstruction from unresectable liver metastases, cholangiocarcinoma, and pancreatic carcinoma with surgical bypass or endoscopic or percutaneous stenting combined with adjuvant radiation and chemotherapy (Smith et al., 1994).
4. Positive psychosocial outcomes have been seen with placement of biliary stents (Ballinger et al., 1994).
5. No survival advantage is seen between palliative surgical bypass and nonsurgical palliation of obstruction in patients with unresectable malignancies. Surgery is associated with greater morbidity and mortality than endoscopic placement of stents (Smith et al., 1994).
6. Long-term patency rates in biliary stenting are difficult to measure because of the high mortality rate among patients with malignant biliary obstruction. However, longer stents with smooth-surfaced polymers or an antibacterial coating show median patency rates of 6 months (polymers) and 5 months (antibacterial coating), an improvement over plastic stents (Seitz et al., 1994).

TEACHING AND EDUCATION

External biliary catheter care: Show the patient and family members how to provide catheter care and how to observe for signs of bile leakage. Instruct them when to notify the physician or nurse about unusual findings during catheter care. Explain the following: The catheter is placed to straight drainage, and daily output is measured. Daily temperature is monitored for the first week, and elevations must be reported to the health care provider. Internal-external catheters can be capped after 24 hours to move the flow of bile into the duodenum. Biliary tubes require flushing three times a week. Catheters should be replaced every 3 to 4 months, because they may break or become occluded over time.

Skin care and products for pruritus: Review these products and provide the patient and family with a list of medications for pruritus; include the name, purpose, dosage, route, frequency, and side effects.

Nausea and vomiting: Explain that nausea and vomiting may occur if obstruction returns and as the disease progresses. Review medications for nausea; list the name, dosage, route, frequency, and side effects.

Palliative and hospice care: For patients who have advanced cancer, introduce the concept of palliative care and explain the hospice care services that are available.

NURSING DIAGNOSES

1. **Acute pain** related to biliary obstruction and/or procedure/surgery
2. **Impaired skin integrity** related to pruritus
3. **Hyperthermia** related to elevated body temperature
4. **Imbalanced nutrition: less than body requirements** related to anorexia and nausea
5. **Ineffective coping** related to acute condition

EVALUATION AND DESIRED OUTCOMES

1. The patient's pain score will be zero or at an acceptable level.
2. The patient's skin will be intact and the level of pruritus will be acceptable.
3. The patient's temperature will be normal.
4. The patient will be able to tolerate oral intake without nausea or vomiting.
5. Jaundice will resolve, and bilirubin levels will return to normal.
6. the patient will be able to set realistic goals with regard to health expectations.

DISCHARGE PLANNING AND FOLLOW-UP CARE

- Signs and symptoms of complications of chronic internal or external drainage need to be reported: right upper quadrant pain, skin infection, bleeding, leakage of bile, rib erosion, and ascites.
- External biliary drainage tubes require regular flushing and dressing changes.
- Routine tube changes usually are necessary at 8- to 12-week intervals to prevent total occlusion.
- Laboratory tests for electrolyte and bicarbonate depletion must be monitored periodically.

GASTRIC OUTLET OBSTRUCTION

PATHOPHYSIOLOGICAL MECHANISMS

Gastric outlet obstruction is complete or partial obstruction of the distal stomach or proximal duodenum, which prevents the stomach contents from emptying completely into the duodenum. The normal physiology of gastric motility consists of peristaltic waves caused by contraction of the smooth muscle of the stomach. Normally the pacemaker cells depolarize the smooth muscle cells at a continual rate, called the *basic electrical rhythm* of the stomach. When food enters the stomach, it stretches, causing further depolarization and strengthening of the peristaltic wave. When the contraction reaches the antrum (the lower part of the stomach), the wave becomes stronger, mixing the food and causing closure of the pyloric sphincter. As peristalsis continues, a small amount of material is forced through the pyloric sphincter into the duodenum. (Corwin, 2000). Hormones released in the small intestine also help to regulate gastric motility. Secretin and cholecystokinin (CCK) are released in response to chyme in the duodenum, which reduces the motility of the stomach. Gastric inhibitory peptide is released in response to fat in the duodenum, which decreases gastric motility (Huether, 2006).

In gastric outlet obstruction, the transport of chyme is partially or completely blocked along the alimentary canal. The obstruction may be caused by a neoplasm growing in the stomach or duodenum, an extramural mass or adhesion, or a tumor in an adjacent organ (e.g., the head of the pancreas), which causes compression. Tumors in the head of the pancreas cause compression of the duodenal C loop, resulting in nausea and vomiting, whereas tumors of the body or tail obstruct the junction of the duodenum and jejunum at the ligament of Treitz (Lillemoe & Barnes, 1995). Other primary tumors that may cause obstruction by direct extension include colon or kidney cancer. As the obstruction persists, gas and chyme accumulate, and gastric motility initially may increase, causing a cramping- or colic-type pain, nausea, and vomiting.

EPIDEMIOLOGY AND ETIOLOGY

The exact incidence of gastric outlet obstruction is not known, but it occurs much less often than intestinal obstruction. Approximately 30% to 50% of patients with advanced gallbladder cancer develop a gastroduodenal obstruction (Jones, 1991). Among patients with pancreatic cancer, 5% have gastric outlet obstruction at the time of diagnosis, and 8% to 25% develop this complication if gastric bypass is not performed (Singh et al., 1990).

RISK PROFILE

- Gastroduodenal obstruction in patients with cancer usually is caused by a primary gastric tumor that is unresectable or by advanced pancreatic cancer.
- Gastric outlet obstruction is a common complication of advanced gastric cancer. Adhesions may contribute to obstruction.
- Malignant conditions that may give rise to gastroduodenal obstruction include gallbladder, pancreatic, colon, and kidney cancers.
- Benign peptic ulcer disease may also be a risk factor.

PROGNOSIS

The prognosis depends on the type and stage of malignancy and the patient's functional status and response to treatment such as chemotherapy, radiation, or surgical bypass. Curative reconstruction of GI continuity is possible in cases of obstruction caused by early stage primary gastric tumors. Resection for cure is possible in only 15% of patients with pancreatic cancer at the time of diagnosis (Waranapa & Williamson, 1992), and fewer than 20% survive for longer than 1 year after diagnosis (Warshaw & Fernandez-del Castillo, 1992).

PROFESSIONAL ASSESSMENT CRITERIA (PAC)

1. A complete history and physical examination should be done. The presenting symptoms of gastric outlet obstruction depend on the degree of occlusion, and they may occur acutely, insidiously, or intermittently. With a partial obstruction, the patient may present with a recent history of early satiety, anorexia, weight loss, nausea, and vomiting. Pain may or may not be present. With a complete obstruction, the patient usually has severe vomiting of large amounts of undigested food. Hematemesis may be present with gastric tumors.
2. The purpose of the diagnostic evaluation is to confirm the site and etiology of the obstruction so that appropriate palliative interventions can be implemented. Barium contrast studies and endoscopy can demonstrate gastric or duodenal obstruction. Supine and abdominal x-ray films may show dilation and fluid levels proximal to the site of the obstruction.

NURSING CARE AND TREATMENT

1. A surgical consult usually is ordered to determine whether resection is indicated. The nurse's role is to make sure that the patient and family understand the surgical options and recommendations and to provide preoperative and postoperative care. The goals of surgery are to re-establish gastrointestinal continuity and to relieve symptoms. The type

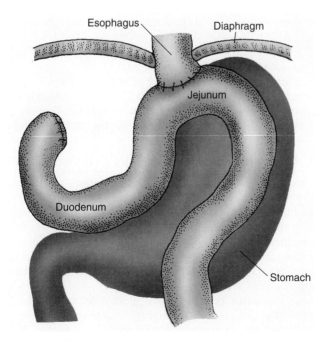

Fig. 17.1 • Total gastrectomy. *(From Ignatavicius, D. D., & Workman, M. L. [2006]. Medical-surgical nursing: Critical thinking for collaborative care. [5th ed.]. St. Louis: Mosby.)*

of palliative surgery performed depends on the disease process and the patient's prognosis and risk factors. Procedures may include subtotal or total gastrectomy (Fig. 17.1), bypass gastrojejunostomy, a Devine antral exclusion procedure (the stomach is transected just proximal to the tumor and a jejunal loop is anastomosed to the proximal stomach), splenectomy, or partial pancreatectomy. During the immediate postoperative period, the patient must be watched for signs of hemorrhage, hypovolemia, hypotension, reflux aspiration, small bowel obstruction, and anastomotic leak. The surgical incision must be examined routinely for signs of infection or fistula formation.

2. A gastrointestinal consult usually is ordered to determine whether procedures to alleviate the obstruction are an option. The nurse's role is to assist in explaining the procedure and providing preprocedural and postprocedural care. Insertion of large-caliber stents (16 to 22 mm) is a nonsurgical alternative for treating gastric outlet obstruction that has minimal risks and high success rates. The success rate for self-expanding metal stents is 80% to 100% in gastroduodenal outlet obstructions (Zollikofer et al, 2000). Although stents placed endoscopically across the obstruction may be helpful for relieving symptoms, recurrent stent occlusion may occur.

3. *Percutaneous* endoscopic *gastrostomy* (PEG): When surgery is not feasible, insertion of a PEG tube can provide symptomatic treatment. Endoscopically, a stoma is created from the abdominal wall into the stomach, and a short feeding tube is inserted percutaneously. In cases of obstruction, these PEG tubes are used for gastric venting and drainage. A low-profile gastrostomy device (LPGD) has a firm or balloon-style internal bumper or retention disk that prevents the GI contents from leaking onto the skin. Attention to skin and wound care is important.

4. A percutaneous jejunostomy (PEJ) tube may also be used for the delivery of enteral nutrition. PEJ tubes bypass the stomach, allowing feeding below the level of obstruction.

5. Palliative chemotherapy and radiation may provide symptomatic relief, and nursing care aimed at managing treatment side effects is necessary in these cases.

6. Pain may be present, especially with pancreatic tumors, and should be treated aggressively (see Chapter 36).

7. Octreotide may reduce gastrointestinal secretions and help control nausea, therefore its use should be considered (Ripamonti et al., 2000).

8. The major nursing interventions described for bowel obstruction also apply to gastric outlet obstruction (see Nursing Care and Treatment for bowel obstruction later in the chapter).

9. Nutritional support and management are aimed at comfort care, to provide adequate nutrients, to preserve body mass, and to minimize and control GI symptoms.

EVIDENCE-BASED PRACTICE UPDATES

1. Qualitative research on patients 3 months after gastrointestinal surgery for tumor found that many patients were unhappy because they did not feel hunger, and eating made them feel full quickly, which caused them to dread eating. Feeling full made them feel nauseous, and many felt that they were being forced to eat by family members and that food was a now a medical treatment and not enjoyable. This led to feels of isolation (Olsson et al., 2002). Nursing care should guide patients and families in ways to help the patient enjoy food after a gastrectomy, such as suggesting new eating and drinking habits that could be integrated into the family's mealtimes and patterns.

2. Glucose levels affect stomach peristalsis. Low glucose levels stimulate the vagus nerve and gastric smooth muscles, causing an increase in peristalsis but not in gastric emptying; this results in the sensation of hunger pain (Smith & Morton, 2001).

3. Aging reduces gastric motility and secretions, and these changes slow gastric digestion and emptying (Huether, 2006).

4. Thirteen percent to 21% of patients with pancreatic cancer who do not undergo a gastrojejunostomy at initial exploration eventually require a the procedure for treatment of gastric outlet obstruction (Waranapa & Williamson, 1992).
5. Gastrojejunostomy does not always achieve palliation of obstructive symptoms, and delayed gastric emptying may occur after this surgery (Jacobs et al., 1989).
6. Laparoscopic gastroenterostomy has been found to be safe and to provide successful palliation of nausea and vomiting (Born et al., 1996).

TEACHING AND EDUCATION

Nutritional decision making: Assist the patient and family in making decisions about the desirability of parenteral or enteral feedings. Review the medical facts about the patient's condition and outline the risks and benefits of artificial nutrition. Ask the patient to explain his or her wishes regarding parenteral or enteral nutrition and what the person hopes to accomplish. Reassure the patient and family that with advanced cancer, not eating or drinking does not lead to suffering, and there is no clear right or wrong answer.

Nutrition: Instruct the patient and family about the enteral or parenteral feeding plan, schedule, and use of equipment (Boxes 17-1 and 17-2). Patients who have undergone a total or partial gastrectomy are at risk for developing dumping syndrome, which is

---

BOX 17-1 TUBE FEEDING CARE AND MAINTENANCE

- If nasogastric or nasoduodenal feeding is ordered, use a soft, flexible, small-bore feeding tube (smaller than 12 French). The initial placement of the tube should be confirmed by x-ray study. Secure the tube with tape or a commercial attachment device after applying a skin protectant; change the tape regularly.
- Check tube placement by x-ray study when the correct position of the tube is in question; an x-ray study is the only reliable method. Checking the pH of the aspirant is a useful adjunct. Other traditional methods for determining tube placement have not proved reliable.
- If a gastrostomy or jejunostomy tube is used, assess the insertion site for signs of infection or excoriation (e.g., excessive redness and drainage). Rotate the tube 360 degrees each day and check for in-and-out play of about {¼}inch (0.5 cm). If the tube cannot be moved, notify the health care provider immediately, because the retention disk may be embedded in the tissue. Cover the site with a dry, sterile dressing and change the dressing at least once a day.
- Check and record the residual volume every 4 hours by aspirating stomach contents into a syringe. If residual feeding is obtained, check the physician's order for the appropriate intervention (usually to slow or stop the feeding for a time).
- Check the feeding pump or controller device (if used) to ensure proper mechanical operation.
- Ensure that the prescribed enteral product is infused at the ordered rate (mL/hr).
- Change the feeding bag and tubing every 24 hours; label the bag with the date and time of the change. Use an irrigation set for no longer than 24 hours.
- For continuous or cyclic feeding, add only 4 hours of product to the bag each time to prevent bacterial growth; a closed system may be used for 24 hours.
- To prevent aspiration, keep the head of the bed elevated at least 30 degrees during the feeding and for 1 hour after the feeding.
- Monitor laboratory values, especially blood urea nitrogen (BUN), serum electrolytes, hematocrit, albumin, prealbumin, and glucose.
- Monitor for complications of tube feeding, especially diarrhea.
- Monitor and carefully record the patient's weight and intake and output.

From Ignatavicius, D. D., & Workman, M. L. (2006). *Medical-surgical nursing:Critical thinking for collaborative care.* (5th ed). St. Louis: Mosby.

> ### BOX 17-2 MAINTAINING A PATENT FEEDING TUBE
>
> - Flush the tube with 30 to 60 mL of water (the amount usually ordered by the health care provider or dietician):
>   - At least every 4 hours during a continuous tube feeding
>   - Before and after each intermittent tube feeding
>   - Before and after medication administration (use warm water)
>   - After checking the residual volume
> - If the tube becomes clogged, use 30 mL of water to flush it, applying gentle pressure with a 50 mL piston syringe.
> - Do not use a carbonated beverage, except for existing clogs, when water is not effective. Also, do not use cranberry juice.
> - Whenever possible, use liquid medications instead of crushed tablets.
> - Do not mix medications with the feeding product. Crush tablets as finely as possible and dissolve them in warm water.
> - Consider use of an automatic flush feeding pump, such as Flexiflo, Quantum, or Kangaroo.
>
> From Ignatavicius, D. D., & Workman, M. L. (2006). *Medical-surgical nursing:Critical thinking for collaborative care.* (5th ed.). St. Louis: Mosby.

characterized by diarrhea 20 to 30 minutes after eating, weakness, dizziness, and palpitations. Instruct the patient to eat small, frequent meals that are high in fat and protein and low in sugar; also instruct the patient to limit juice, avoid very hot or very cold liquids, and avoid eating solids and liquids at the same time.

Vitamin B$_{12}$: Monthly injections of vitamin B$_{12}$ may be indicated to prevent pernicious anemia in patients who have a reasonable prognosis.

NURSING DIAGNOSES

1. **Deficient knowledge** related to medical treatment
2. **Risk for loneliness** related to cancer/inability to eat
3. **Imbalanced nutrition: less than body requirements** related to inadequate oral intake
4. **Diarrhea** related to solute tube feedings or dumping syndrome
5. **Risk for infection** related to invasive procedures/malnutrition

EVALUATION AND DESIRED OUTCOMES

1. The patient and family will be able to verbalize the benefits and risks of surgical and interventional procedures.
2. The patient and family will be able to identify goals of medical care and make a decision on artificial nutrition based on the prognosis for the disease.
3. The patient will be able to identify social support systems.
4. The patient and family will be able to identify social activities that do not involve food.
5. The patient's weight will remain within 5 pounds of the desired weight.
6. The patient will have normal bowel patterns, without cramping or diarrhea.
7. The patient's body temperature will be 36.1° to 37.5° C (97° to 99.6° F)

DISCHARGE PLANNING AND FOLLOW-UP CARE

- Provide instruction on enteral tube feedings (see Boxes 17-1 and 17-2).
- Provide instruction on surgical or tube placement wound care.

- Arrange home nutritional support service for patients with parenteral nutrition.
- Provide a home care nursing referral.
- Arrange a follow-up appointment with the physician or nurse practitioner.
- Provide the name and phone number of an emergency contact person in the event of fever or pain.

BOWEL OBSTRUCTION

PATHOPHYSIOLOGICAL MECHANISMS

Intestinal or bowel obstruction occurs when the passage of intestinal contents is hindered by an occlusion or by lack of normal bowel propulsion. Occlusions may occur at any site in the intestines. The obstruction may be partial or complete and occurs with impairment, failure, or reversal of movement. Mechanical obstruction causes the accumulation of fluid and gas proximal to the obstruction, producing distention of the intestine and resultant symptoms.

The specific types of malignancies that tend to cause obstruction in later stages include colon, ovarian, uterine, stomach, and pancreatic cancers. Bowel obstruction from extraabdominal malignancies is common with metastatic lung or breast cancer and melanoma. The most common cause of nonmalignant obstruction is surgical-related adhesions. Numerous nonmalignant causes of obstruction may coexist, leading to a range of obstructive problems.

The normal physiology of intestinal motility is quite complex, but the main mechanisms involve neural regulation of the musculature of the gut, as well as hormonal influences. The gastroenteric reflex causes slow contractions of the circular smooth muscle of the small intestine to move chyme (digested food) forward and backward with pancreatic enzymes and bile. In response to chyme in the duodenum, the mucosal cells of the small intestine secrete the hormonal peptides secretin, cholecystokinin, and gastric inhibitory peptide. These hormones reduce the motility of the stomach and intestine to allow the digestive enzymes time to break down chyme. Neurotransmitters and inflammatory mediators act on secretomotor receptors to stimulate the intestine to secrete fluid. The small bowel intestinal mucosa absorbs most of the electrolytes. The large intestine absorbs most of the fluid.

Mechanical stretching of the bowel or neural stimulation causes peristalsis. *Peristalsis* is the contraction of circular and longitudinal smooth muscles behind the bolus of chyme, which allows the propulsive movements to push the intestinal contents forward through the bowel. Chyme collects in the terminal ileum, causing increased pressure; this opens the ileocecal valve, allowing the movement of fecal matter into the cecum. The sensation of needing to defecate is perceived when a large section of the colon contracts as a unit. These propulsive mass movements occur several times a day. They last 10 to 30 minutes and are strongest in the morning. Perception of the need to defecate is also initiated by a mass of feces in the rectum, which stimulates the stretch receptors in the anus. Regular bowel function depends on normal neurologic function, appropriate hormonal regulation, adequate fecal mass to stretch the bowel wall, sensory awareness of the need to defecate, and the ability of the abdominal muscle to contract (Huether, 2006).

Several mechanisms are involved in the process of intestinal obstruction, depending on the specific etiology. When the bowel is obstructed, the intestinal wall continues to contract with increased, uncoordinated peristaltic activity; this results in a cycle of distension and secretion motor activity. The hyperactive state leads to intestinal lumen hypertension, damaging the epithelium, which releases prostaglandins and initiates an inflammatory response. During this chemically mediated inflammatory response, vasoactive intestinal polypeptide (VIP) is released into the portal and peripheral circulation, disturbing systemic hemodynamic homeostasis. VIP causes hyperemia and edema of the intestinal wall, with accumulation of fluid in the lumen, and high portal pressures, leading to hypersecretion and splanchnic (gut circulation) vasodilation. The altered hemodynamic process that occurs during obstruction may cause systemic hypotension (Ripamonti, 1998). During vasodilation, fluids and electrolytes are sequestered in the gut wall and lumen, contributing to hypotension, and the combination of these problems can lead to multiorgan system failure, the leading cause of death in bowel obstruction. Sepsis occurs as the bacteria and the toxins produced by the intestinal contents pass through the intestinal wall into the lymphatic and systemic circulation. Metabolic disorders occur as a result of dehydration, electrolyte losses, and acid-base imbalances (Mercadante, 1997).

Malignancy-related obstructive processes may arise from an intraluminal, intramural, or extramural obstruction, a motility disorder, or multiple metastatic lesions. The pathologic process of obstruction in patients with cancer often is multifactorial. Intraluminal obstruction can occur when primary tumors of the right colon form lesions that occlude the lumen or create a point where intussusception can occur. They may also be caused by extension of metastatic tumors into the bowel lumen. Intramural obstruction occurs when the tumor spreads laterally and coats the inner bowel wall, forming a thickened, indurated, and contracted lumen. Extramural obstruction is caused by mesenteric or omental masses or adhesions, which cause extrinsic compression of the intestinal wall. Motility disorders are caused by impaired motility of a segment of the intestine without occlusion of the lumen. Metastatic disease processes such as ovarian cancer infiltrate the mesentery or bowel muscle and may reduce motility. Paraneoplastic neuropathy associated with lung cancer may also impair motility. Disease invasion of the autonomic nerves may stop motility. The use of opioids may significantly slow intestinal motility, leading to constipation and obstruction. Multiple metastatic lesions may cause obstruction at several sites, a condition commonly seen in advanced ovarian cancer. Other processes that cause obstruction include adhesions, inflammatory edema, fecal impaction, fibrosis, inelasticity, change of fecal flora, and hernias (Ripamonti & Mercadante, 2004).

RISK PROFILE/ETIOLOGIES

Obstruction is the presenting symptom in up to 40% of patients with colorectal cancer (Arnell et al., 1998). The incidence of obstruction in colon cancer ranges from 4% to 24% of cases. In ovarian carcinoma, the incidence is 5.5% to 42% (Ripamonti, 1994), and obstruction is the major cause of death in patients with ovarian cancer (Ripamonti, 1998). As mentioned, the most common cause of nonmalignant obstruction is surgical-related adhesions; 20% of hospital admissions for acute abdomen are for treatment of intestinal obstruction (Hirsch & Caswell, 1999).

Numerous conditions put the patient with cancer at risk for obstruction. The malignancy, its treatment, or other factors may lead to obstruction. Motility disorders caused by malignant involvement of the intestinal muscle or autonomic nerves, as well as intraluminal tumors or annular narrowing caused by disease dissemination, place the patient with cancer at high risk for developing intraluminal occlusion. Tumor progression or recurrence may lead to extrinsic compression of the lumen. Malignant involvement of the intestinal muscle wall may cause intramural occlusion or pseudo-obstruction. Treatment-related risk factors include irradiation of the abdomen, resulting in fibrosis and strictures, and adhesions arising from previous cancer surgery.

Many conditions other than active disease that are common to patients with cancer put them at risk for developing an obstruction. Constipation and fecal impaction arising from immobility and a limited oral intake may lead to mechanical obstruction. Some medications can cause severe constipation, which may lead to obstruction if left untreated. These drugs include opioids, anticholinergics, antihypertensives, and general anesthesia. Antibiotics and a poor oral intake can alter the intestinal flora and may cause a decline in bowel motility. Adhesions arising from previous abdominal surgery can cause extrinsic occlusion of the lumen. Inflammatory edema, inflammatory bowel disease, diverticular conditions, and injury or trauma to the abdomen or pelvis also are risk factors. Gallstones, intestinal worms, bezoars (a mass of undigested material such as hair or vegetable matter), and hernias may cause an obstruction. Neurologic disorders that cause vagal dysfunction or autonomic neuropathy, such as paraneoplastic syndromes or diabetic neuropathy with chronic intestinal pseudo-obstruction, are other risk factors (Mercadante, 1997). Mechanical problems such as intussusception or volvulus are motility problems that may lead to full or partial obstruction.

PROGNOSIS

The prognosis depends on the type and stage of malignancy and the patient's functional status and response to treatment, such as chemotherapy, radiation, surgical bypass, or stent placement. Patients with intraabdominal recurrent disease have limited survival, and surgery may fail to resolve the obstruction. Successful palliation after surgery is associated with absence of palpable abdominal or pelvic masses, a volume of ascites less than 3 L, unifocal obstruction, and preoperative weight loss of less than 9 kg (Jong et al., 1995). Prognostic indicators of low likelihood of clinical benefit from surgery for malignant bowel obstruction include obstruction secondary to cancer; intestinal motility problems caused by diffuse intraperitoneal carcinomatosis; widespread tumor; patient over 65 years of age with cachexia; ascites requiring frequent paracentesis; low serum albumin level; previous radiotherapy of the abdomen or pelvis; nutritional deficits; diffuse, palpable intraabdominal masses and liver involvement; distant metastasis; pleural effusion or pulmonary metastases; multiple partial bowel obstructions with prolonged passage time on radiographic examination; elevated blood urea nitrogen level; elevated alkaline phosphatase levels; advanced tumor stage; short diagnosis-to-obstruction interval; poor performance status; involvement of proximal stomach; and extraabdominal metastases that produce symptoms that are difficult to control (Ripamonti & Mercadante, 2004).

PROFESSIONAL ASSESSMENT CRITERIA (PAC)

1. Obtain and document a complete history when a patient is admitted with a suspected bowel obstruction. The following information should be obtained:
   - Type of cancer and previous treatment
   - Previous radiation
   - Previous surgery
   - History of abdominal trauma
   - History of previous obstruction
   - History of chronic constipation
   - Medical history of hernia, gallstones, or inflammatory bowel or diverticular disease
   - Current medications, especially opioids
   - Normal bowel habits and last bowel movement
   - Current symptoms and management of pain, nausea, vomiting, constipation, or diarrhea

2. Presenting symptoms of obstruction depend on the level of the occlusion and may occur acutely, insidiously, or intermittently. Abdominal pain initially may be an intermittent, colicky, cramping sensation in the periumbilical region. The pain typically progresses to a continuous, diffuse discomfort. Jejunoileal obstruction tends to cause an intense, periumbilical, intermittent pain. Large bowel obstruction tends to cause a less intense but deeper, longer-lasting pain. Perforation or strangulation tends to cause an intense, acute pain that worsens or becomes localized. Peritoneal irritation causes pain that increases with palpation or rebound tenderness.

3. Nausea may be chronic or acute. Vomiting occurs sporadically but increases as the obstruction progresses. In gastric outlet or small intestinal obstruction, vomiting develops early after the onset of pain and usually consists of a large volume of biliary, odorless emesis. In contrast, with a large bowel obstruction, nausea usually occurs several hours after the pain starts. Colonic or ileal obstruction may cause a foul, feculent emesis.

4. A history of constipation or a recent history of a change in bowel habits may be seen in obstruction. Obstipation (failure to pass flatus or stool) is seen in lower obstructive disorders. If the obstruction is high in the jejunum, the contents may pass through. Diarrhea may occur from liquefaction of blocked stool in the sigmoid colon or rectum. A partial obstruction may present with a cramping pain followed by explosive diarrhea.

5. Physical findings in bowel obstruction vary, depending on the time, location, intensity, and presence of complications. The patient's general appearance may range from normal to acute distress. The skin may be pale and diaphoretic because of shock. The mouth may be dry with poor skin turgor because of dehydration. Fever and hypotension may occur in sepsis, shock, strangulation, or perforation. Frequent abdominal examination and accurate recording of findings are important in assessing the progression of obstruction. Distention is the most common physical finding, and visible peristaltic waves may be noted. Bowel sounds may be absent in paralytic ileus. Borborygmi (hyperactive sounds), frequently high pitched and intermittent, are noted in early or partial obstruction. Tenderness, especially localized, may be present in bowel strangulation. A mass or rigidity often is noted if the distention is not too severe. The patient should be assessed or peritoneal signs such as Blumberg's sign (rebound tenderness), involuntary rigidity, tenderness with palpation, and costovertebral tenderness. The rectal exam may demonstrate a palpable fecal mass, impaction, or occult fecal blood.

6. Diagnostic evaluation is undertaken to differentiate severe constipation from obstruction and, in a patient who is a candidate for surgery, to confirm the site and nature of the obstruction. Patients with advanced disease and those who are in a terminal phase should not undergo diagnostic testing if the treatment does not depend on it. These patients should be treated palliatively.

7. Laboratory tests are important in the evaluation process. A complete blood count may reveal leukocytosis in cases of infection, perforation, or strangulation. An elevated hematocrit, oliguria, and hyperazotemia may indicate dehydration, and a low hematocrit may reflect internal bleeding. Electrolytes and chemistry data should also be considered. An elevated BUN, specific gravity, and proteinuria are caused by decreased urine flow. Hyponatremia and a low total protein are commonly seen with obstruction (Fainsinger et al., 1994). With distal obstruction, chloride, sodium, potassium, and bicarbonate may be low; with high obstruction, metabolic alkalosis, hypochloremia, and hypokalemia occur from loss of gastric secretions and hypoventilation (Mercadante, 1997). Respiratory acidosis may occur as a result of shallow respirations if abdominal distention elevates the diaphragm significantly.

8. Radiographic tests are the most diagnostic in determining the location and degree of the obstruction. Abdominal supine and upright plain x-ray films show dilated loops of

bowel and air-fluid levels in obstruction, and free air beneath the diaphragm in perforation. Barium swallow with small bowel follow-through may distinguish obstruction from metastasis, radiation injury, or adhesions. Slow passage of barium through undilated bowel is seen in motility disorders. Distended, gas-filled loops of the small and large intestine, or air-fluid levels, may occur in partial small bowel obstruction or ileus. A barium enema may confirm the presence and location of bowel obstruction. Risks associated with a barium enema include perforation of an inflamed lesion and conversion of a partial obstruction to a complete obstruction. Gastrografin, a water-soluble medium, should used instead of barium if a perforation is suspected or if complete obstruction is suspected in an inoperable patient. Computed tomography (non-contrast) of the abdomen may be helpful in documenting a small bowel obstruction, especially when extraluminal abnormalities are suspected, or when immediate surgical intervention is considered. Colonoscopy may be useful for evaluating large bowel obstructions.

NURSING CARE AND TREATMENT

1. Nursing care of the patient with a GI obstruction requires skills in detailed assessment, critical thinking, patient and family education, and counseling. Often the GI obstruction represents a turning point into the transition of the last phase of life. The nurse is responsible for providing sensitive anticipatory guidance on what to expect. Referrals and consultation with other professionals, such as the wound, ostomy, continence nurse (WOCN) or the enterostomal therapy (ET) nurse, social worker, pastoral care, psychologist, and palliative care nurse practitioner are helpful in meeting the multidimensional needs of the patient and family.

2. Initially, a surgical consult should be obtained to evaluate the possible need for surgical intervention. The goal of surgery is to provide symptomatic relief and to restore normal bowel function when the bowel has become necrotic. In patients who have advanced disease, the decision to undergo surgery versus less invasive treatment needs to be discussed with the patient and family in detail. Surgical risk factors include advanced age, poor medical condition or nutritional status, ascites, distant metastasis, peritoneal carcinomatosis, previous abdominal or pelvic radiotherapy, multiple small bowel obstructions, and presence of a small bowel obstruction (Bains, 1998). Surgical procedures are aimed at restoring normal bowel functioning. They include resection and reanastomosis, decompression with colostomy or ileostomy, bypass, and lysis of adhesions. A combination of methods may be used, depending on the underlying process.

3. Colonic stents are an effective, nonsurgical alternative to treatment of acute obstruction of the gastric outlet, duodenum, or large bowel. This new procedure relieves the acute symptoms of ileus in many cases. Large-caliber stents are placed by an endoscopist under fluoroscopic and endoscopic guidance. The use of stents represents an excellent palliative option for a terminally ill patient who wants to resume enteral nutrition.

4. Bowel rest should be initiated, and the patient should be placed on nothing by mouth (NPO) status. Nasogastric tube insertion with suctioning is done for decompression and to alleviate the symptoms of nausea, vomiting, and pain. A PEG decompression/venting gastrostomy tube should be inserted in inoperable patients who need prolonged gastric suctioning. The PEG tube provides comfort by relieving gastric distention; it should never be used for feeding. Once the acute condition has resolved, the patient may be placed on a liquid diet, and the gastrostomy tube may be clamped at meals and for 30 minutes afterward. If the obstruction is not alleviated, a jejunostomy tube placed percutaneously is sometimes used to provide nutrition, medication, and fluids.

5. Administration of parenteral fluids with electrolyte replacement, such as normal saline with 10 to 20 mEq/L of potassium at 75 mL/hr or greater, is useful for maintaining electrolyte balance and preventing dehydration.

6. Pharmacologic treatment includes medications for nausea and pain, often requiring the rectal, sublingual, or parenteral route of administration. Agents useful for nausea include neuroleptics, such as haloperidol 5-15 mg/day SC, or prochlorperazine 25 mg q8h rectally. Prokinetics can be used, such as metoclopramide 60-240 mg/day SC (do not use with complete obstruction). Antihistamines also can be given, such as diphenhydramine 50-100 mg q6h PRN, as can anticholinergics, such as scopolamine (antisecretory agents) 0.3-0.65 mg/day SC or 1.5 mg transdermal patch every 3 days. The somatostatin analog (antisecretory agent) currently used is octreotide 0.2-0.9 mg/day SC. Octreotide has been used successfully to reduce GI secretions, sometimes eliminating the need for nasogastric tube placement. Corticosteroids, such as dexamethasone 20-40 mg/day PO or IV, may be given to reduce inflammation. Pain medications frequently used include opioids such as morphine or hydromorphone, with gradual dosage increases until the pain is controlled.

7. *Psychological support:* For most patients, experiencing a bowel obstruction is a time of anxiety and crisis. Physically the patient may be highly symptomatic with nausea, vomiting, diarrhea, and pain. Often the onset of obstruction coincides with diagnosis or with learning that the cancer is progressing and not curable. It is important to assess the patient's and family's understanding of the situation and to clarify any misconceptions. The explanation may need to be repeated and the treatment options reviewed. This often is a time of profound grief, and providing supportive interventions with which to work through the grief becomes a nursing priority. The nurse should assist the terminally ill person in the decision-making process, in considering the uncertainty of survival, and in assessing the benefits versus the risks of invasive interventions, as well as in defining the goals of palliative care.

8. Frequent mouth care is required to minimize dryness and discomfort; ice chips or hard candy or gum should be offered when appropriate.

9. Intake and output and daily weights should be monitored.

10. The patient should be assessed for signs and symptoms of electrolyte imbalance, and lab values should be monitored.

11. The pain management plan includes assessment, evaluation, and treatment of the pain. Explain the plan to the patient and family, and continually re-evaluate the patient's level of pain, documenting, and medicating accordingly.

EVIDENCE-BASED PRACTICE UPDATES

1. A review of five studies involving 309 patients found that, of those with a history of previous malignancy who presented with bowel obstruction, approximately 25% of those who required laparotomy were found to have benign disease and 4% had a new primary tumor (Diehl & Chang, 2004).

2. In one study, the operative mortality rate for bowel obstruction surgery was 44% in patients with ovarian cancer who had two or more of the following factors: widespread tumor, over age 65 with cachexia, ascites, or previous radiotherapy (Krebs & Goplerud, 1983).

3. A review of 13 studies by Ripamonti and Mercadante (2004) found that the type of obstruction not the surgical procedure had significant effect on the outcome, and survival was related to the response to postoperative chemotherapy. Improvements in surgical techniques and perioperative care have not influenced outcomes.

4. In one study, successful palliation after surgery (survival for longer than 60 postoperative days) was associated with four factors: absence of palpable abdominal or pelvic masses; a volume of ascites less than 3 L; unifocal obstruction; and a preoperative weight loss less than 9 kg (Jong et al., 1995).
5. An open study by Davis and Furste (1999) found that anticholinergic drugs (glycopyrrolate) was effective in controlling GI symptoms in inoperable malignant bowel obstruction.
6. The clinical benefits of octreotide have been documented by numerous studies. Preoperative use of octreotide has improved surgical conditions, resulting in less edema, vessel congestion, and necrosis of the bowel (Mercadante et al., 1996). Prophylactic use of octreotide in patients with cancer who had recurrent episodes of obstruction was helpful for maintaining or restoring the intestinal tract for prolonged periods (Mercadante et al., 1997).

TEACHING AND EDUCATION

1. Explain the diagnosis to the patient and family and communicate the treatment options. Outline the purpose and procedure for all diagnostic tests.
2. Teach the patient who is to undergo surgery the purpose of the intervention, the risks, benefits, and postoperative care.
3. Provide ostomy teaching if an ostomy will be performed.
4. Assess for barriers to pain management in the patient, family, and medical and nursing staff, and educate accordingly. Explain the side effects and how to counteract these. Constipation should be prevented at the onset of opioid administration through the use of a scheduled, stepwise bowel protocol. Cathartics and other GI stimulants should not be used proximal to a complete bowel obstruction because they may cause perforation. Enemas must be used with caution, and the use of stool softeners and suppositories should be considered. Drowsiness from the opioid will subside after several days. Dry mouth can be treated with ice chips, hard candy, sugarless gum, frequent mouth care, and lip lubrication.
5. Explain the purpose of the nasogastric or PEG tube and the general procedure before inserting the tube. Check tube placement before irrigating with normal saline. Assess the quantity and quality of the NG drainage every few hours initially and then every shift. Teach the patient and family the care involved with the tube. Start with simple steps and written materials and have them perform a return demonstration when they feel comfortable handling the equipment. The procedure for feeding the patient using a jejunostomy tube should be explained early in the course of hospitalization so that the patient and family can practice it. Review the function of the pump and equipment. Explain the flushing techniques. Stress the importance of feeding at the prescribed rate with the head of the bed elevated 45 degrees. Teach the caregiver how to crush, mix, and administer medications through the tube. The nurse is responsible for making a referral for home nursing service and for setting up the appropriate equipment before discharge.

NURSING DIAGNOSES

1. **Acute pain** related to bowel obstruction/surgery
2. **Impaired physical mobility** related to pain and weakness
3. **Self-care deficit: toileting** related to pain and immobility
4. **Fear** related to cancer recurrence
5. **Decisional conflict** related to end-of-life decision making

DISCHARGE PLANNING AND FOLLOW-UP CARE

The advanced practice nurse or case manager is in the ideal position to coordinate care with other services such as home care, hospice, and long-term care facilities.

- Review the home situation to aid in arranging for home nursing care.
- Explain NG or gastrostomy/jejunostomy care.
- Provide a list of the medications the patient is taking (i.e., name, dosage, purpose, frequency, and side effects); explain the physical signs and symptoms to report to the health care provider.
- Provide a written pain management plan.
- Order ostomy products and refer the patient to an enterostomal therapist.
- Assess the patient's knowledge of strategies to prevent recurrent obstruction and his or her ability to carry out a bowel regimen independently.
- Teach the patient who has had surgery about incision care, drug therapy, and activity limitations.
- List the signs and symptoms of recurrent obstruction; provide the name and phone number of a contact person who can be called if these are noted.
- Arrange a follow-up appointment with the physician or nurse practitioner.
- Arrange a home hospice referral for patients with a limited prognosis.

REVIEW QUESTIONS

QUESTIONS

1. Susan, a 43-year-old female diagnosed 3 months ago with unresectable pancreatic cancer, has been taking escalating doses of opioids for abdominal and back pain since her diagnosis. She is admitted with acute right upper quadrant pain, nausea, vomiting, and weakness. Her laboratory results show elevated liver enzymes, elevated total bilirubin, elevated direct bilirubin, and a normal indirect bilirubin. Other signs of hyperbilirubinemia that the nurse would find on physical examination include:
   1. Dry, yellow skin and sclera
   2. Dark urine
   3. Right upper quadrant pain extending to the back
   4. All of the above

2. Based on the information in question 1, the most likely cause of Susan's hyperbilirubinemia is:
   1. Bowel obstruction
   2. Opioid-induced hyperbilirubinemia
   3. Biliary obstruction caused by tumor compression
   4. Gastric outlet obstruction

3. Susan has been unable to eat, and she vomited several times a day for the past week before admission. She is lightheaded when standing. The nurse suspects dehydration. Which of the following will provide the quickest information about Susan's volume status:
   1. Liver enzymes and bilirubin level
   2. Serum sodium and potassium, blood urea nitrogen, and creatinine
   3. Orthostatic blood pressure readings
   4. Urine osmolality

4. Susan is found to have orthostatic hypotension with tachycardia. Based on her history of vomiting and of not taking in oral fluids or food, which lab abnormality would you expect:
   1. Hyperkalemia
   2. Metabolic acidosis
   3. Hypokalemia
   4. Hypermagnesemia

5. John is a 68-year-old male with a 2-year history of colon cancer, status post colon resection, and chemotherapy. He calls the clinic nurse to report brisk diarrhea and is

seen later that day by the nurse practitioner, who notes that he has increased bowel sounds, no tenderness or guarding. The condition you suspect is:
1. Dehydration
2. Peritonitis
3. Ileus
4. Early intestinal obstruction

6. **All of the following are common signs and symptoms of intestinal obstruction *except*:**
   1. Pain in the abdomen
   2. Nausea and vomiting
   3. Fever and confusion
   4. Leg swelling

7. **John's abdominal x-ray film shows a dilated and gas-filled colon. No gas is visualized in the colon distally, and there is no free air under the diaphragm. He is diagnosed with a bowel obstruction. Priority nursing care should include:**
   1. Treatment with antibiotics
   2. Neurologic assessment
   3. Instillation of enemas
   4. Nasogastric tube placement and suction

8. **John's bowel obstruction does not resolve, and the etiology is found to be recurrent disease. He is scheduled for a diverting sigmoid colostomy. Preoperative nursing care should focus on:**
   1. Care of the colostomy
   2. Obtaining advance directives for power of attorney for health care decisions
   3. Instruction in postoperative pain management with patient-controlled analgesia
   4. All of the above

9. **Christopher is a 51-year-old male with gastric outlet obstruction caused by advanced cancer. He has been told that he had a limited prognosis of weeks to months. He is unable to eat, and his family is asking for artificial nutrition. The palliative care nurse practitioner is asked to meet with the patient and family to address their concerns. Supportive care for patients with end-stage cancer who are not**
able eat should include which of the following:
1. Suggesting jejunostomy tube feeding and teaching the family how to administer tube feedings, as this will prolong the patient's life.
2. Suggesting total parental nutrition, because this is easier for the family than tube feedings.
3. Discussing the pros and cons of artificial nutrition and letting the patient choose what he wants.
4. Telling the family that nutrition needs to be implemented at this time to keep Christopher from starving to death.

10. **Christopher decides to forgo artificial nutrition. He wants to go home to die in peace surrounded by his family. He is only able to take in sips of water. The pain he experiences is described as continuous and severe, but it is controlled by a continuous intravenous infusion of morphine sulfate. The best plan for home pain management is:**
    1. Continue Christopher on his current dose of IV morphine sulfate because it is providing excellent pain control.
    2. Convert the medication to a long-acting oral form of morphine because it is less expensive.
    3. Convert the medication to a transdermal fentanyl patch with a short-acting agent (given mucosally, sublingually, or rectally) for breakthrough pain.
    4. Convert the medication to sublingual morphine and instruct the family to give it around the clock.

ANSWERS

1. **Answer: 4**
   Rationale: All of the signs listed are signs of hyperbilirubinemia.

2. **Answer: 3**
   Rationale: Biliary obstruction caused by a pancreatic tumor compressing the biliary tract is the most likely cause of her hyperbilirubinemia. Bowel obstruction and

gastric outlet obstruction do not cause biliary obstruction except with metastatic disease to the biliary tract, as is seen with liver metastasis.

3. **Answer: 3**
   Rationale: Orthostatic blood pressure (lying, sitting, and standing positions) is the fastest way to gain information about her hydration status. Tachycardia with mild or moderate hypotension is a common sign of dehydration with cardiac compensation. If the blood pressure is low, the heart rate should be tachycardic to compensate for the decreased pressure. Bradycardia could be associated with severe hypokalemia and needs to be addressed.

4. **Answer: 3**
   Rationale: She is most likely to have hypokalemia. Most body potassium is intracellular, and in the event of dehydration, loss of gastrointestinal fluids, metabolic alkalosis, and elevated glucose levels cause potassium to move into the cells, lowering the serum potassium. Metabolic alkalosis and hypomagnesemia are also seen in dehydration.

5. **Answer: 4**
   Rationale: Early intestinal obstruction often produces increased bowel sounds and brisk diarrhea. With ileus there is an absence of peristalsis and therefore absent or decreased bowel sounds. Peritonitis would have signs of peritoneal irritation, including rebound tenderness, tenderness to light percussion, and guarding.

6. **Answer: 4**
   Rationale: Leg swelling is not associated with bowel obstruction.

7. **Answer: 4**
   Rationale: A nasogastric tube must be inserted to alleviate the pressure above the obstruction.

8. **Answer: 4**
   Rationale: All the choices presented are important issues in patient and family education that should be addressed before the surgical procedure.

9. **Answer: 3**
   Rationale: No evidence indicates that artificial nutrition during end-stage cancer will prolong life. It is important to stress the goal of comfort measures, with pain management as a priority. Often patients at the end of life do not feel hungry, and feedings do not always add to comfort. It is important to educate the family on the progressive nature of the disease.

10. **Answer: 3**
    Rationale: Converting the medication to a transdermal route with a short-acting agent for breakthrough pain is the easiest method for the family to manage and is less expensive than home IV administration. Because the patient's ability to swallow is declining, relying on that ability is not advisable. Using fentanyl citrate (mucosal route) or morphine (sublingually or rectally) for breakthrough pain is helpful and is a route by which the family can be taught to administer the medication.

REFERENCES

Anderson, J. R., Sorensen, S. M., & Kruse, A., et al. (1989). Randomized trial of endoscopic endoprosthesis versus operative bypass in malignant obstructive jaundice. *Gut, 30*:1132-1135.

Arnell, T., Stamos, M. J., & Takahashi, P., et al. (1998). Colonic stents in colorectal obstruction. *American Surgeon, 64*(10):986-988.

Baines, M. (1998). The pathophysiology and management of malignant intestinal obstruction. In G. Doyle, G. Hanks, & N. MacDonald (Eds.), *Oxford textbook of palliative medicine* (pp. 557-571). (2nd ed.). Oxford: Oxford University Press.

Ballinger, A., McHugh, M., & Catnach, S., et al. Symptom relief and quality of life after stenting for malignant biliary obstruction. *Gut, 35*:467-470.

Bonheur, J., Ells, P., & Kamenetz, F. (2006). Biliary obstruction. eMedicine WebMD (June 20, 2006). Retrieved [month day, year,] from http://www.emedicine.com/med/topics 3426.htm.

Born, P., Neuhaus, H., & Rosch, T., et al. (1996). A minimally invasive palliative approach to advanced pancreatic and papillary cancer causing both biliary and duodenal obstruction. *Gastroenterology, 34*(7):416-420.

Corwin, E. (2000). The gastrointestinal system. In *Handbook of pathophysiology* (pp. 536-566). Philadelphia: Lippincott Williams & Wilkins.

Davis, M., & Furste, A. (1999). Glycopyrrolate: A useful drug in the palliation of mechanical bowel obstruction. *Journal of Pain and Symptom Management, 18*:153-154.

Diehl, K., & Chang, A. (2004). Acute abdomen, bowel obstruction, and fistula. In M. Abeloff, J. Armitage, & J. Niederhuber, et al. (Eds.), *Clinical oncology* (pp. 1025-1045). (3rd ed.). St. Louis: Mosby.

Drane, W. (1991). Nuclear medicine techniques for the liver and biliary system: Update for the 1990s. *Radiologic Clinics of North America: Imaging of the Liver and Biliary Tree, 29*:1129-1150.

Earnshaw, J., Hayter, J., & Teasdale, C., et al. (1992). Should endoscopic stenting be the initial treatment of malignant biliary obstruction? *Annals of the Royal College of Surgeons of England, 74*:338-341.

Fainsinger, R., Spachynski, K., & Hanson, J., et al. (1994). Symptom control in terminally ill patients with malignant bowel obstruction (MBO). *Journal of Pain and Symptom Management, 9*(1):12-18.

Frakes, J., Johanson, J., & Stake, J. (1993). Optimal timing for stent replacement in malignant biliary tract obstruction. *Gastrointestinal Endoscopy, 39*:164-167.

Hirsch, C., & Caswell, D. (1999). Gastrointestinal disorders. In A. Gawlinski, & D. Hamwi (Eds.), *Acute care nurse practitioner: Clinical curriculum and certification review* (pp. 624-626). Philadelphia: W. B. Saunders.

Huether, S. (2006). Structure and function of the digestive system. In K. McCance, & S. Huether (Eds.), *Pathophysiology: The biologic basis for disease in adults and children* (pp. 1353-1383). (5th ed.). St. Louis: Mosby.

Jacobs, P., van der Sluis, R., & Wobbes, T. (1989). Role of gastroenterostomy in the palliative surgical treatment of pancreatic cancer. *Journal of Surgical Oncology, 42*(3):145-149.

Jones, R. S. (1991). Palliative operative procedures for carcinoma of the gallbladder. *World Health Journal of Surgery, 15*(3):348-351.

Jong, P., Sturgeon, J., & Jamieson, C. (1995). Benefit of palliative surgery for bowel obstruction in advanced ovarian cancer. *Canadian Journal of Surgery, 38*(5):454-457.

Joseph, P., Bizer, F., & Sprayregen, S., et al. (1986). Percutaneous transhepatic biliary drainage: Results and complications in 81 patients. *Journal of the American Medical Association, 255*:2763-2767.

Khandelwal, M., & Malet, P. F. (1994). Pruritus associated with cholestasis: A review of pathogenesis and management. *Digestive Diseases and Sciences, 39*:1-8.

Kichian, K., & Bain, V. (2004). Jaundice, ascites and hepatic encephalopathy. In D. Doyle, G. Hanks, & N. Cherney, et al. (Eds.), *Oxford textbook of palliative medicine* (3rd ed). (pp. 507-520). Oxford: University Press.

Krebs, H., & Goplerud, D. (1983). Surgical management of bowel obstruction in advanced ovarian carcinoma. *Obstetrics and Gynecology, 61*:327-330.

Lee, H., Choe, H., & Lee, H., et al. (1997). Metallic stents in malignant biliary obstruction: Prospective long-term clinical result. *American Journal of Roentgenology, 168*:741-745.

Lillemoe, K. (1999). Preoperative biliary drainage and surgical outcome. *Annals of Surgery, 230*(2):143-144.

Lillemoe, K. D., & Barnes, S. A. (1995). Surgical palliation of unresectable pancreatic carcinoma. *Surgical Clinics of North America, 75*:953-968.

Mercadante, S. (1997). Assessment and management of mechanical bowel obstruction. In R. K. Portenoy, & E. Bruera (Eds.), *Topics in palliative care* (pp. 113-130). New York, Oxford: Oxford University Press.

Mercadante, S., Avola, G., & Maddaloni, S., et al. (1996). Octreotide prevents the pathological alterations of bowel obstruction in cancer patients. *Supportive Care in Cancer, 4*:393-394.

Mercadante, S., Kargar, J., & Nicolosi, G. (1997). Octreotide may prevent definitive intestinal obstruction. *Journal of Pain and Symptom Management, 13*:352-355.

Olsson, U., Bergbom, I., & Bosaeus, I. (2002). Patients' experiences of their intake of food and fluid following gastrectomy due to tumor. *Gastroenterology Nursing, 25*(4):146-153.

Raderer, M., Muller, C., & Scheithauer, W. (1994). Ondanestron for pruritus due to cholestasis. *New England Journal of Medicine 330*(21):1540 .

Ripamonti, C. (1998). Bowel obstruction. In A. Berger, R. Portenoy, & D. Weissman (Eds.), *Principles and practice of supportive oncology* (pp. 207-214). Philadelphia: Lippincott-Raven.

Ripamonti, C. (1994). Malignant bowel obstruction in advanced and terminal cancer patients. *European Journal of Palliative Care, 1*:16-19.

Ripamonti, C., & Mercadante, S. (2004). Pathophysiology and management of malignant bowel obstruction. In D. Doyle, G. Hanks, & N. Cherney, et al. (Eds.), *Oxford textbook of palliative medicine* (pp. 496-507). (3rd ed.). Oxford: University Press.

Ripamonti, C., Mercadante, S., & Groff, L., et al. (2000). Role of octreotide, scopolamine butylbromide, and hydration in symptom control of patients with inoperable bowel obstruction and nasogastric tubes: A prospective randomized trial. *Journal of Pain and Symptom Management, 19*(1):23-34.

Seitz, U., Vadyeyar, H., & Soehendra, N. (1994). Prolonged patency with a new design Teflon biliary prosthesis. *Endoscopy, 26*(5):478-482.

Shea, W. J., Demas, B. E., & Goldberg, H. I., et al. (1986). Sclerosing cholangitis associated with hepatic arterial FUDR: Chemotheraphy: Radiographic-histologic correlation. *American Journal of Roentgenology, 146*:717-721.

Singh, S. M., Longmire, W. P., & Reber, H. A. (1990). Surgical palliation for pancreatic cancer. *Annals of Surgery, 212*:132-139.

Smith, A., Dowsett, J., & Russell, R., et al. (1994). Randomised trial of endoscopic stenting versus surgical bypass in malignant low bile duct obstruction. *Lancet* 344(3938):1655-1660.

Smith, M., & Morton, D. (2001). *The digestive system*. St. Louis: Mosby.

Stellato, T., Sollinger, R. M. Jr., & Shuck, J. M. (1987). Metastatic malignant biliary obstruction. *American Surgeon, 53*:385.

Waranapa, P., & Williamson, R. (1992). Surgical palliation for pancreatic cancer: Developments during the past two decades. *British Journal of Surgery, 79*(1):8-20.

Warshaw, A., & Fernandez-del Castillo, C. (1992). Pancreatic carcinoma. *New England Journal of Medicine, 326*:455-465.

Zollikofer, C. L., Jost, R., & Schoch, E., et al. (2000). Gastrointestinal stenting. *European Radiology, 10*(2):329-341.

GRAFT VERSUS HOST DISEASE

JILL K. BURLESON

PATHOPHYSIOLOGICAL MECHANISMS

Graft versus host disease (GVHD) is a frequent complication of allogeneic stem cell transplantation and a much rarer complication of blood transfusions. The conditions for GVHD are met when immunocompetent donor cells are introduced into an immuno-compromised recipient, or host, which expresses tissue antigens that are not present in the donor. The donor cells recognize the recipient antigens as being foreign and react by attempting to destroy the tissue. The recipient, by virtue of being immunocompromised, is unable to mount an effective response to this attack and therefore is unable to destroy the donor cells, leading to the manifestation of clinical symptoms. The GVHD reaction was first reported when irradiated mice were injected with spleen cells. Although they recovered from treatment and began engraftment, they eventually died of a secondary disease that manifested in symptoms of diarrhea, weight loss, and skin and liver abnorm-alities (Jaksch & Mattson, 2005).

The mediators of GVHD are the donor T cells and the human leukocyte antigens (HLAs) in the host. HLA typing of a patient is a type of genetic fingerprint and is segregated in families in a Mendelian codominant manner. With the exception of identical twins, no two sets of HLA markers are completely the same. The genes on the HLA locus hold two dif-ferent classes of cell surface molecules. Class I molecules are present on the surface of most nucleated cells, whereas class II molecules are more commonly expressed on the cells specific to the immune system. The class I antigens are HLA-A, HLA-B, and HLA-C; class II antigens include HLA-DQ, HLA-DR, and HLA-DP. Other antigens, called *minor antigens*, also exist, but these are less active mediators in the GVHD response.

Research has shown that the most important antigens involved in determining whether donor cells initiate a graft versus host response are HLA-A, HLA-B, and HLA-DR (Prasad et al., 1999). The major HLA molecules of the host are expressed on many of the host tissue cells. These molecules are seen by the immunocompetent donor T cells either as foreign or as "self." If the molecules match the receptors on the donor T cells, they are seen as self and no response if mediated. If, however, the receptors do not match, the T cells understand the host cells to be foreign and mount an inflammatory reaction to them, eventually causing cell death and tissue destruction. Therefore the goal in stem cell transplantation is to match the donor cells and recipient cells as closely as possible. This is discussed in terms of "5/6 or 6/6" matching; this means that of the six HLA major molecules, the donor matches the host with 5 or 6 of the molecules. By closely matching these antigens on both the donor and recipient stem cells, the chance that the donor T cells will recognize the HLA molecules expressed on the recipient tissue as "self" increases, reducing the risk for GVHD. However, if the donor T cells recognize the host tissue cells as foreign, as may happen with a mis-matched or a less than 6/6 matched donor transplant, the donor T cells mount a response against the host tissue; they produce a variety of cytokines that cause the inflammatory response. Some of these cytokines are tumor necrosis factor (TNF), interleukin-1 (IL-1), and interleukin-2 (IL-2).

GVHD can be categorized into two subtypes, acute and chronic. Patients may develop either type or even both. Acute GVHD is distinguished from chronic GVHD by the different clinical manifestations and time of onset. Most practitioners consider acute GVHD to be GVHD symptoms that develop before day +100 from transplantation, and chronic GVHD usually is classified as occurring after day +100. However, more current studies use the clinical symptoms, rather than the time of onset, as defining characteristics (Chao, 2006b & c).

The targeted organs in GVHD most often are the skin, liver, GI tract and, in chronic GVHD, the lungs and complete immune system. The overall result of this "attack on self" can range from mild manifestations (i.e., a slight skin rash) to overwhelming desquamation of cells, resulting in the patient's death. The severity of the GVHD is categorized into different stages. Acute GVHD may be mild, moderate, severe, or life-threatening. For skin manifestations, stage 1 (mild) involves a skin rash over less than 25% of the body. Stage 2 (moderate) involves a rash over more than 25% of the body, along with mild liver involvement and/or mild diarrhea (not exceeding 1 L/day). Stage 3 (severe) involves severe rash over more than 50% of the body and moderate liver involvement and diarrhea. Stage 4 (life-threatening) involves blistering of the skin, bullous lesions, and severe liver disease and/or voluminous amounts of diarrhea (Stewart, 1992).

For liver manifestations, stage 1 is marked by a bilirubin level of 2 to 3 mg/dL; stage 2 by a level of 3.1 to 6 mg/dL; stage 3 by a level of 6.1 to 15 mg/dL; and stage 4 by a bilirubin level greater than 15 mg/dL.

For enteritis manifestations, stage 1 is considered to be diarrhea greater than 30 mL/kg or 500 mL/day; stage 2 is diarrhea greater than 60 mL/kg or 1000 mL/day; stage 3 is diarrhea greater than 90 mL/kg or 1500 mL/day; and stage 4 is diarrhea of 2 L or more per day and/or severe abdominal pain. The mortality rate for stage 4 acute GVHD is almost 100% (Alexander & Wong, 2000). Researchers are continuing to search for the ability to separate the graft versus leukemia from GVHD by depleting T cells that mediate GVHD, while sparing the T cells that are specific from tumor destruction (Chen et al, 2002).

Many providers use the IBMTR grading system. This system is broken up into grades A, B, C, and D. Grade A is grade 1 skin GVHD with no other systems involved. Grade B is grade 2 skin, and grade 1 or 2 liver. Grade C is a combination of grade 3 skin, gut, and liver. Grade D is a combination of grade 4 skin, gut, and liver.

As our understanding of the immune system has expanded and new treatments for GVHD have been found, a new concept has appeared, the *graft versus tumor effect*. This is the possibility that the donor cells may see malignant cells as foreign and thus react in the same manner as seen with GVHD: creating an actual immune response to the malignancy and preventing the cancer cells from proliferating; in fact, treating the cancer (Alexander & Wong, 2000).

The nurse's main roles in treating and preventing GVHD include early detection and prompt attention to provide treatment; educating the patient about signs and symptoms, as well as preventive measures; providing symptom management for the patient with active GVHD; and helping the patient with chronic GVHD gain a better quality of life or, in some cases, come to an acceptance and a peaceful end of life.

EPIDEMIOLOGY AND ETIOLOGY

The incidence of acute GVHD varies but is inversely proportional to the number of HLA matches. The more major antigens that are matched, the less likely it is that acute GVHD will occur. In the case of two or three mismatched HLA antigens, the incidence increases to 80%; it is closer to 40% to 50% in fully matched siblings (Alexander & Wong, 2000). The severity of GVHD correlates directly with the amount of T cells infused. Therefore it is important to strike a balance between providing the patient with enough stem cells to stimulate adequate engraftment and not stepping over the boundaries and giving too many donor T cells, which would tip the scales in favor of development of GVHD. Acute GVHD accounts for 50% of nonrelapsed deaths. The onset of clinical symptoms occurs, on average, between day +19 and day +25 after transplantation, or during the time of significant WBC engraftment. If acute GVHD occurs, the estimated 100-day survival rate is as follows:

Grade 1: 78% to 90%
Grade 2: 66% to 92%
Grade 3: 29% to 62%
Grade 4: 23% to 25%

Chronic GVHD occurs in up to 50% of long-term survivors of fully matched (6/6) sibling transplants (Chao, 2006c). The incidence increases with certain risk factors, such as prior acute GVHD, and is reduced by other factors, such as the administration of GVHD prophylaxis with methotrexate and tacrolimus.

Transfusion-related GVHD is very rare; the incidence is estimated at 0.1% to 1% in immunocompromised patients. However, the mortality rate with this type of GVHD is 80% to 90% (Silvergleid, 2006).

RISK PROFILE

Acute GVHD

- HLA disparity, particularly one or more of the major antigens in class I or class II
- Advanced age
- Donor and recipient gender disparity (female to male transplantation increases likelihood of GVHD)
- *Status of underlying disease*: The more disease that is present on treatment, the more likely the patient is to have acute GVHD.
- *Amount of radiation delivered*: Larger amounts of total body irradiation are more likely to cause acute GVHD. The greater the amount of radiation, the greater the tissue damage and, in turn, the greater the amount of T-cell proliferation.
- The risk is reduced with prophylactic use of methotrexate and cyclosporine or tacrolimus.
- The risk also is reduced by the presence of a sterile environment (i.e., gut decontamination with Flagyl and ciprofloxacin).
- There is no difference between patients receiving peripheral blood progenitor cells or cells harvested directly from bone marrow (Brown et al, 1999).

Chronic GVHD

- HLA disparity or mismatching
- Advanced age
- Subacute GVHD, usually detected by skin biopsy or buccal mucosal biopsy
- History of moderate to severe acute GVHD
- Previous splenectomy
- Cytomegalovirus seropositivity, either donor or recipient
- Second bone marrow infusions with boosts of donor leukocytes
- Previous herpes virus infection

PROGNOSIS

The prognosis is directly related to the stage of GVHD. Patients with mild disease (stage 1 or stage 2) have a low mortality rate. In patients with stage 4 disease, the mortality rate approaches 100% (Ferrara & Deeg, 1991). The prognosis also depends on the response to treatment. Refractory GVHD has a higher mortality rate, because it often progresses to a more severe stage. Transfusion-related GVHD carries a mortality rate of 80% to 90%. With chronic GVHD, the prognosis is better if the patient has not had a previous episode of acute GVHD; a poorer prognosis is associated with advancing age. A combination of liver and skin GVHD with lichenoid findings carries a poor prognosis.

PROFESSIONAL ASSESSMENT CRITERIA (PAC)

Acute GVHD

1. A maculopapular rash may develop around day + 19 to + 25, (Przepiorka et al, 1995) or around the time of white blood cell engraftment. This is the first and most common manifestation of acute GVHD. The rash usually involves the neck, back of the ears, shoulders, palms, and soles of the feet. It often is described as a "sunburn" and can be painful or pruritic (Chao, 2006b,i). If left untreated, the rash may spread, eventually involving the entire integument, and in severe cases may form causing bullous lesions and peeling of the skin.

2. Skin biopsies are often performed, although treatment is initiated on the basis of the clinical picture. Findings consistent with GVHD include dyskeratotic epidermal keratinocytes and apaptosis at the base of crypts (Chao, 2006f,g,h). The initial treatment for these skin rashes is application of topical steroid creams.

3. An abnormal rise in liver function tests may be seen. The liver is the second most commonly involved organ. A rise in the serum levels of conjugated bilirubin and alkaline phosphatase are often the first signs reported. Other differentials to consider with this finding are hepatic veno-occlusive disease (see Chapter 21), viral hepatitis, and drug effects.

4. Liver biopsy is the only means of definitively diagnosing GVHD of the liver. Most often a transjugular hepatic biopsy is preferred because it poses a lower risk of bleeding. Findings consistent with GVHD are extensive bile duct damage, bile duct atypia and degeneration, and lymphocytic infiltration of small bile ducts with cholestasis. In some cases, Actigall may be beneficial in reducing the liver function values.

5. Jaundice, by assessing color of skin and sclera and liver function laboratory tests (AST, ALT). A yellowing tint to the skin and/or sclerae is another manifestation of liver damage from GVHD.

6. Ascites, by assessing weight and abdominal girth. Ascites may also accompany a rise in liver function values, suggests a differential of GVHD.

7. Diarrhea is seen, distinguished by large volumes (up to 10 L/day) and a consistency that is mostly water and occasionally bloody. Diagnosis is clinical, but a definitive diagnosis can be made through colon biopsy. Another differential to consider is cytomegalovirus (CMV) infection, because its presentation is almost identical.

8. Colon biopsy findings consistent with GVHD show crypt cell necrosis; with severe disease, large areas of the colon may be denuded and show total loss of the epithelium, leading to malabsorption (Chao, 2006e).

9. Malabsorption is often seen in labs with low levels of oral medications, hypomagnesemia, hypokalemia, and other electrolyte abnormalities.
10. An increased risk of infections exists as a result of pancytopenia and a drop in serum concentrations of immunoglobulins.
11. A reduction in precursor cells is seen, leading to thrombocytopenia.

Chronic GVHD

1. Organ fibrosis with collagen deposits and atrophy are hallmark signs. Chronic GVHD is staged as either limited or extensive (Alexander & Wong, 2000).
2. Skin changes in the form of thickening or lichen planus are seen. Histologic findings include epidermal atrophy and dermal fibrosis. The onset may be marked by general erythema or plaques, often with a history of photoactivation. Areas of hyperpigmentation may alternate with hypopigmentation.
3. The skin may become fixed to underlying fascia, causing joint contractures (Chao, 2006c).
4. Serum alkaline phosphatase and bilirubin are elevated. Biopsy may show chronic persistent hepatitis.
5. Changes occur in the oral mucosa. Dry mouth and pain secondary to ulcerations may be presenting complaints. Physical findings include an erythematous mucosa with lichenoid lesions.
6. BOOP (bronchiolitis obliterans see Chapter 7) may be present. Patients present with dyspnea and a nonproductive cough. BOOP is a nonspecific inflammatory reaction that mostly affects the small airways. It is characterized by an organizing intraluminal exudate.
   • The hallmark sign of BOOP is the presence of intraluminal fibrotic buds, called Masson bodies, which are found in bronchioles and alveoli. Inflammatory changes occur around alveolar walls with macrophages present and are considered the organizing pneumonias.
   • Chest x-ray film (CXR) changes noted with BOOP include diffuse infiltrates, and restrictive ventilation is seen on pulmonary function tests (PFTs).
   • A bronchoscopy commonly is performed to try to obtain a biopsy sample from the affected lung. Bronchoscopy may show destruction of the small airways, with fibrous obliteration of the bronchioles.
   • Bronchodilators and cough suppressants are used to control cough. Macrolide antibiotics, such as erythromycin, are used because their mechanism of action reduces the circulating T lymphocytes. Steroids are also used to treat BOOP, as they are for skin, intestine, and liver GVHD (King, 2006).
   • BOOP is often associated with decreased serum IgG levels.
   • Risk factors include advanced age; therefore this is seen more often in the adult transplant population (Kaner, 2006).
7. Recurrent infections are seen in chronic GVHD as a result of prolonged and profound immunosuppression.
8. Pancytopenia, abnormal liver function tests, and electrolyte abnormalities are the most common laboratory results.

Transfusion-Associated GVHD

1. The patient may have a history of blood transfusion in the past 4 to 30 days.
2. Presenting symptoms of transfusion-related GVHD are fever; an erythematous, maculopapular rash; vomiting; diarrhea; and cough (Silvergleid, 2006).
3. Laboratory findings show profound pancytopenia, abnormal liver function tests, and electrolyte abnormalities.

4. Transfusion-related GVHD is most often associated with administration of nonirradiated blood products (Sliverglied, 2006).
5. Prevention is the best treatment. All blood products given to immunocompromised patients should be irradiated with 25 Gy and leukocyte reduced.
6. Currently no adequate treatment exists for this type of GVHD. Steroids, ultraviolet radiation, TNF inhibitors, and thalidomide all have been tried, to no avail.

NURSING CARE AND TREATMENT

1. Recognize the patients at risk for GVHD (i.e., allogeneic patients with any risk factors).
2. Administer preventive measures. The most frequently used prophylactic regimen is methotrexate and cyclosporine (Chao, 2006f). Cyclosporine is administered beginning at day 2 and continues through day +90, when weaning the dose can begin if no GVHD exists. Cyclosporine is also given intravenously for the first several weeks to ensure adequate absorption. Remember to assess liver function tests and creatinine before administering methotrexate, because this drug can cause kidney and liver toxicities. Methotrexate is most often administered IV on days +1, +3, +6, and +11.
3. The patient's urine should be alkalinized with sodium bicarbonate, and the patient should not receive methotrexate until the urine pH is greater than 8.
4. Obtain levels of cyclosporine or tacrolimus per program policy and anticipate adjustments, because there is a therapeutic target serum level. Levels are usually kept at 100 to 300ng/mL for cyclosporine and 10 to 20ng/mL for tacrolimus. NOTE: Interaction is possible between tacrolimus and CYP3AY inhibitors (e.g., erythromycin, itraconazole, ketoconazole, fluconazole, calcium channel blockers, and cimetidine).
5. Recognize possible rashes, changes in bowel habits, and increasing liver function tests that may be indicative of beginning GVHD.
6. Assess mucosal integrity for breakdown or inflammation associated with methotrexate dosing.
7. Monitor for airway protection if mucosal breakdown becomes severe.
8. Administer pain management for mucosal breakdown or abdominal pain associated with GVHD. Patient-controlled analgesia (PCA) may be required for adequate control.
9. Monitor for adverse reactions to tacrolimus or cyclosporine, such as renal insufficiency, hypertension, hyperglycemia, headache and neurotoxicity.
10. Obtain a biopsy sample of the affected organ: colon, skin, liver.
11. Once a diagnosis has been confirmed, administer corticosteroids. There is uncertainty about the drugs' mechanism of action, but some believe that they suppress cytokine activity. Begin with application of a topical steroid cream if the affected organ is the skin; usually 1% triamcinolone is applied to the affected area TID. If other organs are affected, the most common steroid used is Solu-Medrol. The usual dosage is 1 to 2 mg/kg/day with a slow taper once symptoms begin resolving (Chao, 2006d).
12. Monitor for adverse effects of steroids.
    • **Increased risk for infection:** Monitor vital signs regularly for fever and hypotension.
    • **Steroid myopathy:** Encourage daily ambulation and physical therapy as needed. Monitor for muscle strength decrease, particularly in the quadriceps.
    • **Steroid psychoses:** Agitation, aggressive behavior or extreme depression; assess for danger to self or others.
    • **Hyperglycemia:** Patient may require larger doses of insulin during this time; likewise, as steroids are tapered, insulin needs will decrease.
13. Maintain skin integrity if affected. Monitor for skin breakdown or thickening. Provide protective barrier for open lesions. Keep skin moist with lotion.

14. **Daily weights:** Any change of 3 pounds in a 24-hour period requires further evaluation.
15. Assess nutritional intake. Patient may require total parental nutrition (TPN) for adequate nutrition.
16. Obtain and assess daily labs: CBC to monitor for blood requirements, chemistry panel to assess for electrolyte imbalances due to malabsorption, liver function tests to monitor changes in bilirubin and alkaline phosphatase.
17. Monitor oxygen saturations and shortness of breath. The patient may require albuterol nebulizers or inhaled steroids for BOOP.
18. Monitor for bowel function; the risk for ileus is high. The patient should have active bowel sounds. If no bowel sounds are present, obtain a KUB to rule out ileus.
19. **Diet:** Neutropenic—if the GI system is affected, the patient may be NPO until symptoms begin resolving. The patient then may advance to a diet of clear liquids, then to a bland diet, and then progress as tolerated.
20. Anticipate the addition of or an increase in the dosage of immunosuppressants.
21. Anticipate the use of additional treatments if no improvement in symptoms is seen within 3 to 5 days of starting steroids. These agents may include CellCept, which is synergistic with cyclosporine, daclizumab, or infliximab.
22. Assess the patient's coping strategies. Many patients will have altered body image due to skin rashes, loss of weight as a result of diarrhea, or abdominal distention and jaundice with liver GVHD.
23. The use of herbs and alternative medicines is not recommended during the time of transplant, while the patient is taking immunosuppressants, because of uncertainty about the products' purity and possible interactions with common medicines used during this time.

EVIDENCE-BASED PRACTICE UPDATES

1. Multiple trials are ongoing to assess new methods of treatment for GVHD.
   - Treatment of steroid-resistant GVHD with monoclonal antibodies directed against IL-2 receptors is under investigation. The drug daclizumab has been associated with an 84% complete response rate (Herve et al., 1990). Another monoclonal antibody under study is OKT3. The mechanism of action is a direct effect against the CD3 antigen, which is associated with the T-cell receptors. Studies that have been completed with OKT3 showed a good initial response, but they also show a recurrence of GVHD. Therefore the long-term efficacy of the drug is in question. Also, the use of OKT3 has been faulted in the development of posttransplantation lymphoproliferative syndrome (Chao, 2006a).
   - Etanercept (Enbrel), a TNF-alpha receptor fusion protein, is being used as treatment for both acute and chronic GVHD, although the data are mostly in case report form (Chiang et al., 2002). Another TNF-alpha blocker is infliximab. In one retrospective study of 134 patients, 67% had a response to infliximab as a single agent, and 62% had a complete response (Couriel et al., 2004). However, several studies suggest that although TNF blockers initially improved GVHD, they are associated with a high incidence of bacterial, viral, and fungal infections (Marty et al., 2003).
   - Extracorporeal phototherapy is being used to treat chronic GVHD. The results have varied widely, ranging from complete responses in 100% of patients to complete responses in only 12% (Dall'Amico & Messina, 2002).
   - Extracorporeal phototherapy is also being paired with leukapheresis as a means of T-cell depletion (Lee et al., 2004).

- Surgery is an option for patients with intestinal chronic GVHD with obstructive manifestations that are refractory to standard immunosuppressants. Resection or stricturoplasty are types of GI surgery used to correct chronic GVHD of the intestine (Herr et al., 2004). However, few attempts at this radical approach have been made, and no long-term data are available on its efficacy.
- Mesenchymal stem cells are being studied as a means of treating acute GVHD. Because these cells are "universal stem cells," specific typing is not necessary (Le Blanc et al., 2004). These cells are undifferentiated pluripotent stem cells, which means they can develop into many types of tissue cells. They are derived from bone marrow–populated peripheral blood via apheresis. These cells migrate to areas of injury and secrete immunosuppressive factors, leading to the inactivation of T cells. Currently this technique is being used in grade 3 and grade 4 severe refractory GVHD.

2. T-cell depletion is another means of preventing GVHD. Most often the T-cell depletion is accomplished with campath given either in vivo or ex vivo (Chao, 2006g). This process is effective in reducing the incidence of GVHD in mice. However, it can also slow engraftment and offers less protection against relapse. Campath has been used in combination with fludarabine and melphalan as a conditioning regimen for a nonmyeloablative stem cell transplant, with positive results. Only one of 43 patients did not engraft, and no grade 3 or grade 4 acute GVHD occurred. Only one patient developed chronic GVHD (Kottaridis et al., 2000).

3. First-line therapy for patients who fail prophylaxis is steroids, most often given IV at a dosage of 1 to 2 mg/kg/day (Chao, 2006d,i).

4. Another treatment for chronic GVHD is Psoralen ultraviolet irradiation (PUVA). PUVA works by exposing circulating T lymphocytes in the patient to a minimal dose of ultraviolet radiation. This reduces the number and decreases the function of the circulating T cells. One study showed a 30% complete response rate (Kapoor et al., 1992).

5. A salvage therapy for chronic GVHD is thalidomide. One study evaluated the efficacy of thalidomide in this population. Approximately 20% of the patients had a good response. However, 36% discontinued the drug because of the side effects of sedation, constipation, and neuropathies (Parker et al., 1995).

TEACHING AND EDUCATION

1. Patients who receive an allogeneic stem cell transplant must be persistently conscious of sun exposure or exposure to tanning beds. No scientific research provides empiric evidence for the avoidance of tanning beds, but any exposure to UV rays poses a risk. A sunscreen of SPF 15 or higher should be applied before any sun exposure and reapplied as needed, because photoactivation is a known cause of GVHD.

2. The patient should wear protective clothing with long sleeves, pants, and a hat to prevent overexposure to the sun; however, this does not prevent the patient from participating in regular outdoor activities.

3. **Nutrition:** The patient may initially be NPO with gut GVHD. As symptoms improve, the diet may be advanced to clear liquids, then a bland diet, and then as tolerated. Patients should not eat dairy products, because many patients are lactose intolerant after chemotherapy. Lactose products may create diarrhea, thus confusing the clinical picture.

4. **Tests and procedures:**
   - Daily labs should be drawn to assess blood transfusion needs, electrolyte replacement needs, and the progress of liver GVHD.

- *Liver biopsy*: Transjugular liver biopsy is the most common means of biopsy, because it has a reduced risk for bleeding. A catheter is inserted into the subclavian vein and passed through to the liver. Under fluoroscopy, a small biopsy is taken of the affected area. Patients are under conscious sedation during the procedure.
- *Skin biopsy*: The affected area is numbed with a subcutaneous injection of lidocaine, and a small, circular blade is then inserted into the skin and removed. The skin piece is then excised and sent for evaluation. One small stitch is usually required to close the biopsy site.
- *Colon biopsy*: The patient is given a colon preparative regimen, often with Fleet's enemas, until the colon is clear. The patient will be NPO 12 hours before the procedure. With the patient under conscious sedation, a scope is passed rectally into the colon. A small biopsy is taken from an affected area.
- *Pulmonary function tests*: The patient blows into a tube, and a machine assesses lung elasticity and lung volumes.

5. **Treatments:** Treatment often begins with intravenous steroids. Educate the patient about possible side effects: irritability, muscle weakness, increased risk of infection, hyperglycemia, and hypertension. If the patient's condition is refractory to this treatment, other drugs may be added. Patients should be aware of the side effects of all medications they are given.

6. **Prophylaxis:** *Medications* such as cyclosporine or tacrolimus are started at the time of transplantation, even though GVHD has not occurred. This is done to prevent GVHD. It is important for the patient not to miss doses, because efficacy depends on adequate, consistent blood levels of these drugs. These levels are assessed periodically per program protocol, and dosages are adjusted accordingly. The patient will also have prophylactic antibiotics to prevent infections such as pneumococcal pneumonia (PCP).

NURSING DIAGNOSES

1. **Imbalanced nutrition: less than body requirements** related to malabsorption and diarrhea
2. **Risk for deficient fluid volume** related to malabsorption and diarrhea
3. **Risk for infection** related to immunocompromised host
4. **Acute pain** related to abdominal pain associated with GVHD of the gut or liver or pruritus associated with skin GVHD
5. **Disturbed body image** related to skin changes with rash, abdominal bloating, or weight loss

EVALUATION AND DESIRED OUTCOMES

1. The skin rash will resolve, and the integument will be re-established.
2. The diarrhea will resolve, and functioning bowel habits will return.
3. The patient will return to an adequate nutritional oral intake with adequate absorption.
4. Electrolyte balance will be restored.
5. Liver function tests will return to baseline with resolution of jaundice and ascites.
6. Hemodynamic stability will be achieved.
7. The patient will maintain his or her weight.
8. If the pulmonary system has been affected, shortness of breath will resolve and pulmonary function will return to baseline.
9. The patient will return to independent activities of daily living.

DISCHARGE PLANNING AND FOLLOW-UP CARE

- Instruct the patient to continue the oral steroid taper over several weeks.
- Instruct the patient to take prophylactic antibiotics as long as the patient continues steroids.
- Advise follow-up visits with a transplant doctor weekly initially to ensure complete resolution of symptoms without flares of GVHD as steroids are tapered. Laboratory results also need to be evaluated to ensure resolution of liver GVHD.
- Educate the patient on the symptoms of recurrent GVHD: new onset of diarrhea, shortness of breath, dry cough, and skin rash. Instruct the patient to contact the transplant doctor with any concerns.

REVIEW QUESTIONS

QUESTIONS

1. **The two mediators of GVHD are:**
   1. Host T cells and macrophages
   2. Donor T cells and host HLA antigens
   3. Host HLA antigens and donor platelets
   4. Donor tissue cells and host lymphocytes

2. **Which manifestation of GVHD is unique to chronic GVHD:**
   1. Excessive diarrhea (greater than 10 L/day)
   2. Rise in liver function tests with jaundice
   3. Maculopapular rash covering 50% of the body
   4. Thickened skin, resulting in dermal fibrosis and joint contractures

3. **Mrs. N is being treated for acute GVHD of the gut with cyclosporine and high-dose steroids. Yesterday she began complaining of a headache, and this morning you notice that she has an unsteady gait. On taking her vital signs, you note a blood pressure of 160/96. You suspect the cause of her symptoms is:**
   1. Steroid myopathy
   2. Transfusion-related toxicity
   3. Cyclosporine toxicity
   4. Subdural hematoma

4. **A patient who had undergone allogeneic stem cell transplantation is preparing to be discharged to his home. During the discharge teaching, the patient comments to the nurse** that he can't wait to get home to sit by his pool. The nurse should provide what education to this patient:
   1. Inform the patient he will no longer be able to participate in pool activities.
   2. Inform the patient that he can enjoy the pool but must wear protective clothing in the form of long sleeves, pants, and a hat.
   3. Instruct the patient not to sit by the pool without wearing a sunscreen of at least SPF 15 and preferably not during the sunniest part of the day.
   4. Inform the patient that he is able to sit by the pool but should not submerse his body underwater.

5. **Ms. N is a 60-year-old African American female who has received an allogeneic stem cell transplant for AML. She received donor cells from her 5/6 HLA-matched sister. In addition, she received methotrexate as part of her regimen. Her other medications are cyclosporine 100 mg PO q12h, ciprofloxacin 500 mg PO q12h, Flagyl 500 mg PO q8h, and Ativan 1 mg PO q4h PRN. Which of the following is a risk factor for acquiring acute GVHD:**
   1. 5/6 HLA matching
   2. Receiving donor cells from a female sibling
   3. Taking methotrexate as part of the regimen
   4. Taking flagyl and ciprofloxacin as antibiotics

6. Mrs. N presents with symptoms of fever to 102° F, macular rash over her upper torso and neck, and diarrhea over the past 24 hours, which she describes as explosive and large volume. She is an immunocompromised patient who received a blood transfusion approximately a week ago. You suspect transfusion-related GVHD. Your next step would be to:
   1. Assess the patient's laboratory values: CBC, liver function tests, and chemistry panel.
   2. Start steroids at 2 mg/kg/day.
   3. Call for a GI consult for biopsy to diagnose GVHD of the gut.
   4. Contact the blood bank to research whether her transfusion was irradiated and leukoreduced.

7. Mr. R has been battling acute GVHD of the gut. He has been on total parental nutrition for several weeks. He is being treated with IV steroids at 2 mg/kg/day. His symptoms have been slowly improving, and his TPN is being cycled so that he can begin reintroducing foods to his GI system. His family is very attentive and concerned about his well-being. While you were in the room, he mentioned that he would love to have a fast-food hamburger and a milkshake. His family immediately grabs the car keys and starts out the door to accommodate his wish. Your response as a nurse is to:
   1. Suggest that he add fries to his order because he needs lots of calories.
   2. Dissuade his family, because although their intentions are good, a burger and a milkshake are not part of his allowed diet.
   3. Dissuade his family from going because fast food has been sitting out and is not fresh; instead you suggest a homemade burger and milkshake.
   4. Suggest starting with a milkshake, because his stomach will have shrunk after many days without use and he may not be able to complete a full meal.

8. Mr. P presented with 3 L of diarrhea output per day. A colonoscopy and biopsy determined that he has gut GVHD. He was started on steroids at 2 mg/kg/day for treatment. It's been 3 days, and his diarrhea output has stayed persistently high (greater than 3 L/day). However, over the course of your shift, you note that his diarrhea has stopped completely. He continues to have some cramping pain, but no output and no bowel sounds. His family is questioning the sudden turnaround. Your response is:
   1. The steroids have started to work and have quieted his gut.
   2. Without food intake, his diarrhea would naturally slow down.
   3. He may have an ileus as a result of the gut GVHD and you are going to notify the care team.
   4. He most likely has an impaction, and the diarrhea is unable to be released.

9. Mrs. S has gut GVHD. She presented 2 weeks ago with voluminous amounts of diarrhea. She was already on cyclosporine for prophylaxis. She began treatment with steroids at 2 mg/kg/day dosing 1 week ago. Her diarrhea output continues high, at 5 L/day. The next step in treatment is to:
   1. Continue current dosing with steroids
   2. Add a monoclonal antibody, such as daclizumab
   3. Add extracorporeal phototherapy
   4. Give a dose of campath for T-cell depletion

10. A common and viable means of preventing GVHD is:
    1. T-cell depletion
    2. TNF alpha blockers
    3. Corticosteroids
    4. Monoclonal antibodies, such as daclizumab

ANSWERS

1. **Answer: 2**
   Rationale: The mediators of GVHD are the donor T cells and the human leukocyte antigens in the host.

2. **Answer: 4**
   Rationale: In chronic GVHD, skin changes occur in the form of thickening, or lichen planus. Histologic findings include dermal fibrosis. The skin may become fixed to underlying fascia, resulting in joint contractures.

3. **Answer: 3**
   Rationale: Cyclosporine toxicity can manifest as headache, hypertension, renal insufficiency, and neurotoxicity, often in the form of altered gait.

4. **Answer: 3**
   Rationale: Photoactivation is a known cause of chronic GVHD. Patients at risk should be made aware that although they can participate in regular activities, they should minimize sun exposure; they should always wear a sunscreen of at least SPF 15 and ideally should not be exposed to sun during the brightest part of the day.

5. **Answer: 1**
   Rationale: The greatest risk factor for acquiring acute GVHD is HLA disparity. Receiving donor cells from a same-sex sibling does not increase risk. Treatment with methotrexate as part of the regimen reduces the risk, because it is prophylaxis for GVHD. Flagyl and ciprofloxacin are taken for gut decontamination, which provides a sterile environment and reduces the risk of acute GVHD.

6. **Answer: 1**
   Rationale: Assessing labs will point to a more definitive diagnosis in a shorter time. If this is transfusion-related GVHD, you will see pancytopenia on the CBC, elevated liver tests, and electrolyte abnormalities.

7. **Answer: 2**
   Rationale: After being treated for acute GVHD of the gut and supported on TPN while being NPO, the next step forward in diet would be clear liquids. Heavy meats, although rich in protein, will be too much for the gut to digest. In addition, milk products, such as milkshakes, contain lactose, and many patients are lactose intolerant after chemotherapy, which would lead to an increase in diarrhea, thus clouding the clinical picture.

8. **Answer: 3**
   Rationale: Gut GVHD can progress to obstruction with an ileus. This is manifested in a clinical picture of no stool production, no bowel sounds, and pain. A KUB can be done to evaluate for this occurrence.

9. **Answer: 2**
   Rationale: Multiple trials are ongoing with monoclonal antibodies, such as daclizumab, for steroid-resistant GVHD. Daclizumab currently is associated with an 84% response rate. Continuing steroid dosing and adding nothing is not an option, because some response to the steroids should have been seen within 5 days. Photopheresis is a treatment used for chronic GVHD, not the acute form. Campath is used for T-cell depletion as a means of preventing GVHD, not treating it.

10. **Answer: 1**
    Rationale: T-cell depletion, usually in the form of campath, is a means of preventing GVHD. Other means include cyclosporine, tacrolimus, and methotrexate. TNF blockers, corticosteroids, and monoclonal antibodies are all means of treatment.

REFERENCES

Alexander, A., & Wong, S. (2000). Graft versus host disease: Pathophysiology and management. *Jacksonville Medicine, 11*:1-8.

Brown, R., Adkins, H., & Khoury, R., et al. (1999). Long-term follow-up of high-risk allogeneic peripheral-blood stem-cell transplant recipients: Graft-versus-host disease and transplant-related mortality. *Journal of Clinical Oncology, 17*(3):806-812.

Chao, N. (2006a). *Treatment of graft-versus-host disease*. Last updated May 10, 2006, pp. 1-8. Retrieved August 3, 2007, from www.uptodate.com/utd/content/topic.do?topicKey=hcell_tr/7404&view=text.

Chao, N. (2006b). *Clinical manifestations and diagnosis of acute graft-versus-host disease*. Last updated May 10, 2006, pp. 1-5. Retrieved August 9, 2007, from www.uptodate.com/utd/content/topic.do?topicKey= hcell_tr/7113&view=text

Chao, N. (2006c). *Clinical manifestations and diagnosis of chronic graft-versus-host disease*. Last updated May 10, 2006, pp. 1-8. Retrieved August 3, 2007, from www.utdol.com/utd/content/topic.do?topicKey=hcell_tr/ 6824&view=text.

Chao, N. (2006d). *Overview of immunosuppressive agents used for prevention and treatment of graft-versus-host disease*. Last updated May 10, 2006, pp. 1-16. Retrieved July 12, 2007, from www.utdol.com/utd/con-tent/topic.do?topicKey=hcell_tr/8306&view=text?topicKey=hcell_tr/8306&view=text.

Chao, N. (2006e). *Pathogenesis of graft-versus-host disease*. Last updated May 10, 2006, pp. 1-10. Retrieved August 6, 2007, from www.utdol.com/utd/content/topic.do?topicKey=hcell_tr/6108&view=text.

Chao, N. (2006f). *Prevention of acute graft-versus-host disease: Trials of pharmacologic therapy*. Last updated May10, 2006, pp. 1-8. Retrieved July 15, 2007,from www.utdol.com/utd/content/topic.do?topicKey= hcell_tr/4509&view=text.

Chao, N. (2006g). *Prevention of acute graft-versus-host disease: Trials of T cell depletion*. Last updated, May 10, 2006, pp. 1-8. Retrieved August 6, 2007, from www.utdol.com/utd/content/topic.do?topicKey=hcell_tr/ 5792&view=text.

Chao, N. (2006h). *Prevention and treatment of acute graft-versus-host disease: Recommendations*. Last updated, May 10, 2006, pp. 1-6. Retrieved August 3, 2007, from www.utdol.com/utd/content/topic.do?topicKey= hcell_tr/5229&view=text.

Chao, N. (2006i). *Treatment of acute graft-versus-host disease: Clinical trials*. Last updated, May 10, 2006, pp. 1-10. Retrieved August 9, 2007, from www.utdol.com/utd/content/topic.do?topicKey=hcell_tr/ 5433&view=text?topicKey=hcell_tr/5433&view=text.

Chen, B., Xiuyu, C., & Congxiao, L., et al. (2002). Prevention of graft-versus-host disease while preserving graft-versus-leukemia effect after selective depletion of host-reactive T cells by photodynamic cell purging process. *Blood, 99*(9):3083-3088.

Chiang, K., Abhyankar, S., & Bridges, K., et al. (2002). Recombinant human tumor necrosis factor receptor fusion protein as complementary treatment for chronic graft-versus-host disease. *Transplantation, 73*:665-667.

Couriel, D., Saliba, R., & Hicks, K., et al. (2004). Tumor necrosis factor-alpha blockade for the treatment of acute GVHD. *Blood, 104*(3):649-654.

Dall'Amico, R., & Messina, C. (2002). Extracorporeal photochemotherapy for the treatment of graft-versus-host disease. *Therapeutic Apheresis, 6*(4):296-304.

Ferrara, J., & Deeg, J. (1991). Graft-versus-host disease. *New England Journal of Medicine, 324*(10):667-674.

Herr, A., Latulippe, J., & Carignan, S., et al. (2004). Is severe intestinal chronic graft-versus-host disease an indication for surgery? A report of two cases. *Transplantation, 77*(10):1617-1620.

Herve, P., Wijdenes, J., & Bergerat, J., et al. (1990). Treatment of corticosteroid resistant acute graft-versus-host disease by in vivo administration of anti-interleukin-2 receptor monoclonal antibody (B-B10). *Blood, 75*(4):1017-1023.

Jaksch, M., & Mattson, J. (2005). The pathophysiology of acute graft-versus-host disease. *Scandinavian Journal of Immunology, 61*(5):3604-3609.

Kaner, R. (2006). *Pulmonary complications after allogeneic hematopoietic cell transplantation*. Last updated, May 10, 2006, pp. 1-12. Retrieved July 12, 2007, from www.utdol.com/utd/content/topic.do?topicKey= int_lung/21689&view=text.

Kapoor, N., Pelligrini, A., & Copelan, E., et al. (1992). Psoralen plus ultraviolet A (PUVA) in the treatment of chronic graft versus host disease: Preliminary experience in standard treatment resistant patients. *Seminars in Hematology, 29*(2):108-112.

King, T. (2006). *Bronchiolitis in adults*. Last updated, May 10, 2006, pp. 1-3. Retrieved July 12, 2007,from www.utdol.com/utd/content/topic.do?topicKey=int_lung/16473&view=text?topicKey=int_lung/ 16473&view=text.

Kottaridis, P., Milligan, D., & Chopra, R., et al. (2000). In vivo CAMPATH-1H prevents graft-versus-host disease following nonmyeloablative stem cell transplantation. *Blood, 96*(7):2419-2425.

Le Blanc, K., Rasmusson, I., & Sundberg, B., et al. (2004). Treatment of severe acute graft-versus-host disease with third party haploidentical mesenchymal stem cells. *Lancet, 363*(9419):1439-1441.

Lee, S., Dorken, B., & Schmitt, C. (2004). Extracorporeal photopheresis in graft-versus-host disease: Ultraviolet radiation mediates T cell senescence in vivo. *Transplantation, 78*(3):484-485.

Marty, F., Lee, S., & Fahey, M., et al. (2003). Infliximab use in patients with severe graft-versus-host disease and other emerging risk factors of non-Candida invasive fungal infections in allogeneic hematopoietic stem cell transplant recipients: A cohort study. *Blood, 102*(8):2768-2776.

Parker, P., Chao, N., & Nadermanee, A., et al. (1995). Thalidomide as salvage therapy for chronic graft-versus-host disease. *Blood, 86*(9):3604-3609.

Prasad, V. K., Kernan, N., & Heller, G., et al. (1999). DNA typing for HLA-A and HLA-B identifies disparities between patients and unrelated donors matched by HLA-A and HLA-B serology and HLA-DRB1. *Blood, 93*(1):399-409.

Przepiorka, D., Weisdorf, D., & Martin, P., et al. (1995). Meeting report: Consensus Conference on Acute GVHD Grading. *Bone Marrow Transplantation, 15*(6):825-828.

Silvergleid, A. (2006). *Transfusion-associated graft-versus-host disease.* Last updated, May 10, 2006, pp. 1-4. Retrieved August 6, 2007, from www.utdol.com/utd/content/topic.do?topicKey=transfus/13622&view=text.

Stewart, S. (1992). Graft versus host disease. *BMT Newsletter,* 13:91-97. www.bmtinfonet.org/newsletters/index.

HEART FAILURE

JACQUELINE R. GANNUSCIO

PATHOPHYSIOLOGICAL MECHANISMS

Cancer chemotherapy has advanced significantly over the past several decades. However, the use of these agents has been limited by significant cardiac toxicities, including, arrhythmias, ischemia, hypertension, myocarditis, pericarditis, cardiomyopathy, and congestive heart failure (Shanholtz, 2001). The most common and well-known toxicity is congestive heart failure. *Congestive heart failure* (*CHF*) is defined as "defective cardiac filling and/or impaired contraction and emptying, resulting in the heart's inability to pump a sufficient amount of blood to meet the needs of the body tissues or to be able to do so only with an elevated filling pressure" (Colucci & Braunwald, 2004).

The contractile units of the heart muscle are the nonmyocytes and the myocytes (Fig. 19.1). Any injury, regardless of mechanism, leads to impaired contractility. Activation of compensatory mechanisms occurs, primarily through neurohormonal stimulation and cytokine activation, in an attempt to maintain adequate cardiac output to tissues. Patients may have asymptomatic left ventricular (LV) dysfunction for months to years (Moser, 1998). Over time, cellular and biochemical changes occur within the heart that are well recognized, including loss of myofilaments, apoptosis, disorganization of the cytoskeleton, disturbances in calcium homeostasis, and alteration in neurohormonal receptor density, signal transduction, and collagen synthesis (Francis, 2001). The term *cardiac remodeling* refers to ventricular hypertrophy and changes in the size and shape of the ventricle; these are the hallmarks of chronic heart failure and lead to the symptoms that patients experience.

Heart failure has many causes, including ischemic heart disease, hypertension, structural abnormalities of the heart, infection, toxins, and idiopathic causes (Box 19-1). In the United States, the most common cause is ischemic heart disease. A recent NHANES epidemiologic study of more than 13,000 patients with no previous history of heart failure estimated that over 60% of heart failure that occurs in the general population can be attributed to coronary artery disease (He et al., 2001). Although toxins, including chemotherapeutic agents, are not a common cause of heart failure in the general population, these drugs have important implications for oncology patients.

In oncology patients, chemotherapeutic agents lead to myocyte damage in specific ways. In anthracycline toxicity, the mechanism of heart failure is thought to be initiated by cell death, or apoptosis, related to the generation of free oxygen radicals (Perik et al., 2004). The free radicals are thought to produce subcellular changes in the myocardium, resulting in myofibril loss with separation of the intercalated disk and dilation of the sarcotubular system, structures essential for normal contraction of the myocyte (Singal & Iliskovic, 1998). Trastuzumab, a monoclonal antibody that binds to the HER2 receptor site, is known to cause heart failure whether used alone or in combination with anthracyclines for metastatic beast cancer. The mechanism is not well understood; however, it is thought to be a complex interaction between inhibition of the cardioprotective effects of the HER2

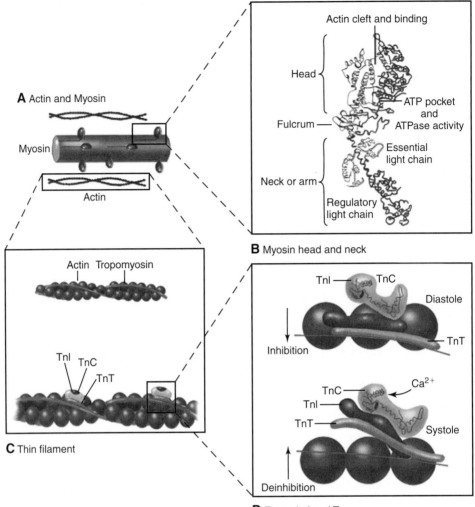

A Actin and Myosin

Myosin

Actin

B Myosin head and neck

Actin cleft and binding

Head

ATP pocket and ATPase activity

Fulcrum

Essential light chain

Neck or arm

Regulatory light chain

Actin Tropomyosin

TnI TnC TnT

C Thin filament

TnI TnC

Diastole

Inhibition

TnT

TnC Ca²⁺

TnI

TnT

Systole

Deinhibition

D Troponin I and T

Fig. 19.1 • Cardiac structure The heart is made up of nonmyocytes and myocytes. **A,** Nonmyocytes include connective tissue (fibroblasts), vascular smooth muscle cells, and endothelial cells. Nonmyocytes comprise most of the cells of the heart. **B,** Myocytes are separated by intercalcated disks, which are important for both structural integrity and electrical conduction. These structures are altered by the presence of free oxygen radicals; contractile force is lost, and cell death occurs. *(From Zipes, D. P., Libby, P., Bonow, R. O., et al. [2005]. Braunwald's heart disease: A textbook of cardiovascular medicine, [7th ed.], Philadelphia, W.B. Saunders.)*

receptors and ligands with additional stressors and the activation of proinflammatory pathways. These events can lead to early cell death and may play a role in cardiac hypertrophy (Feldman et al. 2000). Although their mechanisms are not understood, other chemotherapeutic agents also can rarely cause cardiotoxicity and ultimately congestive heart failure, including alkylating agents, mitomycin, paclitaxel, and vinca alkaloids (Pai & Nahato, 2000).

BOX 19-1	CAUSES OF HEART FAILURE

Most Common Causes
Coronary artery disease
Hypertension
Valvular heart disease (especially aortic and mitral disease)
Other Causes
Infections: Viruses (including the human immunodeficiency virus), bacteria, parasites
Pericardial diseases
Drugs (e.g., doxorubicin [Adriamycin], cyclophosphamide [Cytoxan], cocaine), alcohol
Connective tissue disease
Infiltrative disease (e.g., amyloidosis, sarcoidosis, hemochromatosis, malignancy)
Tachycardia
Obstructive cardiomyopathy
Neuromuscular disease (e.g., muscular or myotonic dystrophy, Friedreich's ataxia)
Metabolic disorders (e.g., glycogen storage disease type 2 [Pompe's disease] and type 5 [McArdle's disease])
Nutritional disorders (e.g., beriberi, kwashiorkor)
Pheochromocytoma
Radiation
Endomyocardial fibrosis
Eosinophilic endomyocardial disease
High-output heart failure (e.g., intracardiac shunt, atrioventricular fistula, beriberi, pregnancy, Paget's disease, hyperthyroidism, anemia)
Peripartum cardiomyopathy
Dilated idiopathic cardiomyopathy

EPIDEMIOLOGY AND ETIOLOGY

In a recent metaanalysis of cardiomyopathy in pediatric patients with cancer, the incidence of anthracycline-induced clinical cardiomyopathy ranged from 0 to 16%, and the condition developed at any time during or after therapy (Kremer et al., 2002a). However, in survivors of childhood cancer, the incidence of late cardiac structural abnormalities can be as high as 65% (Lipschultz et al., 1991, 2005). The incidence of left ventricular dysfunction with the use of trastuzumab alone is 7%; however, when the drug is combined with anthracycline and cyclophosphamide, the incidence can be as high as 28% (Feldman et al., 2000). The combination of anthracycline and mitomycin can result in a 10% incidence of heart failure (Yahalom & Portlock, 2004). Rarely, cardiac tumors can impair ventricular contraction or ventricular filling, leading to symptoms of heart failure.

RISK PROFILE

- **Chemotherapy:** Single or combination (Table 19-1).
- **Mediastinal radiation** (Clements et al., 2002).
- **Gender:** Females are at higher risk (Kremer et al., 2002a), although one study found that males who received concomitant mediastinal radiation also were at higher risk (Clements et al., 2002).
- **Higher cumulative dose** (Kremer et al., 2002a): A gradual rise in incidence is noted with increased doses; a rate as high as 36% is seen with cumulative doses of doxorubicin over 550 mg/m^2 body surface area (Shanholtz, 2001). However, there does not appear to be any absolutely safe dose of anthracycline (Lipshultz et al., 2005)

Table 19-1	CHEMOTHERAPEUTIC AGENTS ASSOCIATED WITH CONGESTIVE HEART FAILURE	
Generic Name	**Trade Name**	
Azacitidine	Vidaza	
Bevacizumab	Avastin	
Bicalutamide	Casodex	
Bortezomib	Velcade	
Cyclophosphamide	Cytoxan	
Doxorubicin	Adriamycin, Doxil	
Estramustine	Emcyt	
Exemestane	Aromasin	
Goserelin	Zoladex	
Idarubicin	Idamycin	
Ifosfamide	Ifex	
Imatinib	Gleevec	
Toremifene	Fareston	

- **Infusion rates:** Continuous infusion over 48 to 96 hours reduces the incidence over standard rapid infusion (Singal & Iliskovic, 1998)
- Earlier age at onset.

PROGNOSIS

In the past, the prognosis for heart failure was linked to the severity of functional limitations. The New York Heart Association (NYHA) Classification has been used to predict survival, tailor therapy, and determine readiness for cardiac transplantation. Class I patients are those with left ventricular dysfunction but no symptoms. Class II patients become symptomatic with moderate exertion. Class III patients are symptomatic with minimal exertion, and Class IV patients are symptomatic at rest. This classification system has been very useful to clinicians; however, it does not emphasize the progressive nature of the disease, because a patient's classification can vary depending on how well controlled the symptoms are. In their most recent guidelines, the American Heart Association and the American College of Cardiology published a staging system for heart failure (HF), which can be summarized as follows (Hunt et al., 2005):

Stage A: High risk for HF without structural heart disease or symptoms
Stage B: Heart disease with asymptomatic left ventricular dysfunction
Stage C: Prior or current symptoms of HF
Stage D: Advanced heart disease and severely symptomatic or refractory HF

In chemotherapy-induced heart failure, three recognized syndromes can occur. The first, acute toxicity causing CHF during the course of chemotherapy, is the rarest. Patients become acutely short of breath with onset of pulmonary edema. This condition is easily reversed with discontinuation of therapy and management of volume overload. However, permanent myocardial injury may have occurred that could lead to late toxicity. (Wouters et al., 2005) The second syndrome, early-chronic progressive heart failure, can occur during therapy or within the first year after completion of therapy. The onset of symptoms is a little more gradual and not as acute. The third syndrome, late-onset chronic progressive heart failure remote, can occur at least 1 year to several years after therapy. Symptoms generally appear gradually. This form has the worst prognosis, because LV dysfunction usually is irreversible and progresses; the 5-year mortality rate is as high as 70%. In women receiving trastuzumab who develop heart failure, the survival rate is 33%

(Kannel, 2000), a rate far worse than the survival rate for women with breast cancer and either regional or no metastases (Reis et al., 2000).

PROFESSIONAL ASSESSMENT CRITERIA (PAC)

Signs and Symptoms

1. Dyspnea on exertion (DOE) and fatigue with exertion are typical symptoms (Coates 1997). Other hallmark symptoms include paroxysmal nocturnal dyspnea, edema of the lower extremities, orthopnea, cough, abdominal fullness or swelling, nausea, anorexia, polyuria at night, weight gain, dizziness, and mental status changes.
2. History of chemotherapy (see Table 19-1) with or without mediastinal radiation
3. Hypoxemia: PaO_2 less than 92%
4. Tachypnea
5. Tachycardia
6. Signs of elevated cardiac filling pressures, as evidenced by elevated jugular venous pressure, presence of S3 gallop, rales on auscultation, hepatojugular reflex, ascites, and edema.
7. Signs of cardiac enlargement, including laterally displaced or prominent apical pulse and/or murmurs indicative of valvular dysfunction.

Diagnostic Testing

1. Chest x-ray (CXR) films show prominent pulmonary vasculature, cephalization of flow, Kerley's B lines, pleural effusions, and cardiomegaly (Fig. 19.2).
2. Labs: B-type natriuretic peptide (BNP) greater than 300 pg/dL, or NT–pro-BNP greater than 900 pg/mL.

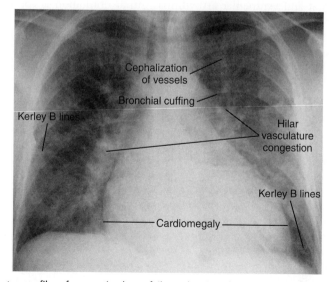

Fig. 19.2 • Chest x-ray film of congestive heart failure, showing characteristic cardiomegaly, cephalization of pulmonary vessels, hilar congestion, and Kerley's B lines. *(From www.med.yale.edu/intmed/ cardio/imaging/findings/pulmonary_edema/index.html. Yale University School of Medicine. Cardiothoracic imaging. [Accessed July 1, 2007.] Copyright 2004, Yale University School of Medicine. All rights reserved.)*

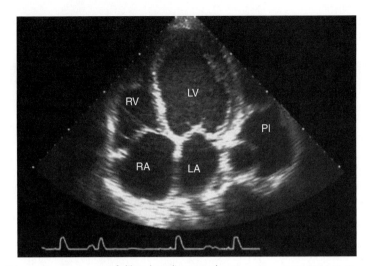

Fig. 19.3 • Echocardiogram image of dilated cardiomyopathy. *(From Zipes, D. P., Libby, P., Bonow, R. O., et al. [2005].* Braunwald's heart disease:A textbook of cardiovascular medicine, *[7th ed.], Philadelphia, W.B. Saunders.)*

3. An echocardiogram may show increased left atrial size, LV dilation, reduced LV ejection fraction, presence and degree of valvular lesions, or presence of pericardial effusions (Fig. 19.3). Serial evaluation of echocardiograms has been shown to be useful.
4. Hemodynamic monitoring indicates increased pulmonary hypertension. Increased PA pressures with increased pulmonary artery occlusion pressure (PAOP). Depending on the presence of cardiogenic shock, MAP < 65 mm Hg.
5. Although an electrocardiogram (ECG) provides no specific indicators of CHF, the ECG may show atrial and ventricular arrhythmias. Atrial fibrillation is common. The ECG may also show evidence of CAD, MI, or left ventricular hypertrophy. QRS voltage may be low as a result of loss of functional myocardium (Young & Mills, 2004).
6. Multigated blood pool scintigraphy (MUGA) is useful in the evaluation of both right and left ventricular size and function (Dae & Botninick, 1997). It has been used for serial evaluation of ventricular function during and after anthracycline therapy (Lu, 2005).

NURSING CARE AND TREATMENT

Acute Therapy (Hobbs, 2004)

1. Hold chemotherapy, radiation therapy if acute onset.
2. Elevate head of bed to high Fowler's position.
3. Vital signs—assess for hypotension, tachycardia, and tachypnea.
4. Obtain and interpret O_2 saturation values (signs of hypoxia include restlessness, dyspnea, anxiety, and cyanosis).
5. Administer oxygen to treat hypoxia.
6. Maintain venous access via peripheral IV (18 gauge in an adult) or with a venous access device (VAD).
7. Auscultate lung fields for crackles and adventitious breath sounds and assess for decreased chest expansion.
8. Obtain and assess laboratory tests: BNP, electrolytes, CBC, ABGs.

9. Obtain and assess chest x-ray film for cardiac size, evaluation of pulmonary vasculature, and presence of pleural effusions.
10. Measure intake and output (I&O) q2-8h.
11. Weigh patient daily on the same scale and compare to previous day's weight; retention of 450 mL of fluid is equal to a 1-pound weight gain.
12. Routine use of pulmonary artery catheters for hemodynamic monitoring in acute heart failure is not recommended except with evidence of cardiogenic shock or resistance to therapy. Pulmonary hypertension causes increased PA pressures, with an elevated PAWP.
13. Administer loop diuretics (e.g., furosemide 40-80 mg twice daily) intravenously to reduce preload. Oral diuretics may be ineffective because of gut edema and decreased absorption. Diurese to the goals of resolution of congestion, improvement in symptoms, and return to dry weight. If hemodynamic monitoring is used, treat to a PWCP less than 15 mm Hg with an SBP greater than 80 mm Hg. Add the thiazide diuretic metolazone, 5 mg given orally daily, if response is inadequate. If resistance to therapy continues, consider continuous infusion of loop diuretics: furosemide 0.1 mg/kg for first dose, then 0.1 mg/kg/hr, then double the dose every 2 hours up to 0.4 mg/kg/hr. Bumetanide or torsemide may be used as alternative.
14. Administer IV vasodilator therapy (nitroglycerin 5 mcg/min, titrating gradually to maximum dose of 200 mcg/min) to reduce afterload. Nitroprusside can be administered as an alternative.
15. Administer low-dose morphine sulfate for anxiety and dyspnea.
16. Administer low-dose angiotensin-converting enzyme inhibitors (ACEIs). Many formulations are available, but those proven to improve survival in heart failure include captopril, enalapril, lisinopril and ramipril. These drugs should be initiated as soon as the systolic blood pressure is greater than 90 mm Hg. They should be titrated to target doses as recommended in guidelines for the management of chronic heart failure. ACEIs are contraindicated in patients with significant renal failure or hyperkalemia or a history of angioedema (Table 19-2).
17. Anticipate initiation of beta-adrenergic blockers (beta blockers) before discharge. Three drugs have shown proven efficacy in heart failure: carvedilol (Coreg), metoprolol succinate (Toprol XL) and bisoprolol (Zebeta). These drugs are contraindicated of there is dyspnea, or significant fluid retention. (Table 19-2)
18. Provide diet of small, frequent, high-calorie meals, limit sodium to 2000 mg/day, and restrict fluids to 2000 mL/day.
19. Monitor activity; ensure bed rest with bathroom privileges as tolerated.

Chronic Therapy

1. Pharmacologic management must include ACEIs and beta-adrenergic blocking agents unless these drugs are specifically contraindicated. The medications should be titrated to doses proven to improve survival (Hunt et al., 2005).
2. Administer adjunctive therapy for chronic heart failure, including digoxin, spironolactone, angiotensin receptor blocers (ARBs), isosorbide dinitrate, and hydralazine in combination (see Table 19-2). These drugs may be started during acute management, but they often are initiated after the patient's condition has stabilized (Hunt et al., 2005).
3. The patient should be referred to a congestive heart failure disease management program that uses a team approach involving nursing specialists, dieticians, home health nurses, hospice, social workers, and/or respiratory therapists. This approach has been shown to improve quality of life, reduce rehospitalizations, and improve survival (Whellan et al., 2005).

Table 19-2 DRUGS USED TO TREAT CHF			
Generic (Trade) Drug	**Starting Dose**	**Target Dose**	**Maximum Dose**
Beta-Adrenergic Blockers			
Bisoprolol (Zebeta)	1.25 mg BID	5 mg QD ($\leq$85kg) 10 mg QD (> 85kg)	20 mg QD
Carvedilol (Coreg)	3.12 mg BID	25 mg BID ($\leq$ 85 kg) 50 mg BID (> 85 kg)	25 mg BID ($\leq$ 85 kg) 50 mg BID (> 85 kg)
Metoprolol succinate (Toprol XL)	12.5 mg QD	200 mg QD	200 mg QD
ACE Inhibitors*			
Lisinopril (Prinivil, Zestril)	5 mg QD	20 mg QD	40 mg QD
Enalapril (Vasotec)	2.5 mg BID	10 mg BID	20 mg BID
Captopril (Capoten)	6.25-12.5 mg TID	50 mg TID	100 mg TID
Ramipril (Altace)	1.25-2.5 mg QD	10 mg QD	10 mg QD
Angiotensin receptor blockers			
Candesartan (Atacand)	4 mg QD	16 to 32 mg QD	32 mg QD
Valsartan (Diovan)	20-40 mg BID	80 mg BID	160 mg BID
Losartan (Cozaar)	25-50 mg QD	100 mg QD	100 mg QD
Aldosterone Antagonists*			
Spironolactone (Aldactone)	12.5-25 mg QD	25 mg QD	25 mg BID
Eplerenone (Inspra)	25 mg QD	50 mg QD	50 mg QD
Vasodilators			
Isosorbide dinitrate (Isordil)	10 mg TID	40 mg TID	
Hydralazine (Apresoline)	10-25 mg TID	75 mg TID	300 mg/day
Others			
Digoxin (Lanoxin)	0.125 mg QD	Target to level 0.5-0.8 ng/mL	Depends on blood level

*Other agents that are not listed are also available.

EVIDENCE-BASED PRACTICE UPDATES

1. Although serial measurement of LVEF by echocardiogram or radionuclide angiocardiography is used widely to monitor patients, newer methods to predict the long-term emergence of clinical cardiac dysfunction are being developed. ANP, BNP, and NT–pro-BNP assays measured during chemotherapy could be indicators of subclinical early cardiotoxicity (Germanakis et al., 2006).
2. Administration of natriuretic peptides (BNP) in the form of nesiritide (Natrecor) has been shown to produce significant diuresis and decreases in wedge pressure, compared to nitroglycerin, in patients with acute decompensated heart failure (VMAC, 2002).
3. Many agents have been studied in an effort to prevent chemotherapy-induced cardiomyopathy, including dexrazoxane, probucol, and amifostine, as have nutritional agents such as vitamins A, C, and E, coenzyme Q10, selenium, and carnitine. The only agent that has shown any benefit in terms of prevention is dexrazoxane (Wouters et al., 2005). Some evidence indicates that higher cumulative doses of doxorubicin can be used; however, this may cause some interference with antitumor activity (Swain, 1998).
4. Cardiac transplantation remains a viable therapy for end-stage CHF related to chemotherapy. The use of immunosuppressive agents does not appear to increase cancer recurrence in these patients (Grande et al., 2003).

TEACHING AND EDUCATION

Discontinuation of chemotherapy, radiation therapy, and interferon alpha: *Rationale:* Explain that (chemo/radiation/interferon) treatment is being discontinued to avoid further damage.

Dyspnea: *Rationale*: Pace your activities during the day to prevent shortness of breath. Please notify your health care provider if you experience increased shortness of breath with exertion or inability to lie flat because of shortness of breath.

Activity: *Rationale*: Stay as active as possible. Increase activities gradually, making sure not to become too tired or short of breath. Walk 5 to 15 minutes, 3 to 5 days a week, with frequent breaks. When resting, rest in bed or in an armchair with your upper body elevated. Avoid extremes of hot or cold, and reduce emotional stress.

Nutrition: *Rationale*: Eat small, frequent meals. A salt-restricted diet is essential for preventing the accumulation of extra fluid. Do not add salt when cooking or to meals. Avoid foods high in sodium, such as ham, bacon, hot dogs, canned foods, frozen foods, cheese, lunch meats, and dry cereals. Follow the prescribed diet as discussed with dietician.

Weight: *Rationale*: Weigh yourself at the same time every day, preferably in the morning after urinating. Call your health care provider if you gain 3 pounds or more overnight or 5 pounds or more in a week.

Symptoms: *Rationale*: Many symptoms may indicate worsening of your heart failure. Call your health care provider if you experience any of these: swelling of your feet or legs, increased fatigue or tiredness, difficulty sleeping at night, a swollen or tender abdomen, loss of appetite, cough, increased nighttime urination, or confusion.

Medications: *Rationale*: You may have to take four or more medications to control your symptoms and improve your survival. It is very important to take all your medications as prescribed. Please notify your health care provider if you should experience any side effects from your medications. Keep a current list of your medications with you at all times. Please refill your prescriptions promptly; missed medications are a common cause of admission to the hospital for your condition.

Anxiety: *Rationale*: When you are short of breath, you sometimes feel anxious and restless, which puts you in a cycle of more anxiety and shortness of breath. To break this cycle, try using guided imagery, watching TV, or listening to music; taking medicine also can help. Yoga exercises may be helpful as well.

Tests and procedures: *Rationale*: You may need several tests. These may include x-ray films, scans of your chest made with a special machine, or placement of a tube in your artery (this is similar to placement of an IV in your vein, but the tube is longer). The tube in your artery is attached to a machine that helps us make sure your heart and lungs are working as they should be. Also, your health care practitioner may prescribe pulmonary rehabilitation for you, because this type of program can benefit individuals with CHF. It includes exercise, air circulation, and oxygen therapies.

Web sites for information:
- Heart Failure Society of America, American Lung Association: www.abouthf.org
- American Heart Association: www.americanheart.org
- National Institutes of Health: www.nlm.nih.gov/medlineplus/heartfailure.html
- Low Sodium Cooking: www.lowsodiumcooking.com

NURSING DIAGNOSES

1. **Excess fluid volume** related to increased sodium and water retention, decreased renal perfusion, compromised regulatory mechanisms, decreased cardiac output
2. **Decreased cardiac output** related to myocardial damage, decreased contractility, alteration in preload and afterload, accumulation of blood in pulmonary and systemic vasculature
3. **Impaired gas exchange** related to ventilation/perfusion imbalance caused by fluid in alveoli
4. **Activity intolerance** related to dyspnea, decreased cardiac output, anxiety
5. **Anxiety** related to change in health status, fear of death, threat to role functioning

EVALUATION AND DESIRED OUTCOMES

1. Dyspnea, cough, fatigue, and anxiety each will be rated less than 3 on a scale of 0 to 10. The patient will be assessed for improvement and medicated accordingly.
2. O_2 saturation will be greater than 92%.
3. The patient will have minimal or no adventitious lung sounds or congestion, pneumonia, productive cough, peripheral edema, or jugular vein distention.
4. The patient will have no nausea or anorexia, and his or her weight will increase by more than 1 pound a week or will remain stable.

DISCHARGE PLANNING AND FOLLOW-UP CARE

- Caregiver to assist with meal preparation, ADLs, and household maintenance (laundry, shopping, housework).
- Home health nursing visits for assessment of pulmonary and cardiac status, medication evaluation, and antianxiety interventions for 1 to 2 months.
- Follow-up visit to physician's office 1 to 2 weeks after discharge.
- Instructions to call health care provider immediately for any of the following: fever higher than 38° C (100.5° F), coughing up blood or blood-tinged mucus, unusual swelling of the hands or feet, weight gain of more than 3 pounds in 1 week, heart palpitations, chest discomfort, increased shortness of breath, and skin rash.

REVIEW QUESTIONS

QUESTIONS

1. **A commonly used imaging test for left ventricular size and function is:**
   1. BNP
   2. Renal ultrasound
   3. MUGA
   4. Head CT

2. **The pathophysiologic process that leads to cell death in anthracycline toxicity is related to:**
   1. Deposition of calcium
   2. Free oxygen radicals
   3. Increased cardiac perfusion
   4. Gastrointestinal bleeding

3. **Which of the following is a common clue to CHF:**
   1. Orthopnea
   2. Weight loss
   3. Unilateral muscle weakness
   4. Increased appetite

4. **You are counseling a patient on a diet for CHF. The most important point to consider is:**
   1. Any foods in any combination are acceptable as long as the patient is eating.

2. The patient should drink at least 8 full glasses of water, in addition to other beverages, during the day.
3. Sodium intake must be limited to a maximum of 2000 mg/day.
4. The patient must eat three large meals daily.

5. **A 56-year-old female with a history of breast cancer presents to the emergency department with a complaint of progressive shortness of breath with exertion. What would you want to know about her past history:**
   1. Presence of allergies
   2. Past surgeries
   3. Chemotherapy regimen
   4. Childhood diseases

6. **The recommended dose of furosemide for acute management of CHF in the hospital is:**
   1. 10 mg given orally
   2. 60 to 80 mg given intravenously
   3. 50 mg given subcutaneously
   4. 400 mg in 50 mL D5W given over 30 minutes

7. **What routine diagnostic procedure is performed to monitor responses to therapy in acute CHF:**
   1. CXR
   2. Pulmonary artery catheterization
   3. BNP
   4. EKG

8. **What effects have comprehensive, multidisciplinary disease management programs had for heart failure patients:**
   1. Fewer hospitalizations
   2. Increased weight and appetite
   3. Lack of medication compliance
   4. 65% of survivors have late cardiac effects

9. **Which pharmacologic agent is contraindicated in patients with severe volume overload:**
   1. Furosemide
   2. Metoprolol
   3. Lisinopril
   4. Valsartan

10. **You are assessing the chest x-ray film of a person who you believe may have congestive heart failure.**

Which description of the x-ray film would indicate CHF:
1. Normal heart size
2. Unilateral pleural effusion
3. Cephalization of vasculature
4. Granulomatous appearance

ANSWERS

1. **Answer: 3**
   Rationale: Multigated blood pool scintigraphy (MUGA) is useful in the evaluation of both right and left ventricular size and function.

2. **Answer: 2**
   Rationale: Cell death, or apoptosis, is related to free oxygen radicals, which produce myofibril loss and loss of contractility after administration of anthracyclines.

3. **Answer: 1**
   Rationale: Orthopnea is a clinical sign of increased pulmonary vascular congestion and alveolar water and a hallmark of CHF.

4. **Answer: 3**
   Rationale: The cornerstone of self-care management strategies is a diet restricted to 2000 mg of sodium. Water retention occurs as sodium intake increases.

5. **Answer: 3**
   Rationale: Anthracyclines are commonly used in breast cancer treatment. A significant risk of cardiotoxicity is associated with these agents. Exertional shortness of breath is the hallmark of CHF.

6. **Answer: 2**
   Rationale: The dose recommended for acute management is 60 to 80 mg given IV two or three times daily until dyspnea improves, weight is reduced, and no orthopnea is present. The maximum daily dose is 400 mg.

7. **Answer: 1**
   Rationale: Chest x-ray films are important in the initial diagnosis and in the evaluation of the effectiveness of therapy.

8. **Answer: 1**
   Rationale: Comprehensive disease management programs have been shown

to have a significant impact on repeat hospitalizations, improved quality of life, and improved survival.

9. **Answer: 2**
Rationale: Beta blockers are contraindicated in patients with volume overload. However, they can and should be initiated before hospital discharge if the dyspnea has improved

and the patient is closer to his or her dry weight.

10. **Answer: 3**
Rationale: Cephalization of vasculature is an indication of pulmonary vascular congestion. Pleural effusions may be present in CHF, but they are bilateral almost all the time and are a nonspecific finding for CHF.

REFERENCES

Clements, I. P., Davis, B. J., & Wiseman, G. A. (2002). Systolic and diastolic cardiac dysfunction early after the initiation of doxorubicin therapy: Significance of gender and concurrent mediastinal radiation. *Nuclear Medicine Communications, 23*(6):521-527.

Coates, A. J. S. (1997). Syndrome of chronic heart failure: Origin of symptoms. In P. Poole-Wilson, W. Colucci, & B. Massie, et al. (Eds.), *Heart failure: Scientific principles and clinical practice* (pp. 297-310). New York: Churchill Livingstone.

Colucci, W. S., & Braunwald, E. (2004). Pathophysiology of heart failure. In (D. Zipes, P. Libby, & R. Bonow, et al. eds.), Braunwald's heart disease: A textbook of cardiovascular medicine (pp. 509–540). (7th ed.). Philadelphia: W. B. Saunders.

Dae, M. W., & Botninick, E. H. (1997). Radionuclide methods. In P. Poole-Wilson, W. Colucci, & B. Massie, et al. (Eds.), *Heart failure: Scientific principles and clinical practice* (pp. 489-498). New York: Churchill Livingstone.

Feldman, A. M., Lorell, B. H., & Reis, S. E. (2000). Trastuzumab in the treatment of metastatic breast cancer: Anticancer therapy versus cardiotoxicity. *Circulation, 102*(3):272-274.

Fisher, N. G., & Marshall, A. J. (1999). Management options: Anthracycline-induced cardiomyopathy. *Postgraduate Medical Journal, 75*(883):265-268.

Francis, G. S. (2001). Pathophysiology of chronic heart failure. *American Journal of Medicine, 110*(7A):37S-46S.

Germanakis, I., Kalmanti, M., & Parthenakis, F., et al. (2006). Correlation of plasma N-terminal pro-brain natriuretic peptide levels with left ventricular mass in children treated with anthracyclines. *International Journal of Cardiology, 108*(2):212-215.

Grande, A. M., Rinaldi, M., & Sinelli, S., et al. (2003). Heart transplantation in chemotherapeutic dilated cardiomyopathy. *Transplant Proceedings, 35*(4):1516-1518.

He, J., Ogden, L. G., & Bazzano, L. A., et al. (2001). Risk factors for congestive heart failure in U. S. men and women: NHANES I epidemiologic follow-up study. *Archives of Internal Medicine, 161*(7):996-1002.

Hobbs, R. E. (2004). Management of decompensated heart failure. *American Journal of Therapeutics, 11*(6):473-479.

Hunt, S. A., Abraham, W. T., & Chin, M. H., et al. (2005). ACC/AHA 2005 guideline update for the diagnosis and management of chronic heart failure in the adult: A report of the American College of Cardiology/American Heart Association Task Force on Practice Guidelines (Writing Committee to Update the 2001 Guidelines for the Evaluation and Management of Heart Failure). *Journal of the American College of Cardiology, 46*:1116-1143.

Kannel, W. B. (2000). Incidence and epidemiology of heart failure. *Heart Failure Review, 5*(2):167-173.

Kremer, L. C. M., van Dalen, E. C., & Offringa M., et al. (2002a). Frequency and risk factors of anthracycline-induced clinical heart failure in children: A systematic review. *Annals of Oncology, 13*:503-512.

Lipshultz, S. E., Colan, S. D., & Gelber, R. D., et al. (1991). Late cardiac effects of doxorubicin therapy for acute lymphoblastic leukemia in the childhood. *New England Journal of Medicine, 324*(12):808-815.

Lipshultz, S. E., Lipsitz, S. R., & Sallen, S. E., et al. (2005). Chronic progressive cardiac dysfunction years after doxorubicin therapy for childhood acute lymphoblastic leukemia. *Journal of Clinical Oncology, 23*(12):2629-2636.

Lu, P. (2005). Monitoring cardiac function in patients receiving doxorubicin. *Seminars in Nuclear Medicine, 35*(3):197-201.

Mann, D. L. (1999). Doxorubicin mechanisms and models in heart failure: A combinatorial approach. *Circulation, 100*(9):999-1008.

Moser, D. K. (1998). Pathophysiology of heart failure update: The role of neurohumoral activation in the progression of heart failure. *AACN Clinical Issues, 9*(2):157-171.

Pai, V. B., & Nahato, M. C. (2000). Cardiotoxicity of chemotherapeutic agents: Incidence, treatment and prevention. *Drug Safety, 22*(4):263-302.

Perik, P. J., van den Berg, M. P., & de Vries, E. G., et al. (2004). Experimental animal model for anthracycline-induced heart failure. *European Journal of Heart Failure, 6*(4):375-376.

Publication Committee for the VMAC Investigators (VMAC). (2002). Intravenous nesiritide vs. nitroglycerin for treatment of decompensated heart failure. *Journal of the American Medical Association, 287*:1531-1540.

Reis, L., Fisher, M., & Kosary, C., et. al. (Eds.) (2000). *SEER cancer statistics review, 1973-1997.* Bethesda, MD: National Cancer Institute.

Shanholtz, C. (2001). Acute life-threatening toxicity of cancer treatment. *Critical Care Clinics, 17*(3):483-502.

Singal, P. K., & Iliskovic, N. (1998). Doxorubicin-induced cardiomyopathy. *New England Journal of Medicine, 339*(13):900-905.

Swain, S. M. (1998). Adult multicenter trials using dexrazoxane to protect against cardiac toxicity. *Seminars in Oncology, 25*(4Suppl 10):43-47.

Whellan, D. J., Hasselblad, V., & Peterson, E. (2005). Meta-analysis and review of heart failure disease management randomized controlled clinical trials. *American Heart Journal, 149*(4):722-729.

Wouters, K. A., Kremer, L. C., & Miller, T. L. (2005). Protecting against anthracycline-induced myocardial damage: A review of the most promising strategies. *British Journal of Haematology, 131*(5):561-578.

Yahalom, J., & Portlock, C. S. (2004). Cardiac toxicities. In V. T. DeVita, S. Hellman, & S. A. Rosenberg (Eds.), *Cancer: Principles and practice of oncology* (pp. 2545-2549). (7th ed.). Philadelphia: Lippincott Williams & Wilkins.

Young, J. B., & Mills, R. M (2004). *Clinical management of heart failure.* West Islip, NY: Professional Communications.

Hemorrhage Secondary to Cervical Cancer

BRENDA K. COBB • CYNTHIA C. CHERNECKY

PATHOPHYSIOLOGICAL MECHANISMS

Cervical cancer is the second most common cancer among women in the world, with about 500,000 cases diagnosed each year. Factors associated with the development of cervical cancer include lack of screening, early sexual intercourse, multiple sexual partners, early pregnancy, oncogenic subtype of HPV, cigarette smoking, and immunocompromised status (Shingleton & Orr, 1995).

One of the first symptoms of cervical cancer is likely to be a thin, blood-tinged vaginal secretion that is not readily noticed by the patient. As the malignancy increases, the abnormal bleeding becomes more readily obvious, more frequent, and lasts longer (Evans-Jones, 2005; DiSaia & Creasman, 2002).

Hemorrhage as a result of cervical cancer is associated with erosion of the cervical surface, which can progress to tissue necrosis. Cancer cells (squamous type [85% to 90%], adenocarcinoma [10% to 20%], and adenosquamous carcinoma) initiate increased vascularity of the cervical microcirculation, and sustained growth occurs as a result of angiogenesis. Subsequent infiltration and expansion of the tumor mass occurs, including to nearby formed blood vessels that supply the tumor with nutrients and oxygen. As more cervical tissue is invaded, the new branching vessels, which arise in the cervical stroma, are pushed to the surface. This makes the contour of the cervix irregular and friable as surface epithelium is lost. Ulceration and exophylic or endophylic lesions then occur.

Ulcerative lesions create a defect of loss of intercellular cohesiveness in the cervix or upper vagina; exophylic lesions protrude from the cervix and replace it; and endophylic lesions protrude from the endocervix. As the tumor becomes more bulky and neovascularization increases, the risk of hemorrhage increases. The end result is increased vascular capillary supply and increased friable and erosive cervical surfaces with large collateral branches of arterial networks, which cause hemorrhage. When the bleeding is chronic, weight loss, extreme fatigue, and anemia occur. Anemia increases hypoxia of cervical carcinomas, which increases iron deprivation, inflammatory reactions, and infections (Marchal et al., 2005) and negates healing. The importance of consistent gynecologic care, including Papanicolaou (PAP) smears, cannot be overstated. PAP smears can detect preinvasive conditions of the surface layers of the cervix before the basement membrane is invaded, increasing the likelihood of cure, survival, and a good quality of life. Preinvasive diagnoses include cervical intraepithelial neoplasia (CIN) and squamous intraepithelial lesions (SILs).

EPIDEMIOLOGY AND ETIOLOGY

The amount of bleeding is directly related to the stage of disease and necrosis of the cervical tumor. The incidence of blood loss greater than 1000 mL during surgery is

0.8% (Cao, 2001); with radical surgery of invasive cervical carcinoma, the incidence is 4.1% (Sliwinski et al., 2003). Although hemorrhage secondary to cervical cancer is rare, it usually is associated with bulky tumor necrosis and advanced stage disease (Bowcutt et al., 2007; Rosenkoetter et al., submitted, 2007). The disease is preceded by a period of cellular abnormality, and whether of low or high grade, these abnormalities are amenable to detection with routine exfoliative sampling by PAP smear (Yoder & Rubin, 1992). The main factor that correlates with development of late-stage disease is absence of routine gynecologic examinations, including a PAP smear, for longer than 5 years. For further validation, a colposcopic examination is conducted (Wiggins et al., 1995). Cigarette smoking is known to increase the cellular incidence of high-grade cervical cancer lesions, and smoking cessation is a necessary intervention of patient care.

RISK PROFILE

- Smoking significantly increases the incidence of high-grade lesions (dos Santos et al., 2004).
- History of abnormal PAP smear, cervical dysplasia or cervical cancer, or squamous cell carcinoma is the most common historical finding, followed by adenocarcinoma (Shintaku et al., 2000), adenosquamous carcinoma, and neuroectodermal tumors (Malpica & Moran, 2002), and lymphoma (Chan et al., 2005).
- Anemia with hemoglobin less than 12g/dL (Marchal et al., 2005).
- As tumor size increases, so does the risk for hemorrhage, especially in FIGO stage III tumors (Sobiczewski et al., 2002).
- Postcoital bleeding (Abu et al., 2006; Jha & Sabharwal, 2002); 11% to 19% of cases are diagnosed as cervical cancer, and 4% are invasive cancer (Rosenthal et al., 2001).
- Factor XI deficiency, primarily in females of Ashkenazi Jewish descent (Kim et al., 2004).
- History of endometrial polyps (Selo-Ojeme et al., 2004); 6.8% are diagnosed with cervical cancer.
- Environmental factors, such as lack of insurance coverage (Edelman & Adams, 2004) and lower socioeconomic status.
- **Medications**: Anticoagulants (heparin, warfarin, ticlopidine, clopidogrel bisulfate [Plavix], aspirin, ibuprofen) and other NSAIDs inhibit platelet aggregation and prolong bleeding time. Herbal medications known to increase bleeding include astragalus root, bilberry, bromelain from pineapple stem, capsicum, cayenne, chamomile, coleus, dong quai, evening primrose, feverfew, flaxseed oil, garlic, ginger, gingko, American ginseng, green tea, hawthorn, horse chestnut, kava kava, licorice, meadowsweet, motherwort, passionflower, poplar, red clover, shepherd's purse, and tumeric; vitamins and supplements include chondroitin, fish oil, and vitamin E (Wren & Norred, 2003).

PROGNOSIS

Control of hemorrhage secondary to cervical cancer through the use of surgery and/or external radiation is successful in 95% of cases. Recurrence of bleeding occurs in 5% of cases, and 3% have uncontrolled bleeding (Sliwinski et al., 2003). Embolized patients have poorer disease-free survival (Kapp et al., 2005). The risk of ovarian metastasis is low for patients with squamous cell carcinoma of the cervix stages IA and IB (L'ubusky et al., 2004). Adenocarcinoma with metrorrhagia has a 5-year survival rate of 68% (Chargui et al., 2006); poor prognostic factors include age over 50 years, tumor larger than 4 cm, later stage, higher tumor grade, and lymph node involvement.

PROFESSIONAL ASSESSMENT CRITERIA (PAC)

For a quick glance at assessment criteria, see Table 20-1.
1. Assess for vaginal bleeding every 15 minutes × 4, then every 1 hour × 24 hours.
2. Assess for intravenous access with at least one 22-gauge catheter.
3. Assess for signs of hypovolemia (CVP less than 8 cm H_2O, tachycardia, hypotension with systolic pressure less than 90 mm Hg, urine output less than 30 mL/hr, Hct less than 30%) every 15 minutes × 2, then every 1 hour × 8 hours.
4. Assess skin: Cold, clammy, diaphoretic, pale.
5. Assess laboratory values: CBC, including Hgb and Hct, chemistry panel for hypokalemia, increased PT/PTT, INR.
6. Pulse oximetry every 1 hour and ABGs as prescribed.
7. Vital signs: Decreased or increased temperature; decreased blood pressure; increased pulse or tachycardia; increased respiratory rate, which may be accompanied by SOB and tachypnea; increased pain.
8. Monitor CVP every 4 hours; if less than 8 cm H_2O or greater than 15 cm H_2O, notify physician.

Table 20-1	ASSESSMENT CRITERIA FOR HEMORRHAGE SECONDARY TO CERVICAL CANCER	
Indicator	**Assessment**	
Vital signs		
Temperature	Subnormal or normal	
Pulse	Tachycardia >100 bpm, weak, thready	
Respirations	Increased, SOB, tachypnea	
Blood pressure	Decreased systolic <90 mm Hg (torr)	
Pain	>5 on 1-10 scale	
CVP	Decreased <8 or >15	
History		
Symptoms, conditions	Lack of routine gynecologic care for longer than 5 years	
	Previously untreated abnormal PAP smear	
	Did not receive HPV vaccine	
	Irregular, intermenstrual, postcoital bleeding	
	Heavier menses	
	Underlying coagulopathy	
	Factor XI deficiency in females of Ashkenazi Jewish descent	
	Increased used of medications or herbals that increase bleeding	
Signs and symptoms	Agitation; anxiety; cold, clammy skin; confusion; diaphoresis; disorientation; fear; pallor; profuse vaginal bleeding; fatigue	
Laboratory values	Hct & Hgb decreased	
	Serum potassium decreased	
	PT, PTT, or INR increased	
Diagnostic tests	Cervical biopsy confirms carcinoma.	
	Pelvic examination positive (may need to be performed under anesthesia).	
	Cystoscopy and/or proctoscopy to evaluate for bladder and bowel invasion.	
	Chest x-ray film indicates lung metastasis.	
	CT scan of abdomen/pelvis indicates obstruction, lymphadenopathy, and/or metastasis and is used to plan for radiation therapy.	

9. Assess for sociologic, cultural, or religious barriers to potential blood transfusions.
10. Assess diagnostic test results: CT pelvic scan for obstruction, lymphadenopathy, or metastasis and CXR for lung metastasis.
11. Assess for fatigue as a sign of anemia, anxiety as a sign of sepsis, and confusion as a sign of hypoxia or sepsis.
12. Assess for adequate renal function by serum creatinine values and hourly urine output values.
13. Assess plasma value of soluble urokinase plasminogen activator receptor (suPAR), as it should be greater than 0.9 mcg/L (Piironen et al., 2006; Riisbro et al., 2001).

NURSING CARE AND TREATMENT

Treatment involves surgery, chemotherapy, radiation therapy, medications, or usually a combination of these. Chemotherapy may include radiosensitization with 5-fluorouracil, cisplatin, or hydroxyurea. External beam radiation to the pelvis may be provided in daily fractions of 300 to 400 cGy for 3 to 4 days, followed by decreased daily fractions of 180 to 200 cGy to maximum dose, to help promote tumor shrinkage and damage to hemorrhagic surface blood vessels. Treatment usually is administered over 5 to 6 weeks and is followed by brachytherapy. Medications are given to treat anemia, volume deficit, infection, and/or hypoxemia (Table 20-2).

1. Placement of a triple lumen intravenous catheter to allow monitoring of CVP and administration of blood products, fluids, and medications (e.g., antibiotics, vasopressors) as prescribed.
2. Placement of a Swan-Ganz catheter for monitoring of cardiovascular status for potential hypovolemic or septic shock.
3. Prepare for vaginal packing or arterial embolization.
4. Insert Foley catheter.
5. Vital signs every 15 minutes × 2, then every 1 hour × 8 hours.
6. I&O every 4 hours.
7. STAT blood work: CBC, Chem-18, PT/PTT, INR, type and crossmatch, ABGs, blood cultures.
8. Oxygen per nasal cannula to maintain oxygen saturation greater than 90%.
9. Monitor for fluid overload: CVP greater than 15 cm H_2O, increased blood pressure, jugular vein distention, bilateral peripheral edema, dyspnea, tachycardia, rales.
10. STAT radiation therapy consult.
11. Monitor for signs and symptoms of sepsis or toxic shock syndrome: CVP less than 8 cm H_2O, tachycardia, decreased blood pressure, increased or decreased temperature, oxygen desaturation, confusion, agitation.

Table 20-2	MEDICATIONS USED TO TREAT HEMORRHAGE SECONDARY TO CERVICAL CANCER
Medication	**Rationale**
Intravenous solutions	Isotonic, crystalloid, and colloid solutions used to treat hypovolemia
Vasopressors	Used to treat hypotension
Oxygen	Used to treat hypoxemia secondary to anemia and/or blood loss
Packed RBCs	Transfusion to maintain Hct >30% and to maximize oxygenation
Fresh frozen plasma or vitamin K	Transfusion or vitamin K to correct coagulopathy
Antibiotics	Broad-spectrum antibiotics to treat infection, sepsis, or toxic shock syndrome
Colony-stimulating factors (CSFs)	Erythropoietin to manage anemia (Marchal et al., 2005)

EVIDENCE-BASED PRACTICE UPDATES

1. Increased endometrial thickening greater than 5 mm, seen in ultrasound, often is overestimated by ultrasound and is not a reliable indicator of cervical cancer, as was once thought (Saha et al., 2004).
2. Although younger women are less likely to develop cervical cancer, women younger than 35 years old have a median time to diagnosis of 9 months; women older than 35 years old have a median time to diagnosis of 2 months (Yu et al., 2005). Younger women who have symptoms suspicious for cervical cancer should be more extensively evaluated.
3. The laparoscopic radical vaginal approach is superior to abdominal radical hysterectomy type II for cervical cancer stages I to III (Malur et al., 2001), and it has a lower rate of blood transfusions, blood loss, and postoperative morbidity.
4. Radical trachelectomy with pelvic lymphadenopathy in stage I cervical cancer involves an estimated blood loss of 203 mL (Schlaerth et al., 2003) and is a feasible treatment to preserve fertility.
5. Many treatments are successful in reducing blood loss (Taylor & Magos, 2006), including medications, laser treatment, surgery, and other procedures (Box 20-1).
6. Radical surgery in women over age 65 is feasible in stages IB or IIA (Choi et al., 2005), with only a 2% rate of massive hemorrhage.
7. Ovarian transposition surgery is used to preserve ovarian function (L'ubusky et al., 2004).
8. A vaccine now exists to prevent the development of cervical cancer caused by the human papillomavirus (HPV), and it should be considered part of health care for women 12 years of age or older (Lowy & Schiller, 2006).

TEACHING AND EDUCATION

Cervical cancer: *Rationale:* You have a cancerous tumor of the cervix, which is the opening to the uterus. This condition needs to be treated, and treatment may include surgery and other types of therapy.

Vaginal packing (if appropriate): *Rationale:* Lots of gauze has been inserted into your vagina to put pressure on the cervix so that it stops bleeding. The gauze needs to stay in place for several days, and then it will be removed by the doctor.

BOX 20-1	SUCCESSFUL TREATMENTS TO REDUCE BLOOD LOSS IN HEMORRHAGE SECONDARY TO CERVICAL CANCER

- Vasopressin administered perioperatively (Martin-Hirsch & Kitchener, 1999)
- Bilateral internal iliac artery ligation (BIIAL) (Gharoro, 2003; Cao, 2001)
- Triple tourniquet technique with open myomectomy (Hatremi et al., 2005)
- Transarterial embolization (Hatremi et al., 2005)
- Embolization or ligation of hypogastric artery (Yalvac et al., 2002)
- Thumbtack to control presacral venous hemorrhage (Harma et al., 2005)
- High-dose ratio cervical ring applicator (Grigsby et al., 2003)
- Cauterization of cone bed (superior to sutures) (Kamat et al., 2004)
- Laser conization (dos Santos et al., 2004)
- Radiofrequency bipolar coagulator therapy (Ercoli et al., 2003)
- Intraabdominal packing with removal of packing in 6 days (Cirese & Larciprete, 2003)
- Vaginal gauze packing (Kim et al., 2002)

Urinary catheter: *Rationale*: A urinary catheter is necessary to keep your bladder small, so that it does not put pressure on the cervix, causing pain and bleeding. We will measure the amount of urine you excrete to assess how well your bladder and kidneys are working.

Central intravenous catheter: *Rationale*: A central intravenous catheter is needed to monitor your heart. It also is used to administer fluids, blood products, and antibiotics and to obtain blood samples for laboratory tests to monitor your progress.

Blood transfusions: *Rationale*: Blood transfusions may be necessary if you lose a lot of blood from your cervix. Blood carries oxygen and contains fluids that are necessary for your comfort and survival. If you have any objections to receiving transfusions, please share those with your physician or nurse.

Radiation therapy: *Rationale*: Radiation therapy may be needed as part of your treatment to shrink the cancer growth. External radiation is given 5 days per week for 5 to 6 weeks. Then a source of internal radiation will be inserted into your vagina, for which you will have to be in the hospital in a special isolation room for a few days.

Oxygen: *Rationale*: You may be given oxygen through small tubes placed in your nose. You will need oxygen if you have lost a lot of blood or if you are having trouble breathing.

Web sites for information:
- www.nlm.nih.gov/medlineplus/cervicalcancer.html (U. S. National Library of Medicine and National Institutes of Health)
- www.cancer.gov/cancertopics/types/cervical (National Cancer Institute)
- www.cancer.org/docroot/CRI/content/CRI_2_4_1X_What_is_cervical_cancer_8.asp (American Cancer Society)
- www.cervicalcancer.com (Merck & Co., Inc.)
- www.chemotherapy.com (Amgen Inc.)
- www.cancer.org (American Cancer Society)
- www.nccc-online.org (National Cervical Cancer Coalition)

NURSING DIAGNOSES

1. **Risk for deficient fluid volume** secondary to blood loss, which may be chronic or acute, regular or irregular, and minimal to profuse
2. **Risk for infection** related to tumor necrosis, which aids bacterial colonization, resulting in localized infection or sepsis
3. **Decreased cardiac output** related to blood loss and fluid volume depletion
4. **Fatigue** related to blood loss and treatment with surgery, radiation, and/or chemotherapy
5. **Fear** related to diagnosis, relapse, recurrent bleeding, and treatment measures

EVALUATION AND DESIRED OUTCOMES

1. No breakthrough bleeding will occur for 72 hours after treatment for hemorrhage.
2. No bleeding will occur for 24 hours after vaginal packing has been removed.
3. Blood pressure, pulse, respirations, CVP, and pain score will be within normal limits within 24 hours.
4. Hematocrit will be stable at greater than 30% within 48 hours.
5. Oxygen saturation will be greater than 90%.

BOX 20-2	AMERICAN CANCER SOCIETY GUIDELINES FOR EARLY DETECTION OF CERVICAL CANCER

1. All women should begin cervical cancer screening about 3 years after they begin having vaginal intercourse, but no later than age 21 years. Screening should be done every year with the regular PAP test or every 2 years with the newer, liquid-based PAP test.
2. Beginning at age 30, women who have had three normal PAP test results in a row may get screened every 2 to 3 years. Another reasonable option for women over age 30 is to get screened every 3 years (but not more frequently) with either the conventional or liquid-based PAP test plus the HPV DNA test. Women who have certain risk factors, such as diethylstilbestrol (DES) exposure before birth, HIV infection, or a weakened immune system as a result of organ transplantation, chemotherapy, or chronic steroid use, should continue to be screened annually.
3. Women 70 years of age or older who have had three or more normal PAP tests in a row and no abnormal PAP test results in the past 10 years may choose to stop having cervical cancer screening. Women with a history of cervical cancer, DES exposure before birth, HIV infection, or a weakened immune system should continue to have screening as long as they are in good health.
4. Women who have had a total hysterectomy (removal of the uterus and cervix) may also choose to stop having cervical cancer screening, unless the surgery was done as a treatment for cervical cancer or precancer. Women who have had a hysterectomy without removal of the cervix should continue to follow the guidelines presented previously.

Modified from American Cancer Society.
http://www.cancer.org/docroot/PED/content/PED_2_3X_ACS_Cancer_Detection_Guidelines_36.asp?sitearea=PED.

6. No evidence of infection, sepsis or toxic shock syndrome will be seen for the duration of vaginal packing.

DISCHARGE PLANNING AND FOLLOW-UP CARE

- Social service consultation for assessment of financial status for further care and discussion of living will and power of attorney.
- Arrangement of transportation daily for outpatient radiation therapy, about 5 to 6 weeks.
- Possible outpatient chemotherapy.
- Possible brachytherapy in hospital.
- Weekly outpatient laboratory blood draw for CBC.
- Weekly office visit and pelvic examination by radiation oncologist.
- Office visit with gynecologic oncologist in 3 to 4 weeks.
- Support group referral.
- Explain parameters for seeking and obtaining preventive care to ensure cervical health (Box 20-2).

REVIEW QUESTIONS

QUESTIONS

1. **Hemorrhage in cervical cancer is:**
   1. Common with preinvasive disease
   2. Associated with advanced-stage disease
   3. Precipitated by PAP smear sampling
   4. Related to normal menstruation

2. **Which factor increases the cellular incidence of high-grade cervical cancer lesions:**
   1. Smoking
   2. Using birth control pills
   3. Using condoms during intercourse
   4. Obesity

3. **Tumor angiogenesis contributes to the potential for hemorrhage in cervical cancer by:**
   1. Releasing polypeptide angiogenic growth factor
   2. Increasing ulceration of the surface of the cervix
   3. Decreasing the vascular supply to the cervix
   4. Increasing the vascular supply to the cervix

4. **The main factor that contributes to the development of advanced cervical cancer is:**
   1. Treatment for a previous abnormal PAP smear
   2. Family history of cervical cancer
   3. Absence of a routine gynecologic exam, including a PAP smear, for longer than 5 years
   4. Dysmenorrhea

5. **Which of the following medications or class of medications can increase bleeding:**
   1. Ibuprofen
   2. Acetaminophen
   3. ACE inhibitors
   4. Proton pump inhibitors

6. **IV antibiotics are administered for the duration of the vaginal packing because:**
   1. Gauze packing is no longer sterile once it is placed in the vagina.
   2. Septic shock may develop secondary to colonization of the vagina with bacteria.
   3. Antibiotics act as radiosensitizers.
   4. Placement of an indwelling urinary catheter may introduce bacteria to the urinary tract.

7. **Which of the following statements is true regarding hemorrhage secondary to cervical cancer:**
   1. The lower the disease stage, the greater the risk of hemorrhage.
   2. The more tumor necrosis, the greater the risk of hemorrhage.
   3. Hemorrhage is common in more than 40% of females with squamous cell carcinoma of the cervix.
   4. PAP smears are 100% effective in diagnosing cervical cancer.

8. ***Initial* nursing interventions for patients with hemorrhage secondary to cervical cancer are directed at:**
   1. Preventing septic shock
   2. Assessment of psychosocial support
   3. Preparing the patient for cervical biopsy
   4. Preventing hypovolemic shock

9. **Follow-up care for the patient with hemorrhage secondary to cervical cancer is most significant for:**
   1. Adherence to the radiation treatment plan
   2. Initiation of chemotherapy and colony-stimulating factor therapy
   3. Continuation of oral antibiotics
   4. Completion of diagnostic procedures to determine the extent of disease

10. **The desired outcome for a hospitalized patient with hemorrhage secondary to cervical cancer is:**
    1. Prevention of thrombolytic events
    2. Absence of bleeding for 24 hours after removal of the vaginal packing
    3. Initiation of radiation therapy and teletherapy within 72 hours of admission
    4. Use of arterial embolization to control venous and arterial bleeding

ANSWERS

1. **Answer: 2**
   Rationale: Spontaneous, profuse bleeding is associated with large, bulky tumors that have metastasized and are in late-stage disease.

2. **Answer: 1**
   Rationale: Smoking is a major risk factor for an increased incidence of high-grade cervical lesions.

3. **Answer: 4**
   Rationale: Angiogenesis is the process whereby blood venules and capillaries in surrounding normal tissue are stimulated to grow and form new vessels. Increased blood vessel growth results in a vascular tumor surface prone to spontaneous bleeding and hemorrhage.

4. **Answer: 3**
    Rationale: Cervical cancer is preceded by a lengthy preinvasive state that is amenable to detection with routine PAP smear screening. Advanced disease is more common in patients who have not had routine gynecologic care.

5. **Answer: 1**
    Rationale: Ibuprofen (Motrin) can cause inhibition of platelet aggregation and prolong bleeding time.

6. **Answer: 2**
    Rationale: In the presence of superabsorbent packing, bacteria that colonize the vagina proliferate. Access to the systemic circulation through erosions in the cervical surface and the process of angiogenesis may lead to the development of sepsis or toxic shock syndrome.

7. **Answer: 2**
    Rationale: Later stage disease and tumor necrosis increase the risk of hemorrhage.

8. **Answer: 4**
    Rationale: Initial nursing interventions in hemorrhage are concerned with correction of sudden volume depletion.

9. **Answer: 1**
    Rationale: The ability to control bleeding is contingent upon reduction of tumor bulk through daily radiation therapy.

10. **Answer: 2**
    Rationale: Spontaneous, profuse bleeding is associated with large, bulky tumors that have spread to surrounding tissues. To stop the bleeding, vaginal packing is inserted and removed when the bleeding has stopped. The goal is absence of bleeding for 24 hours after removal of the vaginal packing, at which time the patient is discharged.

REFERENCES

Abu, J., Davies, Q., & Ireland, D. (2006). Should women with postcoital bleeding be referred for colposcopy?. *Journal of Obstetrics & Gynaecology, 26*(1):45-47.

Bowcutt, M., Rosenkoetter, M., & Chernecky, C., et al. (2007). Implementation of an intravenous infusion pump system-implications for nursing. *Journal of Nursing Management* (accepted and in press).

Cao, Z. (2001). Prevention and management of severe hemorrhage during gynecological operations (Chinese). *Chung-Hua Fu Chan Ko Tsa Chih (Chinese Journal of Obstetrics & Gynecology), 36*(6):355-359.

Chan, J. K., Loizzi, V., & Magistris, A., et al. (2005). Clinicopathologic features of six cases of primary cervical lymphoma. *American Journal of Obstetrics and Gynecology, 193*(3 Pt 1):866-872.

Chargui, R., Damak, T., & Khomsi, F., et al. (2006). Prognostic factors and clinicopathologic characteristics of invasive adenocarcinoma of the uterine cervix. *American Journal of Obstetrics and Gynecology, 194*(1):43-48.

Choi, Y. S., Kim, Y. H., & Kang, S., et al. (2005). Feasibility of radical surgery in the management of elderly patients with uterine cervical cancer in Korea. *Gynecologic & Obstetric Investigation, 59*(3):165-170.

Cirese, E., & Larciprete, G. (2003). Emergency pelvic packing to control intraoperative bleeding after a Piver type-3 procedure: An unusual way to control gynaecological hemorrhage. *European Journal of Gynaecological Oncology, 24*(1):99-100.

DiSaia, P. J., & Creasman, W. T. (2002). *Clinical Gynecologic Oncology*. (6th ed.). Philadelphia: Mosby.

dos Santos, L., Odunsi, K., & Lele, S. (2004). Clinicopathologic outcomes of laser conization for high-grade cervical dysplasia. *European Journal of Gynaecological Oncology, 25*(3):305-307.

Edelman, A., & Adams, K. E. (2004). Ethics surrounding the impoverished patient. *Journal of the American Medical Women's Association, 59*(1):14-16.

Ercoli, A., Fagotti, A., & Maizoni, M., et al. (2003). Radiofrequency bipolar coagulation for radical hysterectomy: Technique, feasibility and complications. *International Journal of Gynecological Cancer, 13*(2):187-191.

Evans-Jones, J. (2005). Gynaecological cancer red flags for physiotherapists. *Journal of the Association of Chartered Physiotherapists in Women's Health. Spring, 96*:60-61.

Gharoro, E. P. (2003). Surgical management of early stages of cervical cancer: The value of internal iliac artery ligation. *Journal of Obstetrics & Gynaecology, 23*(1):44-47.

Grigsby, P. W., Portelance, L., & Williamson, J. F. (2003). High dose ratio (HDR) cervical ring applicator to control bleeding from cervical carcinoma. *International Journal of Gynecological Cancer, 12*(1):18-21.

Harma, M., Marma, M., & Ozturk, A., et al. (2005). The use of thumbtacks to stop severe presacral bleeding. *European Journal of Gynaecological Oncology, 26*(2):233-235.

Hatremi, R., Sameh, A., & Azza, S., et al. (2005). Emergency embolization in gynaecological bleeding: Two case reports (French). *Tunisie Medicale, 83*(8):492-494.

Jha, S., & Sabharwal, S. (2002). Outcome of colposcopy in women presenting with postcoital bleeding and negative or no cytology: Results of a 1-year audit. *Journal of Obstetrics & Gynaecology, 22*(3):299-301.

Kamat, A. A., Kramer, P., & Soisson, A. A. P. (2004). Superiority of electrocautery over the suture method for achieving cervical cone bed hemostasis. *Obstetrics & Gynecology, 102*(4):726-730.

Kapp, K. S., Poschauko, J., & Tauss, J., et al. (2005). Analysis of the prognostic impact of tumor embolization before definitive radiotherapy for cervical carcinoma. *International Journal of Radiation Oncology, Biology, Physics, 62*(5):1399-1404.

Kim, R. Y., Pareek, P., & Duan, J., et al. (2002). Postoperative intravaginal brachytherapy for endometrial cancer: Dosimetric analysis of vaginal colpostats and cylinder applicators. *Brachytherapy,, 1*(3):138-144.

Kim, S. H., Srinivas, S. K., & Rubin, S. C., et al. (2004). Delayed hemorrhage after cervical conization unmasking severe factor XI deficiency. *Obstetrics & Gynecology, 104*(5 Part 2, Suppl):1189-1192.

Lowy, D. R., & Schiller, J. T. (2006). Prophylactic human papillomavirus vaccines. *Journal of Clinical Investigation, 116*(5):1167-1173.

L'ubusky, M., Kudela, M., & L'ubusky, D., et al. (2004). The effectiveness and complications of ovarian transposition in young women with cervical cancer (Czech). *Ceska Gynekologie, 69*(4):283-286.

Malpica, A., & Moran, C. A. (2002). Primitive neuroectodermal tumor of the cervix: A clinicopathologic and immunohistochemical study of two cases. *Annals of Diagnostic Pathology, 6*(5):281-287.

Malur, S., Possover, M., & Schneider, A. (2001). Laparoscopically assisted radical vaginal versus radical abdominal hysterectomy type II in patients with cervical cancer. *Surgical Endoscopy, 15*(3):289-292.

Marchal, C., Rangeard, L., & Brunaud, C. (2005). Anemia impact on treatments of cervical carcinoma (French). *Cancer Radiotherapie, 9*(2):87-95.

Martin-Hirsch, P. L., & Kitchener, H. (1999). Interventions for preventing blood loss during the treatment of cervical intraepithelial neoplasa. *Cochrane Database of Sytematic Reviews*, Issue 1. Art. No.: CD001421. DOI: 10.1002/14651858.CD001421.

Piironen, T., Haese, A., & Huland, H., et al. (2006). Enhanced discrimination of benign from malignant prostatic disease by selective measurements of cleaved forms of urokinase receptor in serum. *Clinical Chemistry, 52*(5):838-844.

Riisbro, R., Stephens, R. W., & Brunner, N., et al. (2001). Soluble urokinase plasminogen activator receptor in preoperatively obtained plasma from patients with gynecological cancer or benign gynecological diseases. *Gynecologic Oncology, 82*(3):523-531.

Rosenkoetter, M. M., Bowcott, M., & Khasanshina, E., et al. (2007). Perceptions of the impact of "smart pumps" on nurses and nursing care provided (submitted).

Rosenthal, A. N., Panoskaitsis, T., & Smith, T., et al. (2001). The frequency of significant pathology in women attending a general gynlogical service for postcoital bleeding. *BJOG: An International Journal of Obstetrics & Gynaecology, 108*(1):103-106.

Saha, T. K., Amer, S. A., & Biss, J., et al. (2004). The validity of transvaginal ultrasound measurement of endometrial thickness: A comparison of ultrasound measurement with direct anatomical measurement. *BJOG: An International Journal of Obstetrics & Gynaecology, 111*(12):1419-1424.

Schlaerth, J. B., Spirtos, N. M., & Schlaerth, A. C. (2003). Radical trachelectomy and pelvic lymphadenectomy with uterine preservation in the treatment of cervical cancer. *American Journal of Obstetrics & Gynecology, 188*(1):29-34.

Selo-Ojeme, D. O., Dayoub, N., & Patel, A., et al. (2004). A clinico-pathological study of postcoital bleeding. *Archives of Gynecology & Obstetrics, 270*(1):34-36.

Shingleton, H. M., & Orr, J. W. (1995). *Cancer of the cervix*. Philadelphia: Lippincott.

Shintaku, M., Kariya, M., & Shime, H., et al. (2000). Adenocarcinoma of the uterine cervix with choriocarcinomatous and hepatoid differentiation: Report of a case. *International Journal of Gynecological Pathology, 19*(2):174-178.

Sliwinski, W., Debniak, J., & Lukaszuk, K., et al. (2003). Surgical complications in patients treated for invasive cervical cancer (Polish). *Ginekologia Polska, 74*(8):577-584.

Sobiczewski, P., Bidzinski, M., & Deriatka, P. (2002). Laparoscopic ligature of the hypogastric artery in the case of bleeding in advanced cervical cancer. *Gynecologic Oncology, 84*(2):344-348.

Taylor, A., & Magos, A. (2006). Reducing blood loss at open myomectomy using triple tourniquet: A randomized controlled trial. *BJOG: An International Journal of Obstetrics & Gynaecology, 113*(5):618-619.

Wiggins, D. L., Granai, C. O., & Steinhoff, M. M., et al. (1995). Tumor angiogenesis as a prognostic factor in cervical carcinoma. *Gynecology Oncology, 56*(3):353-356.

Wren, K. R., & Norred, C. L. (2003). *Complementary and alternative therapies.* St. Louis: Mosby.

Yalvac, S., Kayikcioglu, F., & Boran, N., et al. (2002). Embolization of uterine artery in terminal stage cervical cancers. *Cancer Investigation, 20*(5–6):754-758.

Yoder, L., & Rubin, M. (1992). The epidemiology of cervical cancer and its precursors. *Oncology Nursing Forum, 19*(3):485-493.

Yu, C. K., Chiu, C., & McCormack, M., et al. (2005). Delayed diagnosis of cervical cancer in young women. *Journal of Obstetrics & Gynaecology, 25*(4):367-370.

HEMORRHAGIC CYSTITIS

CATHY FORTENBAUGH

PATHOPHYSIOLOGICAL MECHANISMS

Hemorrhagic cystitis (HC) is an irritation of the endothelial lining of the bladder characterized by mucosal inflammation and ulceration with bleeding, clotting, or hemorrhage. The severity of bleeding (Table 21-1) can range from microscopic hematuria (5 to 50 RBCs per high-power field) to death from exsanguinating hematuria (Polovich et al., 2005). HC is considered a urologic emergency.

The three main causes of HC in patients with cancer are treatment with chemotherapy, hematopoietic stem cell transplantation (HSCT), and treatment with radiation, either external beam or brachytherapy.

Signs and symptoms of HC include microscopic or frank hematuria with or without clots; dysuria; urgency; nocturia; frequent urination in small volumes; burning on urination; suprapubic, flank, or back pain; and bladder pain or spasm. Men may experience penile pain, which is referred pain caused by bladder spasm (Polovich et al., 2005; Bramble & Morley, 1997).

Chemotherapy-related HC occurs as a result of drug metabolites or byproducts binding to the bladder lining. A second, more unusual, cause of chemotherapy-related HC is instillation of the chemotherapeutic agent directly into the bladder (intravesically) to treat bladder cancer. The two main chemotherapeutic agents responsible for HC are cyclophosphamide and ifosfamide. Cyclophosphamide breaks down into acrolein, and ifosfamide breaks down into acrolein and chloroacetaldehyde. Other intravenous chemotherapeutic agents (e.g., bortezomib) can cause HC in rare cases. Gemcitabine and irinotecan can cause HC after repeated cycles (Polovich et al., 2005).

HC after radiation therapy (RT) is rare. When it does occur, it causes either early damage or late damage. Early damage can take 4 to 6 weeks to develop after completion of RT. It does not occur immediately unless precipitated by another injury, such as chemotherapy-induced toxicity, because of the slow turnover time of the bladder epithelium. Early damage is characterized by epithelial inflammation and edema. As normal tissue repair occurs, early HC resolves (Crew et al., 2001). Late damage starts 6 months to 2 years after completion of RT. In these cases, the bladder tissue undergoes radiation-related changes. Bladder wall epithelial changes may progress to necrosis of the vascular endothelium. The result is fibrosis and vessel wall thickening. The tissue becomes hypovascular, hypoxic, and ischemic, and further fibrosis results. The damage is progressive and can lead to poorly healing ulcers, superficial bladder epithelial denudation, occasional bladder perforation, and fistula formation. Fibrosis of the bladder, with reduced urine capacity, can occur up to 10 years after RT (Nehman et al., 2005; Crew et al., 2001).

Two types of HSCT-related HC can occur, early onset and late onset. HC that occurs within 72 hours after treatment with high-dose cyclophosphamide is known as *early onset HC*. *Late onset HC* usually is virally mediated. Viral infections usually are caused by polyomavirus BK (BK), adenovirus, and cytomegalovirus (CMV). These viral infections occur

Table 21-1 SEVERITY OF BLEEDING IN HEMORRHAGIC CYSTITIS

Adverse Event	Short Name	Grade 1	Grade 2	Grade 3	Grade 4	Grade 5
Hemorrhage GU Select Bladder Fallopian tube Kidney Ovary Prostate Retroperitoneum Spermatic cord Stoma Testes Ureter Urethra Urinary NOS Uterus Vagina Vas deferens	Hemorrhage GU—Select	Minimal or microscopic bleeding; no intervention indicated	Gross bleeding; medical intervention or urinary tract irrigation indicated	Transfusion,* interventional radiation therapy (i.e., hemostasis of bleeding site), or endoscopic or operative intervention indicated	Life-threatening consequences; major urgent intervention indicated	Death

*Transfusion implies pRBCs.
Also consider: fibrinogen; international normalized ratio of prothrombin time (INR); platelets; partial thromboplastin time (PTT).

weeks to months after the conditioning therapy. Virally mediated HC is thought to be due to reactivation of a latent form of the virus that is already present in the patient's system. The BK virus infects the patient during childhood and remains latent in the kidney until immunocompromise occurs (Azzi et al., 1999). Adenovirus type II has an affinity for the bladder. CMV affects many areas of the body, including the bladder. Graft versus host disease is another cause of late onset HC in patients who have received transplants, but its role is not clearly understood (Ezzone, 2004).

EPIDEMIOLOGY AND ETIOLOGY

Symptomatic or asymptomatic hematuria occurs in 6% to 10% of adults treated with standard low-dose cyclophosphamide (less than 1000 mg). Microscopic or frank hematuria with clotting occurs in up to 40% of adults treated with high-dose cyclophosphamide. Up to 50% of adults treated with ifosfamide develop HC ranging from microscopic to frank hematuria; 18% to 40% of adults treated with this drug develop frank hematuria (Polovich et al., 2005).

HC-related symptoms occur in children within a few weeks after treatment with cyclophosphamide or ifosfamide. Five percent to 10% of children treated with low-dose cyclophosphamide experience HC ranging from mild dysuria to severe hemorrhage. Children treated with ifosfamide have a higher incidence of HC; 20% to 40% experience mild dysuria to severe hemorrhage (Polovich et al., 2005). One third of patients treated with intravesical thiotepa or mitomycin develop hematuria. Most patients treated with bacilli Calmette-Guerin develop irritative voiding symptoms that are not severe enough to warrant discontinuation of therapy (DeVita et al., 2001). The incidence of HC in all patients treated with RT is less than 5% (Moy & Joyce, 2006). The incidence of HC in patients who receive HSCT is about 30% (Ezzone, 2004).

RISK PROFILE

Because cyclophosphamide and ifosfamide are the main causes of chemotherapy-related HC, patients treated with either of these agents are at risk. Patients treated with high-dose cyclophosphamide and any dosage of ifosfamide have the highest risk. Patients treated with bortezomib, or with repeated doses of gemcitabine or irinotecan, are also at risk (Polovich et al., 2005). Previous treatment with busulfan also increases the risk, because busulfan is excreted in the urine and causes bladder damage (Ezzone, 2004).

Patients with prostate, cervical, or bladder cancer who are being treated with radiation are at the greatest risk of developing radiation-related HC, because the radiation field could be in the area of the bladder. The risk of developing HC depends on the total radiation dose, volume irradiated, fractionation schedule, and method (i.e., external beam or brachytherapy). The higher the dose of radiation, the greater the risk of developing HC (Moy & Joyce, 2006).

With HSCT, patients treated with high-dose cyclophosphamide are at the greatest risk of developing early onset HC. Patients who are expected to have or who already have had long periods of immunocompromise are at increased risk of developing virally mediated, late onset HC. Patients with a known previous infection with the BK virus, adenovirus, or CMV are at additional risk (Ezzone, 2004).

PROGNOSIS

Severe HC across all treatment modalities, including HSCT, occurs in fewer than 10% of patients. HC is associated with a 2% to 4% mortality rate across all treatment modalities (Moy & Joyce, 2006).

PROFESSIONAL ASSESSMENT CRITERIA (PAC)

1. CBC with differential to assess for and/or rule out anemia, neutropenia, and thrombo-cytopenia (Moy & Joyce, 2006).
2. BUN and creatinine to assess for and/or rule out renal pathology (Moy & Joyce, 2006).
3. Coagulation parameters, including PT/APTT, INR, to assess for and/or rule out coagu-lopathy (Moy & Joyce, 2006).
4. Monitor vital signs as appropriate to assess hemodynamic stability, specifically pulse, pulse pressure, and temperature, because HC can be life-threatening (Moy & Joyce, 2006).
5. Ensure strict intake and output to monitor fluid status; instruct patient and family in how to participate in this process (Polovich et al., 2005).
6. Obtain baseline urinalysis before beginning therapy and continue to monitor regularly throughout treatment, including subjective reports (Polovich et al., 2005).
7. Visually inspect urine for blood, and instruct the patient and family in this process (Polovich et al., 2005).
8. Test with urine dipstick for blood to monitor for bleeding.
9. Obtain urine cultures at baseline and as needed to rule out urinary tract infection (Moy & Joyce, 2006).
10. Note previous medication history, including previous chemotherapy to assess the patient's risk of developing HC. Include over-the-counter and herbal medications (Moy & Joyce, 2006), especially those known to increase bleeding, such as bilberry, bromelain from pineapple stem, cayenne, chamomile, coleus, dong quai, feverfew, flaxseed oil, garlic, ginger, ginkgo, American ginseng, green tea, horse chestnut, meadowsweet, motherwort, poplar, shepherd's purse, and tumeric (Kumar et al., 2002).
11. Note previous radiation treatment to assess the patient's risk of developing HC (Moy & Joyce, 2006).
12. Use pelvic ultrasound to rule out urinary flow obstruction if the patient is experiencing clots. (Ezzone, 2004).
13. Cystoscopy is done to confirm the diagnosis of HC; it can pinpoint a bleeding source in severe cases (Ezzone, 2004).
14. Bladder biopsy is done to assess for tumor invasion or direct tumor extension into the bladder (Moy & Joyce, 2006).
15. Evaluate for infection with CMV or BK virus by PCR if patient is undergoing HSCT and is symptomatic (Ezzone, 2004).
16. Evaluate for adenovirus with urine culture if patient is undergoing transplantation and is symptomatic (Ezzone, 2004).

NURSING CARE AND TREATMENT

Prevention

The best treatment of HC is to prevent it from occurring. The initial focus of nursing care is on prevention.

Chemotherapy-Induced HC

For chemotherapy-induced HC, preventive measures center around assessment and mon-itoring, forced hydration, diuresis, free voiding, and treatment with mesna (Strohl, 2000).

1. Have the patient urinate every 2 to 4 hours (Polovich et al., 2005; West, 1997).
2. Maintain strict intake and output, and instruct the patient and family in the process (Polovich et al., 2005; West, 1997).
3. Weigh the patient daily (Polovich et al., 2005; West, 1997).
4. Report urine output that is less than 100 mL/hr (Polovich et al., 2005; West, 1997).
5. Instruct the patient to increase oral intake to 2 to 3 L a day. Increased fluid intake should begin 12 to 24 hours before chemotherapy and continue for 2 to 3 days after chemotherapy (Polovich et al., 2005; West, 1997).
6. If the patient is unable to drink an adequate amount of fluids, before and after chemotherapy administration, begin intravenous hydration (Polovich et al., 2005; West, 1997).
7. Forced saline hydration and diuresis are necessary for high-dose cyclophosphamide and ifosfamide to minimize the contact metabolites have with the bladder (Polovich et al., 2005; West, 1997).
8. Inspect the patient's urine at each void to detect frank blood.
9. Administer cyclophosphamide or ifosfamide early in the day so that metabolites do not sit in the bladder during the night (Wilkes & Barton-Burke, 2005).
10. Administer mesna as prescribed. Mesna is a bladder protectant that is administered with high doses of cyclophosphamide and all doses of ifosfamide. Mesna works by binding to the drug metabolites, allowing them to be inactivated and detoxified. NOTE: *Never administer ifosfamide without mesna* (Polovich et al., 2005).
11. Mesna can be administered by several different methods, depending on the dose of cyclophosphamide and ifosfamide and the route of mesna administration.
    * For adult patients receiving standard-dose ifosfamide, the total dose of mesna is equal to 60% of the total ifosfamide dose. The IV bolus doses of mesna are divided into 15 minutes before and 4 and 8 hours after ifosfamide administration (Polovich et al., 2005).
    * Another method of mesna administration in adults receiving standard-dose ifosfamide is to give an IV bolus dose of mesna equal to 20% of the total daily ifosfamide dosage before starting the ifosfamide infusion. Then, give a continuous mesna infusion at 50% to 100% of the daily ifosfamide dosage while the ifosfamide is infusing. This allows continuous contact of mesna with metabolites traveling through the bladder (Polovich et al., 2005).
    * A third method of mesna administration in adults receiving standard-dose ifosfamide is to begin with an IV bolus dose of 20% of the total daily dose of ifosfamide; this is followed by a continuous infusion of mesna of up to 40% of the total daily ifosfamide dose, which is continued for 12 to 24 hours after ifosfamide infusion is complete (Polovich et al., 2005).
12. For patients who are to be treated with oral mesna, the first dose is still given intravenously, in an amount equal to 20% of the daily ifosfamide dose; this is followed at 2 and 6 hours by a dose equal to 40% of the total daily ifosfamide dose. Oral mesna can be used only if the ifosfamide regimen calls for a total daily ifosfamide dose of less than 2 g/m^2 (Schucnter et al., 2002).
13. No clinical evidence supports the administration of mesna at doses greater than 60% of the total daily ifosfamide dose. Higher doses of mesna are associated with increased gastrointestinal toxicity (Polovich et al., 2005).
14. No guidelines have been established for mesna dosing with high-dose ifosfamide in adults. However, it is known that in these patients, more frequent and prolonged mesna dosing than is used for standard-dose ifosfamide is necessary to prevent HC (Polovich et al., 2005).
15. Total mesna doses for high-dose cyclophosphamide in adults should be 40% of the total cyclophosphamide dose administered intravenously 15 minutes before and 4 and 8 hours after cyclophosphamide in bolus doses (Polovich et al., 2005).

16. The IV mesna dose in children usually is 60% of the total daily dose of either the cyclophosphamide or ifosfamide. A 1:1 ratio sometimes is used. The most common mesna administration schedule is an IV bolus dose given 15 minutes before and 4 and 8 hours after cyclophosphamide or ifosfamide. The prechemotherapy bolus dose is given intravenously, but the subsequent doses may be administered orally. Note: The oral dose is higher than the IV dose (Polovich et al., 2005).
17. Monitor the patient for side effects of mesna, including nausea, vomiting, diarrhea, abdominal pain, taste changes, rash, urticaria, headache, and hypotension (SLOCR, 2004).

HSCT-Related HC

Prevention of early onset HC in HSCT is also the initial focus of nursing management in patients receiving transplants. Preventive measures center on assessment and monitoring, hyperhydration, diuresis, free voiding, continuous bladder irrigation, and treatment with mesna.

1. Maintain IV hydration of 3 L/m^2/day (Ezzone, 2004).
2. Encourage the patient to increase oral intake (Ezzone, 2004).
3. Administer continuous-infusion mesna as prescribed at 100% to 160% of the total daily dose of either cyclophosphamide or ifosfamide (Ezzone, 2004).
4. Continuous bladder irrigation of 300 to 1000 mL/hr (Ezzone, 2004).
5. Hourly voids if no bladder irrigation (Ezzone, 2004).
6. Diuretics as needed to keep urine flowing through the bladder (Ezzone, 2004).
7. Strict intake and output, and instruct the patient and family in the process (Ezzone, 2004).
8. Daily weights (Ezzone, 2004).
9. Report any urine output that is less than 100 mL/hr (Ezzone, 2004).
10. Inspect urine at each void or at least every 2 hours to detect frank blood (Ezzone, 2004).
11. Administer cyclophosphamide early in the day so that urine containing metabolites does not sit in the bladder during the night (Ezzone, 2004).

RT-Related HC

Prevention of HC in patients receiving RT is based on recent advances in radiation techniques that allow patients to receive the maximum radiation dose possible to the tumor with minimal damage to surrounding tissues. The radiation planning process is crucial to preventing either early or late onset radiation-induced HC. Three-dimensional computerized tomography (CT) planning systems can accurately calculate the radiation dose to an area, such as the bladder, and ensure that normal tissue tolerance is not exceeded.

Emergency Care

Once HC occurs, it is considered a urologic emergency. Treatment plans differ, depending on the cause and severity of the HC.

Chemotherapy-Induced and Early Onset HSCT–Related HC

1. If gross hematuria or cystitis is present, discontinue the cyclophosphamide or ifosfamide and notify the physician (Polovich et al., 2005).
2. Insert a three-way Foley catheter if continuous bladder irrigation is indicated (Polovich et al., 2005).
3. Start continuous irrigation with saline or acetylcysteine as prescribed. If clots are obstructing urine flow, a large-bore Foley catheter, along with aggressive saline irrigation, will be necessary (Polovich et al., 2005).

4. Give aminocaproic acid as ordered to promote clotting. This drug is an antifibrinolytic agent (Polovich et al., 2005).
5. Saline, potassium aluminum sulfate, silver nitrate, and formalin all work by forming a protein precipitate over bleeding surfaces (Polovich et al., 2005).
6. Administer topical analgesics as prescribed (e.g., phenazopyridine 100-200 mg TID) for symptoms of dysuria, urgency, and frequency (Russo, 2000).
7. Administer antispasmodics (e.g., oxybutynin) as ordered for bladder spasm (Russo, 2000).
8. For intravesical chemotherapy with bacilli Calmette-Guerin, isoniazid, acetaminophen, or ibuprofen is given to relieve irritative symptoms.
9. Blood transfusions are given as prescribed based on hemoglobin and hematocrit laboratory values and the patient's symptoms. One unit of packed RBCs increases the hemoglobin by 1 g and the hematocrit by 3% (George-Gay & Chernecky, 2002).
10. Obtain a urology consult.
11. Cystoscopy with electrocautery and cryosurgery are used to stop bleeding (Moy & Joyce, 2006).
12. Cystectomy is performed in rare cases when bleeding cannot be stopped (Moy & Joyce, 2006).
13. Long-term urologic follow-up is needed because the inflammation, bleeding, and irritation associated with HC can lead to permanent changes, such as cystitis, fibrosis, and an increased risk of bladder cancer (Polovich et al., 2005).

Late Onset HSCT–Related HC

1. If the HC is related to CMV infection, administer gancyclovir as prescribed (Ezzone, 2004).
2. No proven treatments are available for BK virus or adenovirus infection (Ezzone, 2004).
3. If persistent bleeding occurs, start saline hydration; also, insert a three-way Foley catheter and begin continuous bladder irrigation. Both hydration and continuous bladder irrigation are less aggressive than for chemotherapy-related HC (Ezzone, 2004).
4. Obtain a urology consult.
5. Perform alum bladder irrigation as prescribed (Ezzone, 2004).
6. Administer topical analgesics as prescribed (e.g., phenazopyridine 100-200 mg TID) for symptoms of dysuria, urgency, and frequency (Russo, 2000).
7. Administer antispasmodics (e.g., oxybutynin) for bladder spasm (Russo, 2000).
8. Blood transfusions are given based on hemoglobin and hematocrit results and the patient's symptoms (Ezzone, 2004). One unit of packed RBCs increases the hemoglobin by 1 g and the hematocrit by 3% (George-Gay & Chernecky, 2002).
9. Cystoscopy with electrocautery and cryosurgery are used to stop bleeding (Ezzone, 2004).
10. Cystectomy is performed in rare cases when bleeding cannot be stopped (Ezzone, 2004).

Radiation-Induced HC

1. Administer topical analgesics as prescribed (e.g., phenazopyridine 100-200 mg TID) for symptoms of dysuria, urgency, and frequency (Russo, 2000).
2. Administer antispasmodics (e.g., oxybutynin) for bladder spasm (Russo, 20004).
3. For mild radiation-related HC, insert a three-way Foley catheter and begin continuous bladder irrigation as ordered (Crew et al., 2001).
4. For mild radiation-related HC, intravenous hydration and diuresis usually are prescribed (Crew et al., 2001).

5. Blood transfusions are given as prescribed based on hemoglobin and hematocrit results and the patient's symptoms (Crew et al., 2001). One unit of packed RBCs increases the hemoglobin by 1 g and the hematocrit by 3% (George-Gay & Chernecky, 2002).
6. Obtain a urology consult.
7. Prepare the patient for hyperbaric oxygen treatment if prescribed. Hyperbaric oxygen improves regional tissue oxygenation, resulting in neovascularization and capillary growth into hypoxic and scarred bladder submucosal tissue. It is most effective when started within 6 months of radiation treatment (Nehman et al., 2005; Chong et al., 2004; Crew et al, 2001).
8. Cystoscopy with electrocautery and cryosurgery are used to stop bleeding (Moy & Joyce, 2006).
9. Cystectomy is performed in rare cases when bleeding cannot be stopped (Moy & Joyce, 2006).

All Patients (Regardless of Treatment Modality)

1. Provide referral to home care, social worker, physical therapist, and chaplain or other spiritual leader as needed.
2. Consider integrative care modalities, such as music therapy, art therapy, massage, and guided imagery, to provide distraction and reduce anxiety (NCCAM, 2002).

EVIDENCE-BASED PRACTICE UPDATES

1. Several studies have reported that vidarabine is effective for treating adenovirus-related HC in patients receiving HSCT (Kurosaki et al., 2004).
2. One case report discussed successful treatment with gancyclovir for HC caused by adenovirus in patients receiving HCST (Chen et al., 1997).
3. One case report found good results with the use of cidofovir to treat HC caused by BK virus in patients receiving HSCT (Held et al., 2000).
4. Several studies have reported that sodium pentosan polysulphate, given orally, can effectively treat either chemotherapy- or radiation-induced HC (Toren & Norman, 2005; Sandhu et al., 2004; Hampson & Woodhouse, 1994, Liu et al., 1994).
5. Several studies have shown that conjugated estrogens are an effective treatment for HC. One case report concerned 10 patients treated with conjugated estrogens for HC in allogeneic HSCT. This report showed positive results in 7 of the 10 patients (Ordemann et al., 2000).
6. A case report demonstrated that hyperbaric oxygen was effective in managing HC in a patient with multiple myeloma treated with HSCT who received cyclophosphamide and busulfan. The patient had BK virus and adenovirus. The HC was refractory to multiple conventional treatments before being effectively treated with hyperbaric oxygen (Hughes et al., 1998).
7. Several studies have been done on internal iliac artery embolization for severe HC; these studies have found mixed results (Crew et al., 2001).
8. Hydrodistention for radiation-induced HC has had disappointing results (Crew et al., 2001).
9. Intravesical prostaglandins were used in 10 patients who developed BK virus–related HC after allogeneic bone marrow transplantation. Gross hematuria was eliminated in all 10 cases (Laszio et al., 1995).
10. Intravesical granulocyte-macrophage colony-stimulating factor (GM-CSF) was used in a small study of six patients who developed HC after receiving cyclophosphamide for

allogeneic bone marrow transplantation. The patients received GM-CSF 400 mcg intravesically for 3 days. The HC resolved completely in three patients and partially in three patients (Vela-Ojeda et al., 1999).

TEACHING AND EDUCATION

1. Inform patients who are receiving cyclophosphamide, ifosfamide, or radiation to the bladder or pelvis, or who are undergoing HSCT that HC could occur (Polovich et al., 2005).
2. Instruct patients receiving cyclophosphamide and ifosfamide to void at the first sensation, even at night, so that drug metabolites will be in contact with the bladder for only a short period. Instruct patients that they will need to wake up at night to void and that they will need to void at least every 2 hours. Instruct patients who received stem cell transplants and who do not have continuous bladder irrigation that they will need to void hourly (Ezzone, 2004).
3. Verify that the patient and family know the signs and symptoms of HC to report and the contact information, so that the disorder can be reported and managed in a timely manner (Moy & Joyce, 2006).
4. Instruct the patient to increase oral fluids to at least 2 L a day for 2 to 3 days after treatment with cyclophosphamide or ifosfamide to keep urine flowing through the bladder; or, describe the plan for intravenous fluids and diuresis as appropriate.
5. Instruct the patient who is required to drink at least 2 L of fluid a day and who is unable to keep fluids down to call the health care provider, because the patient may need to receive intravenous hydration.
6. Instruct the patient and family to check for pink-tinged urine, frank blood, or clots in the urine each time the patient voids.
7. Emphasize that the patient must take every dose of mesna prescribed to reduce the chance of HC.
8. If the patient is to receive oral mesna at home, encourage the family to fill the prescription before discharge or to telephone the pharmacy to make sure that the drug is available.
9. Encourage the patient who will be taking oral cyclophosphamide at home to take it early in the day and to take the final dose no later than 4 pm, or 1600 hours (Polovich et al., 2005).
10. Instruct the patient with a three-way Foley catheter in catheter self-care.

NURSING DIAGNOSES

1. **Impaired urinary elimination** related to HC
2. **Deficient knowledge** related to prevention, diagnosis, treatment, and impact on quality of life related to HC
3. **Acute pain** related to HC
4. **Risk for decreased cardiac output, deficient fluid volume, and ineffective tissue perfusion** related to bleeding due to HC
5. **Deficient fluid volume** related to hemorrhage

EVALUATION AND DESIRED OUTCOMES

1. Toxins will be in contact with the bladder for a minimal period of time.
2. Mesna will be given as prescribed to all patients receiving any dose of ifosfamide and high-dose cyclophosphamide.

3. HC-related symptoms will resolve, including microscopic or frank hematuria with or without clots; dysuria; urgency; nocturia; frequent urination in small volumes; burning on urination; suprapubic, flank, or back pain; and bladder pain or spasm.
4. Late effects of HC (i.e., cystitis and fibrosis) will be reduced because inflammation, bleeding, and irritation associated with HC will have been aggressively managed.

DISCHARGE PLANNING AND FOLLOW-UP CARE

- Home care to administer ifosfamide or high-dose cyclophosphamide post hydration, diuretics, and mesna if patient will be discharged to home after chemotherapy. Home care will teach the patient and family how to self-administer post hydration, diuretics and/or post mesna.
- Home care to assess signs and symptoms of HC as appropriate.
- Follow-up with an urologist for patients who have had HC. Follow-up is periodic and involves at least annual urinalysis, urine cytology, and cystoscopy. Periodic excretory urograms are necessary for patients with gross hematuria, new microhematuria, abnormal urine cytologic findings, and persistent irritative voiding.
- Patient to call the health care provider if he or she has new or more severe hematuria; microscopic or frank bleeding; clots; and new or increased symptoms of dysuria, nocturia, urgency, frequency, or burning on urination; suprapubic, flank, penile, or back pain; and bladder pain or spasm.

REVIEW QUESTIONS

QUESTIONS

1. **Which of the following patients is at greatest risk for developing HC:**
   1. The patient starting low-dose oral cyclophosphamide.
   2. The patient receiving RT to the mediastinum.
   3. The patient receiving the first dose of ifosfamide.
   4. The patient receiving the second dose of gemcitabine.

2. **What blood tests are most appropriate for patients experiencing HC:**
   1. CBC, PT/INR, creatinine
   2. Hgb, LFTs, ANC
   3. ANC, PT/INR, LFTs
   4. PT/INR, LFTs, creatinine

3. **The initial focus of care for patients at risk for developing HC is:**
   1. Administration of fibrinolytic agents (e.g., aminocaproic acid) to promote clotting
   2. Prevention of the development of HC
   3. Blood transfusion to increase hemoglobin

   4. Cystoscopy to visualize the bladder and localize bleeding

4. **Metabolites of ifosfamide responsible for HC are:**
   1. Formulin and acrolein
   2. Alum and acrolein
   3. Acrolein and chloroacetaldehyde
   4. Chloroacetaldehyde and formulin

5. **Mrs. Smith received high-dose cyclophosphamide 24 hours ago in your outpatient area. She received aggressive hydration and mesna 4 and 8 hours after cyclophosphamide. She calls to tell you that she is nauseous and unable to keep fluids down. Your response is to:**
   1. Call in a prescription for additional antiemetics to her local pharmacy and ask her to call you in the morning if the nausea does not resolve.
   2. Ask her to try bland foods and to call back in several hours if the nausea does not resolve.
   3. Instruct her to take two additional doses of oral mesna to reduce the risk of HC.

4. Ask her to return to the office to receive intravenous hydration and to have her antiemetic regimen adjusted.

6. Your patient is receiving high-dose ifosfamide daily for 5 days every 3 weeks. On day 3, midway through the infusion, she returns from the bathroom and tells you she is experiencing severe urinary frequency, urgency, and burning. She tells you that her urine appears red. Your immediate nursing actions are to:
   1. Increase the amount of mesna that you will give 4 and 8 hours after ifosfamide.
   2. Insert a three-way Foley catheter and call the physician for further instructions.
   3. Discontinue the ifosfamide, maintain intravenous hydration, and contact the physician for further instructions.
   4. Call 911, because this is a life-threatening urologic emergency.

7. Mr. Smith is a 67-year-old male who was diagnosed with prostate cancer 9 months ago. He was treated with 6 weeks of radiation followed by hormonal therapy. He comes in for a follow-up visit complaining of urinary frequency, urgency, flank pain, penile pain, and bladder spasms. He reports that all of these symptoms have been getting progressively worse over the past several months. He is experiencing:
   1. Early onset RT-related HC
   2. HC related to hormonal therapy
   3. Idiopathic HC
   4. Late onset RT-related HC

8. Ms. R. is a 42-year-old female who is 3 months status post allogenic peripheral stem cell transplant (PSCT). She underwent a conditioning regimen that included cyclophosphamide. She has returned for a follow-up visit complaining of urgency, burning on urination, and nocturia. Urinalysis reveals a trace amount of blood in the urine. Urine cultures are negative. What information will be helpful for determining the cause of Ms. R's urinary symptoms:
   1. Ms. R. is hepatitis B positive.
   2. Ms. R. is CMV positive.
   3. Ms. R is HSV positive.
   4. Ms. R. is hepatitis C positive.

9. For children receiving ifosfamide, the incidence of HC ranging from mild dysuria to severe hemorrhage is:
   1. 5% to 10%
   2. 3% to 5%
   3. 20% to 40%
   4. 40% to 80%

10. The physician writes the following prescriptions for an adult patient with sarcoma:
    Palanosetron 0.25 mg IV ×
      1 pre-chemotherapy day 1
    Dexamethasone 10 mg IV ×
      1 pre-chemotherapy
    Ifosfamide 300 mg/day days 1-3
    Carboplatin 600 mg/day days 1-3
    Etoposide 200 mg/day days 1-3
    Neulasta 6 mg SQ × 1 day 4 and
      every 21 days

    The drug that is missing from the prescribed chemotherapy is:
    1. Mesna
    2. Ganciclovir
    3. Ciprofloxacin
    4. Lorazepam

ANSWERS

1. *Answer: 3*
   Rationale: The incidence of combined microscopic and frank hematuria in patients receiving ifosfamide can run as high as 50%.

2. *Answer: 1*
   Rationale: Patients with HC are monitored for anemia, neutropenia, and thrombocytopenia, coagulation abnormalities, and renal function.

3. *Answer: 2*
   Rationale: The best treatment of HC is to prevent it before it occurs.

4. *Answer: 3*
   Rationale: Acrolein and chloroacetaldehyde are metabolites of ifosfamide that cause HC.

5. *Answer: 4*
Rationale: A patient who has received high-dose cyclophosphamide must drink at least 2 L of fluid a day for 48 to 72 hours after chemotherapy to help minimize contact with metabolites in the bladder. Because the patient is nauseous and not drinking, she is unable to receive adequate oral hydration. Too much time could lapse if she waited for the antiemetics to work without starting hydration. She could also receive intravenous fluids at home with home care if her insurance covers the treatment.

6. *Answer: 3*
Rationale: The first step in the management of gross hematuria or cystitis is to discontinue ifosfamide to minimize further damage.

7. *Answer: 4*
Rationale: Patients with prostate cancer who have received RT to the pelvis are at increased risk of developing HC. Late onset radiation—related HC begins around 6 months after treatment.

8. *Answer: 2*
Rationale: Ms. R. may be experiencing late onset HC after PSCT, possibly as a result of infection with the CMV virus.

9. *Answer: 3*
Rationale: For children receiving ifosfamide, the incidence of HC ranging from mild dysuria to severe hemorrhage is 20% to 40%.

10. *Answer: 1*
Rationale: Mesna must always be given with ifosfamide to prevent HC.

REFERENCES

Azzi, A., Cesaro, S., & Laszio, D., et al. (1999). Human polyomavirus bk (bkv) load and hemorrhagic cystitis in bone marrow transplantation patients. *Journal of Clinical Virology, 14*(2):79-86.

Bramble, F. J., & Morley, R. (1997). Drug-induced cystitis: The need for vigilance. *British Journal of Urology, 79*:3-7.

Chen, F. E., Liang, R. H., & Lo, J. Y., et al. (1997). Treatment of adenovirus-associated hemorrhagic cystitis with ganciclovir. *Bone Marrow Transplantation, 20*(11):997-999.

Chong, K. T., Hampson, N. B., & Bostwick, D. G., et al. (2004). Hyperbaric oxygen does not accelerate in vivo prostate cancer: Implications for the treatment of radiation-induced haemorrhagic cystitis. *BJU International, 94*(9):1275-1278.

Crew, J. P., Jephcott, C. R., & Reynard, J. M. (2001). Radiation-induced hemorrhagic cystitis. *European Urology, 40*:111-123.

DeVita, V. T., Hellman, S., & Rosenberg, S. A. (Eds.). (2001). *Cancer principles and practice of oncology* (pp. 2645-2649). (6th ed.). Philadelphia: Lippincott Williams & Wilkins.

Ezzone, S. (Ed.). (2004). *Hematopoietic stem cell transplantation: A manual for nursing practice* (pp. 172-174). Pittsburgh: Oncology Nursing Society.

George-Gay, B., & Chernecky, C. (2002). *Clinical medical-surgical nursing: A decision-making reference.* Philadelphia: W. B. Saunders.

Hampson, S. J., & Woodhouse, C. R. (1994). Sodium pentosan polysulphate in the management of hemorrhagic cystitis: Experience with 14 patients. *European Urology, 25*:40-42.

Held, T. K., Beil, S. S., & Nitsche, A., et al. (2000). Treatment of BK virus—associated hemorrhagic cystitis and simultaneous CMV reactivation with cidofovir. *Bone Marrow Transplantation, 26*:347-350.

Hughes, A. J., Schwarer, A. P., & Miller, I. L. (1998). Hyperbaric oxygen in the treatment of refractory haemorrhagic cystitis. *Bone Marrow Transplantation, 22*(6):585-586.

Kumar, N. K., Moyers, S., & Allen, K., et al. (2002). *Integrative nutritional therapies for cancer* (pp. 155-160). St. Louis: Wolters Kluwer, Facts and Comparisons.

Kurosaki, K., Miwa, N., & Yoshida, Y., et al. (2004). Therapeutic basis of vidarabine on adenovirus-induced hemorrhagic cystitis. *Antiviral Chemistry and Chemotherapy, 15*(5):281-285.

Laszlo, D., Bosi, A., & Guidi, S., et al. (1995). Prostaglandin E2 bladder instillation for the treatment of hemorrhagic cystitis after allogenic bone marrow transplantation. *Haematologica, 80*(5):421-425.

Liu, Y. K., Harty, T. L., & Steinbock, G. S., et al. (1994). Treatment of radiation or cyclophosphamide induced hemorrhagic cystitis using conjugated estrogen. *Journal of Urology, 144*:41-43.

Moy, B., & Joyce, R. M. (2006). Cystitis in patients with cancer. Retrieved April 24, 2006, from http://www.uptodateonline.com/utd/content/topic.do?topicKey=genl_onc/7757&view=text.

NCCAM. (2002). Get the facts: What is complementary and alternative medicine? Retrieved May 30, 2006, from http://nccam.nih.gov/health/whatiscam/.

Nehman, A., Nativ, O., & Moskovitz, B., et al. (2005). Hyperbaric oxygen therapy for radiation-induced haemorrhagic cystitis. *BJU International, 96:*107-109.

Ordemann, R., Naumann, R., & Geissler, G., et al. (2000). Encouraging results in the treatment of hemorrhagic cystitis with estrogen: Report of 10 cases and review of the literature. *Bone Marrow Transplantation, 25*(9):981-985.

Polovich, M., White, J. M., & Keller, L. O. (Eds.). (2005) *Chemotherapy and biotherapy guidelines and recommendations for practice* (pp. 180-182). (2nd ed.). Pittsburgh: Oncology Nursing Press.

Russo, P. (2000). Urologic emergencies in cancer patients. *Seminars in Oncology, 27*(3):284-298.

Sandhu, S. S., Goldstraw, M., & Woodhouse, C. R. (2004). The management of hemorrhagic cystitis with sodium pentostatin. *BJU International, 94*(6):845-847.

Schucnter, L. M., Hensley, M. L., & Meropol, J., et al. (2002). 2002 Update of recommendations for the use of chemotherapy and radiotherapy protectants: Clinical practice guidelines of the American Society of Clinical Oncology. *Journal of Clinical Oncology, 20*(12):2895-2903.

SLOCR Pharmaceuticals. (2004). Mesna [package insert]. Irvine, CA: SLOCR.

Strohl, R. (2000). Hemorrhagic cystitis. In D. Camp-Sorrell, & R. A. Hawkins (Eds.). *Clinical manual for the oncology advanced practice nurse* (pp. 547-549). Pittsburgh: Oncology Nursing Society.

Toren, P. J., & Norman, R. W. (2005). Cyclophosphamide induced hemorrhagic cystitis successfully treated with pentosanpolysulphate. *Journal of Urology, 173*(1):103.

Vela-Ojeda, J., Tripp-Villanueva, F., & Sanchez-Cortes, E., et al. (1999). Intravesical rhGM-CSF for the treatment of late onset hemorrhagic cystitis after bone marrow transplant. *Bone Marrow Transplantation 24*(12):1307-1310.

West, N. J. (1997). Prevention and treatment of hemorrhagic cystitis. *Pharmacotherapy, 17*(4):696-706.

Wilkes, G. M., & Barton-Burke, M. (2005). *2005 Oncology nursing drug handbook.* Sudbury, MA: Jones & Bartlett.

HEPATIC ENCEPHALOPATHY

KATHLEEN MURPHY-ENDE

PATHOPHYSIOLOGICAL MECHANISMS

Hepatic encephalopathy (HE) is a complex neuropsychiatric syndrome marked by disturbances in consciousness, personality, intellect, and neuromuscular coordination and control; a diminishing level of consciousness; and electroencephalographic changes. End-stage cirrhosis and extensive hepatic metastases are the common underlying diseases that lead to this condition. Fulminant hepatic failure, characterized by the development of acute liver failure over several weeks, may be followed by hepatic encephalopathy. In reversible liver disease, the encephalopathy may be acute and reversible with early intervention; however, in end-stage liver disease, it has a grave prognosis.

The complete physiology of hepatic encephalopathy is not precisely known. It is thought to involve a combination of shunted liver circulation and biochemical alterations that ultimately alter neurotransmission. In liver dysfunction, collateral blood vessels form and shunt blood from the portal circulation to the systemic circulation, allowing neurotoxins absorbed from the gastrointestinal (GI) tract to bypass the liver and circulate to the brain. (A transjugular intrahepatic portosystemic stent shunt procedure can also alter the portal circulation.) The gastrointestinal (GI) tract normally absorbs toxic substances, which are broken down or detoxified by the liver before being released into the central circulatory system. If the process of detoxification is eliminated because of shunting, these toxic substances are released directly into the general circulation and may cross the blood-brain barrier. In liver failure, the permeability of the blood-brain barrier may also be increased.

The best known hazardous substance is ammonia, the end product of intestinal protein digestion or digestion of blood from GI bleeding. Bacteria in the colon also form ammonia, which contributes to raising the ammonia level, resulting in hyperammonemia. When ammonia comes in contact with the central nervous system, it interferes with neurotransmitters, alters cerebral energy, and causes cerebral edema. Massive cerebral edema may cause brain herniation and death (Huether, 2006). Ammonia also inhibits cellular chloride channels, additionally contributing to depression of the central nervous system (Haussinger et al., 2002). The correlation between the level of ammonia and the severity of encephalopathy is not definitively understood.

An accumulation of gamma-aminobutyric acid (GABA), an inhibitory neurotransmitter, may be responsible for the decreased level of consciousness. Endogenous benzodiazepine substances in the central nervous system of individuals with liver failure may increase GABA's inhibitory transmission function, ultimately causing a decrease in neurotransmission (Jones et al., 1993). Benzodiazepine levels are higher in hepatic encephalopathy, but they show only a weak correlation with the stage of encephalopathy (Basile et al., 1993).

Glutamine, which is synthesized from glutamate and ammonia, is an excitatory neurotransmitter. In hepatic encephalopathy, the reuptake of glutamate into cells may be inhibited, because brain tissue levels of glutamate are decreased, whereas extracellular levels are increased. The reason for these shifts is thought to be the hyperammonemia. The main center for the synthesis of glutamine from glutamate and ammonia is the astrocytes, and it may be that the hyperammonemia causes swelling of the astrocytes, preventing this process (Norenberg, 1998).

Other toxins that alter neuropsychiatric functioning include false neurotransmitters, accumulation of short-chain fatty acids, elevated manganese, hypokalemia, and alkalosis. False neurotransmitters are molecules similar to neurotransmitters which can inhibit the transmission of neural messages. In liver failure, branched-chain amino acids (BCAAs) are decreased and aromatic amino acids (AAAs) are increased. The AAAs travel to the brain, where they are metabolized into false neurotransmitters. Hyperammonemia may increase the breakdown of BCAAs. However, not enough is known yet about this pathway to use BCAAs to guide treatment (Als-Nielson et al., 2003).

Manganese may play a role in the pathogenesis of HE, because 80% of patients with cirrhosis in hepatic coma have increased concentrations of manganese. Prolonged exposure to manganese results in extrapyramidal symptoms and Alzheimer type II astrocytosis. Manganese and ammonia may act synergistically in causing HE symptoms (Weissenborn et al., 1995).

Other factors can aggravate HE, include vomiting and diarrhea, which can lead to hypokalemia and alkalosis. Alkalosis may increase the amount of the gaseous form of ammonia in the blood (Yurdaydin, 2003). Renal impairment may contribute to alkalosis, and if urea synthesis is impaired, more ammonia is formed. GI bleeding, transfusions, and an excessive protein intake may potentially cause hyperammonemia. Infection may worsen encephalopathy in individuals with acute liver failure (Rolando et al., 2000). Certain medications, especially sedatives, also can contribute to worsening symptoms.

The pathogenesis of hepatic encephalopathy is multifactorial, with ammonia being the predominant causative agent. Astrocytic changes in the brain and decreased glucose utilization in the cerebral cortex, with increased glucose utilization in the thalamus, caudate lobe, and cerebellum, suggest that hypometabolism explains the neuropsychiatric abnormalities seen in hepatic encephalopathy.

There are many variants of HE. The acute form is caused by fulminant liver failure with rapid progression to coma, seizures, and decerebrate rigidity; this form is associated with a high mortality rate from cerebral herniation and hypoxia. The slower onset form has milder symptoms and a longer duration and is reversible if the precipitating factors can be treated. The chronic form of HE is characterized by persistence of neuropsychiatric symptoms that do not resolve with adequate treatment. In rare cases, progressive, irreversible neurologic changes occur, including dementia, extrapyramidal manifestations, cerebellar degeneration, transverse cordal myelopathy, and peripheral neuropathy. The subclinical form of HE does not produce overt neuropsychiatric symptoms, but subtle changes can be detected with psychomotor testing; this form usually is reversible with treatment (Abou-Assi & Vlahcevic, 2001).

EPIDEMIOLOGY AND ETIOLOGY

Because the clinical manifestations of HE can range from subtle abnormalities to coma, the epidemiology is difficult to estimate. HE is seen most often with cirrhosis, the excessive scarring of the liver caused by a chronic. irreversible reaction to hepatic inflammation and necrosis. In the United States, the most common causes of cirrhosis are alcoholic liver disease and hepatitis C, whereas worldwide, hepatitis B is the leading cause of cirrhosis (Murphy, 2006). Estimates of the incidence of HE in cirrhosis run as high as 50% to 70%.

Subclinical HE occurs in 50% to 80% of patients with cirrhosis; the most common symptoms are difficulty sleeping and altered concentration and hand-eye coordination (Friedman & Schiano, 2004). All patients with fulminant hepatic failure have HE (Gitlin et al., 1986). HE also occurs in patients with extensive hepatic metastasis.

RISK PROFILE

- Acute or chronic liver disease
- Cirrhosis
- Hepatitis
- Primary malignant liver tumors
- Cholangiocarcinoma
- Metastasis of GI malignancies. GI malignancies are prone to spread to the liver because of the portal venous drainage. Metastasis can reach the liver from any organ, but the passage of blood from the GI tract to the liver via the portal circulation explains the high rate of metastasis from GI primary tumors. Fifteen percent of colorectal cancers present with liver metastasis, and 60% develop liver metastasis (Kemeny et al., 2004).
- Breast cancer, lung cancer, and melanoma with liver metastasis, or any malignancy with widespread hepatic metastasis
- Inherited errors of the urea cycle
- Spontaneous or iatrogenic portosystemic venous shunting
- Precipitating factors (Box 22-1)

BOX 22-1	PRECIPITATING CONDITIONS IN HEPATIC ENCEPHALOPATHY

- Alkalosis
- Anemia
- Azotemia/uremia
- Constipation
- Dehydration
- Excessive protein intake
- Gastrointestinal bleeding
- Hepatocellular cancer
- Hypoglycemia
- Hypokalemia
- Hyponatremia
- Hypothyroidism
- Hypovolemia
- Hypoxia
- Infection (*Helicobacter pylori* infection in the stomach)
- Liver metastasis (widespread)
- Medications (opioids, benzodiazepines, sedatives)
- Noncompliance with treatment
- Portosystemic shunts
- Surgery
- Transjugular intrahepatic portosystemic shunt (TIPS)
- Vascular occlusion

PROGNOSIS

The 1-year survival rate for hepatic encephalopathy in cirrhosis is 40% (Friedman & Schiano, 2004). The prognosis for HE in patients with cancer depends on the extent of liver metastasis and the patient's response to cancer treatment. In gastric and pancreatic cancer, metastasis to the liver correlates with a short survival. In colorectal cancer, if the liver is the sole site of metastatic disease and treatment is effective, survival may be extended (Kemeny et al., 2004). Extensive liver metastasis may cause malabsorption, electrolyte disturbances, hepatic encephalopathy, and liver failure progressing to death. HE in individuals with massive liver metastasis, disseminated disease, and poor response to treatment has a limited prognosis.

PROFESSIONAL ASSESSMENT CRITERIA (PAC)

1. The clinical features of hepatic encephalopathy tend to vary, because all parts of the brain may be affected, and the condition may manifest differently in the acute and chronic forms of liver failure. The acute form of HE is associated with fulminant liver failure characterized by rapid progression to profound coma, seizures, and decerebrate rigidity. Chronic HE is characterized by persistence of neuropsychiatric symptoms. Subclinical HE involves subtle changes detectable by psychomotor testing and is usually reversible. Box 22-2 presents the four stages of portosystemic encephalopathy.
2. Assess airway.
3. **Neurologic status:** Level of consciousness (ranges from slightly altered to coma), pupils, and ability to follow commands. In acute liver failure, seizures and lateralizing signs may be observed.
4. **Neuromuscular symptoms:** Range from tremor and asterixis to hyperreflexia, rigidity, myoclonus and, ultimately, decerebrate posture.
5. **Dietary history:** Excessive protein intake may precipitate HE by increasing the nitrogen load in the GI tract.
6. **Medication history:** Recent use of opioids, sedatives, or diuretics may precipitate HE.
7. **Bowel history:** Constipation may increase nitrogen absorption from the gut, and could precipitate HE.
8. **Laboratory data:** There is no biochemical test for HE. Blood tests are used to help rule out precipitating factors or other causes of encephalopathy.
   - CBC may be decreased.
   - Electrolytes: May have hyponatremia, hypokalemia, or metabolic alkalosis/acidosis.
   - Glucose: Hypoglycemia can be a lethal complication of HE and should be monitored every 4 hours.
   - Renal function may be abnormal
   - PT/PTT and INR may be increased.
   - Plasma ammonia level may be elevated in 90% of patients with HE, but levels do not correlate with the course or severity of HE (Kichian & Bain, 2004).
   - Liver function values may be elevated.
   - Stool may be positive for blood with GI bleeding.
   - Culture of body fluids: Urine, blood, and ascitic fluid should be cultured if infection is suspected.

BOX 22-2	STAGES OF PORTOSYSTEMIC ENCEPHALOPATHY

Stage 1: Prodromal
- Subtle manifestations that may not be recognized immediately
- Personality changes
- Behavior changes (agitation, belligerence)
- Emotional lability (euphoria, depression)
- Impaired thinking
- Inability to concentrate
- Fatigue, drowsiness
- Slurred or slowed speech
- Sleep pattern disturbances

Stage II: Impending
- Continuing mental changes
- Mental confusion
- Disorientation to time, place, or person
- Asterixis

Stage III: Stuporous
- Progressive deterioration
- Marked mental confusion
- Stuporous, drowsy, but arousable
- Abnormal electroencephalogram tracing
- Muscle twitching
- Hyperreflexia
- Asterixis

Stage IV: Comatose
- Unresponsiveness, leading to death in 85% of patients progressing to this stage
- Unarousable, obtunded
- Response to painful stimulus
- No asterixis
- Positive Babinski's sign
- Muscle rigidity
- Fetor hepaticus (characteristic liver breath; musty, sweet odor)
- Seizures

From Ignatavicius, D. D., & Workman, M. L. (2006). *Medical-surgical nursing: Critical thinking for collaborative care.* (5th ed.). Philadelphia: W. B. Saunders.

- Cerebrospinal fluid: May be normal or may show increased protein and increased GABA levels. Lumbar puncture is done only to rule out other, concomitant CNS pathologic conditions.
9. **Nonbiochemical tests:**
   - Reitan trail-marking or number connection: Patient connects a series of scattered numbers from 1 to 50 while being timed.
   - Neuropsychiatric testing
   - Electroencephalogram (EEG) may show nonspecific abnormalities, such as low-frequency or slow triphasic wave activity over the frontal areas.
10. **Diagnostics:** Advances in the detection and treatment of liver metastasis have led to more effective therapies. With some malignancies, hepatic metastases represent disseminated disease, and diagnostic testing may not be undertaken.
    - Computed tomography: Non-contrast CT, contrast CT, CT angiography, CT portography, delayed CT
    - Magnetic resonance imaging (MRI) scan

- Intraoperative ultrasonography
- Positron emission tomography (PET) scan

NURSING CARE AND TREATMENT

Nursing care is presented as a prioritized list.
1. Maintain the airway and administer oxygen to keep oxygen saturation above 90%. Keep airway at bedside.
2. **Aspiration precautions:** Assist with feeding and drinking and elevate head of bed.
3. Seizure precautions.
4. **Promote safety and prevent self-harm:** Assist with ambulation, keep call bell within reach, remove potentially dangerous equipment or devices from room, and frequently monitor patient activity. Prevent falls.
5. Assess and document neurologic status every 4 hours while awake.
6. Review current medications and suggest discontinuation of drugs that can potentiate hepatotoxicity, such as benzodiazepines, chemotherapeutic agents, and medications that are metabolized in the liver.
7. **Diet:** Lower the level of toxic substances by reducing or excluding protein from the diet. Initially limit protein to 20 g/day; this can be increased by 10 g every 3 to 5 days as tolerance allows. Vegetable protein may be advantageous in improving nitrogen balance without precipitating or worsening hepatic encephalopathy, and the fiber content may be beneficial (Wolf, 2006).
8. Assist in identifying and eliminating any precipitating factors (see Box 22-1).
9. Cancer treatment aimed at treating liver metastasis may be initiated. These procedures and treatments include hepatic resection, systemic chemotherapy, hepatic artery infusion of chemotherapy, hepatic artery embolization, ablative cryosurgery, radiofrequency ablation, absolute ethanol injection, and radiation therapy.
10. Medication is aimed at controlling the generation of neuroactive toxins. In acute liver failure with rapid onset and progression toward cerebral edema, mannitol intervenous injection (0.5 g/kg given over 10 minutes) is the main pharmacologic treatment. Treatment with acetylcysteine by continuous infusion improves cerebral blood flow and cerebral oxygen metabolism. Epoprostenol (prostaglandin I-2) improves cerebral oxygen utilization (Riordan & Williams, 1997). In urgent cases of HE, cleansing of the gut with an enema or colonic lavage may be indicated. Nonabsorbable disaccharides act as laxatives and reduce both ammoniagenesis and ammonia absorption from the GI tract. Lactulose is a synthetic disaccharide that is degraded by intestinal bacteria to produce acidification and an osmotic diarrhea. This acidification of colonic contents reduces ammonia absorption by trapping nitrogenous compounds in the lumen. The dosage of lactulose should be titrated to the patient, with the goal of two to four loose stools per day; an average daily dosage is 45 to 90 g in divided doses (Worobetz, 2006). Monitor for too much diarrhea and electrolyte abnormalities. Antibiotics alter colonic acidity and inhibit urea splitting and deaminating bacteria, reducing the production of ammonia; they may be use instead of or in conjunction with nonabsorbable disaccharides (e.g., neomycin 1-3 g daily or metronidazole 250 mg four times daily).
11. Pruritus may be improved with emollients, lotion with menthol, soft clothing, air humidification, and tepid cool baths using unperfumed, mild soap. Trim and file nails short to prevent injury from scratching. Nighttime sedation with antihistamines or a hypnotic can promote sleep. If the pruritus has an obstructive cause, biliary stenting provides relief. If the cause is intrahepatic cholestasis and obstructive jaundice, bile acid sequestrants (e.g., cholestyramine 4 g PO QID) may be helpful (Yarbro & Seiz, 2004). Topical corticosteroids have antiinflammatory and vasoconstrictive actions.

12. **Procedures:** Patients with spontaneous or surgically created portosystemic shunts or transjugular intrahepatic portosystemic shunts (TIPS) who have refractory HE may benefit from transhepatic embolization or surgical ligation of the portosystemic shunt. Refractory hepatic encephalopathy as a complication of TIPS can be managed with a reducing stent (Riordan & Williams, 1997). Orthotopic liver transplantation may be used in the treatment of patients with end-stage cirrhosis.

EVIDENCE-BASED PRACTICE UPDATES

1. Seventy percent of patients receiving scheduled lactulose showed improvement in their encephalopathy over a 4-week period (Loguercio et al., 1995); however this study did not have a control group. A Cochrane systematic review by Als-Nielson and colleagues (2004) concluded that not enough quality evidence is available to support the use of nonabsorbable disaccharides.
2. The use of synbiotics was found to reduce hepatic encephalopathy and ammonia levels by increasing the fecal content of non-urase-producing bacteria (Liu et al., 2004).
3. Significant reductions in ammonia levels and a decrease in the level of encephalopathy were found with the administration of L-ornithine–L-asparate (OA) (Kircheis & Haussinger, 2002).
4. Flumazenil, a benzodiazepine antagonist, improved clinical symptoms in patients with hepatic encephalopathy (Kircheis & Haussinger 2002; Butterworth, 2000); 30% showed some improvement (Als-Nielson et al., 2003).

TEACHING AND EDUCATION

1. Teach the patient and family to watch for the signs and symptoms of hepatic encephalopathy, including confusion, hand tremors, and sedation. Emphasize the importance of calling the physician or nurse practitioner immediately if these symptoms occur.
2. Explain the purpose of the low-protein diet, which is to reduce the conversion of protein into ammonia in the gut.
3. Provide information about the patient's medications: name, purpose, dosage, route, frequency, and side effects.
4. For patients with progressive liver failure, provide information about end of life care. Help the patient and family identify issues that require decision making.
5. **Web sites for information:**
   - Centers for Disease Control and Prevention (2002): Hepatitis fact sheet: http://www.cdc.gov/ncidod/diseases/hepatitis.htm
   - Hepatitis Liver Cirrhosis/HCC: http://www.extremehealthusa.com/hepatitis.html

NURSING DIAGNOSES

1. **Risk for injury** related to altered neurologic function.
2. **Risk for deficient fluid volume** related to treatment.
3. **Bowel incontinence** related to diarrhea secondary to lactulose treatment.
4. **Impaired verbal communication** related to altered level of consciousness.
5. **Risk for impaired skin integrity** related to diarrhea, immobility, and low protein intake.

EVALUATION AND DESIRED OUTCOMES

1. The patient will be free of physical injury.
2. The patient will be comfortable and have an acceptable level of pain.

3. The patient's cognition will return to his or her baseline level.
4. The patient will regain the previous physical functional status.
5. Bleeding will be controlled.
6. The patient's skin will remain intact.
7. Pruritus will resolve or will be at a level acceptable to the patient.
8. The patient and family will be able to identify the early signs and symptoms of hepatic encephalopathy and will know whom to call if these occur.
9. For patients with terminal disease, the patient and family will be prepared for death.

DISCHARGE PLANNING AND FOLLOW-UP CARE

- Home health care referral, with possible need for equipment such as hospital bed, wheelchair, walker, and beside commode.
- Hospice referral for patients with a prognosis of 6 months or less.
- Follow-up appointments for labs and with the physician or nurse practitioner.
- For patients with progressive liver failure, provide anticipatory guidance on the progressive nature of the symptoms.

REVIEW QUESTIONS

QUESTIONS

1. **The initial nursing assessment for a patient with acute liver failure should include:**
   1. Obtain a list of patient medications
   2. Obtain laboratory data from previous admissions
   3. Assess the patient's mental status
   4. All of the above

2. **A common condition in oncology patients with hepatic metastases that may precipitate hepatic encephalopathy is:**
   1. Constipation
   2. Rash
   3. Pleural effusion
   4. Opioid use

3. **The common symptoms of HE include all of the following *except*:**
   1. Asterixis
   2. Pain
   3. Decreased level of consciousness
   4. Apraxia

4. **Pain from liver capsule distention is best treated with:**
   1. Radiation
   2. Stenting of the portal obstruction
   3. Aspirin
   4. Antiinflammatory agents

5. **The lab result(s) most useful in evaluating hepatic encephalopathy is/are:**
   1. CBC
   2. Ammonia level
   3. Electrolytes
   4. All of the above

6. **Mary is a 52-year-old female with breast cancer who has extensive liver metastasis with liver failure. She went into a hepatic coma last night. She has advanced cancer and signed up for hospice a month ago. The family asks when the patient will wake up. Your best response is:**
   1. "In a few days, after the treatment starts to take effect."
   2. "There is always hope that she will wake up; let's try to wake her up now."
   3. "It is unlikely that she will wake up completely because her liver is failing, but you can still talk to her, and she may be able to hear you."
   4. "Once a person has entered a hepatic coma, she almost never wakes up."

7. **The purpose of antibiotics in HE is to:**
   1. Prevent an infection
   2. Lower the bacterial count in the GI tract

3. Treat pneumonia
4. Treat a hepatic infection

8. **The purpose of lactulose is to:**
   1. Cause diarrhea
   2. Increase the absorption of ammonia
   3. Cleanse the liver of toxins
   4. None of the above

9. **Patients treated with lactulose are at risk for skin breakdown because:**
   1. Lactulose tends to cause a pruritic rash.
   2. Lactulose alters protein absorption, leading to poor wound healing.
   3. Lactulose causes diarrhea, which may be very irritating to the skin.
   4. Lactulose causes sedation, which leaves the patient immobile.

10. **Patients with advanced cancer and end-stage liver failure need what type of information:**
    1. Liver transplant options
    2. Experimental chemotherapy options
    3. Palliative care options
    4. Massive doses of opioids

ANSWERS

1. *Answer: 4*
   Rationale: All the information listed is important for developing a nursing care plan.

2. *Answer: 1*
   Rationale: Constipation can precipitate HE by increasing the length of time that bacteria, which break down protein into ammonia, are in the gut.

3. *Answer: 2*
   Rationale: Pain may be present as a result of liver capsule distention or from metastatic sites, but it is not a symptom of HE.

4. *Answer: 4*
   Rationale: Antiinflammatory agents, such as NSAIDs or steroids, may be useful. Aspirin may cause bleeding. Stents are used for portal shunts that have failed and not for pain. Radiation would be indicated only for radiosensitive tumors of the liver.

5. *Answer: 4*
   Rationale: All of the laboratory data listed are used together to evaluate the patient's' condition and response. No single test is useful by itself.

6. *Answer: 3*
   Rationale: End-stage liver disease tends to progress, and hepatic coma is an end-stage irreversible condition. Answer 3 is honest, yet provides some comfort to the family by encouraging them to continue to communicate with the patient. Answer 4 is rather abrupt.

7. *Answer: 2*
   Rationale: The bacteria break down protein into ammonia.

8. *Answer: 1*
   Rationale: The purpose of lactulose is to decrease GI transit time in order ultimately to diminish the ability of the bacteria in the gut to convert substances into ammonia.

9. *Answer: 3*
   Rationale: The diarrhea from lactulose can cause skin breakdown.

10. *Answer: 3*
    Rationale: Patients who have terminal cancer and develop hepatic encephalopathy have a poor prognosis, and the goal of care is comfort and palliation of symptoms. Curative measures, such as liver transplantation, are not appropriate in these patients. Clinical trials tend not to accept patients in end-stage liver disease. Pain should always be treated, but high doses of opioids may not be needed. Patients with hepatic encephalopathy often are comfortable, because the altered level of consciousness caused by the neurotoxic substances tends to be sedating.

REFERENCES

Abou-Assi, S., & Vlahcevic, R. (2001). Hepatic encephalopathy: Metabolic consequences of cirrhosis often are reversible. *Postgraduate Medicine, 109*(2):52-70.

Als-Nielson, B., Gluud, L., & Gluud, C. (2004). Nonabsorbable disaccharides for hepatic encephalopathy. *Chochrane Review,* (3).

Als-Nielson, B., Kjaergard, L. L., & Gludd, C. (2003). Benzodiazepine receptor antagonists for acute and chronic encephalopathy. *Cochrane Review,* (4).

Basile, A. S., Harrison, P. M., & Hughes, R. D., et al. (1993). Relationship between plasma benzodiazepine receptor ligand concentrations and severity of hepatic encephalopathy. *Hepatology, 19*:122.

Butterworth, R. (2000). Complications of cirrhosis. III. Hepatic encephalopathy. *Journal of Hepatology, 32*:171-180.

Friedman, S., & Schiano, T. (2004). Cirrhosis and its sequelae. In L. Goldman, & D Ausiello (Eds.), *Cecil textbook of medicine* (pp. 936-944). (22nd ed.). W. B. Saunders.

Gitlin, N., Lewis, D. C., & Hinkley, L. (1986). The diagnosis and prevalence of sub-clinical hepatic encephalopathy in apparently healthy, ambulant, non-shunted patients with cirrhosis. *Journal of Hepatology, 3*:75-82.

Haussinger, D., Schleiss, F., & Kirches, G. (2002). Pathogenesis of hepatic encephalopathy. *Journal of Gastroenterology and Hepatology, 17*:S256-S259.

Huether, S. (2006). Alterations of digestive function. In K. McCance & S. Huether (Eds.), *Pathophysiology: The biologic basis for disease in adults and children* (pp. 1385-1445). (5th ed.). St. Louis: Mosby.

Jones, E. A., Basile, A. S., & Yurdaydin, D., et al. (1993). Do benzodiazepine ligands contribute to hepatic encephalopathy? *Advances in Experimental Biology and Medicine, 341*:57-69.

Kemeny, N., Kemeny, M., & Lawrence. (2004). Liver metastases. In J Abeloff, J. Armitage, & J Neiderhuber, et al. (Eds.), *Clinical Oncology* (pp. 1141-1178). (3rd ed.). Elsevier.

Kircheis, G., & Haussinger, D. (2002). Management of hepatic encephalopathy. *Journal of Gastroenterology and Hepatology, 17*:S2660-S2667.

Kichian, K., & Bain, V. (2004). Jaundice, ascites, and hepatic encephalopathy. In D Doyle, G Hanks, & N Cherney, et al. (Eds.), *Oxford textbook of palliative medicine* (pp. 507-520). (3rd ed.). Oxford: University Press.

Liu, Q., Duan, Z., & Ha, D., et al. (2004). Symbiotic modulation of gut flora: Effect on minimal hepatic encephalopathy in patients with cirrhosis. *Hepatology, 39*:1441-1449.

Loguercio, C., Abbiati, R., & Rinaldi, R., et al. (1995). Long term effects of *Enterococcus faecium* SF68 versus lactulose in the treatment of patients with cirrhosis and grade 1-2 hepatic encephalopathy. *Journal of Hepatology, 23*:39-46.

Murphy, M. (2006). Interventions for patients with liver problems. In (D. Ignatavicus & L. Workman Eds.), *Medical surgical nursing* (pp. 1368-1395). (5th ed.). Elsevier. St. Louis.

Norenberg, M. M. D. (1998). Astroglial dysfunction in hepatic encephalopathy. *Metabolic Brain Disease, 13*:319-328.

Riordan, S., & Williams, R. (1997). Treatment of hepatic encephalopathy. *New England Journal of Medicine, 337*(7):473-479.

Rolando, N., Wade, J., & Davalos, M., et al. (2000). The systemic inflammatory response in acute liver failure. *Hepatology, 32*:739-743.

Weissenborn, K., Ehrenhein, C., & Hori, A., et al. (1995). Pallidal lesions in patients with liver cirrhosis: Clinical and MRI evaluations. *Metabolic Brain Disorders, 10*(3):219-231.

Wolf, D. (2006). Encephalopathy, Hepatic. From WebMD:emedicine.http://www.emedicnie,com/med/topic3185.htm. Retrieved October 17, 2006.

Worobetz, L. J. (2006). Hepatic encephalopathy. In A. B. R. Thompson, & E. A. Shaffer. (Eds.), *First principles of gastroenterology* (p. 537).

Yabro, C., & Seiz, A. (2004). Pruritus. In C. Yarro, M. Frogge, & M. Goodman (Eds.), *Cancer symptom management* (pp. 97-108). Boston: Jones & Bartlett.

Yurdaydin, D. (2003). Blood ammonia determination in cirrhosis: Still confusing after all these years? *Hepatology, 38*.

TUMOR-INDUCED HYPERCALCEMIA

KATHRYN E. PEARSON

PATHOPHYSIOLOGICAL MECHANISMS

Approximately 99% of calcium in the body is bound to bones and teeth. The remaining 1% is found in the serum. Serum calcium exists in an ionized form, a protein-bound form, and a complexed fraction. About half of the total extracellular calcium is ionized, and half is bound mainly to albumin or, to a lesser degree, to other proteins and anions. The ionized form is the biologic component active in the regulation of intracellular and extracellular functions (McDonnell Keenan & Wickham, 2005).

Hypercalcemia occurs when calcium is mobilized from the bone storage areas to the circulation, where it is reflected in total serum calcium values. Serum calcium values are affected by serum protein levels in that every change of total serum albumin of 1 g/dL is associated with a 0.8 mg/dL change in total calcium (Body, 2004). Therefore, because cancer patients frequently have low albumin levels which, in turn, yield falsely low serum calcium measurements, the serum calcium values may need to be corrected for protein concentration to reflect true serum calcium (Table 23-1).

Another strategy in these patients is to obtain an ionized calcium measurement, which more accurately denotes hypercalcemia (values greater than 1.35 mmol/L are considered hypercalcemic), but the test is more expensive and less readily available (McDonnell Keenan & Wickham, 2005). In adults, a total serum calcium level (adjusted for protein concentration) greater than 10.5/dL is considered hypercalcemic (Stewart, 2005; Guise & Mundy, 1998). There is no standard hypercalcemia severity scale, but a calcium level greater than 10.5 mg/dL but less than 12 mg/dL may be classified as mild hypercalcemia. Hypercalcemia is considered severe when the calcium level is above 13.5 to 15 mg/dL (Stewart, 2005; Shuey & Brant, 2004; Davidson, 2001).

Normal calcium homeostasis is maintained by negative feedback loop interactions between parathyroid hormone (PTH), calcitriol, an active metabolite of vitamin D (1,25-dihydroxycholecalciferol), and calcitonin. PTH stimulates osteoclastic bone resorption and the release of calcium and phosphate from bone. It stimulates calcium reabsorption and inhibits phosphate reabsorption from the renal tubules. It also stimulates 1,25-dihydroxycholecalciferol production from the kidney, which plays a role in intestinal calcium and phosphate absorption. Calcitonin directly inhibits osteoclastic bone resorption (Guise & Mundy, 1998).

Normal bone undergoes continual and dynamic remodeling by osteoclasts and osteoblasts, which interact in a balance of bone resorption and rebuilding in response to the normal mechanical stressors placed on the bone. The process is orchestrated by numerous growth factors, hormones, and cytokines (Lipton, 2004).

Table 23-1 CORRECTION OF SERUM CALCIUM LEVELS

Step 1	Step 2	Step 3	Step 4
Sample lab reports: $Ca^{++} = 10$ mg/dL Albumin $= 1.6$ g/dL Increase calcium by 0.8 mg/dL for each 1 g/dL of albumin below normal $\dfrac{0.8}{1} = \dfrac{X}{\text{Corrected albumin}}$	Correct albumin: Subtract low normal serum albumin level from report level: Normal 4.0 g/dL minus −1.6 g/dL reported 2.4 g/dL	To correct underreported Ca^{++}: $\dfrac{Ca^{++}}{\text{Albumin}} = \dfrac{X}{\text{Corrected albumin}}$ $\dfrac{0.8}{1} = \dfrac{X}{2.4}$ $X = 1.92$ mg/dL	Corrected Ca^{++} = Reported Ca^{++} + Correction factor: $10.00\text{mg/dL} + \dfrac{1.92\text{mg/dL}}{11.92\text{mg/dL}}$

Four primary biologic pathways have been identified in the development of tumor-induced hypercalcemia (TIH). Each pathway may be solely responsible for TIH, or they may interact with varying degrees of complexity (Guise & Mundy, 1998).

Most commonly (in about 80% to 90% of occurrences), TIH is related to the secretion of parathyroid hormone–related protein (PTHrP) by cancer cells (Stewart, 2005; Saunders et al., 2004; Guise & Mundy, 1998). PTHrP is distinctly different from but behaves in a biologically similar manner to PTH (Guise & Mundy, 1998). PTHrP is increased in the presence of factors such as epidermal growth factor, insulin, IGF-I and IGF-II, TGF alpha and beta, angiotensin II, and the *src* protooncogene. It is decreased by glucocorticoids and 1,25-dihydroxycholecalciferol (Guise & Mundy, 1998). Although PTHrP has been identified in normal tissue and in normal human physiology, tumor-produced PTHrP interacts with PTH receptors in bone and kidney to cause enhanced renal retention of calcium, osteoclast-mediated bone resorption, and increased phosphate excretion in patients with malignancy (Guise & Mundy, 1998). Tumor-secreted PTHrP has been identified in a variety of solid and hematologic malignancies. About 60% of breast cancers secrete PTHrP which, in addition to being a mediator of hypercalcemia, may also play an important part in the pathophysiology of breast cancer metastasis to bone (Guise & Mundy, 1998).

About 20% of TIHs result from factors that increase osteoclastic bone resorption in areas of the bone infiltrated with malignant cells (Stewart, 2005; Saunders et al., 2004). IL-1, IL-6, TNF alpha, and tumor necrosis factor have been identified as agents with the ability to stimulate osteoclastic resorption, with resultant hypercalcemia. Prostaglandin E may play a minor part in metastatic tumor–related bone resorption and hypercalcemia (Guise & Mundy, 1998).

In fewer than 1% of occurrences, TIH may be related to ectopic production of true PTH (Stewart, 2005). Also, some hematologic malignancies (e.g., lymphomas) secrete 1,25-dihydroxycholecalciferol, thereby enhancing osteoclastic bone resorption and increasing intestinal absorption of calcium (Stewart, 2005; Saunders et al., 2004).

EPIDEMIOLOGY AND ETIOLOGY

Malignancy has been reported as the most common cause of hypercalcemia in hospitalized patients. It has also been cited as a frequently undiagnosed and undertreated condition

(Lamy et al., 2001). TIH is most commonly observed in breast, lung, and hematologic malignancies, but it has been seen with virtually all malignancies, including melanoma and vulvar, renal, ovarian, aerodigestive, and prostate cancers (Bilenchi et al., 2005; Penel et al., 2005; Wu et al., 2004; des Grottes et al., 2001; Lamy et al., 2001; Guise & Mundy, 1998). Classically, TIH has been observed in 10% to 20% of patients with malignancies (Saunders et al., 2004). However, with the use of bisphosphonates in patients with bone involvement of multiple myeloma and breast cancer, the incidence of hypercalcemia has been empirically observed to be decreasing (although this has not fully been documented by evidence) (Maxwell et al., 2003; Body, 2004; McCloskey et al., 2001).

RISK PROFILE

- TIH occurs in advanced malignancies, most commonly lung, breast, aerodigestive, and hematologic malignancies.
- TIH can be further complicated or influenced by conditions of primary hyperparathyroidism, immobility, dehydration, hyperthyroidism, renal dysfunction, skeletal fracture, acute osteoporosis, vitamin D intoxication, Paget's disease, tuberculosis, coccidioidomycosis, human immunodeficiency virus (HIV) infection, adrenal insufficiency, and granulomatous disease.
- Infantile hyperphosphatasia can contribute to hypercalcemia in pediatric patients.
- Age and concomitant administration of sedatives or narcotics may enhance the neurologic symptoms associated with hypercalcemia (Stewart, 2005).
- Drugs that can contribute to hypercalcemia include all-transretinoic acid, estrogens and antiestrogens (e.g., tamoxifen), antacids containing calcium, calcium supplements, lithium, and thiazide diuretics.
- An excessive intake of calcium and vitamin D can contribute to TIH in patients whose tumors produce 1,25-dihydroxycholecalciferol (e.g., lymphomas) (Davidson, 2001). Foods rich in calcium and vitamin D include almonds, broccoli, collards, dairy products, fortified orange juice, leafy green vegetables, salmon, sardines, shrimp, tofu, soy beans, and parenteral feedings.

PROGNOSIS

TIH occurs most frequently in patients with advanced malignancies and is considered to be an indicator of a poor prognosis (Penel et al., 2005; Stewart, 2005; Lamy et al., 2001). Treatment of the underlying malignancy is the most important factor in determining the prognosis (Kristensen et al., 1998). In a retrospective study of 84 patients, Siddiqui and colleagues (2002) found that age, presenting symptoms, hemoglobin, platelets, creatinine, and albumin did not predict mortality. Male gender, an underlying diagnosis other than multiple myeloma, and a higher initial serum calcium level at presentation predicted early mortality. Penel and colleagues (2005) found a 72% mortality rate, with a median overall survival of 35 days, in a population of patients with aerodigestive cancers and TIH. Kristensen and coworkers (1998) determined an overall median survival in breast cancer patients of 6.7 months after the first episode of TIH, with higher initial calcium levels being predictive of decreased survival time. Higher calcium levels at presentation may reflect increased severity of the underlying malignancy, which partly explains why successful return to normocalcemia does not seem to improve the prognosis (Kristensen et al., 1998).

PROFESSIONAL ASSESSMENT CRITERIA (PAC)

Presenting symptoms vary according to the serum calcium level and the rate at which the serum calcium became elevated (Clines & Guise, 2005; Stewart, 2005; Body, 2004). For example, a patient who has a rapid rise in calcium to a moderate level of 12.5 mg/dL may show obvious neurologic changes, whereas a patient with a chronic rise in calcium to greater than 14 mg/dL may be relatively symptom free. The symptoms of hypercalcemia and the underlying cause of the TIH may create a cycle effect (Fig. 23.1).

Classic Symptoms

1. Anorexia
2. Confusion
3. Polydipsia
4. Polyuria
5. Weakness

History

1. Advancing malignant disease
2. Primary parathyroid condition and/or immobility
3. More rarely, history of recent initiation of tamoxifen therapy in breast cancer patients with bone metastasis, creating a "flare" hypercalcemia (Nikolic-Tomasevic et al., 2001)

Vital Signs and Physical Exam

1. Temperature may be elevated.
2. Pulse may be rapid and weak.

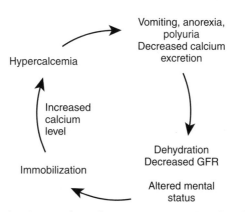

Fig. 23.1 • Cycle of hypercalcemia. Data from Clines, G. A, & Guise, T. A. (2005). Hypercalcaemia of malignancy and basic research on mechanisms responsible for osteolytic and osteoblastic metastasis to bone. *Endocrine-Related Cancer*, 12:549-583; Stewart, A. F. (2005). Hypercalcemia associated with cancer. *New England Journal of Medicine*, 352(4):373-379.

3. Respirations may be tachypneic or normal.
4. Hypotension and postural hypotension may be present with dehydration.
5. Weight loss of 1 to 2 kg/day may occur in association with dehydration.

Neurologic and Psychological Changes

A study by Siddiqui and colleagues (2002) found neurologic and psychological changes in about one third of patients at presentation.
1. Altered cognition
2. Disorientation
3. Lethargy
4. Bone pain
5. Muscle fatigue and weakness
6. Hypotonia
7. Nightmares, disturbed sleep
8. Decreased or absent deep tendon reflexes
9. Late symptoms: stupor, coma, and seizures

Renal and Urinary Elimination Symptoms

The same study by Siddiqui and coworkers (2002) found that two thirds of the patients presented with acute renal failure associated with volume depletion.
1. Polyuria
2. Renal calculi
3. Renal failure

Cardiovascular Symptoms

1. Prolonged P-R interval
2. Widened QRS
3. Shortened QT, ST intervals
4. Bradycardia (in rapidly escalating hypercalcemia)
5. Late symptoms: Widened T waves, heart block, ventricular arrhythmias, cardiac arrest, and enhanced sensitivity to digitalis

Gastrointestinal Symptoms

1. Nausea and vomiting
2. Anorexia
3. Polydipsia
4. Increased secretion of gastric acid
5. Constipation/ileus

Diagnostic Tests

1. ECG to detect dysrhythmias
2. Bone scintigraphic scan to determine burden of bony metastasis

Laboratory Tests

1. BUN
2. Creatinine
3. Serum calcium
4. Albumin
5. Total protein
6. Ionized calcium (if doubt exists about validity of total calcium results) (Stewart, 2005)
7. PTH (to rule out co-morbid hyperparathyroidism) (Stewart, 2005)

8. Plasma 1,25(OH)$_2$D (1,25-dihydroxycholecalciferol) in sarcoidosis, granulomatous disorders, and hematologic malignancies (Stewart, 2005)
9. Phosphorus (low with TIH)
10. Potassium (low with TIH)
11. Magnesium (low with TIH) (Milionis et al., 2002)
12. PTHrP (if available)

NURSING CARE AND TREATMENT

The goals of treatment include correction of dehydration, inhibition of bone resorption, an increase in renal excretion of calcium, and treatment of the underlying malignancy. Because antihypercalcemic therapy is considered a palliative therapy that has no ultimate effect on survival (Stewart, 2005), prompt treatment of the malignancy is imperative. However, in cases of advanced, symptomatic malignancy for which no effective cancer treatment is available, a humane approach may be no treatment. Left untreated, patients experience a rapid rise in calcium and resultant unawareness of their condition because of increasing encephalopathy.

1. The most effective approach to long-term management of TIH is medical treatment of the underlying malignancy (surgery, chemotherapy, and/or radiation therapy). Nursing interventions that support these therapies are necessary.
2. **Assess vital signs, mental status, neurologic status, hydration status, and GI system status.** The frequency of reassessment is determined by the severity of the TIH and the patient's symptoms. In severe TIH, assessment may need to be done every hour until the patient's condition becomes stable; frequency then can be reduced to every 4 hours.
3. **Obtain baseline body weight.** Monitor daily until normocalcemia and fluid balance are achieved.
4. **Institute safety precautions.** Include seizure precautions if severe TIH is suspected or known.
5. **Establish intravenous access suitable for high-volume flow.** Assess intravenous access site routinely for signs of infection, infiltration, and pain.
6. Send laboratory specimens needed to complete patient workup as listed in Professional Assessment Criteria.
7. **Obtain an ECG.** If severe TIH is suspected, place the patient on continuous cardiac monitoring.
8. **Maintain strict intake and output monitoring.** Institute hourly measurement with severe TIH. Insert an indwelling urinary catheter if necessary.
9. Volume repletion improves the patient's clinical status and interrupts the vicious cycle of TIH by expanding fluid volume, correcting dehydration, and reducing tubular reabsorption of calcium by increasing the glomerular filtration rate and promoting renal calcium excretion (Body, 2004; Davidson, 2001).
   - Increasing oral fluids to 3 to 4 L/day may correct fluid deficit in mild or asymptomatic TIH.
   - In patients with moderate to severe TIH and those unable to tolerate oral fluids to the required volume, intravenous normal saline should be administered until normocalcemia is achieved. The rate of infusion depends on the degree of hypercalcemia, the patient's cardiovascular status, the degree of mental impairment, renal status, and the degree of dehydration (Stewart, 2005; Davidson, 2001).
10. **Administer bisphosphonate.** Bisphosphonates are synthetic analogs of pyrophosphate compounds that inhibit calcification. Bone resorption is inhibited by inhibiting

osteoclast recruitment and adhesion and through modulation of the osteoclast-osteoblast interaction. One group of bisphosphonates acts as an analog of ATP and therefore inhibits ATP-dependent intracellular enzymes. A second group of bisphosphonates inhibits enzymes of the mevalonate pathway, disrupting the signaling functions of key regulatory proteins (Saunders et al., 2004). In contrast to previous pharmaceutical methods used to control hypercalcemia, bisphosphonates have increased the number of patients who achieve normocalcemia and increased the interval before relapse (Saunders et al., 2004). With IV administration of bisphosphonates, serum calcium begins to fall in 12 hours, and the calcium nadir is reached within 4 to 7 days. The mean time to normal calcium ranges from 2 to 6 days after administration of bisphosphonates (Saunders et al., 2004). For these reasons, bisphosphonates are the standard treatment for TIH. However, in select situations, other antihypercalcemic agents may be used (Table 23-2).

11. Avoid salt restriction.
12. Avoid overhydration in patients with compromised cardiovascular status.
13. **Monitor for signs of fluid overload.** If present, reduce the hydration rate and consider furosemide 20-40 mg every 12 hours.
14. Diuretic therapy should not be instituted before correction of the hypovolemia. Some consider forced saline diuresis an outdated procedure (Body, 2004).
15. A loop diuretic (furosemide) may be used only after rehydration has been achieved. Caution is advised with its use. Loop diuretics are meant to control volume overload and promote sodium and calcium diuresis. However, they may have a stronger effect on sodium excretion than on calcium. If sodium excretion exceeds sodium replacement, normal physiologic renal sodium–conserving mechanisms are activated, causing a decrease in sodium and calcium excretion (Stewart, 2005).
16. Thiazide diuretics should be avoided, because they decrease calcium excretion and contribute to calcium elevation (Stewart, 2005).
17. Patients with pre-existing renal compromise who therefore are unable to tolerate aggressive hydration require dialysis with a calcium-free or low-calcium solution.
18. Discontinue use of oral calcium supplements (Stewart, 2005).
19. Discontinue lithium, calcitriol, vitamin D, and thiazides.
20. Reduce use of sedatives and analgesics if possible (Stewart, 2005).
21. Monitor electrolytes and renal function daily.
22. **Monitor for hypophosphatemia.** If it occurs, administer supplements as needed. Phosphorus replacement ideally should be achieved via the oral route or by enteral feeding. Intravenous phosphorus replacement is associated with hypocalcemia, seizures, and renal failure (Stewart, 2005).
23. **Encourage weight-bearing ambulation.** In patients with mild TIH, increasing ambulation, which encourages normal bone resorption, may be efficacious enough to restore normal calcium homeostasis.
24. Monitor serum and urinary calcium daily until normocalcemia is achieved.
25. Reduce doses of digoxin.
26. Administer analgesics for bone pain.
27. Administer antiemetics as indicated for nausea and vomiting.
28. Administer laxatives and stool softeners as needed to correct constipation.
29. Restrict dietary calcium in patients with 1,25-dihydroxycholecalciferol pathway TIH (e.g., hematologic malignancies).
30. When the patient is able to tolerate oral fluids, encourage an oral intake of 2 to 3 L/day.
31. Refer the patient to case management, physical therapy, clinical nurse specialist, clinical social worker, home health/palliative care team, spiritual care professional, or hospice services as indicated.

Table 23-2	ANTIHYPERCALCEMIC AGENTS	
Drug	**Action**	**Comments**
Calcitonin	Inhibits osteoclastic bone resorption	Safe in dehydrated or renal compromised patients.
	Moderate calciuric effect	Rapid onset of action (4-6 hours), but short duration of response (1-4 days). Useful in life-threatening symptomatic TIH. Maximum treatment time of 8 days.
Plicamycin	Inhibits RNA synthesis in osteoclasts, thereby inhibiting bone resorption	One of the first recognized hypocalcemia agents. Rapid onset but has a variable and unpredictable duration of response. May cause nephrotoxicity, hepatotoxicity, and platelet defects. Avoid extravasation.
Gallium nitrate	Inhibits bone resorption by inhibiting PTHrP	Potent, sustained hypocalcemic effect. Should not be administered to patients with severe renal impairment (serum creatinine > 2.5 mg/dL) Risk of dose-related nephrotoxicity characterized by renal tubular necrosis and obstruction of the tubular lumen. Infused over 24 hours for up to 5 days; requires hospitalization. May be more efficacious in patients with high PTHrP (Leyland-Jones, 2004).
Bisphosphonates	Inhibit osteoclastic bone resorption (bone breakdown), thereby decreasing calcium release and the serum calcium level	Highest recommended dose should be used, regardless of baseline calcium level, to achieve normocalcemia and to increase time to relapse (Saunders et al., 2004).
Etidronate		Administered as a 4-hour infusion every day for a minimum of 3 days. Duration of action is variable. Dose must be adjusted in patients with renal compromise.
Clodronate		Not approved in United States. Has been administered subcutaneously in palliative care settings (Roemer-Becuwe et al., 2003).
Pamidronate		Very effective and has low toxicity profile. Shown to be superior in duration to clodronate (Purohit et al., 1995).
Alendronate		Efficacy in TIH has not been established. (Body, 2004).
Zoledronic acid		Agent of choice to treat TIH; superior efficacy, short infusion time. Use with caution in patients with renal insufficiency.
Ibandronate		Not commercially available in the United States
Investigational anti-RANKL agents anti-PTHrP antibodies		
Phosphorusrepletion	Inhibits bone resorption	Should be administered orally. Do not give intravenously (Stewart, 2005).

Continued

Table 23-2 ANTIHYPERCALCEMIC AGENTS—cont'd		
Drug	**Action**	**Comments**
Glucocorticoids	Reduces 1,25-dihydroxycholecalciferol and inhibits gastrointestinal absorption of calcium Increased urinary excretion of calcium	Used in treatment of TIH with tumor-induced 1,25-dihydroxycholecalciferol production (e.g., multiple myeloma, lymphoma). Maximum effect in days to weeks after initiation of therapy. May be used in combination with calcitonin to increase duration of effect (Davidson, 2001).

Data from McDonnell Keenan, A. K., & Wickham, R. S. (2005). Hypercalcemia. In C. H. Yarbro, M. H. Frogge, & M. Goodman (Eds.), Cancer nursing principles and practice (pp. 791–807). (6th ed.). Sudbury, MA: Jones & Bartlett; Stewart, A. F. (2005). Hypercalcemia associated with cancer. *New England Journal of Medicine* 352(4):373–379; Davidson, T. G. (2001). Conventional treatment of hypercalcemia of malignancy. Amer*ican Journal of Health-System Pharmacy*, 58(Suppl 3):8-15; Body, J. J. (2004). Hypercalcemia of malignancy. *Seminars in Nephrology* 24(1):48–54; Purohit, O. P., Radstone, C. R., & Anthony, C., et al. (1995). A randomized double-blind comparison of intravenous pamidronate and clodronate in the hypercalcemia of malignancy. *British Journal of Cancer*, 72:1289-1293; and Leyland-Jones, B. (2004). Treating cancer-related hypercalcemia with gallium nitrate. *Journal of Supportive Oncology*, 2(6):509–520.

EVIDENCE-BASED PRACTICE UPDATES

1. The mean time to normocalcemia after administration of bisphosphonates ranges from 2 to 6 days (Saunders et al., 2004).
2. Treatment of underlying malignancy is the most important factor in determining the prognosis for patients with hypercalcemia.(Kristensen et al., 1998).
3. Zoledronic acid produces a higher rate of normocalcemia more quickly and for a longer duration than pamidronate. Fever, hypophosphatemia, and asymptomatic hypocalcemia are the most common adverse drug reactions. Zoledronic acid has replaced pamidronate as the standard of care for moderate to severe TIH (Major & Coleman, 2001).
4. Pamidronate gives a longer time to relapse than clodronate or etidronate (Saunders et al., 2004). Zoledronic acid achieves a longer mean time to relapse than pamidronate (Major et al., 2001).
5. High initial levels of PTHrP are associated with a worse prognosis and a shorter duration of normocalcemia after pamidronate administration (Saunders et al., 2004).
6. Clodronate can be given subcutaneously, which may be useful in select palliative care settings (Walker et al., 1997).
7. Patients who become resistant to one bisphosphonate may achieve normocalcemia with another bisphosphonate (e.g., pamidronate-resistant patients may respond to clodronate (Kristensen et al., 1998).
8. The presence of hypokalemia must be considered when treating TIH with loop diuretics to avoid further reduction of the potassium level and resultant arrhythmias (Milionis et al., 2002).
9. Restrict sun exposure in patients with 1,25-dihydroxyvitamin D pathway–related hypercalcemias (Papapetrou et al., 2003).
10. Metabolic alkalosis and hypomagnesemia are more common in TIH than hyperparathyroid–related hypercalcemia (Milionis et al., 2002).

TEACHING AND EDUCATION

Maintain hydration: *Rationale*: You can become dehydrated if you do not maintain an intake of 2 to 3 L of fluid per day. You will need to increase your intake if you are experiencing diarrhea, vomiting, or increased urination or if you are sweating. If you become or may become unable to maintain your hydration, notify your doctor or nurse.

Management of nausea and vomiting: *Rationale*: Inability to control nausea and vomiting contributes to dehydration. It is important that you use preventive measures to control nausea and vomiting. These include taking your prescribed medication and avoiding situations and foods that may trigger your nausea and vomiting. Your doctor, nurse, and/or dietician can help you develop a plan for preventing or managing nausea and vomiting.

Weight-bearing exercise and mobility: *Rationale*: Walking and other weight-bearing activities help to keep calcium in the bones. If you are unsteady on your feet, be sure to use assistive devices and/or ask for assistance to avoid falling. If you are feeling weak and deconditioned, ask a nurse or physical therapist to help you develop a plan for increasing your strength.

Medications: *Rationale*: Some of your medications may be discontinued, or the dose may be adjusted, to help prevent hypercalcemia.

Early recognition of symptoms: *Rationale*: Report any changes such as dry mouth, excessive urination, changes in mental status, constipation, weight changes, dizziness, and increasing fatigue to your doctor or nurse.

Safety: *Rationale*: You may be at risk for falling and breaking a bone if you are dizzy, weak, or are feeling disoriented. If you have had dizzy or weak spells, ask for assistance when going to the bathroom or walking. High calcium can affect your ability to think clearly, cause drowsiness, and cause changes in your behavior. You or your family members should report these changes to your doctor or nurse.

Heart rate changes: *Rationale*: Calcium can affect your heart muscle. Notify your doctor or nurse if you become aware that your heart is beating too fast or too slowly.

Diet: You may continue your usual diet. You do not need to restrict the calcium from your diet. (Exception: If you have hypercalcemia that is related to vitamin D imbalance, you need to restrict calcium-rich foods.)

Follow-up testing and appointments. *Rationale*: High calcium can return. Your doctor or nurse can better manage any changes in your condition if you are seen routinely.

NURSING DIAGNOSES

1. **Risk for injury** related to confusion and mental status changes, blurred vision, fatigue, muscle weakness
2. **Deficient fluid volume** related to dehydration related to polyuria, nausea, and vomiting, anorexia
3. **Excess fluid volume** related to rehydration intervention
4. **Impaired urinary elimination** related to polyuria, renal failure
5. **Constipation** related to dehydration, hypotonia

EVALUATION AND DESIRED OUTCOMES

1. Serum Ca^{++} will decrease to 2 to 3 mg/dL within the first 24 to 48 hours.
2. Serum Ca^{++} will return to normal range within 5 to 7 days.
3. Serum electrolytes will return to and be maintained within the normal range.
4. Normal fluid balance will be achieved.

5. The patient will be free of injury.
6. The patient will be free of symptoms related to abnormal calcium levels.
7. The patient's activity and mobilization will be maximized to the patient's tolerance.
8. Constipation will resolve within 3 days.
9. The patient and/or caregiver will understand the signs and symptoms of hypercalcemia and will be knowledgeable about preventive measures before the patient is discharged.
10. The patient and/or caregiver will understand the outpatient plan of care, including physician/clinic appointments, necessary laboratory testing, and referrals to outpatient support services, such as home care.

DISCHARGE PLANNING AND FOLLOW-UP CARE

A hypercalcemic patient may need home health/palliative care services for:
- Monitoring and management of hypercalcemia-related symptoms
- Physical and/or occupational therapy for mobility and self-care
- Pain management
- Patient and family education for self-care
- Management of psychosocial/spiritual responses to the severity of the illness and the threat to survival

Follow-up care should include:
- Visit to physician's office within 1 week
- Outpatient testing for serum electrolytes and renal function in 1 week
- Plan for potential emergent changes in the patient's condition (e.g., call 911, call palliative care nurse, go to emergency department or urgent care center)

REVIEW QUESTIONS

QUESTIONS

1. **The most common etiology of tumor-induced hypercalcemia is:**
   1. Tumor-produced PTHrP
   2. Bone metastasis
   3. Overexpression of PTH
   4. Tumor-produced 1,25-dihydroxyvitamin D

2. **Classic symptoms of TIH include:**
   1. Polydipsia, polyuria, nausea, vomiting, altered mental status
   2. Polyphagia, disorientation, hypertension
   3. Stupor, muscle twitching, anorexia
   4. Muscle cramping, arrhythmias, diarrhea

3. **The first therapeutic intervention for the patient presenting with TIH and hypotension should be:**
   1. Administer a bisphosphonate
   2. Administer a loop diuretic
   3. Hydrate with normal saline 200-300 mL/hr
   4. Start dopamine drip

4. **The most rapid onset of action with an antihypercalcemic agent is obtained by using:**
   1. High-dose pamidronate
   2. Calcitonin given subcutaneously every 12 hours
   3. Zoledronic acid
   4. Plicamycin

5. **Mr. A. is a 65-year-old man admitted for moderate TIH. His symptoms include polydipsia, polyuria, constipation, and irritability. He has co-morbid cardiac disease. He takes digoxin, cimetidine, sertraline hydrochloride, and morphine sulfate sustained and immediate release. The nurse should:**
   1. Plan for dialysis because he is at risk for fluid overload.

2. Consult with the physician to reduce or hold the digoxin dose.
3. Hold the antidepressants and morphine.
4. Request a thiazide diuretic to be given during rehydration.

6. **Serum chemistry alterations that can be expected in TIH include:**
   1. Hypermagnesemia
   2. Hypokalemia
   3. Hyperphosphatemia
   4. Hyponatremia

7. **Mr. J. presents with a history of lung cancer, a calcium level of 11 mg/dL, and an albumin level of 1.8 g/dL. His corrected calcium level is:**
   1. 14 mg/dL
   2. 12.8 mg/dL
   3. 8.8 mg/dL
   4. 13.2 mg/dL

8. **Mr. J. has:**
   1. Normocalcemia
   2. Mild TIH
   3. Moderate TIH
   4. Severe TIH

9. **Nursing management of the patient being treated for severe TIH should include:**
   1. Frequent monitoring of vital signs, daily weights, and safety precautions.
   2. Restriction of fluids and foods containing calcium and monitoring for CHF.
   3. Maintenance of bed rest and seizure precautions.
   4. Intravenous administration of phosphorus.

10. **Discharge planning for the patient who has been treated for TIH should include:**
    1. Referral to hospice.
    2. Referral to home health for continued bisphosphonate infusions.
    3. Physician or nurse practitioner office appointment within 1 week and education about the signs and symptoms that should be reported and whom to call on an emergency basis.
    4. Dietician follow-up regarding calcium restrictions in the diet.

ANSWERS

1. *Answer: 1*
   Rationale: About 80% to 90% of TIH is related to the secretion of PTHrP.

2. *Answer: 1*
   Rationale: Additional symptoms may be hypotonia, hypotension, and constipation.

3. *Answer: 3*
   Rationale: Repletion of fluid volume increases the GFR, thereby increasing calcium excretion and also allowing bisphosphonate to be given safely. Diuretics are contraindicated with dehydrated status.

4. *Answer: 2*
   Rationale: Although bisphosphonates are the anticalcemic agents of choice, calcitonin has a faster onset of action.

5. *Answer: 2*
   Rationale: Digoxin toxicity increases with high calcium levels. Thiazide diuretics are contraindicated in patients with hypercalcemia. Holding sedatives and analgesics could be considered, but not at the expense of pain symptom management.

6. *Answer: 2*
   Rationale: Magnesium, phosphorus, and potassium levels may decrease in patients with hypercalcemia.

7. *Answer: 2*
   Rationale: (Normal albumin [4 g/dL] ÷ actual albumin [1.8 g/dL] = 2.2) × 0.8 = 1.76 + calcium level [11 mg/dL] = 12.76, or 12.8 mg/dL.

8. *Answer: 3*
   Rationale: Patients with a corrected calcium level greater than 12 mg/dL but less than 13.5 to 15 mg/dL are considered to have moderate hypercalcemia.

9. *Answer: 1*
   Rationale: Patients with severe TIH are volume depleted; vigorous rehydration is indicated. Weight-bearing activities (within the realm of safety) reduce calcium exit from bone storage areas. Intravenous phosphorus is contraindicated.

10. *Answer: 3*

Rationale: Recurrent TIH is common unless the malignant process is controlled. Frequent monitoring by health care professionals and prompt reporting of symptoms assist in early intervention.

Bisphosphonate infusions are intermittent and periodic. Dietary calcium restrictions are indicated in rare cases. Hospice may be indicated, but the TIH was treated, indicating that palliation of hypercalcemic symptoms is the goal.

REFERENCES

Bilenchi, R., Poggiali, S., & Pisani, C., et al. (2005). Malignant hypercalcemia in vulvar cancer. *Minerva Ginecologica, 57*:569-574.

Body, J. J.(2004). Hypercalcemia of malignancy. *Seminars in Nephrology, 24*(1):48-54.

Clines, G. A, & Guise, T. A.(2005). Hypercalcaemia of malignancy and basic research on mechanisms responsible for osteolytic and osteoblastic metastasis to bone. *Endocrine-Related Cancer, 12*:549-583.

Davidson, T. G.(2001). Conventional treatment of hypercalcemia of malignancy. *American Journal of Health-System Pharmacy, 58*(Suppl 3):8-15.

des Grottes, J. M., Dumon, J. C, & Body, J. J.(2001). Hypercalcaemia of melanoma: Incidence, pathogenesis, and therapy with bisphosphonates. *Melanoma Research, 11*:477-482.

Guise, T. A., & Mundy, G.(1998). Cancer and bone. *Endocrine Reviews, 19*(1):18-54.

Kristensen, B., Ejlertsen, B., & Mouridsen, T., et al. (1998). Survival in breast cancer patients after the first episode of hypercalcaemia. *Journal of Internal Medicine, 244*:189-198.

Lamy, O., Jenzer-Closuit, A., & Burckhardt, P.(2001). Hypercalcaemia of malignancy: An undiagnosed and undertreated disease. *Journal of Internal Medicine, 250*:73-79.

Leyland-Jones, B.(2004). Treating cancer-related hypercalcemia with gallium nitrate. *Journal of Supportive Oncology, 2*(6):509-520.

Lipton, A.(2004). Pathophysiology of bone metastases: How this knowledge may lead to therapeutic intervention. *Supportive Oncology, 2*:(3):205-213.

Major, P., & Coleman, R.(2001). Zoledronic acid in the treatment of hypercalcemia of malignancy: Results of the international clinical development program. *Seminars in Oncology, 28*(2):17-24.

Major, P., Lortholary, A., & Hon, J., et al. (2001). Zoledronic acid is superior to pamidronate in the treatment of hypercalcemia of malignancy: A pooled analysis of two randomized, controlled clinical trials. *Journal of Clinical Oncology, 19*(2):558-567.

Maxwell, C., Swift, R., & Goode, M., et al. (2003). Advances in supportive care of patients with cancer and bone metastases: Nursing implications of zoledronic acid. *Clinical Journal of Oncology Nursing, 7*(4):403-408.

McCloskey, E. V., Guest, J. F., & Kanis, J.(2001). The clinical and cost considerations of bisphosphonates in preventing bone complications in patients with metastatic breast cancer or multiple myeloma. *Drugs 61*:1253-1274.

McDonnell Keenan, A. K., & Wickham, R. S.(2005). Hypercalcemia. In C. H. Yarbro, M. H. Frogge, & M. Goodman (Eds.), *Cancer nursing principles and practice* (pp. 791-807). (6th ed.). Sudbury, MA: Jones & Bartlett.

Milionis, I. J., Rizos, E., & Liamis, G., et al. (2002). Acid-base and electrolyte disturbances in patients with hypercalcemia. *Southern Medical Journal, 95*(11):1280-1287.

Nikolic-Tomasevic, Z., Jelic, S., & Popov, I., et al. (2001). Tumor "flare" hypercalcemia: An additional indication for bisphosphonates? *Oncology, 60*:123-126.

Papapetrou, P. D., Bergi-Stamatelou, M., & Karga, H., et al. (2003). Hypercalcemia due to sun exposure in a patient with multiple myeloma and elevated parathyroid hormone–related protein. *European Journal of Endocrinology, 148*:351-355.

Penel, N., Berthon, C., & Everard, F., et al. (2005). Prognosis of hypercalcemia in aerodigestive tract cancers: Study of 136 recent cases. *Oral Oncology, 41*:884-889.

Purohit, O. P., Radstone, C. R., & Anthony, C., et al. (1995). A randomized double-blind comparison of intravenous pamidronate and clodronate in the hypercalcemia of malignancy. *British Journal of Cancer, 72*:1289-1293.

Roemer-Becuwe, C., Vigano, A., & Romano, F., et al. (2003). Safety of subcutaneous clodronate and efficacy in hypercalcemia of malignancy: A novel route of administration. *Journal of Pain and Symptom Management, 26*(3):843-848.

Saunders, Y., Ross, J. R., & Broadley, K. E.(2004). Systematic review of bisphosphonates for hypercalcaemia of malignancy. *Palliative Medicine, 18*:418-431.

Shuey, K. M., & Brant, J. M.(2004). Hypercalcemia of malignancy. *Part II. Clinical Journal of Oncology Nursing, 8*(3):321-323.

Siddiqui, I., Bhally, H.S., & Niaz, Q., et al. (2002). Tumor-induced hypercalcemia: Predictors of early mortality. *Journal of the Pakistan Medical Association, 52*(8):361-364.

Stewart, A. F.(2005). Hypercalcemia associated with cancer. *New England Journal of Medicine, 352*(4):373-379.

Walker, P., Watanabe, S., & Lawlor, P., et al. (1997). Subcutaneous clodronate: A study evaluating efficacy in hypercalcemia of malignancy and local toxicity. *Annals of Oncology, 8*:915-916.

Wu, C. H., Lan, Y. J., & Wang, C. H., et al. (2004). Hypercalcemia in cancer with positive neuron-specific enolase stain. *Renal Failure, 26*(3):325-327.

HYPERKALEMIA

MARY PAT LYNCH

PATHOPHYSIOLOGICAL MECHANISMS

Hyperkalemia is a potentially life-threatening metabolic problem caused by the inability of the kidneys to excrete potassium, impairment of the mechanisms that transfer potassium from the circulation into the cells, or a combination of these factors (Hollander-Rodriguez & Calvert, 2006). Hyperkalemia in patients with or without cancer usually occurs as a consequence of renal failure.

Normal serum potassium (K+) ranges from 3.5 to 5.5 mEq/L. *Hyperkalemia* is defined as a serum potassium level greater than 5.5 mEq/L (Smith, 2000; Wallach, 2000). Potassium is the most common intracellular cation, and only a small percentage is found in the extracellular fluids. Potassium plays a critical role in cellular function, neuromuscular activity, and cardiac conduction, including maintenance of intracellular osmolality, maintenance of a balance between hydrogen and sodium within the cell, and maintenance of a stable resting membrane potential for transmitting and conducting nerve impulses. Potassium also plays a role in glycogen deposition in skeletal and liver cells in response to insulin (Smith, 2000).

The body does not store potassium, therecfore a minimum daily intake of 40 to 60 mEq is required. The typical Western diet provides an average of 50 to 100 mEq a day (Murphy-Ende, 2006). Most potassium (80%) is excreted through the kidneys in response to hyperkalemia and/or aldosterone. Fifteen percent is excreted through the gastrointestinal tract, and 5% is lost through the skin (Smith, 2000).

Potassium levels normally are regulated by two mechanisms, which are activated in response to variation in potassium intake. In the first mechanism, ingested potassium enters the hepatic portal circulation, which stimulates the pancreas to release insulin. The elevated levels of insulin cause the rapid transport of potassium from the extracellular space into cells. In the second mechanism, increased potassium in the circulation causes the release of rennin from the renal juxtaglomerular cells; this stimulates hepatic activation of angiotensin I, which is converted to angiotensin II in the lungs (Hollander-Rodriguez & Calvert, 2006). Angiotensin II causes the secretion of aldosterone from the kidney, and elevated aldosterone causes the kidney to excrete potassium and retain sodium, thereby lowering the serum potassium. A balance of GI intake and renal excretion results in long-term potassium balance (Garth, 2006).

EPIDEMIOLOGY AND ETIOLOGY

Disorders of potassium are the most commonly encountered electrolyte abnormalities in hospitalized patients. Hyperkalemia occurs in up to 8% of hospitalized patients (Garth, 2006; Gennari, 2006) as a result of an imbalance in normal potassium handling. It most often occurs when potassium excretion is impaired by a medical condition or by medications taken by a patient with some degree of underlying renal dysfunction (Schaeffer & Wolford, 2005). The most common causes of hyperkalemia are kidney dysfunction, adrenal gland disease, shifting of potassium out of the cells into the circulation, and medication side effects (Stoppler, 2005). Hyperkalemia can result from:

- Decreased or impaired potassium excretion (e.g., acute or chronic renal disease, use of diuretics)
- Addition of potassium into the extracellular space (e.g., potassium supplements, hemolysis)
- Transmembrane shifts (e.g., use of beta blockers, acute digitalis toxicity)
- Pseudohyperkalemia (e.g. improper blood collection, laboratory error, leukocytosis, and thrombocytosis) (Garth, 2006)

RISK PROFILE

- Acute or chronic renal failure, particularly in patients on dialysis.
- Trauma, including crush injuries and burns.
- Ingestion of foods high in potassium (e.g., bananas, oranges) and high-protein diets.
- **Medications:** Potassium supplements, potassium-sparing diuretics, nonsteroidal anti-inflammatory drugs (NSAIDs), beta blockers, digoxin, succinylcholine, digitalis, ACE inhibitors, trimethoprim-sulfamethoxazole (NOTE: Severe hyperkalemia does not usually occur with these medications unless they are given to a patient with kidney dysfunction.) (Stoppler, 2005)
- **Redistribution of potassium:** Metabolic acidosis (DKA), catabolic states (Garth, 2006).
- Rapid tumor lysis after therapy, particularly in patients with Burkitt's lymphoma (Casciato, 2004).
- **Adrenal metastases:** Clinical adrenal insufficiency from metastases is unusual (Casciato, 2004).
- **Pseudohyperkalemia:** This disorder can occur in patients with persistent thrombocytosis, especially in the myeloproliferative disorders (Casciato, 2004). When thrombocytosis, hemolysis, or extremely high white blood cell counts occur, lysis of the cells in the test tube releases potassium into the serum, increasing the measured value (Gennari, 2002).

PROGNOSIS

The primary cause of mortality with hyperkalemia is potassium's effect on cardiac function. The mortality rate can exceed 65% if severe hyperkalemia is not treated rapidly and effectively (Garth, 2006). Most patients can expect a full resolution with correction of the underlying etiology (Garth, 2006).

PROFESSIONAL ASSESSMENT CRITERIA (PAC)

1. Hyperkalemia can be difficult to diagnose clinically, because the patient may have no or only vague complaints. Hyperkalemia frequently is an incidental laboratory finding.
2. Elevated serum potassium.
3. Check the BUN and creatinine to evaluate renal status.
4. Check the calcium level; in patients with renal failure, hyperkalemia can exacerbate cardiac arrhythmias.
5. Check the digoxin level if the patient is taking a digitalis medication.
6. Check the arterial blood gases if acidosis is suspected.
7. The patient may be asymptomatic or may report:

- Generalized fatigue
- Weakness
- Paresthesias
- Muscular paralysis and hypoventilation (rare)
- Palpitations

8. Cardiac examination may reveal extrasystoles, pauses, or bradycardia.
9. Neurologic examination may reveal diminished deep tendon reflexes or decreased motor strength.
10. Severe cellular injury can cause tumor lysis syndrome:
    - Most common in cancers such as leukemia and lymphoma (especially Burkitt's lymphoma)
    - Rare in solid tumors
11. Acidosis
12. Marked thrombocytosis or leukocytosis
13. Improper handling of blood specimen:
    - Tourniquet applied too tightly, or blood sample taken from the arm into which potassium is infusing.
14. The severity of ECG abnormalities corresponds with the severity of the hyperkalemia. As hyperkalemia worsens, the ECG shows increased T-wave amplitude, decreased R-wave amplitude, increased S-wave depth, depressed ST segment, prolongation of P-R intervals, and widening of the QRS complex, then a sine wave pattern, and finally asystole or ventricular tachyarrhythmias (Fig. 24.1) (Casciato, 2004).

NURSING CARE AND TREATMENT

1. Verify that the potassium level is truly elevated (repeat serum potassium, measure plasma potassium; avoid treating pseudohyperkalemia).
2. Treat the underlying cause (e.g., tumor lysis syndrome, acidosis, adrenocortical insufficiency).
3. Review all medications for contribution to hyperkalemia; adjust as needed (e.g., discontinue potassium supplements, salt substitutes, ACE inhibitors, NSAIDs, potassium-sparing diuretics).
4. Mild to moderate hyperkalemia (5.5 to 6 mEq/L) may require only dietary restrictions or medication adjustment if the patient's condition is stable (Smith, 2000).
5. Mild to moderate hyperkalemia can also be treated with furosemide 40-160 mg IV or PO daily. (Garth, 2006; Smith, 2000).
6. Moderate hyperkalemia (5.5 to 6.5 mEq/L) can be treated with sodium polystyrene sulfonate (Kayexalate) 15 g given orally 1-4 times per day or rectally 30-50 g every 6 hours (contraindicated with diarrhea). Mix with 100 mL of 20% sorbitol. When potassium normalizes, maintenance doses of 15 g/day may be needed (Garth, 2006; Smith, 2000).
7. Severe hyperkalemia (6.5 to 7 mEq/L) can be life-threatening. The potassium level can be lowered immediately by IV administration of 10 units of regular insulin plus 50 to 100 mL of 50% dextrose solution. If the patient is acidotic, 150-300 mEq of sodium bicarbonate is given IV (Garth, 2006; Hollander-Rodriguez & Calvert, 2006; Casciato, 2004, Smith, 2000). Administration of glucose and insulin shifts potassium into cells within 10 to 20 minutes and lowers the serum potassium by 0.5 to 1.5 mEq/L, an effect that is sustained for 2 to 3 hours (Gennari, 2002).
8. Calcium gluconate 10 mL of a 10% solution given IV over 5 to 10 minutes may be necessary to protect the heart and muscles from severe hyperkalemia (Garth, 2006; Smith, 2000). Intravenous calcium can rapidly reverse cardiac conduction abnormalities and should be used without delay in this setting, except when the hyperkalemia is

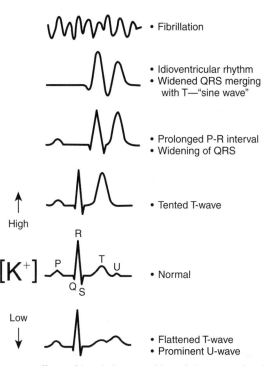

- Fibrillation

- Idioventricular rhythm
- Widened QRS merging
  with T—"sine wave"

- Prolonged P-R interval
- Widening of QRS

- Tented T-wave

High

- Normal

Low

- Flattened T-wave
- Prominent U-wave

Fig. 24.1 • Characteristic effects of hypokalemia and hyperkalemia on the electrocardiogram. *(From Gennari, F. J. [2002]. Disorders of potassium homeostasis: Hypokalemia and hyperkalemia. Critical Care Clinics, 18[2]:273–288.)*

caused by digoxin toxicity, because acute hypercalcemia can potentiate the toxic effects of this drug (Gennari, 2002).

9. Nebulized albuterol 10-20 mg in 4 mL of normal saline, nebulized over 10 minutes, may help shift potassium into the intracellular space when intravenous access is a problem.(Garth, 2006, Gennari, 2002; Smith, 2000). Inhaled beta agonists (albuterol) have a rapid onset of action, and the effect is additive to that of administered insulin; the two drugs can be taken together (Hollander-Rodriguez & Calvert, 2006).

10. Hemodialysis may be necessary to manage chronic or refractory hyperkalemia, especially in patients with acute or chronic renal failure.

EVIDENCE-BASED PRACTICE UPDATES

1. Patients with hyperkalemia who show ECG changes, a rapid rise in serum potassium, decreased renal function, or significant acidosis should be urgently treated (evidence rating: consensus) (Hollander-Rodriguez & Calvert, 2006).

2. Patients with hyperkalemia and characteristic ECG changes should be given intravenous calcium gluconate (evidence rating: consensus) (Hollander-Rodriguez & Calvert, 2006).

3. The potassium level should be acutely lowered by giving intravenous insulin with glucose, a beta-2 antagonist by nebulizer, or both (evidence rating: consensus). (Hollander-Rodriguez & Calvert, 2006).

4. The total body potassium usually should be lowered with sodium polystyrene sulfonate (Kayexelate) (evidence rating: consensus). (Hollander-Rodriguez & Calvert, 2006).

5. No clear guidelines have been established regarding the appropriate setting for the treatment of hyperkalemia. The decision for hospital admission for continuous ECG monitoring is a matter of clinical judgment in each case (Hollander-Rodriguez & Calvert, 2006).
6. Patients believed to have a rapid rise in potassium usually need inpatient care, whereas patients whose hyperkalemia has developed over a period of time often can be managed in an outpatient setting with close follow-up (Hollander-Rodriguez & Calvert, 2006).
7. Intravenous beta agonists (albuterol) have been used in Europe but have not been approved by the U.S. Food and Drug Administration (Hollander-Rodriguez & Calvert, 2006).

TEACHING AND EDUCATION

1. Instruct the patient to adjust the diet to reduce potassium intake through foods by avoiding foods that are high in potassium. Review high- and low-potassium foods and dietary supplements.
2. Instruct the patient to avoid all medications that may cause hyperkalemia, such as potassium-sparing diuretics, ACE inhibitors, NSAIDs, beta blockers, digitalis, digoxin, and potassium supplements.
3. Treatment of hyperkalemia is individualized based on the underlying cause of the hyperkalemia, the severity of the symptoms, the cardiac effects of the hyperkalemia, and the overall health status of the patient.
4. Hyperkalemia is diagnosed by a blood test, and the potassium level in the blood is determined in the laboratory.
5. If hyperkalemia is suspected, an ECG often is performed, because the ECG may show changes typical for hyperkalemia.
6. Emergency treatment may be needed if hyperkalemia is severe and has caused changes in the ECG. Severe hyperkalemia is best treated in the hospital, often in the intensive care unit with continuous heart monitoring.
7. Severe hyperkalemia may require intravenous administration of glucose and insulin, which promotes the movement of potassium from the extracellular space back into the cells. It may also require intravenous calcium to temporarily protect the heart and muscles from the effects of hyperkalemia.
8. If hyperkalemia is mild to moderate, it may require the administration of a diuretic, either intravenously or by mouth, to reduce the total potassium stores by increasing excretion of potassium in the urine.
9. Mild to moderate hyperkalemia may also be treated with medications known as cation-exchange resins, which bind potassium and lead to its excretion through the gastrointestinal tract.
10. If other measures have failed or if the patient has renal failure, dialysis may be required.
11. Most patients make a full recovery with correction of the underlying problem that led to hyperkalemia. However, if hyperkalemia is not treated promptly, life-threatening cardiac arrhythmias may occur.

NURSING DIAGNOSES

1. **Decreased cardiac output** related to effect of elevated potassium level on cardiac muscle
2. **Risk for excess fluid volume** related to underlying disease, medications or diet

3. **Anxiety** related to severity of illness and hospitalization
4. **Deficient knowledge** related to low potassium foods and medications
5. **Imbalanced nutrition: less than body requirements** related to dehydration or diarrhea from treatment with diuretics or Kayexelate

EVALUATION AND DESIRED OUTCOMES

1. The potassium level will normalize, and the underlying cause will be resolved.
2. ECG abnormalities will normalize.
3. For severe hyperkalemia, patients usually are monitored in the ICU or telemetry unit, and potassium levels are checked every 3 to 5 hours until stabilized.
4. Once the patient's condition has stabilized, acid-base problems have been resolved, and coexistent electrolyte problems have been corrected, the patient usually is moved to a regular unit or discharged with follow-up in 2 or 3 days for serum potassium levels.
5. Potassium excretion can be augmented with loop or thiazide diuretics or chronic Kayexelate therapy.
6. Insulin therapy should begin to work within 15 to 30 minutes, and the duration of effect is 2 to 6 hours. Potassium levels should be monitored serially until stable.
7. Calcium gluconate has an immediate onset and a 30-minute duration of effect in protecting the myocardium from the toxic effects of calcium; however, it does not affect the serum potassium level.
8. Furosemide has an onset of 15 minutes to 1 hour and a 4-hour duration of effect.
9. Kayexelate has a 1- to 2-hour onset and a 4- to 6-hour duration of effect.

DISCHARGE PLANNING AND FOLLOW UP CARE

- For mild to moderate asymptomatic hyperkalemia, outpatient care and follow-up are appropriate. If the patient is stable, is treated with dietary or medication changes, and has good renal function, and if acute changes are unlikely, the serum potassium can be checked weekly for 1 to 3 weeks.
- Adjust the diet to reduce the dietary potassium load.
- Adjust medications that predispose the patient to or exacerbate hyperkalemia.
- Hyperkalemia caused by the use of ACE inhibitors or angiotensin receptor blockers in patients with chronic renal failure and metabolic acidosis may respond to sodium bicarbonate supplementation, 25-50 mEq daily (Hollander-Rodriguez & Calvert, 2006).
- Re-evaluate renal function if signs of renal insufficiency are present.
- Refer the patient to a nephrologist if ongoing dialysis is indicated.

REVIEW QUESTIONS

QUESTIONS

1. **Which co-morbid condition is most likely to increase the risk of hyperkalemia significantly:**
   1. Hepatic insufficiency
   2. Renal insufficiency
   3. Cancer

4. Diabetes

2. **All of the following ECG changes are associated with severe hyperkalemia *except*:**
   1. Prolonged P-R interval
   2. Widened QRS complex
   3. Tented T wave

4. Elevated ST segment

3. **All of the following medications are associated with elevated potassium levels *except*:**
   1. ACE inhibitors
   2. Beta blockers
   3. Penicillin
   4. Potassium-sparing diuretics

4. **Which of the following cancers poses the highest risk of hyperkalemia developing:**
   1. Burkitt's lymphoma
   2. Breast cancer
   3. Leukemia
   4. Renal cell cancer

5. **A patient presents to the office with an incidental finding of a potassium level of 6 mEq/L. The ECG shows no changes. A review of the patient's recent labs shows that the potassium level has been increasing gradually over the past 6 months. Which of the following is the most appropriate course of action for this patient:**
   1. Admit him to the critical care unit for continuous cardiac monitoring.
   2. Start calcium gluconate IV for cardiac protection.
   3. Start nebulized albuterol.
   4. Discontinue the potassium-sparing diuretic and start furosemide 40 mg PO daily. Recheck the potassium level in 2 days.

6. **A patient presents with a potassium level of 7 mEq/L, an increase of 1.5 mEq over 2 days. Which of the following is the most appropriate action for this patient:**
   1. Admit her to the critical care unit for continuous cardiac monitoring.

2. Start calcium gluconate IV for cardiac protection.
3. Start insulin 5-10 units IV with 50 L of 50% dextrose.
4. All of the above

ANSWERS

1. *Answer: 2*
   Rationale: Potassium is normally excreted by the kidneys, therefore disorders that decrease the function of the kidneys can result in hyperkalemia.

2. *Answer: 4*
   Rationale: Severe hyperkalemia causes a depressed ST segment.

3. *Answer: 3*
   Rationale: Penicillin is not associated with elevated potassium levels.

4. *Answer: 1*
   Rationale: Burkitt's lymphoma poses a high risk of tumor lysis syndrome; when the tumor cells are lysed and their contents released, the level of potassium and other electrolytes can rise significantly.

5. *Answer: 4*
   Rationale: A potassium level of 6 mEq/L, with a gradual rise in potassium, is considered mild to moderate hyperkalemia and can be treated in the outpatient setting with medication adjustment and diuretics.

6. *Answer: 4*
   Rationale: All the options are appropriate for a patient with severe hyperkalemia with a rapid onset.

REFERENCES

Casciato, D. A. (2004). Metabolic complications. In *Manual of clinical oncology*. (5th ed.). Philadelphia: Lippincott Williams & Wilkins.

Garth, D. (2006). Hyperkalemia. Retrieved October 1, 2006 from http://www.emedicine.com/emerg/topic 261.htm.

Gennari, F. J. (2002). Disorders of potassium homeostasis: Hypokalemia and hyperkalemia. *Critical Care Clinics, 18*(2):273-288.

Hollander-Rodriguez, J. C., & Calvert, J. F. (2006). Hyperkalemia. *American Family Physician, 73*(2):283-290.

Murphy-Ende, K. (2006). Potassium. In C. Chernecky, D. Macklin, & K. Murphy-Ende (Eds.), *Fluids and electrolytes* (pp. 79-103). (2nd ed.). St. Louis: Mosby.

Schaefer, T. J., & Wolford, R. W. (2005). Disorders of potassium. *Emergency Medicine Clinics of North America,* *23*(3):723-747.

Smith, W. J. (2000). Hypokalemia/hyperkalemia. In D. Camp-Sorrel, & R. Hawkins (Eds.), *Clinical manual for the oncology advanced practice nurse.* Pittsburgh: Oncology Nursing Press.

Stoppler, M. C. (2005). Hyperkalemia. http://www.medicinenet.com.

Wallach, J. (2000). Interpretation of diagnostic tests. (7th ed.). Philadelphia: Lippincott Williams & Wilkins.

Hyperleukocytosis in Childhood Leukemia

KRISTIN CASEY

PATHOPHYSIOLOGICAL MECHANISMS

Hyperleukocytosis is a life-threatening phenomenon that occurs when a peripheral leukocyte count exceeds 100,000/mL. An increase in the absolute number of one or more of the white blood cells is generically referred to as *leukocytosis*. This can be further differentiated by the breakdown of each cell lineage. Leukocytosis can be caused by normal inflammatory and immunologic responses, autoimmune diseases, myeloproliferative disorders, and hematopoietic malignancies. Elevated white blood cell counts can be seen in septicemia and leukemoid reactions, particularly those caused by *Staphylococcus aureus, Haemophilus influenzae* type b, *Neisseria meningitidis*, and *Salmonella* organisms (Pizzo & Poplack, 2002). Evaluation of the peripheral smear can help determine whether these cells represent acute leukemia (blasts), chronic leukemia (myeloid lineage cells in all phases of differentiation; may include early blasts), or a leukemoid reaction (Hastings, 2002). This chapter focuses specifically on leukocytosis in childhood leukemia.

The presence of excessive white blood cells in the circulation increases the viscosity of the blood and is associated with aggregation of leukemic cells in the microcirculation. The viscosity depends on the packed erythrocyte and packed lymphoblast volumes. A myeloblast is relatively large (350 to 450 mm^3), whereas a lymphoblast is relatively small (250 to 349 mm^3) (Pizzo & Poplack, 2002). Blast cells do not change shape readily, and they tend to trap plasma between them. This results in poor perfusion and anaerobic metabolism of blasts in the circulation, leading to accumulation of these cells, which contributes to lactic acidosis (Pizzo & Poplack, 2002). A packed cell volume of leukocytes that exceeds 20% to 35% increases the bulk viscosity of blood (Pizzo & Poplack, 2002; Nathan & Orkin, 1998). The effects of trapped plasma and high leukocyte counts become apparent in the microcirculation at lower volumes of packed cells.

A hematologic emergency is described as an acute, life-threatening event that occurs either directly or indirectly because of alterations in total white blood cells, red blood cell volume, platelets, and/or coagulation factors (Baggott et al., 2002). These events occur as a secondary result of chemotherapy, bone marrow replacement with cancerous cells, or marrow aplasia. Hyperleukocytosis is considered a hematologic emergency and requires immediate attention.

A number of events can occur as a consequence of a high white blood cell count. Hyperleukocytosis increases blood viscosity as the number of leukocytes increases. An excessive number of white blood cells may obstruct the microcirculation, causing damage to vessel walls. Severe metabolic disturbances may occur when cytotoxic therapy is initiated as a result of rapid destruction of white blood cells (Baggott et al., 2002).

Obstruction of a blood vessel can lead to intracranial or pulmonary hemorrhage, renal failure, disseminated intravascular coagulation (DIC) and, with chemotherapy, acute tumor lysis syndrome (ATLS) (Wilson et al., 2002). Hemorrhage and leukostasis are more prevalent in acute nonlymphocytic leukemia (ANLL), because the myeloblasts are larger than the lymphoblasts and therefore more easily trapped in circulation. This medical emergency occurs when clumps of leukemic blasts accumulate in the small circulatory vessels, leading to hypoxia, infarction, and hemorrhage. At very high white blood cell counts, leukemic aggregates proliferate into the cerebral vasculature and into the brain itself, leading to damage to blood vessels and hemorrhage (Pizzo & Poplack, 2002). CNS involvement may cause confusion, headache, somnolence, coma, and stroke.

Another phenomenon seen with hyperleukocytosis is pulmonary leukostasis or hemorrhage. This occurs when degenerating aggregates of leukemic blasts in the vessels and then the interstitium release their intracellular contents, damaging the alveoli. Leukemia-associated respiratory failure is exacerbated by possible toxins released from the blast cells, which damage the pulmonary endothelium and cause pulmonary hemorrhage (Pizzo & Poplack, 2002). Lung involvement can result in significant tachypnea and eventually lead to respiratory failure (Pizzo & Poplack, 2002).

Patients presenting with hyperleukocytosis are also at increased risk of cerebrovascular accidents (CVAs) and DIC. Leukemic promyelocytes enhance thrombin activation and express high levels of annexin II, which increases production of plasmin, a fibrolytic protein, causing DIC and CVA (Pizzo & Poplack, 2002) (see Chapter 11). Metabolic alterations occur as a result of the hypermetabolic state produced as the leukocytes cause pseudohypoglycemia and pseudohyperkalemia.

Tumor lysis syndrome results when massive lysis of tumor cells occurs after initiation of chemotherapy. Tumor lysis syndrome is seen almost exclusively in acute lymphocytic leukemia (ALL), because lymphoblasts are more sensitive then myeloblasts to chemotherapy (Lanzkowsky, 1995). The cause seems to arise from the release of large amounts of phosphate from lysed blasts; the phosphate co-precipitates with calcium in the kidneys, leading to hypocalcemia and sometimes renal failure. Hyperphosphatemia and secondary hypocalcemia could potentially lead to a seizure. Hyperuricemia may occur as a result of metabolism of the excess amounts of nucleic acid released. This may complicate the situation even more by impairing the body's ability to excrete other metabolites. Hyperkalemia may cause alterations in the echocardiogram, such as an increase in T-wave amplitude, arrhythmias, and possibly cardiac arrest.

Lactic acidosis has been a metabolic accompaniment of the leukemia. The mechanism is unclear, but this condition is thought to be related to anaerobic metabolism by the leukemic cells at sites of leukostasis (Flombaum, 2000; Lester et al., 1985). Hyperuricemia, hyperkalemia, hyperphosphatemia, and hypocalcemia may be mild to severe, depending on the leukemic burden and the rate of leukemic cell turnover (see Chapter 48).

EPIDEMIOLOGY AND ETIOLOGY

Hyperleukocytosis occurs in approximately 9% to 13% of children with acute lymphoblastic leukemia, in 5% to 20% of children with acute nonlymphoblastic leukemia, and in virtually all children with chronic myelogenous leukemia (CML) (Altman, 2004). It is more common in infant ALL, acute myeloid leukemia (AML), T-cell ALL with a mediastinal mass, and hypodiploid ALL (Pizzo & Poplack, 2002).

RISK PROFILE

- Newly diagnosed or recurrent leukemia is a risk factor.
- Patients with markedly elevated white blood cell counts have a higher risk of leukocytosis.

- The risk of complications increases as the white blood cell count increases over $100,000/mL^3$.
- A higher risk of leukocytosis is seen with infant ALL, AML, T-cell ALL with a mediastinal mass, and hypodiploid ALL (Pizzo & Poplack 2002).
- Extramedullary organ involvement at diagnosis indicates a higher risk.

PROGNOSIS

Hyperleukocytosis is associated with a 23% mortality rate in ANLL and a 5% mortality rate in ALL (Lanzkowsky, 1995). Hyperleukocytosis can lead to death by CNS hemorrhage or thrombosis, metabolic complications of tumor lysis syndrome, and pulmonary leukostasis. An increase in the white blood cell count greater than $250,000/mL^3$ increases the risk of intracranial bleeding and death (Basade et al., 1995).

PROFESSIONAL ASSESSMENT CRITERIA (PAC)

1. Patients may be asymptomatic on presentation.
2. A patient with a complete blood count (CBC) that shows a white blood cell (WBC) count exceeding $100,000/mL^3$ should be evaluated for hyperleukocytosis.
3. The patient may present with mental status changes, headaches, fever, vomiting, blurred vision, tinnitus, oliguria, or anuria. The symptoms depend on where leukemic infiltration occurs (Tomlinson & Kline, 2005).
4. Seizures; coma; symptoms of stroke; papilledema; retinal artery or retinal vein distention; diminished lung sounds; rales; tachycardia; signs of respiratory distress; and hepatosplenomegaly may be seen (Baggott et al., 2002).
5. Pulmonary leukocytosis causes dyspnea, hypoxia, acidosis, and cyanosis.
6. Priapism, clitoral engorgement, and dactylitis have been described with hyperleukocytosis (Baggott et al., 2002).
7. Additional labs that may indicate complications include serum electrolytes, uric acid, renal function tests, glucose, and a coagulation panel. Tumor lysis syndrome causes hyperuricemia, hyperkalemia, hyperphosphatemia, and hypocalcemia. The glucose level is decreased because the hypermetabolic state creates a pseudohypoglycemia. The coagulation panel is abnormal and shows a prolonged prothrombin time and partial prothrombin time and decreased fibrinogen, which suggest DIC.
8. A chest x-ray film may show a mediastinal mass, diffuse interstitial infiltrates, or cardiomegaly.
9. A CT scan or MRI may be needed to detect CNS lesions in the white matter of the brain surrounded by hemorrhage.
10. Bone marrow biopsy may be done to confirm the diagnosis and type of leukemia.

NURSING CARE AND TREATMENT

The following nursing care is prioritized.
1. Monitor pulse, respirations, and blood pressure every hour, temperature every 4 hours; once vital signs are stable, every 4 hours.

2. Establish IV access.
3. Start intravenous hydration of 5% dextrose 0.45% NaCl at two to four times the maintenance volume with alkalinization using 1 ampule of sodium bicarbonate.
4. Start allopurinol 10 mg/kg PO daily to reduce the likelihood of tumor lysis syndrome (Holmes, 1998).
5. Patients with a platelet count less than 20,000/mm^3 should receive platelet transfusions to prevent cerebral hemorrhage. Platelets do not worsen blood viscosity.
6. Maintain oxygenation; assess oxygen saturation and administer oxygen using a non-rebreather mask to maintain oxygen saturation above 90%. Be prepared for emergency endotracheal intubation in event of respiratory failure.
7. Prepare the room for seizure precautions. Keep the patient safe from falls, pad the sides of the bed appropriately, ensure access to antiepileptic medications and keep at bedside if ordered, set up oxygen and suction at bedside.
8. Prepare for lumbar puncture; have supplies ready and prepare the patient.
9. Obtain a baseline neurologic assessment; document and reassess for changes in behavior, level of consciousness, speech, strength, coordination, and gait.
10. Maintain adequate pain management.
11. The hemoglobin level should not exceed 10 g/dL. Red blood cell transfusions should be given cautiously to avoid increasing whole blood viscosity and worsening symptoms.
12. Exchange transfusions or leukapheresis and initiation of cytotoxic chemotherapy can rapidly lower the WBC count and leukemic cells.
13. Measure I&O and maintain urine output at 1 to 2 mL/kg/hr.
14. Obtain baseline weight and weigh patient daily.
15. Ensure aggressive correction of metabolic abnormalities.
16. Cranial irradiation has been performed to prevent CNS hemorrhage. However, the risk of CNS hemorrhage is relatively small in ALL patients, and most pediatric oncologists do not use prophylactic irradiation (Basade et al. 1995).
17. Leukapheresis and exchange transfusions may be treatment options. Prepare the patient and monitor appropriately.
18. Teach the family about chemotherapy administration. Review chemotherapy safety, side effects, and home precautions.

EVIDENCE-BASED PRACTICE UPDATES

1. Cranial irradiation is associated with significant complications and therefore is used less frequently. Children who undergo cranial irradiation are at risk of growth impairment and central nervous system deficits. Follow-up analyses from a study of 201 children treated with a total dose of 18 Gy found that after a median of 9.1 years, IQ and memory were normal, but the ability to draw a complex figure was impaired. Children treated before 3 years of age had an average overall IQ but compromised verbal skills (Meyers et al., 2004; Pizzo & Poplack 2002; Bleyer & Poplack, 1985).

2. Exchange transfusion or leukapheresis can rapidly lower the WBC count and may improve coagulopathy. Pediatric studies found a 52% to 66% mean reduction in WBCs with exchange transfusion and a 48% to 62% reduction with leukapheresis (Pizzo & Poplack, 2002).

3. Maurer and colleagues (1988) noted a significantly lower incidence of tumor lysis syndrome in patients with ALL who had a WBC count over 200,000/mL^3 and who underwent leukapheresis, compared to patients who did not undergo leukapheresis.

4. Neurologic abnormalities, respiratory distress, and priapism have improved after leukapheresis in patients with AML, ALL, and CML (Bunin et al., 1987).

TEACHING AND EDUCATION

1. Reduce the number of WBCs by exchange transfusion or leukapheresis, before initiating cytotoxic chemotherapy to reduce the chance of secondary complications. Induction chemotherapy causes cell death and the release of toxic substances, causing bleeding or cardiac arrhythmias.
2. Provide intravenous hydration at 3000 mL/m^2/day, alkalinization, and allopurinol to reduce the risk of tumor lysis syndrome.
3. Maintain urine output at 1 to 2 mL/kg/hr and keep track of accurate input and output. Report if output is decreased, because renal failure is a potential complication of hyperleukocytosis.
4. Report symptoms such as headache, respiratory difficulties, fever, vomiting, ringing in the ears, intense thirst, or weakness immediately. These changes may indicate secondary complications from the hyperleukocytosis.
5. If metabolic errors occur, supplements may be required in the diet. Failure to correct the electrolyte balance could lead to further renal damage and complications.
6. Establish central venous access to allow easy access for blood samples, administration of chemotherapeutic drugs, blood, IV fluids, nutrition, and medications.
7. Chemotherapy (induction therapy) is started immediately to put the child into remission. Chemotherapy usually is continued, depending on the type of leukemia.

NURSING DIAGNOSES

1. **Acute pain** related to the clumping of leukemic aggregates leading to decreased blood supply and thus may cause pain. Bone pain related to high cellular turnover
2. **Decreased cardiac output and respiratory failure** related to high number of WBC leukemic infiltrates in the pulmonary vessels and the interstitium releasing intracellular contents resulting in alveolar and pulmonary endothelium damage
3. **Acute confusion** related to the hyperviscosity in the cerebral vessels, resulting in damage to the vessels and hemorrhage; may lead to headaches, mental status changes, blurred vision, seizures, coma, and papilledema
4. **Risk for imbalanced fluid volume** related to leukemic aggregates proliferating in the cerebral vasculature
5. **Deficient knowledge** related to early diagnosis, intervention, and complications

EVALUATION AND DESIRED OUTCOMES

1. Pain assessment will show acceptable pain scores.
2. The patient will rate the pain at less than or equal to 2 on a 5-point pain scale.
3. The patient will remain afebrile and other vital signs will be stable.
4. Abnormal lab values will be reported, and steps will be taken to correct abnormalities:
   - CBC with differential
     - Blast count will decrease.
     - White blood cell count will decrease.
     - Differential will show a decreased neutrophil count.
   - Platelet count
     - Will be within normal range or slightly decreased (keep greater then 20,000 mm^3).
   - LDH
     - Will be decreased (this value is elevated at the time of diagnosis with ALL or CML).
   - Glucose
     - Will be maintained at 70 to 110 mg/dL fasting.

- Electrolytes
  - Will be watched closely and corrected if necessary.
  - Patient will be monitored for hyperuricemia, hyperkalemia, hyperphosphatemia, and hypocalcemia (these are seen with tumor lysis syndrome).
5. Tumor lysis syndrome will be prevented.

DISCHARGE PLANNING AND FOLLOW-UP CARE

- Follow-up with physician or pediatric nurse practitioner 5 to 7 days after discharge.
- Chemotherapy appointments and lab tests.
- Call appropriate health care provider immediately for fever greater than 38° C, nausea, vomiting, pain, headache, blurred vision, decreased urine output, shortness of breath or cough, restlessness, mental status changes, dizziness, and signs of infection or bleeding.
- Medication list (i.e., name, purpose, dosage, frequency, and side effects) given to patient and family.
- Central venous access care reviewed with patient and family.

REVIEW QUESTIONS

QUESTIONS

1. **Hyperleukocytosis is *most* likely to occur in which patient:**
   1. A 3-year-old with a hepatoblastoma
   2. An 11-year-old recently diagnosed with chronic myelogenous leukemia
   3. A 5-year-old in the maintenance phase of chemotherapy for ALL
   4. A 15-year-old with osteogenic sarcoma

2. **Which of the following factors puts a patient at higher risk for developing thrombosis:**
   1. Hemoglobin level of 9.5 g/dL
   2. White blood cell count of 120,000 mm^3
   3. Platelet count of 100,000 mm^3
   4. Absolute neutrophil count of 1000 mm^3

3. **Which of these symptoms may be *most* indicative of hyperleukocytosis:**
   1. Hypotension
   2. Bradycardia
   3. Polyuria
   4. Headache

4. **When caring for a patient with a white blood cell count of 236,000 mm^3, the nurse should give highest priority to:**
   1. Administering a blood transfusion
   2. Preparing a patient for cranial irradiation
   3. Transfusing platelets
   4. Initiating hydration fluids at two to four times maintenance

5. **A patient newly diagnosed with CML is experiencing headache, nausea, decreased urine output, and shortness of breath. The *most* likely cause of these symptoms is:**
   1. Side effects of chemotherapy
   2. An infectious process
   3. Hyperleukocytosis
   4. A kidney stone

6. **The *most* likely cause of the complications related to hyperleukocytosis is:**
   1. Decreased platelet function
   2. Increased blood viscosity
   3. Increased hepatic flow
   4. Decreased neutrophil count

7. **In assessing a patient with hyperleukocytosis, the highest priority should be given to assessing:**
   1. Hourly intake and output
   2. Abdominal girth
   3. Pitting edema
   4. Bowel sounds

8. **Patients who present with hyperleukocytosis are at greatest risk of also developing:**
   1. Disseminated intravascular coagulation
   2. Septic emboli

3. Diabetes insipidus
4. Adrenal insufficiency

9. **Which of the following lab results *most* likely indicates a patient with tumor lysis syndrome:**
   1. Potassium, 4.9 mEqL; uric acid, 2.6 mg/dL; calcium, 10.3 mg/dL; phosphate, 4.2 mg/dL
   2. Potassium, 5.3 mEqL; uric acid, 1.9 mg/dL; calcium, 10.6 mg/dL; phosphate, 4 mg/dL
   3. Potassium, 5.2 mEqL; uric acid, 7 mg/dL; calcium, 6.5 mg/dL; phosphate, 8.6 mg/dL
   4. Potassium, 6 mEqL; uric acid, 5.8 mg/dL; calcium, 8.7 mg/dL; phosphate, 4.2 mg/dL

10. **A patient with hyperleukocytosis with a secondary complication of DIC might show which of the following lab values:**
    1. Prothrombin time, 1.6; partial prothrombin time, 28 sec; fibrinogen, 400 mg/dL
    2. Prothrombin time, 1.6; partial prothrombin time, 39 sec; fibrinogen, 145 mg/dL
    3. Prothrombin time, 1.6; partial prothrombin time, 22 sec; fibrinogen, 450 mg/dL
    4. Prothrombin time, 1.1; partial prothrombin time, 22 sec; fibrinogen, 401 mg/dL

ANSWERS

1. *Answer: 2*
   Rationale: The incidence of hyperleukocytosis is 50% to 100% during the acute phase of chronic myelogenous leukemia.

2. *Answer: 2*
   Rationale: The risk of thrombosis increases as the white blood cell count rises above 100,000.

3. *Answer: 4*
   Rationale: Headache is a sign of CNS involvement. Expected symptoms are hypertension, tachycardia, and signs of renal failure (e.g., oliguria) (Baggott et al., 2002).

4. *Answer: 4*
   Rationale: Starting hydration fluids should be the first step in managing hyperleukocytosis. Administering hydration fluids at high volume reduces viscosity, helps correct metabolic abnormalities, and reduces the likelihood of tumor lysis syndrome.

5. *Answer: 3*
   Rationale: The symptoms described are all classic symptoms of hyperleukocytosis. Hyperleukocytosis is seen in nearly all patients presenting with CML (Altman, 2004).

6. *Answer: 2*
   Rationale: As a result of an excess of white blood cells in the circulation, blood viscosity increases. This is associated with aggregation of leukemic cells in the microcirculation. Blast cells do not change shape readily, and they tend to trap plasma between them. The result is poor perfusion and anaerobic metabolism of the blasts in the circulation, leading to accumulation of these cells, which contributes to lactic acidosis (Pizzo & Poplack, 2002).

7. *Answer: 1*
   Rationale: Initially some patients present with mental status changes, headache, fever, vomiting, blurred vision, tinnitus, oliguria, and aniridia. Symptoms depend on where leukemic infiltration occurs. (Tomlinson & Kline, 2005). Urine output should be maintained at 1 to 2 mL/kg/hr, and input and output must be measured accurately, because renal failure is a potential complication of hyperleukocytosis.

8. *Answer: 1*
   Rationale: The presence of an excessive number of white blood cells may result in obstruct of the microcirculation, causing damage to vessel walls. Severe metabolic disturbances related to rapid destruction of white blood cells may occur when cytotoxic therapy is initiated (Baggott et al., 2002). Obstruction of a blood vessel can lead to intracranial or pulmonary hemorrhage, renal failure, DIC, and acute tumor lysis syndrome.

9. *Answer: 3*
Rationale: Tumor lysis syndrome is marked by hyperkalemia, hyperuricemia, hypocalcemia, and hyperphosphatemia.

10. *Answer: 2*
Rationale: Patients presenting with hyperleukocytosis are also at increased risk of CVA and DIC. Leukemic promyelocytes enhance thrombin activation and express high levels of annexin II, which increases production of plasmin, a fibrolytic protein, causing DIC and CVA (Pizzo & Poplack, 2002). The coagulation panel would show a prolonged prothrombin time and partial prothrombin time and decreased fibrinogen, suggesting DIC.

REFERENCES

Altman, A. J. (2004). *Supportive care of children with cancer.* (3rd ed.). Baltimore: John Hopkins University Press.

Baggott, C. R., Kelly, K. P., & Fochtman, D., et al. (2002). *Nursing care of children and adolescents with cancer.* (3rd ed.). Philadelphia: W.B. Saunders.

Basade, M., Dhar, A., & Kulkarni, S. M., et al. (1995). Rapid cytoreduction in childhood leukemic hyperleukocytosis by conservative therapy. *Medical and Pediatric Oncology, 25:*204-207.

Bleyer, W. A., & Poplack, D. G. (1985). Prophylaxis and treatment of leukemia in the central nervous system and other sanctuaries. *Seminars in Oncology, 12:*131-133.

Bunin, N. J., Kunkel, K., & Callihan, T. R. (1987). Cytoreductive procedures in the early management in cases of leukemia and hyperleukocytosis in children. *Medical and Pediatric Oncology, 15:*232-235.

Flombaum, C. D. (2000). Metabolic emergencies in the cancer patient. *Seminars in Oncology, 27:*322-324.

Hastings, C. (2002). *The Children's Hospital Oakland: Hematology/oncology handbook.* St. Louis: Mosby.

Holmes, W. (1998). Hyperleukocytosis in childhood leukemia. In C. Chernecky, & B. Berger (Eds.), *Advanced and critical care oncology nursing: Managing primary complications* (pp. 283-297). Philadelphia: W.B. Saunders.

Lanzkowsky, P. (1995). *Manual of pediatric hematology and oncology.* (2nd ed.). New York: Churchill Livingstone.

Lester, T. J., Johnson, J. W., & Cuttner, J. (1985). Pulmonary leukostasis as the single worst prognostic factor in patients with acute myeloid leukemia and hyperleukocytosis. *American Journal of Medicine, 79:*43-45.

Maurer, H. S., Steinherz, P. G., & Gaynon, P. S., et al. (1988). Management of hyperleukocytosis (HL) in childhood with acute lymphoblastic leukemia. *Journal of Clinical Oncology, 6:*1425-1426.

Meyers, C. A., Smith, J. A., & Bezjak, A., et al. (2004). Neurocognitive function and progression in patients with brain metastases treated with whole brain irradiation. *Journal of Clinical Oncology, 22:*157-160.

Nathan, D. G., & Orkin, S. H. (1998). *Nathan and Oski's hematology of infancy and childhood.* (5th ed.). Philadelphia: W.B. Saunders.

Pizzo, P. A., & Poplack, D. G. (2002). *Principles and practice of pediatric oncology.* (4th ed.). Philadelphia: Lippincott Williams & Wilkins.

Tomlinson, D., & Kline, N. E. (Eds.). (2005). *Pediatric oncology nursing: Advanced clinical handbook.* New York: Springer Berlin Heidelberg.

Wilson, K., Secola, R., & Reid, D. (2002). Oncologic emergencies. In N. Kline, (Ed.), *Essentials of pediatric oncology nursing: A core curriculum* (pp. 147-149). (2nd ed). Glenview, IL: Association of Pediatric Oncology Nurses.

HYPERNATREMIA

MADY STOVALL

PATHOPHYSIOLOGICAL MECHANISMS

Homeostatic alteration in water and sodium is frequently encountered in patients with cancer (Fojo, 2005), and hyponatremia (see Chapter 29) occurs more frequently than hypernatremia (Murphy-Ende, 2006a). Sodium, the major extracellular cation, is crucial for maintaining volume stability. A normal serum sodium level for adults and children is 135 to 145 mEq/L (or mmol/L). The term *hypernatremia* refers to a serum sodium level greater than 145 mEq/L. Hypernatremia is an infrequent electrolyte abnormality.

Body water and electrolyte balance is the result of numerous physiologic mechanisms. Two major fluid and electrolyte transport systems support sodium and water balance and serum osmolality; passive transport systems and active transport systems. Passive transport systems do not expend energy; these are composed of the processes of diffusion, filtration, and osmosis. *Diffusion* is based on the principle that molecules and ions flow freely, but randomly, from an area of higher concentration to an area of lower concentration across a biologic membrane. Diffusion depends on the concentration gradients of solutes and is permitted or enhanced by the permeability of a cell membrane. *Filtration* is the movement of a solute and a solvent from one side of a membrane to another side caused by hydrostatic pressure differences between the two sides of the membrane. This is most noticeable when a patient develops right-side heart failure and blood backs up into the systemic venous circulation, causing venous and capillary hydrostatic pressures to rise. As a result, water moves from the capillaries into the interstitial spaces in the periphery, causing visible edema, or *third spacing*. *Osmosis* is the movement of a solvent from an area of lower concentration to an area of higher concentration through a semipermeable membrane that separates the solutions. In this process, fluids move into and out of the cell. The concentration of solutes dissolved in body fluids, therefore, affects the movement of water. This is known as *osmotic pressure* or *water pulling pressure* (Metheny, 2000).

The intracellular sodium level is 10 mEq/L, a stark contrast to the extracellular sodium concentration of 135 to 145 mEq/L. Therefore, maintaining sodium in its proper intracellular fluid (ICF) and extracellular fluid (ECF) concentrations requires an active transport system. Energy is constantly expended using cellular adenosine triphosphate (ATP) to power the sodium-potassium pump in every body cell to maintain homeostasis by moving sodium out of the cell and potassium into the cell, against their respective concentrations gradients (Metheny, 2000).

Increased serum sodium is always synonymous with increased serum osmolality. The osmolality of a solution is determined by the number of solute particles per kilogram of water. The following equation defines serum osmolality:

$$\text{Serum osmolality} = (2 \times \text{Na}) + (\text{Glucose} \div 18) + (\text{Urea} \div 2.8)$$

Serum osmolality is regulated tightly between 275 and 290 mOsm/kg, primarily through the influence of vasopressin. Extracellular fluid primarily consists of sodium salts, glucose, and urea. Therefore an increased serum osmolality is not always related to increased sodium levels, because the osmolality may be increased as a result of an increase in other serum solutes. However, under normal conditions, glucose and urea solutes contribute minimally to serum osmolality (Fall, 2000).

$$\uparrow Na = \uparrow Osmolality$$

$$\uparrow Osmolality = \uparrow Serum\ solute(i.e.,\ sodium,\ glucose,\ or\ urea)$$

Numerous mechanisms work to maintain body water and sodium balance. Because sodium is largely restricted to the ECF, deficits or excesses of total body sodium are characterized by signs of ECF volume depletion or overload, respectively. The serum sodium concentration does not necessarily change with deficits or excesses of total body sodium. The main determinant of the plasma sodium concentration is plasma water content, which itself is determined by water intake, insensible losses, and urinary dilution (Reynolds et al., 2006). The plasma water, or ECF volume, is regulated by four major control mechanisms: arginine vasopressin (antidiuretic hormone [ADH]), the renin-angiotensin-aldosterone system, the baroreceptor reflex, and volume receptors (Murphy-Ende, 2006a).

Vasopressin system malfunction can produce observable problems, specifically central diabetes insipidus (DI), nephrogenic DI, and syndrome of inappropriate antidiuretic hormone (SIADH). Central and nephrogenic DI may lead to hypernatremia, whereas SIADH leads to hyponatremia.

Under normal conditions, ADH is released from the posterior pituitary when osmoreceptors in the hypothalamus sense an increased serum osmolality. ADH tends to reduce diuresis and increase water retention at the distal tubules of the kidneys, so that fluid will move (by osmosis) from inside the cell into the extracellular spaces; this leaves the cell dehydrated, and the plasma more dilute. Cells in the central nervous system are especially vulnerable to a sudden shift in fluid, which may manifest as neurologic signs or symptoms in the patient (Box 26-1).

The thirst center plays an important role in the regulation of serum sodium. The thirst center, which is located in the hypothalamus, consists of neuronal cells, which function as osmoreceptors. Thirst is promoted when the osmotic pressure in the cerebrospinal fluid of the third ventricle or in the circulating extracellular fluid increases. Intracellular dehydration in hypernatremia, and hypercalcemia, causes increased osmolar concentration of the extracellular fluid. Another stimulus that causes thirst is increased production of angiotensin II (Murphy-Ende, 2006a). Thirst is a common symptom in cancer patients and may be related to decreased fluid intake, increased

---

BOX 26-1   NEUROLOGIC SIGNS AND SYMPTOMS OF HYPERNATREMIA

- Thirst
- Hypertension
- Low-grade fever
- Mental confusion, disorientation
- Tremors, seizures
- Muscle rigidity and weakness
- CNS irritability: restlessness, agitation
- Muscle cramps, muscle twitching, increased deep tendon reflexes (DTRs)

fluid output, poor fluid transport, medications, and mouth breathing. Pathologic conditions that can cause thirst include aldosteronism, chronic glomerulonephritis, DM, DI, hyperparathyroidism, hyperthyroidism, multiple sclerosis, SIADH, primary polydipsia, and terminal condition. (Murphy-Ende, 2006b).

An excess of aldosterone leads to hypernatremia through the complex interaction of hormones and renal function. Under normal conditions the renin-angiotensin-aldosterone system plays an important role in regulating blood volume. Sympathetic stimulation (acting via beta-1 adrenoceptors), renal artery hypotension, and decreased sodium delivery to the distal tubules stimulates the release of renin by the juxtaglomerular cells of the kidney. Renin then travels to the liver and is converted to angiotensin I, which is converted to angiotensin II in the lungs. Angiotensin II travels to the adrenal glands and stimulates the production of aldosterone. Aldosterone is a steroid hormone that acts on the kidneys to increase reabsorption of sodium, which leads to water retention and ultimately to increases in fluid volume and sodium levels. Angiotensin II also stimulates the release of ADH to further enhance fluid retention. The renin-angiotensin-aldosterone cycle is crucial for responding to a low serum sodium level; however, disease states and treatments that lead to an excess of aldosterone may also lead to an excess of sodium. In fact, 65% of patients with primary hyperaldosteronism have solitary aldosterone-producing adrenal adenomas (White, 1994).

EPIDEMIOLOGY AND ETIOLOGY

Four major age-related changes predispose the elderly to dehydration and hypernatremia: a decrease in total body water, an altered sense of thirst, a decrease in the renal urine concentrating ability, and a decrease in the effectiveness of antidiuretic hormone (Arinzon et al., 2005). Frail nursing home residents and hospitalized patients are prone to hypernatremia, because they often depend on others to meet their water requirements (Androgué & Madias, 2000). Hypernatremia occurs in about 1% of all hospitalized patients and in 9% of patients in intensive care (Tisdall et al., 2006). For this reason, monitoring for hypernatremia has been recommended as a measure for ICU quality of care (Polderman et al., 1999), and it may be an indicator of nursing home neglect (Himmelstein et al., 1983).

Sustained hypernatremia can occur only when thirst or access to water is impaired; therefore the groups at highest risk are individuals with altered mental status, intubated patients, infants, and the elderly (Adrogué & Madias, 2000). Oncology patients often have significant water losses, caused by febrile illness, respiratory distress, or gastrointestinal losses, which increase their risk of dehydration and fluid and electrolyte abnormalities.

In the acute care setting, the most common cause of hypernatremia is excessive parenteral administration of sodium solutions (Palevsky et al., 1996). In most patients outside the acute care setting, hypernatremia is caused by water loss in excess of solute where recent fluid loss history may be significant for fevers, sweating, or recent respiratory infection in the setting of altered thirst or altered ability to self-quench a thirst (Fall, 2000). Other causes of hypernatremia include saltwater near-drowning, extreme salt ingestion, and excessive amounts of adrenocortical hormones, such as occurs in Cushing's syndrome and hyperaldosteronism. Primary hypodipsia may result from destruction of the thirst center or osmoreceptors in the hypothalamus. Central DI also results from a defect in the secretion of ADH and presents in the same scenarios as primary hypodipsia. These conditions have been described in a variety of disorders, including craniopharyngiomas, hypophysectomy, primary or metastatic tumors (most commonly breast and lung) of the hypothalamus, CNS infections or other primary or metastatic brain tumors, cerebrovascular disease/vascular lesions, granulomatous diseases, and head trauma (Kugler & Hustead, 2000; Palevsky et al., 1996).

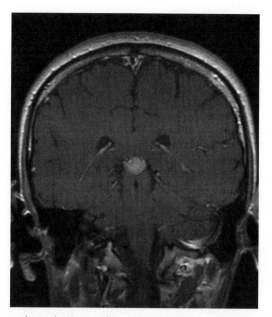

Fig. 26.1 • A gadolinium-enhanced MRI revealing a pineal tumor (contrast-enhancing lesion seen in the center of the brain) with enlargement of the pituitary stalk. This 23-year-old man's initial symptom was diabetes insipidus, which appeared 4 months before his diagnosis of germ cell tumor. He has had episodic hypernatremia from his initial presentation and throughout his chemotherapy and radiation. His central DI is managed with DDAVP.

Essential hypernatremia, a variant of primary hypodipsia, can be seen with tumors that invade the lateral hypothalamus. In this disorder, ADH release as a result of osmotic stimuli is impaired, but ADH response to volume and other nonosmotic stimuli is normal. Patients are euvolemic and asymptomatic (Fig. 26.1) (Kapoor & Chan, 2001).

Hypokalemia and hypercalcemia are the two electrolyte disorders most likely to affect sodium homeostasis, because these conditions reduce the water permeability of the renal collecting ducts by inhibiting adenylate cyclase activation in response to ADH (Kapoor & Chan, 2001). Diseases that may lead to chronic tubulointerstitial disease (e.g., systemic lupus erythematosus, sickle cell anemia, multiple myeloma) and congenital defects may cause nephrogenic DI (Kugler & Hustead, 2000; Palevsky et al., 1996).

Numerous medications may be associated with hypernatremia, including antacids with sodium bicarbonate, antibiotics (e.g., ticarcillin disodium-clavulanate potassium [Timentin]), salt tablets, sodium bicarbonate injections (e.g., during cardiac arrest), intravenous sodium chloride solutions, and sodium polystyrene sulfonate (Kayexalate). Medications that specifically may cause NDI include lithium, amphotericin B, demeclocycline, methoxyflurane, and foscarnet (Kugler & Hustead, 2000; Palevsky et al., 1996). In addition, ingestion of large amounts of licorice leads to increased secretion of aldosterone, causing retention of sodium and water (Shibata, 2000).

RISK PROFILE

- **Cancers involving the brain:** Hypothalamic (craniopharyngioma, germinoma, meningioma), pituitary (suprasellar extension); other primary or metastatic tumors (i.e., lung, breast, leukemia, lymphoma) of the brain involving the supraoptic or para-ventricular nuclei. Malignancy of the kidney or adrenal glands (i.e., renal cell carci-noma, sarcoma), multiple myeloma, and malignant ascites (Reynolds et al., 2006; Kapoor & Chan, 2001; Kugler & Hustead, 2000; Shulz, 1998; Palevsky et al., 1996; White, 1994).

- **Conditions:** Infants and elderly individuals unable to ingest fluids at will. Congestive heart failure; kidney damage; coma; Cushing's syndrome; excessive fluid losses; uncon-trolled diabetes mellitus that causes solute diuresis; fever; head injury; neurosurgery; chronic hypokalemia or hypercalcemia; pregnancy; psychosis; diabetes insipidus that causes urine-concentrating defects; mental or physical disability; sickle cell nephropa-thy; central nervous system infections, such as TB, syphilis, mycoses, toxoplasmosis, encephalitis, and chronic meningitis; granulomas (neurosarcoid, histiocytosis, Wegener's disease); hypertonic dialysis; and electrolyte abnormalities (hypercalcemia, hypokalemia) (Reynolds et al., 2006; Kugler & Hustead, 2000; Schulz, 1998; Palevsky et al., 1996;).
- **Environmental factors:** Near-drowning in saltwater, residence in nursing home, severe burns (Schulz, 1998; Himmelstein et al., 1983).
- **Foods:** Licorice, high-sodium foods, high-protein tube feedings (Achinger et al., 2006; Shibata, 2000; Schulz, 1998; Palevsky et al., 1996).
- **Medications:** Catecholamines; ethanol; reserpine; morphine; chlorpromazine; pheny-toin; lithium carbonate; demeclocycline; methoxyflurane; cisplatin; sodium bicarbo-nate; sodium chloride; Aldomet; Apresoline; sodium-containing antibiotics/antifungals (e.g., carbenicillin, ticarcillin, and amphotericin B); hypertonic saline administration; foscarnet; clozapine; aminoglycosides; ifosfamide; and analgesics (i.e., analgesic nephropathy) (Reynolds et al., 2006; Kugler & Hustead, 2000; Schulz, 1998; Palevsky et al., 1996;).

PROGNOSIS

The mortality rate associated with hypernatremia varies widely, depending on the severity of the condition and the rapidity of onset. However, differentiating the contribution of hypernatremia to mortality from the contribution of underlying illnesses is difficult (Adrogué & Madias, 2000). For example, coexisting medical conditions, such as hyperosmolar hyperglycemic nonketotic syndrome, negatively affect mortality. Mortality rates vary from 16% to 60%, depending on the patient population (Palevsky et al., 1996). A retrospective study by Polderman and colleagues (1999) found that hospital-acquired hypernatremia was associated with a higher mortality rate (32%) than hypernatremia present on admission to the ICU (20.3%). This mortality rate may be worse because of delays in diagnosis or inappropriate treatment (Chassagne et al., 2006).

Arinzon and colleagues (2005) evaluated elderly patients in long-term care who developed acute illness. They found that disturbances in sodium concentrations were predictors of bad outcomes. However, in this study the bad outcomes were related to the underlying disease burden and not to the underlying changes in plasma sodium, the time of its development, advanced age, gender, or coexisting changes in the plasma potassium level.

Additional research is needed to further identify the individual contribution of hyper-natremia to increased morbidity and mortality, often in the setting of numerous confounders.

PROFESSIONAL ASSESSMENT CRITERIA (PAC)

	Hypovolemic State	Euvolemic State	Hypervolemic State
Vital Signs			
Temperature	Normal or elevated	Normal	Normal
Blood pressure	Decreased	Normal	Increased
Pulse	Elevated	Normal	Elevated
Respiratory rate	Normal	Normal	Tachypneic
Central venous pressure	<2 mm Hg	2-6 mm Hg	>6 mm Hg
History	• Extremely excessive oral and/or IV intake • Fluid losses from GI tract • Intubation or coma, limiting intake • Tumors or trauma to hypothalamus, pituitary, or adrenal glands • Kidney disease or trauma • Mental impairment (psychosis, inability to advocate for self) • Increased serum osmolality (hyperglycemia, high-protein tube feedings)	• Excessive oral and/or IV sodium intake • Medication administration (see Risk Profile)	• Excessive adrenocortical secretion (i.e., adenomas, Cushing's syndrome, steroid administration, abnormally large ingestion of licorice) • Congestive heart failure
Hallmark Physical Signs and Symptoms	• Thirst, lethargy, dry mucous membranes, decreased skin turgor	• Thirst	• Weight gain, jugular vein distention
Urine Output	• DI: High urine output with low specific gravity	• Normal to slightly increased urine output	• Decreased urine output with normal to low specific gravity
Other Physical Signs and Symptoms	• Hypercalcemia, malignant ascites, fever	• Malignant ascites	• Restlessness, dyspnea, agitation, S3 heart sound, generalized edema with heart failure, possible hypokalemia
Psychological Signs and Symptoms	• Confusion, disorientation, apprehension		
Blood and Urine Laboratory Values			
Sodium, serum	High	High	High
Potassium, serum	Normal	Normal	Normal or low

Continued

Aldosterone, serum	Decreased	Low	High in conditions that increase adrenocortical secretion
ADH, serum	Increased to compensate for fluid volume losses

Decreased if fluid volume is low due to DI | Increased | Normal or may be decreased if fluid volume is high due to condition causing excessive aldosterone release |
Osmolality, serum	High	High	High
Creatinine and urea nitrogen, blood	Volume depletion associated with adipsia causes elevations in BUN and creatinine and an increase in the BUN/creatinine ratio.	Normal	Decreased or normal
Osmolarity, urine	Low	Normal or low	High
Specific gravity, urine	High
Low in DI	High	High
Low in conditions that cause excessive aldosterone release
Sodium, urine	Decreased in DI
Increased in response to aldosterone in other types of hypernatremia	Increased	Increased or decreased in conditions that cause excessive aldosterone release
Creatinine, urine	Normal or high in renal damage	Normal	Normal

Diagnostic Exams

Deep tendon reflexes	Hyperreactive	Hyperreactive	Hyperreactive
Water deprivation test	If due to DI: a twofold increase in urine osmolality after administration of vasopressin	No response to vasopressin	No response to vasopressin
Computed tomography (CT) scans or magnetic resonance imaging (MRI)	• *Brain*: May reveal intracranial lesion or hemorrhage involving hypothalamic or pituitary region; cerebral edema (see Fig. 26.1). **NOTE**: CT scans (with and without contrast) may not be sensitive to all intracranial tumors, although they generally are adequate for evaluation of suspected intracranial hemorrhage or hydrocephalus. Currently the best modality for evaluation of suspected intracranial lesions is MRI, with and without gadolinium. Brain images may be useful for evaluating adipsia or in ruling out complications of hypernatremia (e.g., IC hemorrhage). • *Body*: Renal or adrenal lesions or trauma		
Positron emission tomography (PET scan, FDG-type)	• May reveal adrenal or renal diseases or intracranial lesions from primary or metastatic disease (e.g., lung cancer, adenomas).		

Other Considerations

• Assess chemotherapeutic drugs and dosing intervals to evaluate chemotherapy-induced nausea and vomiting or diarrhea. Also assess antiemetic regimen and optimization of antiemetic or antidiarrheal regimen.

- Assess content and rate of IV fluids.
- Assess for medications high in sodium or for those that reduce renal responsiveness to ADH.

1. **Neurologic status:** May have acute confusion, lethargy, coma, or seizures.
2. **Fluid status:** Poor skin turgor, dry eyes and mouth in dehydration, edema and jugular vein distention in fluid overload.
3. **History:** The cause of the hypernatremia often is evident from the history (Reynolds et al., 2006). Signs and symptoms include lethargy, altered mental status, irritability, hyperreflexia, and spasticity (Kapoor & Chan, 2001). The patient progresses from feeling thirsty, with a slightly increased serum sodium (138 to 139 mEq/L), to becoming increasingly lethargic as levels increase. Eventually coma sets in, and with extreme hypernatremia, the patient may suffer generalized seizures and death.
4. **Sodium levels:** Check the labs and compare the sodium level to previous levels (see table, above). A rapid change in levels requires prompt attention.
5. **Urine osmolarity and sodium concentration:** Measuring the urine osmolarity and urine sodium concentration can be helpful in establishing the cause of hypernatremia and in guiding therapy (Fall, 2000). If defense mechanisms are intact, namely ADH secretion and thirst, and the renal concentrating mechanism is normal, the patient should have a maximally concentrated urine and a urine osmolality of greater then 800 mOsm/kg (Fall, 2000). This normal response is seen in patients with salt overload, insensible or gastrointestinal water losses, or primary hypodipsia (Fall, 2000). A high urine osmolality (greater than 700 mOsm/kg) with a low urine sodium level usually indicates an extrarenal hypotonic loss of free water (i.e., excessive sweating, diarrhea, respiratory loss). That same urine osmolality with a higher urinary sodium level suggests renal free water loss (i.e., osmotic diuresis, diuretics, interstitial renal disease) (Healy & Jacobson, 1994). Patients with a urine osmolality of less than 150 to 200 mOsm/kg with hypernatremia and polyuria usually have some form of diabetes insipidus.

NURSING CARE AND TREATMENT

1. Treatment of hypernatremia involves identifying and treating the underlying cause and water administration. If the patient is hypovolemic, sodium must also be replaced; this is followed by isotonic saline replacement and then photonic saline or oral free water administration. To correct the water deficit, the existing deficit and ongoing losses must be replaced. Correction of the osmolar imbalance is accomplished by replacing what was lost (water, hypotonic fluids with or without electrolytes) or by ridding the body of excess sodium (Table 26-1).
2. In acute hypernatremia (develops in less than 24 hours), water can be replaced rapidly. In chronic hypernatremia or hypernatremia of unknown duration, the rate of correction should not exceed 0.5 mEq/L/hr or 10 mEq/L/24 hr (Kapoor & Chan, 2001). Worsening neurologic status during free water replacement may indicate the development of cerebral edema and requires prompt re-evaluation and temporary discontinuation of water replacement. Volume depletion should be corrected before replacement therapy is initiated to correct the deficit.

Table 26-1	VOLUME STATUS GUIDE FOR SODIUM CORRECTION		
Type of Hypernatremia	Common Oncologic Settings	State of Body Sodium	Treatment
Hypovolemic hypernatremia	Uncontrolled DM, DI, uncontrolled nausea/vomiting/diarrhea or inability to consume fluids because of mucositis, high-protein tube feedings	Low total body sodium	Restore hemodynamics with NS, then change to D5W or ½ NS
Hypervolemic hypernatremia	Adenomas, Cushing's syndrome, administration of steroids	Excess total body sodium	Give loop diuretics to increase Na excretion and then replace D5W to correct hypertonicity. Dialyze if kidneys are not working.
Euvolemic hypernatremia	Elderly, CHF, kidney damaged	Normal total body sodium	Give D5W

3. In patients with hypovolemic hypernatremia, normal saline solution is indicated initially to correct the intravascular volume deficit. When that has been accomplished, more hypotonic fluids (e.g., 0.45% NS) can be used. In patients with hypervolemic hypernatremia, removing the source of salt excess, administering diuretics, and replacing water are important to successful therapy

4. **Medications:** Acute corrections may be managed with IV desmopressin (DDAVP) given over 2 to 3 days. Intranasal desmopressin may be used in chronic cases of hypernatremia (Robertson, 2001). In hypervolemic hypernatremia and euvolemic hypernatremia, diuretics may be used (Fall, 2000). In nephrogenic DI, discontinue drugs that inhibit renal response to ADH, such as catecholamines or phenytoin (Reynolds et al., 2006).

5. Assess vital signs and neurologic status every 4 hours until the sodium level is normal.

6. Maintain the airway; keep resuscitation and suction and seizure precaution equipment at the bedside until the serum sodium level is normal.

7. Measure intake and output every 4 hours. Weigh the patient daily.

8. Encourage oral fluids if the patient is dehydrated.

9. Provide a low-sodium diet.

10. Prepare the patient for surgery if intracerebral or adrenal tumors are to be removed.

11. Prepare the patient for chemotherapy if he or she will be receiving adjuvant treatment.

12. Prepare the patient for radiation therapy if the individual will be undergoing radiation treatment for brain tumors that affect pituitary ADH secretion.

EVIDENCE-BASED PRACTICE UPDATES

1. Patients with euvolemic hypernatremia usually require water replacement alone, either free water orally or an infusion of 5% dextrose in water (Fall, 2000).

2. Overly rapid correction of the sodium level may result in cerebral edema (Kapoor & Chan, 2001; Androgué & Madias, 2000).

3. Hypernatremia that occurs acutely (in less than 24 hours) may result in rapid brain shrinkage and can lead to intracranial hemorrhage from traction on dural veins and venous sinuses. Chronic hypernatremia manifests with milder symptoms because the brain has had time to adapt by accumulating intracellular solutes, thus restoring intracellular volume toward normal (Kapoor & Chan, 2001).

4. Severe symptoms of hypernatremia usually are evident only with acute and large increases in the plasma sodium concentration (i.e., above 158 to 160 mEq/L) (Reynolds et al., 2006).
5. Thirst may be absent in two thirds of elderly patients with hypernatremia (Chassagne et al., 2006).

TEACHING AND EDUCATION

1. Explain the individual patient's known cause of hypernatremia or the importance of determining the cause to prevent further episodes.
2. Explain the treatment goal of reducing the serum sodium level to normal and the need for frequent monitoring of the patient's vital signs, neurologic status, and blood tests.
3. Teach the patient and family about the patient's medications (i.e., name, dosage, route, frequency, purpose, and side effects).
4. Explain the need for restricting sodium in both dietary intake and over-the-counter medications (e.g., antacids). Major dietary sources of sodium are canned soups and vegetables, processed meats, salt, salty snack foods, cheese, ketchup, and seafood.
5. Teach the patient and family the signs and symptoms of hypernatremia: altered mental status, irritability, restlessness, lethargy, muscular twitching, spasticity, hyperreflexia, and abnormal thirst (see Box 26-1).
6. Educate cancer patients about the proper use of antiemetics and how and when to notify the health care provider if their nausea or vomiting is uncontrolled.
7. Teach the patient and family the proper use of antidiarrheals; this is imperative, especially for patients treated with diarrhea-inducing drugs (e.g. irinotecan) to prevent dehydration.

NURSING DIAGNOSES

1. **Deficient fluid volume** related to fluid loss from osmotic diuresis or DI; specific oncology patient confounders may include uncontrolled nausea and vomiting, diarrhea, or decreased fluid intake
2. **Excess fluid volume** related to fluid retention secondary to excessive ADH secretion; specific concerns in oncology patients (in whom excessive ADH secretion may cause hypernatremia) include Cushing's syndrome, high doses of glucocorticoids, and adenomas
3. **Risk for injury** related to altered mental status or neurologic decline; specific oncologic settings in which hypernatremia could lead to injury include uncontrolled seizures, lethargy or confusion, or intensive care areas, where the patient relies on others for fluids or is unable to communicate verbally
4. **Acute confusion** related to dehydration or fluid overload; oncology patients are at high risk for fluid volume shifts related to GI loss of fluid volume or fluid retention as a result of treatment or tumor effects
5. **Deficient knowledge** related to (1) hypernatremia (cause of and signs and symptoms); (2) medication management; and (3) potential for recurrence; oncology patient and caregiver education should be directed at safe medication management and follow-up

EVALUATION AND DESIRED OUTCOMES

1. With acute hypernatremia, the serum sodium level will be reduced at a maximum rate of 1 mEq/L every 2 hours, with the goal of obtaining a normal serum sodium level.

2. With nonacute hypernatremia, IV fluids and medication treatment will be initiated within the first few hours of diagnosis, with a normal serum sodium level achieved within a few days.
3. Complications from hypernatremia will be prevented.
4. Nurses will realize that hypernatremia is best prevented by recognizing patients at risk for the disorder. Memorizing a list of conditions that place a person at risk for hypernatremia is not necessary, as long as nurses understand that hypernatremia requires at least one of the following to occur: impaired access to water or a massive sodium load (Achinger et al., 2006).
5. Hyperglycemia will be corrected, and the glucose level will be stabilized.

DISCHARGE PLANNING AND FOLLOW-UP CARE

- **Medications:** The patient and caregivers need education about medications prescribed to treat the underlying condition, including the name, purpose, dosage, route, frequency, and expected and possible side effects.
- **Laboratory evaluation:** The patient should be discharged with a follow-up plan to have blood drawn to evaluate sodium and hydration status.
- **Home care:** If the patient is leaving the acute care setting but still needs nursing assistance (e.g., cognitive impairment, physical or social situation inadequate to offer a safe home environment), arrangements need to be established and communicated for ongoing health maintenance.
- **Referrals:** If an underlying condition is discovered during the evaluation and management of hypernatremia, outpatient referrals needs to be arranged for follow up. For example, setting appointments with an oncologist or surgeon after discharge facilitates ongoing care and follow up. Patients who have hyperaldosteronism or central DI may need referral to an endocrinologist. Patients with renal failure or nephrotic syndrome or those in need of dialysis will need referral to a nephrologist.
- **Nursing care for evaluation and symptom management:** Patients may need frequent assessment and intravenous fluid intervention if they are having large fluid volume losses secondary to chemotherapies (e.g., irinotecan-induced diarrhea). Nurses perform most telephone triage for outpatient cancer patients and have a unique opportunity to provide symptom evaluation and management (e.g., intervention for chemotherapy-induced nausea and vomiting or early evaluation for fever).
- **Nutritional evaluation and education:** Patients and caregivers need strategies for managing salt restrictions (making food choices that are lower in salt), ensuring an adequate fluid intake (especially patients receiving tube feedings or those with limited mobility), and facilitating free access to water for patients who are immobile (e.g., placing water within reach) or who do not have a thirst mechanism.

REVIEW QUESTIONS

QUESTIONS

1. **Hypernatremia is defined as:**
   1. Serum sodium greater than 150 mEq/L
   2. Serum sodium greater than 135 mEq/L
   3. Serum sodium greater than 145 mEq/L
   4. Serum sodium greater than 160 mEq/L

2. Severe neurologic symptoms of hypernatremia are most evident at which measured serum sodium level:
   1. Na >160 mEq/L
   2. Na >145 mEq/L
   3. Na >170 mEq/L
   4. Na >135 mEq/L

3. Differential diagnosis of hypernatremia does *not* include which of the following:
   1. Dehydration
   2. CNS malignancy
   3. Hypoaldosteronism
   4. None of the above

4. An increased plasma osmolality always exists with which of the following:
   1. Hyperglycemia
   2. Hypernatremia
   3. Hypokalemia
   4. All of the above

5. The most likely cause of hypernatremia in an otherwise clinically stable patient with no IV access who relies on tube feedings for nutrition is:
   1. Decreased renal urinary concentrating ability
   2. Lack of free-water intake
   3. Impaired neurologic status
   4. Lack of intravenous fluid management

6. Improper acute correction of hypernatremia in a patient who has had hypernatremia for a long period of time may result in:
   1. Brain herniation and death
   2. Seizures
   3. Permanent neurologic impairment from brain damage
   4. All of the above

7. A young woman is in your care in the postsurgical setting after having a craniopharyngioma resection less than 24 hours ago. The patient is intubated, febrile, and agitated and has a serum sodium level of 160 mEq/L.

Her serum sodium 12 hours ago was 145 mEq/L. Which intravenous fluid do you anticipate hanging:
   1. D5W
   2. 0.9% NS
   3. 0.45% NS
   4. 0.3% NS

8. A young woman has a large germ cell tumor involving the pineal gland. She is status post 4 cycles of cisplatin + etoposide and is currently undergoing regional radiation therapy. She presents to your clinic reporting intermittent polyuria and polydipsia for the past 2 weeks. Her sodium level is 148 mEq/L. Which condition is the primary cause of her symptoms:
   1. Nephrogenic DI
   2. Hypernatremia
   3. Central DI
   4. Hyperaldosteronism

9. The two main mechanisms of defense against hypernatremia are:
   1. ADH secretion and the conversion of angiotensin I to angiotensin II
   2. ADH release and increased urine output
   3. ADH release and thirst
   4. Aldosterone suppression and thirst

10. Which cluster of age-related changes predisposes the elderly to hypernatremia:
   1. Decrease in total body water, decreased effectiveness of ADH, increased urine concentrating ability, and altered sense of thirst
   2. Decreased mobility, decreased urine concentrating ability, and increase in total body water
   3. Decrease in total body water, altered sense of thirst, decreased effectiveness of ADH, and decrease in renal urine concentrating ability
   4. Confusion, increased sense of thirst, and decreased effectiveness of ADH

ANSWERS

1. *Answer: 3*
   Rationale: A normal serum sodium range is 135 to 145 mEq/L. Therefore a serum sodium level greater than 145 mEq/L defines hypernatremia.

2. *Answer: 1*
   Rationale: Severe neurologic symptoms are evident with acute and large increases in plasma sodium greater than 160 mEq/L.

3. *Answer: 3*
   Rationale: Hypoaldosteronism may actually lead to hyponatremia. Aldosterone is a steroid hormone that increases sodium and fluid retention at the distal tubule of the kidney. With a deficiency of aldosterone, sodium and water are not adequately retained.

4. *Answer: 2*
   Rationale: Although glucose is a contributor to osmolality, only extreme cases of hyperglycemia (i.e., HHNK) directly contribute to increased plasma osmolality. Sodium is the major extracellular solute and is the main plasma osmolality contributor, over urea and glucose.

5. *Answer: 2*
   Rationale: Patients who receive high-protein tube feedings that are not supplemented with water may have decreased urinary concentrating ability as a result of damage to the renal tubules; administration of free water may help protect the kidneys in this setting of decreased plasma volume.

6. *Answer: 4*
   Rationale: Overly rapid correction of chronic hypernatremia results in swelling of brain cells, intracranial edema, and possibly extreme and irreversible brain damage or even death. If a patient develops new or worsening neurologic symptoms during free water replacement, the replacement should be promptly discontinued and the patient re-evaluated.

7. *Answer: 1*
   Rationale: The young woman's hypernatremia is acute (<24 hours in onset), and although she did have a cranial surgical procedure, the sodium overload is most likely related to fluid administration by the health care team. D5W would be indicated first to carefully correct the fluid (water to sodium) balance.

8. *Answer: 3*
   Rationale: Her symptoms are due to central diabetes insipidus caused by tumor and/or treatment effects (i.e., radiation therapy) involving the hypothalamic region. This leads to an inability to secrete ADH adequately in response to systemic needs.

9. *Answer: 3*
   Rationale: ADH release and thirst are the two main defense mechanisms against hypernatremia. ADH results in maximal urinary concentration (thereby increasing sodium and water reabsorption). Increased plasma osmolality stimulates osmoreceptors in the hypothalamus, which triggers the powerful thirst sensation. This sensation is so strong that rarely will an alert person who is able to consume water at will develop hypernatremia.

10. *Answer: 3*
    Rationale: The four major age-related changes that predispose the elderly to dehydration and hypernatremia are a decrease in total body water, an altered sense of thirst, decreased effectiveness of ADH, and a decrease in renal urine concentrating ability.

REFERENCES

Achinger, S., Moritz, M., & Ayus, J. (2006). Dysnatremias: Why are patients still dying? *Southern Medical Journal, 99*(4):353-362.

Androgué, H., & Madias, N. (2000). Hypernatremia. *New England Journal of Medicine, 342*(20):1581-1599.

Arinzon, Z., Feldman, J., & Peisakh, A., et al. (2005). Water and sodium disturbances predict prognosis of acute diseases in long term cared frail elderly. *Archives of Gerontology & Geriatrics, 40*(30):317-326.

Chassagne, P., Druesne, L., & Capet, C., et al. (2006). Clinical presentation of hypernatremia in elderly patients: A case control study. *Journal of the American Geriatrics Society, 54*(8):1225-1230.

Fall, P. (2000). Hyponatremia and hypernatremia: A systematic approach to causes and their correction. *Postgraduate Medicine, 107*(5):75-82.

Fojo, A. (2005). Metabolic emergencies. In V. DeVita, S. Hellman, & S. Rosenberg (Eds.), *Cancer: Principles and practice of oncology* (pp. 2295-2296). (7th ed.). Philadelphia: Lippincott Williams & Wilkins.

Healy, P., & Jacobson, E. (1994). *Common medical diagnosis: An algorithmic approach.* (2nd ed.). Philadelphia: W.B. Saunders.

Himmelstein, D., Jones, A., & Woolhandler, S. (1983). Hypernatremic dehydration in nursing home patients: An indicator of neglect. *Journal of the American Geriatrics Society, 31*(8):466-471.

Kapoor, M., & Chan, G. (2001). Fluid and electrolyte abnormalities. *Critical Care Clinics, 17*(3):503-529.

Kugler, J., & Hustead, T. (2000). Hyponatremia and hypernatremia in the elderly. *American Family Physician, 61*(12):3623-3630.

Metheny, N. (2000). *Fluid and electrolyte balance: Nursing considerations.* (4th ed.). Philadelphia: Lippincott Williams & Wilkins.

Murphy-Ende, K. (2006a). Dynamics of fluids and electrolytes. In C. Chernecky, D. Maclin, & K. Murphy-Ende (Eds.), *Fluid and electrolytes* (pp. 8, 12, 56-57). (2nd ed.). Philadelphia: W.B. Saunders.

Murphy-Ende, K. (2006b). Thirst. In D. Camp-Sorrell, & R. Hawkins (Eds.), *Clinical manual for the oncology advanced practice nurse* (pp. 997-1001). (2nd ed.). Pittsburgh: Oncology Nursing Society.

Palevsky, P., Bhagrath, R., & Greenberg, A. (1996). Hypernatremia in hospitalized patients. *Annals of Internal Medicine, 124*(2):197-203.

Polderman, K., Schreuder, W., & van Schijndel, R., et al. (1999). Hypernatremia in the intensive care unit: An indicator of quality of care? *Critical Care Medicine, 27*(6):1105-1108.

Reynolds, R., Padfield, P., & Seckl, J. (2006). Disorders of sodium balance. *British Medical Journal, 332*(7543):702-705.

Robertson, G. (2001). Antidiuretic hormone: Normal and disordered function. *Endocrinology and Metabolism Clinics, 30*(3):671-694.

Schulz, K. (1998). Hypernatremia. In C. Chernecky, & B. Berger (Eds.), *Advanced and critical care oncology nursing* (pp. 298-313). Philadelphia: W.B. Saunders.

Shibata, S. (2000). A drug over the millennia: pharmacognosy, chemistry, and pharmacology of licorice. *Journal of the Pharmaceutical Society of Japan, 120*(10):849-862.

Tisdall, M., Crocker, M., & Watkiss, J., et al. (2006). Disturbances of sodium in critically ill adult neurologic patients. *Journal of Neurosurgical Anesthesiology, 18*(1):57-63.

White, P. (1994). Disorders of aldosterone biosynthesis and action. *New England Journal of Medicine, 331*(4):250-258.

HYPERSENSITIVITY REACTIONS TO CHEMOTHERAPY

TERESA KUNTZSCH • CASSIE A. VOGE

PATHOPHYSIOLOGICAL MECHANISMS

A hypersensitivity reaction (HSR) is defined as "an exaggerated immune response that results in local tissue injury or changes throughout the body in response to an antigen or foreign substance" (Gobel, 2005). HSRs are divided into four categories of HSRs (Table 27-1). Anaphylactic reactions (IgE mediated) and anaphylactoid reactions (not IgE mediated) are regarded as type I HSRs. Anaphylaxis occurs on subsequent exposure to the antigen after the previous exposure causes the formation of gamma E immunoglobulin antibodies (Held-Warmkessel, 2005). Most reactions to antineoplastic agents are thought to be type I reactions, because the signs and symptoms seen are clinically consistent with this type of reaction.

Regardless of the specific type of reaction, a rapid release of mediators occurs, including histamine, prostaglandins, and leukotrienes. This mediator release is responsible for the clinical manifestations of the HSR. Mast cells contain immunoglobulin E (IgE) receptors on the cell surface and store histamine, heparin, and serotonin. IgE is produced by the B lymphocytes in response to exposure to an antigen. Antigen IgE binds mast cells sensitizing to the antigen. When the sensitized mast cell is exposed a second time to the antigen, the mast cell receives a message to degranulate, releasing the above-mentioned chemical mediators. All these mediators cause the signs and symptoms of anaphylaxis, namely, vasodilation, capillary permeability, and contraction of smooth muscles (Sheffer & Horan, 1993). These physiologic changes cause edema, decreased volume, hypotension, and constricted bronchial airway passages. Patients show signs and symptoms ranging from mild discomfort to respiratory arrest, circulatory collapse, and death.

Although it is important that oncology nurses understand the physiologic mechanisms underlying the different HSRs (anaphylactic and anaphylactoid), the treatment of HSRs is the same.

EPIDEMIOLOGY AND ETIOLOGY

The incidence of HSRs associated with the administration of antineoplastic agents has been estimated at 5% to 15% (Weiss, 1997; Labovich, 1999). However, incidence rates are often underreported, and much of the current literature and the case reports are anecdotal.

Table 27-1	**HYPERSENSITIVITY REACTIONS TO CHEMOTHERAPY**		
Reaction Type	**Cells Involved**	**Pathophysiologic Response**	**Examples**
I	IgE mediated, mast cells, and basophils	Immediate, IgE mediated	Bee stings, penicillin allergy, most HSRs to antineoplastic agents
II	IgG or IgM mediated	Antibody mediated	Blood product transfusion reaction
III	Antigen-antibody	Immune-complex mediated	Systemic lupus erythematosus (SLE), serum sickness
IV	Cell mediated; T cells react with antigen to release lymphokines	Delayed	Graft rejection, contact dermatitis

The incidence varies depending on specific drug classification, individual patient sensitivity, and drug formulation (excipient), and no common pathway is known.

RISK PROFILE

All medications have the potential to cause an HSR. Certain drugs, drug-specific characteristics, and patient risk factors influence the severity and occurrence of HSRs. The most commonly implicated antineoplastic agents are taxanes, platinum compounds, monoclonal antibodies, epipodophyllotoxins, asparaginase, bleomycin, and liposomal preparations (Box 27-1). Drug characteristics that influence the development of anaphylaxis include the route of entry and the rate of antigen absorption. Therefore, administering a highly concentrated intravenous drug presents a greater likelihood of an HSR than administration of an oral preparation (Labovich, 1999). Preparation-related risk factors that increase the likelihood of an HSR include medications derived from live organisms (i.e., bacteria) or animal sources (i.e., murine) and the presence of an excipient (Cremophor EL) (Gobel, 2005).

Patient-related risk factors can help delineate a population that may be more susceptible to developing an HSR. A thorough patient history is necessary, including past reactions to other medications, foods, radiographic contrast dye, and bee stings. Research seems to suggest that patients who have environmental (bee sting) or medication allergies and who undergo platinum- or taxane-based chemotherapy regimens may be at increased risk of developing an HSR (Markman et al., 2003a; Grosen et al., 2000).

If a medication has a predictable high probability of initiating an HSR, premedication is indicated (Box 27-2). Premedication typically includes a histamine-2 (H_2) receptor antagonist (ranitidine or cimetidine), a corticosteroid (dexamethasone), and a histamine-1 (H_1) receptor antagonist (diphenhydramine). Although premedication reduces the overall incidence of HSRs, reactions do still occur. Gathering and evaluating data to assess a patient's overall risk profile are vital; however, it is important to note that no reliable method exists for predicting which patients will experience a hypersensitivity reaction.

All HSRs express similar clinical manifestations. However, individual drugs or drug classes have unique characteristics that should be considered in preparing for and managing a hypersensitivity event (e.g., time of onset, severity, recommended premedication drugs, mechanism responsible for precipitating the HSR). In the following sections these unique characteristics are highlighted for the drug categories responsible for most antineoplastic HSRs.

BOX 27-1	MEDICATIONS THAT MAY CAUSE A HYPERSENSITIVITY REACTION

High Probability
Carboplatin (especially more than 6 cycles)
Oxaliplatin (in heavily pretreated patients)
Cisplatin
Paclitaxel (especially in cycles 1 and 2)
Docetaxel
Murine monoclonal antibodies
Etoposide
Teniposide
L-asparaginase
Moderate Probability
Doxorubicin
Daunorubicin
Idarubicin
Epirubicin
Low Probability
Bleomycin
Mercaptopurine
Azathioprine
Chlorambucil
Melphalan
Cyclophosphamide
Ifosfamide
Cytarabine
Fludarabine
Dacarbazine
Dactinomycin
Fluorouracil
Hydroxyurea
Methotrexate
Vincristine
Vinblastine

Taxanes

Taxanes often are one of the first classes of chemotherapeutic drugs mentioned with regard to chemotherapy and HSRs. The incidence rate for HSRs with paclitaxel and docetaxel ranges from 2% to 4% with appropriate premedication (Shepherd, 2003). The excipients in which these chemotherapeutic drugs are dissolved are thought to be the likely culprits in taxane-related HSRs. Cremophor EL is used to formulate paclitaxel, and polysorbate 80 (Tween 80) is the diluent for docetaxel. ONS guidelines recommend premedication for paclitaxel and docetaxel as follows:

BOX 27-2	POSSIBLE PREMEDICATION REGIMEN FOR PACLITAXEL THERAPY

- Dexamethasone 20 mg PO 12 hours and 6 hours before start of paclitaxel infusion *OR* dexamethasone 20 mg IV immediately before start of infusion.
- Ranitidine 50 mg IV 30 minutes before start of infusion.
- Diphenhydramine 50 mg IV 30 minutes before start of infusion.

- *Paclitaxel:* Premedicate to help prevent HSRs, including anaphylaxis: cimetidine 300 mg IV 30-60 minutes before treatment, and diphenhydramine 50 mg IV 30-60 minutes before treatment; also (unless contraindicated) dexamethasone 20 mg IV 30-60 minutes before treatment (Polovich et al., 2005).
- *Docetaxel:* Premedicate to reduce the severity of HSRs and fluid retention: dexamethasone 8 mg PO BID, beginning 1 day before docetaxel treatment and continuing for the day of treatment and 1 day after (Polovich et al., 2005).

As mentioned, even with appropriate premedication, HSRs can occur. In these cases, the patient and medical staff need to discuss whether rechallenge is appropriate (i.e., infusing the same or a similar compound after an HSR, usually with additional drugs used in the premedication regimen). It is important to note that a patient who has a reaction to one of the taxanes is not any more likely to react to the other (Gobel, 2005). Increasing the infusion time or titrating the start of these medications may aid successful desensitization.

Platinum Compounds

Platinum-induced HSRs tend to occur in heavily pretreated patients. Platinum compounds as a group are associated with an HSR incidence rate of 10% to 27% (Gobel, 2005). The success rate for rechallenge varies and likely depends on the premedication regimen, time of infusion, and concentration of the agent.

Although carboplatin is used in a variety of patient populations, most research related to HSRs is reported in the gynecologic oncology literature (typically patients with ovarian carcinoma). Studies report an HSR incidence rate of 5% to 34% in this patient population (Dizon et al., 2002). A significant point of interest with carboplatin HSRs is that they are far more likely to occur after at least 6 cycles of the drug (Markman et al., 2004; Jones et al., 2003; Rose et al., 2003), which suggests that sensitization to the agent plays a role in the development of the reaction. Some studies report that reactions can occur within minutes of administration, but they also can occur days after the exposure (Dizon et al., 2002). Other studies state that HSRs to carboplatin usually occur after approximately 50% of the agent has been administered (Rose et al., 2003; Markman et al., 1999).

Most of the literature describing rechallenges involves patients with documented HSRs to carboplatin. One study describes a successful crossover rechallenge with cisplatin in 5 of 7 (71%) patients who initially developed HSRs to carboplatin (Dizon et al., 2002). A similar crossover study reports an initial successful rechallenge in five patients after full desensitization. The desensitization protocol included daily dexamethasone and diphenhydramine for 4 days before the day of treatment; diphenhydramine on the morning of treatment; an intradermal skin test; premedication with ranitidine, dexamethasone, and ondansetron; and then a titrated schedule of cisplatin (starting at 50 mL of {1/1000} of a full dose of the drug over 30 minutes and subsequently increasing the concentration while reducing the infusion time) (Jones et al., 2003). Later cycles ultimately were discontinued because three patients had disease progression and two developed HSRs (Jones et al., 2003).

Another study reported an 88% success rate (29 of 33 patients) on initial rechallenge with the same agent (carboplatin) (Rose et al., 2003). This prolonged desensitization protocol, as detailed by Rose and colleagues (2003), involved a 15- to 16-hour gradually increase in the concentration of the chemotherapeutic agent, with premedication. However, three more patients (of the initial 29 who were successfully rechallenged) developed HSRs to carboplatin during subsequent cycles 2 through 6 (Rose et al., 2003).

Markman and colleagues (2003a) found that intradermal skin testing (at initiation of second-line therapy/cycle 6 and above) may help predict the probability that a patient will *not* react to carboplatin. They stated, "A negative carboplatin skin test seems to predict with reasonable reliability for the absence of a severe hypersensitivity reaction with the subsequent drug infusion. The implications of a positive test remain less certain." The authors also reported a 1.5% false positive rate. In another study, Markman and coworkers (2004) built on previous research and developed a novel desensitization strategy for patients with positive skin tests or documented HSRs to carboplatin. Theorizing that the underlying mechanisms responsible for the carboplatin-related HSRs are complex and multifactorial, the authors developed a multipronged approach. Cisplatin was substituted for carboplatin for most of the patients with positive skin test results to carboplatin. Patients also received an extensive multidrug premedication regimen aimed at preventing an HSR. The drugs used for premedication included oral prednisone, histamine receptor antagonists (H_1 and H_2 blockers), indomethacin, albuterol sulfate, montelukast, Zileuton, diphenhydramine, and dexamethasone. Skin testing with cisplatin or carboplatin was done immediately before infusion of the first dilution of the agent. Then, escalating concentrations of cisplatin or carboplatin were infused. Four of the five patients in the study were successfully rechallenged. One patient had a positive skin test result immediately before the infusion and therefore was not rechallenged.

Although carboplatin is the platinum agent of choice in most circumstances because of its greater efficacy and more desirable side effect profile, cisplatin is still used in a number of patient populations. The incidence of IV cisplatin–related HSRs is reported to be 5% (Koren et al., 2002). Recent evidence suggests that concurrent pelvic radiation therapy increases a patient's risk of developing an HSR threefold (4 out of 25, or 16%) (Koren et al., 2002). Researchers theorize that this is due to increased cytokine release from the tumor.

One approach to cisplatin-related HSRs is crossover to carboplatin, although cross-sensitivity has been reported (Zanotti & Markman, 2001). Some case reports in the HSR literature cite an association with intraperitoneal administration of cisplatin (Ozguroologes et al., 1999). With the recent resurgence of intraperitoneal administration of cisplatin (Armstrong et al., 2006), additional information may become available regarding the incidence rate, premedication regimens, and treatment for these specific HSRs.

Oxaliplatin is a third-generation platinum compound that is effective in treating advanced colorectal cancer (Brandi et al., 2002), as well as pancreatic, ovarian, and non-small cell lung cancer (Lenz et al., 2003). The incidence of HSRs to oxaliplatin is reported to be 0.5% to 13% (Brandi et al., 2002). Patients may have an HSR upon first exposure or after a number of cycles (Brandi et al., 2002), which suggests differing underlying mechanisms (anaphylactoid versus anaphylactic). Symptoms generally occur within minutes of starting the infusion (Lenz et al., 2003; Brandi et al., 2002) but have been known to occur after the infusion is complete (Mis et al., 2005). Rechallenge was unsuccessful in one study (Lenz et al., 2003) but successful in another with the addition of dexamethasone, cimetidine, diphenhydramine, acetaminophen, and granisetron (Dold et al., 2002). Some studies suggest that extending the infusion time from 2 hours to 6 hours may reduce the incidence of oxaliplatin-induced HSRs to 1% (Maindrault-Goebel et al., 2001; Giacchetti et al., 2000). A more recent study describes a variety of desensitization protocols involving histamine blockade, serial dilutions of oxaliplatin, and lengthening the infusion time up to 8 hours (Mis et al., 2005).

Monoclonal Antibodies

The incidence of HSRs caused by monoclonal antibodies is directly related to how humanized the medication is (Polovich et al., 2005). The oncology nurse should be fully prepared for a reaction to murine and chimeric (a combination of murine and humanized antibodies) preparations. These reactions can occur on first exposure and on subsequent exposures. Within 30 minutes of the start of the infusion, many patients show symptoms such as rigor, chills, and temperature elevation. Fever and chills are common side effects of monoclonal antibodies that would not be expected in other chemotherapy-related HSRs (Carr & Burke, 2001). Standard protocols for these medications should include premedication, emergency medications (including meperidine to ameliorate rigors), a titration schedule, and monitoring requirements (Polovich et al., 2005).

Epipodophyllotoxins

HSRs to etoposide and teniposide have been reported, although the incidence rate may be as low as 6% (Gobel, 2005). These reactions appear within the first 10 minutes of the infusion and can occur on initial or repeated exposure (Siderov et al., 2002). The underlying mechanism of these HSRs is thought to be related to the excipient used to dissolve the drug into an aqueous solution. Etoposide HSRs are related to the polysorbate 80 (Tween 80) used to dissolve the drug (Weiss, 1997). This assumption is supported by the evidence that there are no reported HSRs to oral etoposide and that patients have been successfully rechallenged with etoposide phosphate (Siderov et al., 2002). Teniposide is solubilized in the excipient Cremophor EL; as with the taxanes (Gobel, 2005), this specific excipient is thought to cause the HSRs seen with this drug. Although these drugs have a low incidence of HSRs, nurses need to remain vigilant in monitoring patients for HSRs throughout the duration of treatment cycles.

Asparaginase

Asparaginase HSRs occur in 10% to 25% of patients (Carr & Burke, 2001). They can occur on first administration, although they are more common with repeated administrations or when the drug is reintroduced after a break in the treatment plan of 1 week or longer (Wilkes & Barton-Burke, 2006). Intravenous administration increases the occurrence and severity of HSRs compared to intramuscular administration (Polovich et al., 2005; Zanotti & Markman, 2001). Also, patients have more HSRs with intermittent dosing than with continuous dosing (Zanotti & Markman, 2001). An HSR to asparaginase can occur immediately after administration or within 1 hour of intravenous or intramuscular administration. The clinical presentation can range from a mild rash to severe and potentially life-threatening complications. Skin testing is recommended before the first dose and if a break of 1 week or longer has occurred since the last exposure (Spratto & Woods, 2005). Because an asparaginase HSR likely is related to the use of a live bacterium (*Escherichia coli*) in the preparation (Skidmore-Roth, 2006; Zanotti & Markman, 2001), when an HSR occurs, the patient potentially can be treated with an alternative preparation of the drug, such as Erwinia carotovora L-asparaginase or polyethylene glycol–modified (PEG) asparaginase. Emergency medications should be readily available with these other preparations as well.

Bleomycin

HSRs to bleomycin are rare (1% of cases) (Shepherd, 2003). This low incidence may be due to the common practice of administering premedication (acetaminophen and diphenhydramine) before administration of bleomycin. However, patients with lymphoma have a higher incidence of HSRs after bleomycin administration (Polovich et al., 2005). These reactions can occur minutes into the infusion or up to several hours after the infusion is complete. The exact underlying mechanisms are unknown, but common characteristics of a bleomycin-related HSR include hypotension, confusion, tachycardia, wheezing, and facial edema. HSRs usually are seen with the first and second doses of bleomycin, and use of a test dose (1 to 2 units given IV, SQ, or IM) should be discussed. A test dose is recommended for patients with lymphoma before the first dose of bleomycin (Polovich et al., 2005). Symptoms generally resolve with the administration of emergency medications (e.g., histamine receptor antagonists).

Liposomal Preparations

Liposomal preparations, including doxorubicin hydrochloride liposomal injection, can precipitate an HSR. The incidence rate for HSRs with this drug is 7% (Wilkes & Barton-Burke, 2005). The common practice is to rechallenge with appropriate premedication (corticosteroids, histamine receptor antagonists), increase the infusion time, and consider slow titration of the infusion.

PROGNOSIS

After an HSR has occurred, the optimal outcome is successful readministration of the agent. The outcomes of HSRs vary depending on the severity of the reaction, the time to initiation of appropriate treatment, and the patient's degree of hypersensitivity. Although fatalities have been reported anecdotally, no published rates are available. With changes in the premedication regimen, infusion time, and chemical formulations, as well as possible use of crossover medications (carboplatin to cisplatin), rechallenge is possible. Skin testing (L-asparaginase) and administration of test doses before the first dose (bleomycin) historically have been used. Newer research suggests that skin testing for carboplatin HSRs may be useful (Zanotti & Markman, 2001).

PROFESSIONAL ASSESSMENT CRITERIA (PAC)

HSRs can manifest within seconds of drug administration, but they also can occur at seemingly random points during therapy. Immediate intervention is required for anaphylaxis. The possible the signs and symptoms of an HSR range from mild to life-threatening.

1. **Preadministration assessment:**
   - Allergy history
   - Previous exposure/recent treatment
   - Disease status/presentation
   - Verify or administer premedication drugs
   - Patient knowledge about reporting symptoms
   - Psychosocial status of patient and family
2. **Assessment during an HSR:**
   - General assessment (rash, facial or whole body flushing, obvious patient discomfort)
   - Subjective patient report (warmth, nausea, shortness of breath, back pain, feeling "different," a sense of impending doom, anxiety/panic)
   - ABC (airway, breathing, circulation) assessment (dyspnea, bronchospasm, laryngospasm, wheezing, angioedema, urticaria)
   - Vital signs (hypotension/hypertension, tachycardia/bradycardia, tachypnea, possible temperature elevation)
   - Initiate emergency protocol.
   - Alert health care provider.
3. **Assessment after an HSR:**
   - Continue to monitor vitals signs and ABCs until return to baseline.
   - Provide patient and family with support and education.

- Anticipate possible rechallenge.
- Make next day phone call in outpatient setting.

NURSING CARE AND TREATMENT

Prevention (the First Treatment)

1. Identification of drug, specific drug characteristics, and patient profile that increases the likelihood of an HSR.
2. Premedication (i.e., histamine receptor antagonists and corticosteroid).
3. Patient and family education to emphasize the importance of adhering to the premedication regimen.

Preparation for Possible HSR

1. Obtain/document baseline vital signs and assessment.
2. Keep emergency medications at bedside (Box 27-3), as well as emergency resuscitation equipment (i.e., crash cart).
3. Situate patient to optimize monitoring and treatment in the event of an HSR (close to nurse's station, near oxygen source and emergency equipment).
4. Assess for resource availability (additional medical/nursing personnel) in case of HSR and need for emergency protocol.
5. Skin test/test dose if indicated (reactions can occur up to 1 hour later or longer); observe for local or systemic reaction (Polovich, et al., 2005).

Assessment and Recognition of HSR

1. Close monitoring of high-risk situations, including continual RN presence, vital signs, and ongoing patient assessment.
2. Patient education about early signs and symptoms of an HSR and the importance of reporting any deviation from baseline.

Intervention for HSR

1. Immediately stop the chemotherapy infusion when an HSR is recognized.
2. Stay with the patient and alert another staff member to contact the health care provider immediately.
3. Keep venous access patent by infusing 0.9% normal saline.
4. Assess ABCs and vital signs (frequency depends on the patient's condition):
   - Airway (A)—angioedema/laryngoedema

BOX 27-3	EMERGENCY KIT FOR A HYPERSENSITIVITY REACTION

- Carpoject TM or Tubex TM
- 0.9% normal saline flushes/syringes
- Extra 0.9% normal saline and primed tubing (preferably connected via Y-site at most proximal port to patient)
- Oxygen tubing/mask
- Pulse oximeter
- Vital signs monitoring equipment (automatic blood pressure machine)
- Epinephrine
- Hydrocortisone
- Dexamethasone
- Diphenhydramine

- Breathing (B)—tachypnea
- Circulation (C)—hypotension/tachycardia/hypoxia
- Oxygen saturation (i.e., pulse oximetry):
  - Obtain and interpret oxygen saturation levels; signs of hypoxia include restlessness, dyspnea, anxiety, cyanosis, and bronchospasm.
  - Administer oxygen as needed.
5. Medications to ameliorate the HSR (medication administration depends on the specific symptoms):
  - Angioedema/laryngoedema/stridor: Epinephrine (1:1000 or 1:10,000) SQ rather than IV.
  - Monitor for cardiac arrhythmias related to use of epinephrine (Burns, 2004):
    - Mild to moderate wheezing: Inhaled bronchodilator and/or corticosteroids.
    - Hypotension: Intravenous fluid resuscitation.
    - Urticaria/rash: Diphenhydramine and/or corticosteroid.
    - Nausea/vomiting: Antiemetic.
    - Positioning: Supine or reverse Trendelenburg position.

Post-HSR Care

1. Continue to monitor vitals signs and ABCs until they return to baseline.
2. Anticipate possible rechallenge (readministration of the same agent).
3. Provide patient and family support and education about follow-up care and possible rechallenge.
4. Document treatment and the patient's response in the medical record.

Rechallenge

Oncology nurses face a number of nursing implications when the decision to rechallenge is made. These include providing the patient and family with education and support, ensuring that appropriate personnel and resources are available, and initiating and completing the chemotherapy infusion. Providing accurate and thorough information to patients and families is the first step in alleviating the natural emotions of fear and anxiety. HSRs often are a new experience for patients and families, at a time when these individuals must incorporate a cancer diagnosis and prognosis into their lives. Once a patient recovers from an HSR, the concern often becomes, "How am I going to be able to get the treatment to alleviate or minimize my cancer?" Patients and families frequently ask how often HSRs occur; however, quoting exact percentages from various articles, reports, and studies is not necessary. General possibilities should be explained. It is imperative that the patient understand the importance of his or her role in reporting *any* abnormal sensations, because these sometimes are the first signs of an HSR. The nurse is in the ideal role to provide ongoing support and reassurance to the patient and family, who may face the rechallenge with feelings of trepidation. Validating the emotions of the patient and family and normalizing their feelings can help put them more at ease and increase their comfort level.

Although it is not the staff nurse's primary responsibility to provide adequate staffing, the nurse probably will want to collaborate with the nurse manager, pharmacist, and responsible physician to make sure that appropriate personnel are available. The nurse must be able to provide one-on-one care and direct nursing supervision during the first 30 minutes of the rechallenge in the event of a second HSR.

The steps in initiating a rechallenge vary, depending on each institution's specific protocol. One commonality that rechallenge protocols are likely to have is the verification and/or administration of premedication drugs. The specific premedication drugs, dosages, routes, and time to be given before chemotherapy infusion will vary.

Defining rechallenge best practice is an interesting area of oncology research and one that continues to generate much professional literature. Currently, most publications available are anecdotes or case reports. Large, randomized, controlled trials are needed to provide evidence that supports the best strategy for developing the ideal protocol in rechallenging patients who have had an HSR to an antineoplastic agent. As always, the risks and benefits of any treatment-related decision must be fully explained to the patient and family so that they can make an informed choice based on the best information available.

EVIDENCE-BASED PRACTICE UPDATES

1. The use of crossover agents (carboplatin to cisplatin), lower concentration admixtures/ solutions, and administering the chemotherapeutic drug at a slower rate of infusion are all strategies reported in recent literature to reduce the likelihood of a second HSR (Gobel, 2005; Mis et al., 2005; Markman et al., 2004; Jones et al., 2003; Lenz et al., 2003; Dizon et al., 2002).
2. Patients who have environmental (bee sting) or medication allergies and who receive platinum- or taxane-based chemotherapy may be at increased risk of developing an HSR (Markman et al., 2003a; Rose et al., 2003; Grosen et al., 2000).

TEACHING AND EDUCATION

1. Before administration of the chemotherapy, provide general chemotherapy information:
   - Inform the patient of the risk profile of specific medications, their side effects and side effect management, and the drug schedule.
   - Ask the patient about his or her allergy history, sensitivities, and medication reactions in the past.
   - Explain the possibility of an allergic reaction with high-risk chemotherapeutic agents.
   - Instruct the patient to notify the nurse immediately if the patient feels anything "different," specifically, if the patient has any trouble breathing, feels flushed or warm, has chest or back pain, or feels anxious.
2. During an HSR:
   - Briefly explain the ongoing treatment to the patient and family.
   - Describe expected sensations and the outcomes of interventions.
3. After an HSR:
   - Discuss the possibility of discontinuing chemotherapy or of a rechallenge.
   - Provide support to the patient and family and provide contact numbers for additional questions and support.

NURSING DIAGNOSES

1. **Ineffective airway clearance** related to laryngeal edema and bronchospasm
2. **Ineffective tissue perfusion** related to hypotension and angioedema
3. **Anxiety** related to ineffective breathing pattern
4. **Fear** related to threat to disease prognosis
5. **Deficient knowledge** related to complexity of therapeutic regime (rechallenge)

EVALUATION AND DESIRED OUTCOMES

1. Vital signs will return to baseline.
2. Oxygenation saturation will return to baseline.
3. Subjective symptoms (e.g., rash, flushing, nausea, SOB) will resolve.
4. The patient's anxiety will be decreased.
5. The patient and family will verbalize the follow-up treatment plan.

6. The patient will not require increased medical intervention (e.g., IMC admission, extended stay).

DISCHARGE PLANNING AND FOLLOW-UP CARE

- Provide patient education on delayed signs and symptoms of an HSR and appropriate plan of action, including the name and phone number of the health care provider to call.
- Offer support and education about rechallenge or alternative therapy.
- Provide standard teaching for chemotherapy discharge, as appropriate.
- Assess safety of transport home and home environment.
- Schedule follow-up appointments for:
  - Rechallenge with premedication, or
  - New treatment regimen
  - Lab tests

REVIEW QUESTIONS

QUESTIONS

1. **An early sign of an HSR is:**
   1. A low oxygen saturation level
   2. Bradycardia
   3. Hypotension
   4. A patient states, "I don't feel right."

2. **When the nurse recognizes that an HSR is occurring, the first nursing action is:**
   1. Administer oxygen
   2. Alert the medical team/physician
   3. Stop the infusion
   4. Administer 0.9% normal saline

3. **Your patient states, "I'm so scared to retry my chemotherapy again. I felt like I was going to die when the reaction happened." Your best response is:**
   1. "It's okay, because reactions very rarely happen twice."
   2. "Most patients are anxious about undergoing a rechallenge. I will be right here with you to make sure you are safe. Please let me know if you feel anything different."
   3. "Don't worry so much, you'll be fine!"
   4. "The important thing is to tell me right away if you feel anything different."

4. **Your patient appears to be having a reaction to cycle 1 paclitaxel, and you** quickly obtain vital signs: BP 94/60, HR 100, RR 28 (no stridor or wheezing as yet), pulse oximetry 89% on room air. You anticipate the physician will order:
   1. Diphenhydramine
   2. Dexamethasone
   3. Epinephrine
   4. Ranitidine

5. **Most HSRs to antineoplastic agents are classified as which type of reaction:**
   1. I
   2. II
   3. III
   4. IV

6. **In your practice, you educate the patient and family about the cycle 1 paclitaxel/cycle 8 carboplatin regimen. As part of your education, you inform them that:**
   1. A hypersensitivity reaction is very likely to occur.
   2. A hypersensitivity reaction is not likely to occur.
   3. Although the possibility of a hypersensitivity reaction exists, many precautions are in place to prevent it. If one does occur, you and your colleagues are competent to ensure a safe outcome for the patient.
   4. A reaction is most likely to occur with cycle 1 of paclitaxel and/or cycle 8 of carboplatin.

7. In which of the following situations would you administer epinephrine:
1. Pulse oximetry of 88%
2. BP of 84/46
3. Severe stridor and obvious difficulty breathing
4. Slight wheezing

8. You are caring for four patients in an outpatient chemotherapy setting. The one most likely to have an HSR is undergoing:
1. Cycle 4 oxaliplatin
2. Cycle 2 paclitaxel
3. Cycle 2 docetaxel
4. Cycle 14 carboplatin

9. You are acting as a preceptor for a registered nurse who is new to the outpatient oncology practice. As you review the emergency protocol for patients having an HSR, she asks about the difference between an anaphylactoid and an anaphylactic reaction. You explain that:
1. It does not matter, because they are both HSRs and are treated the same.
2. An anaphylactic reaction occurs with a prior exposure, whereas an anaphylactoid response occurs without prior exposure.
3. They are the same.
4. An anaphylactoid response occurs with a prior exposure, and an anaphylactic reaction occurs without prior exposure.

10. An optimal outcome of HSR teaching for a patient would be:
1. The patient refuses treatment.
2. The patient states that he is not afraid of a reaction.
3. The patient has no reaction.
4. The patient can state the signs and symptoms of an HSR and knows the appropriate action to take (i.e., alert the nurse).

ANSWERS

1. *Answer: 4*
Rationale: The *earliest* sign (subjective) is often a patient stating that he or she feels different, "off," or "not right."

2. *Answer: 3*
Rationale: All the answer choices are important interventions during an HSR. However, the top priority is to prevent any further antigen exposure (i.e., introduction of the chemotherapeutic drug into the patient's bloodstream) in hopes of limiting the severity of the reaction.

3. *Answer: 2*
Rationale: This response validates and normalizes the patient's emotions with regard to the rechallenge while reassuring the patient and educating the individual about the most important part of his or her role in reporting subjective sensations.

4. *Answer: 1*
Rationale: The histamine receptor antagonist will block any further binding at the histamine site, thereby ameliorating a further reaction. A corticosteroid may be given next, because it helps to down-regulate the inflammatory response. Epinephrine is given only when a patient's airway is severely compromised (stridor, severe wheezing).

5. *Answer: 1*
Rationale: See Table 27-1.

6. *Answer: 3*
Rationale: This response informs the patient and family of the possibility of an HSR without causing undue concern. It also reassures the patient that systems are in place to prevent and ameliorate such a reaction.

7. *Answer: 3*
Rationale: Epinephrine has a number of side effects (e.g., arrhythmias, tachycardia, palpitations) (Skidmore-Roth, 2006) and should be given with caution in certain patients (e.g., those taking digitalis or tricyclic antidepressants). Therefore it is given only in emergency situations, when a patient's airway is severely compromised.

8. *Answer: 2*
Rationale: An HSR to paclitaxel is an example of a typical anaphylactic response in which a patient has had previous exposure to an antigen.

9. *Answer: 2*
Rationale: Although the two types of reactions are treated in the same way, anaphylaxis requires prior exposure to an antigen.

10. *Answer: 4*
Rationale: Because prevention and early detection are the best treatment for an HSR, it is imperative that the patient have the ability to be an active participant in the identification of such a reaction.

REFERENCES

Armstong, D. K., Bundy, B., & Wenzel, L., et al. (2006). Intrapertioneal Cisplatin and paclitaxel in ovarian cancer. *New England Journal of Medicine, 354:*34-43.

Brandi, G., Pantaleo, M. A., & Galli, C., et al. (2002). Hypersensitivity reactions related to oxaliplatin (OHP). *British Journal of Cancer, 89:*477-481.

Burns, A. (2004). Action stat: Anaphylaxis. *Nursing2004, 34*(3):88.

Carr, B. W., & Burke, C. (2001). Outpatient chemotherapy: Hypersensitivity and anaphylaxis. *American Journal of Nursing,* April 27-30.

Dizon, D. S., Sabbatini, P. J., & Aghajanian, C., et al. (2002). Analysis of patients with epithelial ovarian cancer or fallopian tube carcinoma retreated with cisplatin after the development of a carboplatin allergy. *Gynecologic Oncology, 84:*378-382.

Dold, F., Hoey, D., & Carbery, M., et al. (2002). Hypersensitivity in patients with metastatic colorectal carcinoma undergoing chemotherapy with oxaliplatin. *Proceedings of the American Society of Clinical Oncology, 38:*21.

Giacchetti, S., Perpoint, B., & Zidani, R., et al. (2000). Phase III randomized trial of oxaliplatin added to chronomodulated fluorouracil-leucovorin as first line treatment of metastatic colorectal cancer. *Journal of Clinical Oncology, 18:*136-147.

Gobel, B. H. (2005). Chemotherapy-induced hypersensitivity reactions. *Oncology Nursing Forum, 32*(5):1027-1055.

Grosen, E., Siitari, E., & Larrison, E., et al. (2000). Paclitaxel hypersensitivity reactions related to bee stings allergy (letter). *Lancet, 354:*288-289.

Held-Warmkessel, J. (2005). Managing three critical cancer complications. *Nursing2005, 35*(1):58-63.

Jones, R., Ryan, M., & Friedlander, M. (2003). Carboplatin hypersensitivity reactions: Re-treatment with cisplatin desensitization. *Gynecologic Oncology, 89:*112-115.

Koren, C., Yerushalmi, R., & Katz, A., et al. (2002). Hypersensitivity reaction to cisplatin during chemoradiation therapy for gynecologic malignancy. *American Journal of Clinical Oncology, 25*(6):625-626.

Labovich, T. M. (1999). Acute hypersensitivity reactions to chemotherapy. *Seminars in Oncology Nursing, 15:*(3):222-231.

Lenz, G., Hacker, U. T., & Kern, W., et al. (2003). Adverse reactions to oxaliplatin: A retrospective study of 25 patients treated in one institution. *Anti-Cancer Drugs, 14*(9):731-733.

Maindrault-Goebel, F., De Gramont, A., & Louvet, C., et al. (2001). High-dose intensity oxaliplatin added to the simplified bimonthly leucovorin and 5-fluorouracil regimens as second-line therapy for metastatic colorectal cancer (FOLFOX-6). *European Journal of Cancer, 35:*1000-1005.

Markman, M., Kennedy, A., & Webster, K., et al. (1999). Clinical features of hypersensitivity reactions to carboplatin. *Journal of Clinical Oncology, 17*(4):1141-1145.

Markman, M., Zanotti, K., & Kulp, B., et al. (2003a). Relationship between a history of systemic allergic reactions and risk of subsequent carboplatin hypersensitivity. *Gynecologic Oncology 89:*514-516.

Markman, M., Zanotti, K., & Peterson, G., et al. (2003b). Expanded experience with an intradermal skin test to predict for the presence or absence of carboplatin hypersensitivity. *Journal of Clinical Oncology, 21*(24):4611-4614.

Markman, M., Hsieh, F., & Zanotti, K., et al. (2004). Initial experience with a novel desensitization strategy for carboplatin-associated hypersensitivity reactions: Carboplatin-hypersensitivity reactions. *Journal of Cancer Research in Clinical Oncology, 130:*25-28.

Mis, L., Fernando, N. H., & Hurwitz, H. I., et al. (2005). Successful desensitization to oxaliplatin. *Annals of Pharmacotherapy, 39:*966-969.

Ozguroologes, M., Demir, G., & Madel, N. M. (1999). Anaphylaxis form intraperitoneal infusion of cisplatin: A case report. *American Journal of Clinical Oncology, 22*(2):172-173.

Polovich, M., White, J. M., & Kelleher, L. O. (2005). *Chemotherapy and biotherapy guidelines and recommendations for practice.* (2nd ed.). Pittsburgh: Oncology Nursing Society.

Porzio, G., et al. (2002). Hypersensitivity reaction to carboplatin: Successful resolution by replacement with cisplatin. *European Journal of Gynecologic Oncology, 23*(4):335-336.

Rose, P. G., Fusco, N., & Smrekar, M., et al. (2003). Successful administration of carboplatin in patients with clinically documented carboplatin hypersensitivity. *Gynecologic Oncology, 89*:429-433.

Sheffer, A. L., & Horan, R. G. (1993). Anaphylaxis. In S. T. Holgate, M. K. Church, (Eds.), *Allergy* (pp. 27.1-27.10). London: 1993, Gower Medical Publishing.

Shepherd, G. M. (2003). Hypersensitivity reactions to chemotherapeutic drugs. *Clinical Reviews in Allergy and Immunology, 24*:253-262.

Siderov, J., Prasad, P., & Boer, R., et al. (2002). Short communication: Safe administration of etoposide phosphate after hypersensitivity reaction to intravenous etoposide. *British Journal of Cancer, 86*:12-13.

Skidmore-Roth, L. (2006). *Drug guide for nurses.* (6th ed.). St. Louis: Mosby.

Spratto, G., & Woods, A. (2005). 2006 Physician's desk reference: A nurses drug handbook. New York: Thomson.

Weiss, R. B. (1997). Miscellaneous toxicities: Hypersensitivity reactions. In V. T. DeVita, S., Hellman, & S. A. Rosenberg (Eds.), *Cancer: Principles and practice of oncology.* (5th ed.). Philadelphia: Lippincott-Raven.

Wilkes, G. M., & Barton-Burke, M. (2005). 2006 Oncology Nursing Drug Handbook. Sudbury, MA: Jones & Bartlett.

Zanotti, K. M., & Markman, M. (2001). Prevention and management of antineoplastic-induced hypersensitivity reactions. *Practical Drug Safety, 24*:(10):767-779.

HYPERURICEMIA

LIBBY MONTOYA

PATHOPHYSIOLOGICAL MECHANISMS

Hyperuricemia, an excessive amount of uric acid in the blood, is a potentially life-threatening metabolic complication that results from overproduction or inefficient elimination of uric acid or from a combination of these processes. Nonmalignant exogenous causes of an increased serum uric acid level may be related to a dietary intake of foods high in nucleic acid (e.g., liver, kidney, anchovies, and "sweetbreads" consisting of thymus and pancreas tissue) (Wartmann, 2004). Overproduction of uric acid may arise from endogenous sources of purine production, such as excessive degradation of skeletal muscle ATP after strenuous physical exercise or status epilepticus. Accelerated ATP breakdown may also explain hyperuricemia related to myocardial infarction, smoke inhalation, and acute respiratory failure. Inefficient elimination of uric acid may result from decreased glomerular filtration, decreased tubular secretion, or enhanced tubular reabsorption. More than 90% of individuals with sustained hyperuricemia have a defect in renal handling of uric acid. Prolonged hyperuricemia predisposes these individuals to gouty arthritis, urolithiasis, and renal dysfunction (Wartmann, 2004; Cairo & Bishop, 2004).

Hyperuricemia may occur in patients with rapidly proliferating malignancies, such as Burkitt's lymphoma or T cell acute lymphoblastic leukemia (ALL), and in patients with a malignancy involving a high tumor burden (Ribeiro & Pui, 2003; Schiffer, 2001). Hyperuricemia may be present when the cancer is diagnosed, or it may occur spontaneously before initiation of therapy, but it usually is present within 12 to 72 hours after initiation of therapy. Historically, it was associated with a high morbidity rate and delays in the delivery of chemotherapy (Rheingold & Lange, 2005; Pui et al., 1997). Early treatment and preventive measures now can prevent this potentially fatal complication.

Hyperuricemia occurs as a result of the release of purine nucleic acids, which are metabolized into hypoxanthine by the liver. The release of these acids may occur spontaneously as the result of ongoing cell death in a rapidly growing tumor, or as the result of cell death induced by chemotherapy. Hypoxanthine is converted into uric acid, a reaction that is catalyzed by xanthine oxidase. Uric acid crystals, in the presence of an acidic pH, precipitate in the renal tubules and obstruct urine flow in the tubules, causing acute obstructive uropathy, which may lead to renal failure (Del Toro et al., 2005; Fojo, 2005; Haut, 2005). Hyperuricemia may occur as an isolated metabolic complication or as one feature of a collection of metabolic derangements recognized as tumor lysis syndrome (see Chapter 48) (Shin et al., 2006).

EPIDEMIOLOGY AND ETIOLOGY

Hyperuricemia is present in approximately 5% of the general population and in up to 25% of hospitalized patients. Many of these individuals are completely asymptomatic with no clinical risk. However, if hyperuricemia is identified, the underlying cause should be determined and corrected (Wartmann, 2004).

The presence of hyperuricemia in the patient with cancer varies, depending on the type of malignancy. It is the direct result of the release of nucleic acids from destroyed malignant cells into the circulating blood system. Hyperuricemia has been reported in up to 50% of patients with acute myeloid leukemia (AML), and it may be associated with tumor lysis, although the full syndrome of tumor lysis is more frequently identified in acute lymphoblastic leukemia (ALL) (Greer et al., 2004). Hyperuricemia is a rare complication of cancer therapy for solid tumors, although reported cases likely underestimate the true incidence (Baeksgaard & Sorensen, 2003). A retrospective chart review of European cancer patients from 17 countries revealed that 13.6% of the reviewed cases had hyperuricemia alone, and an additional 5.3% had full tumor lysis syndrome (Annemans et al., 2003b).

If hyperuricemia is not prevented or goes untreated, the incidence of acute renal failure associated with the precipitation of uric acid crystals in the renal tubules may be as high as 30% in patients with Burkett's lymphoma, and renal sequelae may be irreversible (Cohen et al., 1980).

RISK PROFILE

- Patients whose neoplastic cells have a very active purine metabolism, have high nucleic acid and phosphorus content, and are highly sensitive to chemotherapy (Ribeiro & Pui, 2003; Brant, 2002).
- Features at presentation include leukocytosis, massive hepatomegaly and splenomegaly, large abdominal mass, extrinsic obstructive uropathy, and decreased urinary flow (Ribeiro & Pui, 2003).
- Pre-existing renal compromise resulting in impaired ability to clear tumor byproducts (Brant, 2002).
- Dehydration
- Infection
- Medications that may increase uric acid, such as thiazide diuretics, probenecid, salicylates, corticosteroids, furosemide, gentamycin, methicillin, niacin, rifampin, propranolol, and phenothiazines (Brant, 2002), or medications that may impair renal function, such as nonsteroidal antiinflammatory agents (NSAIDs) (Cantril & Haylock, 2004).
- Male gender (Tsimberidou & Keating, 2005)
- Age under 25 years (Tsimberidou & Keating, 2005)

PROGNOSIS

Prevention and management of hyperuricemia usually are successful in lowering patient morbidity (Brant, 2002). The formation of uric acid crystals in the renal tubules and subsequent renal dysfunction can occur with uric acid levels near 8.3 mg/dL. If significant renal dysfunction develops before or during other electrolyte abnormalities accompanying tumor lysis syndrome, preventing those abnormalities from becoming life-threatening is much more difficult (Hutcherson et al., 2006). Approximately 15% of patients with acute lymphoid malignancies, mainly those with a high tumor burden at diagnosis, develop renal failure requiring dialysis, which may compromise the optimal delivery of chemotherapy (Ribeiro & Pui, 2003). Approximately 19% of patients with leukemia or lymphoma receiving induction therapy and 12.9% of patients receiving salvage therapies developed hyperuricemia (Annemans et al., 2003a).

PROFESSIONAL ASSESSMENT CRITERIA (PAC)

1. **History of present illness:** Time of onset of symptoms in relation to malignancy, abdominal pain or fullness, back pain, vomiting, diarrhea, lethargy, dehydration, and anorexia.
2. **Past medical history and lifestyle:** Dietary intake focusing on foods high in nucleic acids, medications taken for chronic conditions that may impair renal function (Rheingold & Lange, 2006; Wartmann, 2005; Cantril & Haylock, 2004). Assess patient for history of asthma, allergies, anaphylactic reaction or history of hypersensitivity reaction with urate oxidase, and history of glucose-6-phosphate dehydrogenase (G6PD) deficiency.
3. **Laboratory studies:** Complete blood count (CBC), sodium, potassium, chloride, calcium, phosphorus, carbon dioxide, blood urea nitrogen (BUN), creatinine, uric acid, and urinalysis.
4. **Physical examination:** If the exam yields an abdominal or pelvic mass, perform ultrasound and/or CT of the abdomen/pelvis to rule out obstructive renal failure. Renal failure from obstructive nephropathy can have the same signs and symptoms as that caused by hyperuricemia (Rheingold & Lange, 2006). If the examination yields signs and symptoms of infection, complete the appropriate diagnostic evaluation (cultures and/or diagnostic imaging as indicated).
5. Monitor the serum uric acid, serum creatinine, and BUN every 4 hours in the initial stage of therapy (Cope, 2004; Murphy-Ende & Chernecky, 2002).
6. Observe for signs of renal failure (e.g., oliguria, nausea, vomiting, lethargy, edema, heart failure, or seizure).
7. Observe for rapid weight gain (more than 2 pounds in 24 hours).
8. If using allopurinol, assess uric acid levels, because the maintenance dose is based on these levels. Observe precautions in patients with impaired renal or hepatic function, heart failure, diabetes, or hypertension.
9. If using rasburicase (urate oxidase enzyme): Assess serum G6PD before starting. Patients at high risk for G6PD deficiency include those of African, Mediterranean, or Asian ancestry (Wang et al., 2006; Cheson & Dutcher, 2005). Assess for hypersensitivity to rasburicase. Onset usually is abrupt and is characterized by bronchospasm, dyspnea, hypoxemia, hypotension, and cutaneous rash as urticaria (Lascombes et al., 1998; Pui et al., 1997). Assess for hemolytic anemia and methemoglobinemia. One of the byproducts of the breakdown of uric acid to allantoin is hydrogen peroxide, which can induce hemolytic anemia or methemoglobinemia in patients with G6PD deficiency. G6PD results in intravascular hemolysis after erythrocytes are subjected to oxidative stress (Pui et al., 2001). Three main symptoms of methemoglobinemia are illness out of proportion to the history of illness, cyanosis that does not resolve with administration of oxygen, and blood that appears darker than usual (Nelson & Hostetler, 2003).

NURSING CARE AND TREATMENT

1. The primary aims of treatment are to prevent hyperuricemia and ensure a high urine flow, because this reduces the likelihood of uric acid precipitation in the renal tissue (Baeksgaard & Sorensen, 2003).
2. The standard prophylaxis for and treatment of malignancy-associated hyperuricemia in the United States has been administration of allopurinol with vigorous hydration,

urinary alkalinization, and osmotic diuresis (Pui et al., 1997). Allopurinol inhibits the enzyme xanthine oxidase, preventing the conversion of hypoxanthine and xanthine to uric acid and thereby reducing the renal load of uric acid. (Fig. 28.1). It may take several days for the uric acid level to normalize.

- If allopurinol is given PO, it may be given with meals. Instruct the patient to drink 10 to 12 8-ounce glasses of water a day.
- If the dosage of allopurinol is greater than 300 mg/day, it should be given in divided doses. The oral dosage is 100 mg/m^2/dose every 8 hours (10 mg/kg/day in 3 divided doses) to a maximum of 800 mg/day.
- For IV administration: Reconstitute a 500 mg dose to a concentration of 20 mg/mL. Infuse over 30 to 60 minutes. The IV dosage is 200-400 mg/m^2/day in 1-3 divided doses to a maximum of 600 mg/day. The maintenance dose is based on the serum uric acid levels.
- Hydration maintains both blood volume and blood pressure, which ensures renal perfusion even with loss of autoregulation (Ronco et al., 2004).
- Vigorous diuresis may also prevent crystallization of xanthine and other purine metabolites, the excretion of which is increased with the use of allopurinol.

3. Rasburicase is a recombinant urate oxidase enzyme that rapidly catalyzes the enzymatic oxidation of uric acid into allantoin and hydrogen peroxide (see Fig. 28.1) (Hutcherson et al., 2006). Rasburicase should *never* be administered as a bolus. It should be infused over 30 minutes, without a filter, in a dedicated intravenous line. If it is not possible to use a line different from that through which other medications are being given, flush the line with 15 mL of normal saline before and after the infusion of rasburicase.

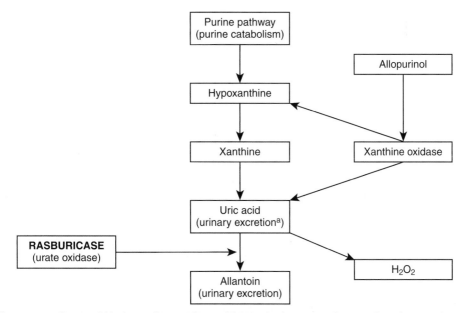

Fig. 28.1 • Allopurinol blocks xanthine oxidase, inhibiting the formation of uric acid. Rasburicase (urate oxidase) metabolizes uric acid to allantoin, a protein five to 10 times more soluble than uric acid that is easily excreted. In the conversion of uric acid to allantoin, hydrogen peroxide is produced. This fact is important, because patients who are deficient in glucose-6-phosphate dehydrogenase should not receive rasburicase. *(From Cheson, B. D., & Dutcher, B. S. [2005]. Managing malignancy-associated hyperuricemia with rasburicase.* Journal of Supportive Oncology, *3:117-124.)*

The recommended dosage is 0.15-0.2 mg/kg daily for 5 consecutive days (Cheson & Dutcher, 2005). Recent studies have shown that less aggressive treatment is successful (see Evidence-Based Practice Updates). Monitor carefully for signs and symptoms of anaphylaxis. Make sure that emergency drugs (epinephrine, diphenhydramine, and steroids), oxygen, and emergency equipment are available before rasburicase is administered (Brant, 2002).

4. Ensure the accuracy of uric acid determinations by collecting the blood samples in prechilled tubes and sending them to the laboratory in an ice bath. Rasburicase causes enzymatic degradation of uric acid in blood samples if they are left at room temperature, resulting in falsely low values (Fojo, 2005; Brant, 2002).

5. Weigh the patient daily, or every 12 hours if fluid retention becomes apparent.

6. Maintain strict intake and output measurement, with accurate documentation every 4 hours (Ribeiro & Pui, 2003).

7. Provide aggressive IV hydration before and during chemotherapy administration; frequent monitoring of electrolytes and uric acid; allopurinol and/or rasburicase or other agents for hyperuricemia; urinary alkalinization with the addition of sodium bicarbonate to IV fluids (Haut, 2005).

8. Monitor urinary pH and notify the physician if it is less than 7 or greater than 8. Maintaining the urinary pH above 7 keeps uric acid ionized, which reduces urate crystal deposition in the renal tubules. If the urine pH becomes too alkaline, the patient may be predisposed to urinary calcium phosphate precipitation, leading to a decreased glomerular filtration rate (Jeha, 2001).

EVIDENCE-BASED PRACTICE UPDATES

1. Therapy for hyperuricemia has progressed over the past three decades. Today's standard for prophylaxis and treatment is allopurinol, initiated at the time of diagnosis; alkalinization; and hydration (Pui et al., 2001; DeConti & Calabresi, 1966; Krakoff & Meyer, 1965). Studies on rasburicase included its use as prophylaxis, and 100% of both children and adults in the clinical trial had a significant decline in uric acid and maintained a normal uric acid level after a median of two and three doses of rasburicase, respectively (Pui et al., 2001).

2. Earlier studies showed that nonrecombinant urate oxidase is a more effective uricolytic agent than allopurinol, but it is associated with acute hypersensitivity reactions, even in patients without allergy. The decrease in the uric acid level not only was more pronounced but also more rapid in the urate oxidase group (119 patients) compared to the allopurinol group (129 patients), all of whom were newly diagnosed with acute lymphoblastic leukemia (either B cell or non-B cell) or stage III or stage IV B-cell non-Hodgkin's lymphoma (Pui et al., 1997).

3. An open, randomized comparison trial of 52 children with leukemia and lymphoma showed more rapid control and lower levels of uric acid in patients with hematologic malignancies who received rasburicase compared to allopurinol. None required assisted renal support in the rasburicase group, whereas one patient in the allopurinol group required hemofiltration (Goldman et al., 2001).

4. Rasburicase (recombinant urate oxidase) is effective in patients with hyperuricemia before the initiation of chemotherapy. Close monitoring of normalized uric acid levels and continued rasburicase treatment is necessary for patients at high risk of hyperuricemia after initiation of chemotherapy. Urinary alkalinization facilitates renal clearance of uric acid (Shin et al., 2006; Wang et al., 2006).

5. Rasburicase has been well tolerated in a wide range of ages, both children and adults, and in patients with a variety of cancer types. Allergic reactions, including anaphylaxis

(less than 1%), rash (1%), hemolysis (less than 1%), and methemoglobinemia (less than 1%), are the most serious complications of treatment. In one study of 1069 patients, only 10 patients (less than 1%) were withdrawn for possible drug-related events (Jeha et al., 2005).

TEACHING AND EDUCATION

Explain to patient:
1. Intravenous fluids should be given to promote hydration and to flush the kidneys of the byproducts of cell destruction.
2. Depending on several factors, sodium bicarbonate may be added to the IV fluids. This will make the urine more alkaline and prevent crystallization of uric acid, which could result in renal damage.
3. Taking allopurinol is necessary to prevent elevation of uric acid. Report nausea and vomiting, or any other reason that would prevent the administration of allopurinol.
4. Report signs and symptoms of increasing uric acid, such as nausea, vomiting, anorexia, flank pain, and pruritus.
5. Maintain strict intake and output with accurate measurement. Obtain daily weights to assess fluid balance and report a weight gain of 2 pounds or more over a 24-hour period.
6. An indwelling catheter may be used during the time of intense IV hydration to maintain accurate urinary output measurement.
7. Frequent collection of blood and urine samples will occur during this period to monitor the body's response to the chemotherapy and interventions to prevent and/or treat the hyperuricemia.

NURSING DIAGNOSES

1. **Impaired urinary elimination** related to urate nephropathy
2. **Deficient fluid volume** related to inadequate fluid intake and/or nausea with vomiting associated with side effects of chemotherapy
3. **Risk for imbalanced fluid volume** related to aggressive hydration with intravenous fluids and/or oliguria secondary to obstruction of renal tubules with urate crystals
4. **Deficient knowledge** related to unfamiliarity with treatment and sequelae of hyperuricemia
5. **Anxiety** related to new diagnosis of cancer

EVALUATION AND DESIRED OUTCOMES

1. The serum uric acid level will be less than 8 mg/dL during initial chemotherapy and at least 48 hours afterward.
2. Renal function will be within normal limits, as evidenced by serum creatinine and BUN at levels normal for age, 48 hours after chemotherapy.
3. The urine pH will be between 7 and 8 during initial chemotherapy.
4. An indwelling urinary catheter (if used) will be removed within 48 to 72 hours of completion of chemotherapy.
5. Physical evidence of disease will reflect a response to chemotherapy, indicating destruction of malignant cells and reflecting a decreased risk of hyperuricemia. Patients with hyperleukocytosis, high blast counts, lymphadenopathy, hepatosplenomegaly, or a large tumor mass will show marked decrease or resolution of these signs and symptoms, reflecting near-completion of malignant cell destruction.
6. The patient will be free of any signs or symptoms of hyperuricemia during and 48 hours after chemotherapy.

7. The patient and family will verbalize an understanding of preventive measures and the treatment plan for hyperuricemia.

DISCHARGE PLANNING AND FOLLOW-UP CARE

- A patient at risk of hyperuricemia is hospitalized during the time this is expected to occur and remains hospitalized until the risk of tumor lysis is past.
- After discharge, follow-up laboratory tests and appointments with the physician or nurse practitioner should be scheduled.

REVIEW QUESTIONS

QUESTIONS

1. **Hyperuricemia is most commonly associated with which of the following malignancies:**
   1. Acute myeloid leukemia
   2. Colon cancer
   3. Pancreatic cancer
   4. Renal cancer

2. **When is the oncology patient most likely to show signs and symptoms of hyperuricemia:**
   1. During anesthesia
   2. After a packed red blood cell transfusion
   3. While receiving a platelet transfusion
   4. Within 12 to 72 hours of initial chemotherapy

3. **Which of the following therapies is *not* usually associated with hyperuricemia:**
   1. Antiemetic therapy
   2. Chemotherapy
   3. Radiation therapy
   4. Steroid therapy

4. **Prevention and management of hyperuricemia are necessary to prevent which of the following complications:**
   1. Congestive heart failure
   2. Diabetes mellitus
   3. Renal failure
   4. Sick sinus syndrome

5. **A priority nursing intervention in the patient with hyperuricemia is to:**
   1. Assess for symptoms of gastric ulceration.
   2. Correlate weight with the chemotherapy dosage.
   3. Monitor intake and output.
   4. Promote successful coping with the diagnosis.

6. **Use of rasburicase to treat hyperuricemia results in normalization of the uric acid:**
   1. After the chemotherapy is complete
   2. Within a few hours
   3. Slowly, over a period of 5 to 7 days
   4. Within the first month of therapy

7. **Rasburicase is administered:**
   1. By a bolus intravenous route
   2. By the intramuscular route in the leg only
   3. By an intravenous route over 30 minutes
   4. By mouth with food

8. **To collect specimens that will accurately reflect the serum uric acid level in a patient treated with rasburicase, the nurse/phlebotomist must:**
   1. Use a carbonated preservative in the tube.
   2. Use florescent lighting to identify venous access.
   3. Use prechilled tubes and send the specimen to the lab in an ice bath.
   4. Use a rapid technique of blood withdrawal.

9. **A patient receiving rasburicase must be monitored carefully for signs of:**
   1. Abnormal clotting
   2. Anaphylaxis
   3. Peripheral nephropathy
   4. Red man's syndrome

10. **Which of the following is an evaluation outcome for a patient with hyperuricemia who is ready for discharge:**
    1. Absence of signs and symptoms of skin infection.
    2. Bronchial washings that are free of bacterial findings.
    3. Liver enzymes that have returned to baseline.
    4. Renal function within age-appropriate normal limits.

ANSWERS

1. *Answer: 1*
   Rationale: Reports of hyperuricemia in patients with acute myeloid leukemia are as high as 50%; the disorder is rare with solid tumors.

2. *Answer: 4*
   Rationale: Although hyperuricemia may be present when the malignancy is diagnosed, it usually develops within 12 to 72 hours of administration of chemotherapy in individuals at risk.

3. *Answer: 1*
   Rationale: All the therapies listed, except for antiemetic therapy, cause cell destruction, which results in the release of nucleic acids and hyperuricemia.

4. *Answer: 3*
   Rationale: The formation of uric acid crystals in the renal tubules may cause renal dysfunction, which progresses to renal failure when uric acid levels are 8.3 mg/dL or higher.

5. *Answer: 3*
   Rationale: Because of the importance of hydration and the risk of renal

dysfunction, accurate intake and output must be maintained to detect changes in renal function.

6. *Answer: 2*
   Rationale: Because rasburicase results in the end product of allantoin, which is five to 10 times more soluble than uric acid, uric acid levels decline within a matter of hours rather than days.

7. *Answer: 3*
   Rationale: Rasburicase should never be given as a bolus; instead, it should be infused over 30 minutes (without a filter) through a dedicated intravenous line. If it is not possible to use a line different from that in which other medications are infusing, the line should be flushed with 15 mL of normal saline before and after infusion of rasburicase.

8. *Answer: 3*
   Rationale: Rasburicase causes enzymatic degradation of uric acid in blood samples left at room temperature, which results in falsely low values.

9. *Answer: 2*
   Rationale: Anaphylaxis is a sign of hypersensitivity, and the onset is usually abrupt. Emergency drugs, oxygen, and emergency equipment should be available before rasburicase is administered.

10. *Answer: 4*
    Rationale: Renal function, as reflected by the serum BUN and creatinine levels, should be within age-appropriate normal limits before discharge.

REFERENCES

Annemans, L., Moeremans, K., & Lamotte, M., et al. (2003a). Incidence, medical resource utilisation and costs of hyperuricemia and tumour lysis syndrome in patients with acute leukemia and non-Hodgkin's lymphoma in four European countries. *Leukemia & Lymphoma, 44*(1):77-83.

Annemans, L., Moeremans, K., & Lamotte, M., et al. (2003b). Pan-European multicenter economic evaluation of recombinant urate oxidase (rasburicase) in prevention and treatment of hyperuricemia and tumor lysis syndrome in haematological cancer patients. *Supportive Care in Cancer, 11*:249.

Baeksgaard, L., & Sorensen, J. B. (2003). Acute tumor lysis syndrome in solid tumors: A case report and review of literature. *Cancer Chemotherapy and Pharmacology, 51*(3):187-192.

Brant, J. M. (2002). Rasburicase: an innovative new treatment for hyperuricemia associated with tumor lysis syndrome. *Clinical Journal of Oncology Nursing, 6*(1):12-16.

Cairo, M. S., & Bishop, M. (2004). Tumour lysis syndrome: New therapeutic strategies and classification. *British Journal of Haematology, 127*:3-11.

Cantril, C. A., & Haylock, P. J. (2004). Tumor lysis syndrome. *American Journal of Nursing, 104*(4):49-53.

Cheson, B. D., & Dutcher, B. S. (2005). Managing malignancy-associated hyperuricemia with rasburicase. *Journal of Supportive Oncology, 3:*117-124.

Cohen, L. F., Balow, J. E., & Magrath, I. T., et al. (1980). Acute tumor lysis syndrome: A review of 37 patients with Burkitt's lymphoma. *American Journal of Medicine, 68*:486-491.

Cope, D. (2004). Tumor lysis syndrome. *Clinical Journal of Oncology Nursing, 8*(4):415-416.

DeConti, R. C., & Calabresi, P. (1966). Use of allopurinol for the prevention and control of hyperuricemia in patients with neoplastic disease. *New England Journal of Medicine, 280*:426-427.

Del Toro, G., Morris, E., & Mitchell, C. S. (2005). Tumor lysis syndrome: Pathophysiology, definition, and alternative treatment approaches. *Clinical Advances in Hematology & Oncology, 3*(1):54-61.

Fojo, A. T. (2005). Oncologic emergencies. In V. T. DeVita, Jr., S. Hellman, & S. A. Rosenberg (Eds.), *Cancer: Principles and practice of oncology* (pp. 2292-2295). (7th ed.). Philadelphia: Lippincott Williams & Wilkins.

Goldman, S. C., Holcenberg, J. S., & Finklestein, J. Z., et al. (2001). A randomized comparison between rasburicase and allopurinol in children with lymphoma or leukemia at high risk for tumor lysis. *Blood, 97*:2998-3003.

Greer, J. P., Foerster, J., & Lukens, J. N., et al. (2004). *Wintrobe's clinical hematology.* (11th ed.). Philadelphia: Lippincott Williams & Wilkins.

Haut, C. (2005). Oncological emergencies in the pediatric intensive care unit. *AACN Clinical Issues, 16*(2):232-245.

Hutcherson, D. A., Gammon, D. C., & Bhatt, M. S., et al. (2006). Reduced dose rasburicase in the treatment of adults with hyperuricemia associated with malignancy. *Pharmacotherapy, 26*(2):242-247.

Jeha, S. (2001). Tumor lysis syndrome. *Seminars in Hematology, 38*(4 Suppl. 10):4-8.

Jeha, S., Kantarjian, H., & Irwin, D., et al. (2005). Efficacy and safety of rasburicase, a recombinant urate oxidase (Elitek), in the management of malignancy-associated hyperuricemia in pediatric and adult patients: Final results of a multicenter compassionate use trial. *Leukemia, 19*:34-35.

Krakoff, I. H., & Meyer, R. L. (1965). Prevention of hyperuricemia in leukemia and lymphoma: Use of allopurinol, a xanthine oxidase inhibitor. *Journal of the American Medical Association, 193*:89-94.

Lascombes, F., Sommelet, D., & Gebhard, F., et al. (1998). High efficacy of recombinant urate oxidase in prevention of renal failure related to tumor lysis syndrome (TLS). *Blood, 92*:237B.

Murphy-Ende, K., & Chernecky, C. (2002). Assessing adults with leukemia. *Nurse Practitioner, 27*(11): 49-56.

Nelson, K., & Hostetler, M. A. (2003). An infant with methemoglobinemia. *Hospital Physician, 39*(2):31-38, 62.

Pui, C. H. (2001). Optimal treatment of malignancies associated with hyperuricemia. *Seminars in Hematology, 38*(4 Suppl. 10):1-3.

Pui, C. H., Jeha, S., & Irwin, D., et al. (2001). Recombinant urate oxidase (rasburicase) in the prevention and treatment of malignancy-associated hyperuricemia in pediatric and adult patients: Results of a compassionate use trial. *Leukemia, 15*(10):1505-1509.

Pui, C. H., Relling, M. V., & Lascombes, F., et al. (1997). Urate oxidase in prevention and treatment of hyperuricemia associated with lymphoid malignancies. *Leukemia, 11*(11):1813-1816.

Rheingold, S. R., & Lange, B. J. (2005). Oncologic emergencies. In P. A. Pizzo, & D. G. Poplack (Eds.), *Principles and practice of pediatric oncology* (pp. 1222-1224). (5th ed.). Philadelphia: Lippincott Williams & Wilkins.

Ribeiro, R. G., & Pui, C. H. (2003). Recombinant urate oxidase for prevention of hyperuricemia and tumor lysis syndrome in lymphoid malignancies. *Clinical Lymphoma, 3*(4):225-232.

Ronco, C., Bellomo, R., & Inguaggiato, P., et al. (2004). Rasburicase therapy in hyperuricemic renal dysfunction. *Contributions to Nephrology, 144:*158-165.

Schiffer, C. A. (2001). Treatment of high-grade lymphoid malignancies in adults. *Seminars in Hematology, 38*(Suppl. 10):22-26.

Shin, H. Y., Hyoung, J. K., & Park, E. S., et al. (2006). Recombinant urate oxidase (rasburicase) for the treatment of hyperuricemia in pediatric patients with hematologic malignancies: Results of a compassionate prospective multicenter study in Korea. *Pediatric Blood Cancer, 46*(4):439-445.

Tsimberidou, A. M., & Keating, M. J. (2005). Hyperuricemic syndromes in cancer patients. *Contributions to Nephrology, 147:*47-60.

Wang, L., Shih, L, & Chang, H., et al. (2006). Recombinant urate oxidase (rasburicase) for the prevention and treatment of tumor lysis syndrome in patients with hematologic malignancies. *Acta Haematologica, 115:*35-38.

Wartmann, R. L. (2004). Disorders of purine and pyrimidine metabolism. In D. L. Kasper, E. Braunwald, & S. Hauser et al. (Eds.), *Harrison's principles of internal medicine* (pp. 2308-2311). (16th ed.). New York: McGraw-Hill.

HYPOKALEMIA

MARY PAT LYNCH

PATHOPHYSIOLOGICAL MECHANISMS

Hypokalemia is a low serum potassium level, which may result from a number of conditions. The normal serum potassium level ranges from 3.5 to 5.5 mEq/L; hypokalemia exists when the potassium level is less than 3.5 mEq/L.

Potassium is the most common intracellular cation, but only a small portion is found in the extracellular fluids. Potassium plays an important role in cellular function, neuromuscular activity, and cardiac conduction. Because the body does not store potassium, it requires a minimum intake of 40 to 60 mEq/day. Most potassium (80%) is excreted through the kidneys in response to hyperkalemia and/or the hormone aldosterone; 15% is excreted through the gastrointestinal tract, and 5% is lost through the skin. (Smith, 2000)

Potassium levels normally are regulated by two mechanisms in response to variation in potassium intake. In the first mechanism, ingested potassium enters the hepatic portal circulation, which stimulates the pancreas to release insulin. The elevated levels of insulin cause the rapid transport of potassium from the extracellular space into cells. In the second mechanism, increased potassium in the circulation causes the release of renin from the renal juxtaglomerular cells; this stimulates hepatic activation of angiotensin I, which is converted to angiotension II in the lungs (Hollander-Rodriguez & Calvert, 2006).

The most common cause of hypokalemia is potassium depletion, which results from an inadequate intake or abnormal losses. Hypokalemia can also occur without actual loss of total body potassium, through processes that result in a shift from the extracellular fluid to the intracellular spaces (e.g., acidosis). In acidosis, potassium moves out of the cell in exchange for hydrogen; as the kidneys continue to excrete potassium, hypokalemia becomes evident. In metabolic acidosis, severe potassium depletion usually is seen as a result of increased bicarbonate reabsorption. Hypovolemia stimulates the rennin-angiotensin system, which leads to the secretion of aldosterone and the excretion of potassium through the kidneys (Smith, 2000).

When trauma or severe injury occurs, anabolic cellular activity increases the demand for intracellular potassium, and this can cause hypokalemia. Pseudohypokalemia can occur with leukocytosis because of an increased uptake of potassium by white blood cells after a specimen has been drawn (Smith, 2000).

EPIDEMIOLOGY AND ETIOLOGY

Hypokalemia is an exceptionally common electrolyte abnormality in clinical practice. More than 20% of hospitalized patients have been reported to have some degree of hypokalemia (Schaefer & Wolford, 2005).

As mentioned, the most common cause of hypokalemia is potassium depletion caused by inadequate intake or abnormal losses. Although loss of electrolytes through vomiting, diarrhea, or nasogastric drainage does not cause potassium depletion, it does cause significant chloride depletion, which alters the renal signals for potassium secretion and promotes renal potassium losses (Gennari, 2002).

Increased excretion of potassium can occur through renal losses caused by diuretics, metabolic alkalosis, mineralocorticoid excess, magnesium depletion, and renal tubular acidosis.

A variety of tumors may ectopically synthesize ACTH and cause Cushing's syndrome; this can be rapidly fatal with fast-growing tumors. The patient may complain of weakness, and hypokalemia and metabolic acidosis may be severe (Casciato, 2004).

RISK PROFILE

- Inadequate dietary intake of potassium due to malnutrition or cachexia.
- Excessive loss of potassium:
  - GI loss through vomiting, diarrhea, nasogastric suctioning, laxative abuse, bulimia
  - Renal loss from diuretics, particularly loop and thiazide diuretics
  - Metabolic acidosis
  - Osmotic diuresis from uncontrolled diabetes
  - Medications (penicillins can cause hypokalemia)
  - Mineralocorticoid excess from primary hyperaldosteronism, glucocorticoid-responsive aldosteronism, congenital adrenal hyperplasia
  - Magnesium depletion
  - Renal tubular acidosis
  - Excessive glucocorticoid effects (Cushing's syndrome, exogenous steroids, ectopic adrenocorticotropic hormone production)
  - Diabetic ketoacidosis (Gennari, 2002; Smith, 2000)
- Tumors that commonly cause ectopic ACTH syndrome:
  - Small cell lung cancer
  - Malignant thymoma
  - Pancreatic cancer, especially islet cell tumors
  - Bronchial carcinoids
- Tumors that uncommonly or rarely cause ectopic ACTH syndrome
  - Ovarian cancer
  - Thyroid cancer (except medullary)
  - Colon cancer
  - Prostate cancer
  - Renal cancer
  - Sarcomas
  - Hematologic malignancies (Casciato, 2004)

PROGNOSIS

The prognosis for hypokalemia depends entirely on the underlying cause. Hypokalemia caused by diarrhea has an excellent prognosis. Hypokalemia caused by a rapidly growing tumor that is producing ACTH has a poor prognosis.

PROFESSIONAL ASSESSMENT CRITERIA (PAC)

1. Patients with hypokalemia usually are asymptomatic. The disorder is identified in most instances by a low serum potassium level.

2. When symptoms are present, they usually are nonspecific and related to muscular or cardiac function.
3. The patient may complain of weakness or fatigue.
4. Worsening of diabetes control and polyuria may be seen.
5. The patient may complain of palpitations.
6. Muscle cramps and pain can occur when rhabdomyolysis is caused by severe hypokalemia.
7. Vital signs usually are normal, but tachycardia and tachypnea can occur as a result of respiratory muscle weakness.
8. With severe hypokalemia, muscle weakness and flaccid paralysis may be found on the physical exam.
9. With severe hypokalemia, depressed or absent deep tendon reflexes may be found on the physical exam.
10. Alteration in mental status (depression, confusion, malaise) may be seen.
11. Dysrhythmias may be found with severe hypokalemia.
12. Laboratory tests should include electrolytes, BUN, creatinine, glucose, and magnesium levels.
13. The urine potassium level should be measured to determine whether the potassium loss is extrarenal or the result of excess renal excretion.
14. An ECG may show changes or arrhythmias. Changes associated with hypokalemia include a depressed ST segment, a flattened T wave, and the presence of a U wave.
15. When ectopic ACTH syndrome is suspected in a patient with cancer, the diagnosis can be made in most cases by demonstrating failure of dexamethasone to suppress ACTH levels (Lederer et al., 2005; Casciato, 2004; Gennari, 2002; Smith, 2000).

NURSING CARE AND TREATMENT

1. The goal of treatment is to normalize the potassium level to a range of 3.5 to 5.5 mEq/L.
2. Because of the risk of hyperkalemia, intensive intravenous potassium is rarely administered or indicated (Gennari, 2002).
3. In patients with cancer, control of the underlying tumor is the most effective treatment, and hypokalemia is often difficult to treat in these patients.
4. For other causes, the primary rule is to treat the underlying cause as well.
5. Dietary replacement can be used for mildly low or asymptomatic potassium levels (3 to 3.5 mEq/L).
6. Encourage the patient to eat a diet rich in potassium (fresh or dried fruits, fruit juice, vegetables, meats, nuts).
7. Adjust medications as needed (e.g., replace a thiazide diuretic with a potassium-sparing diuretic).
8. For patients with moderate hypokalemia, oral supplements are preferred over intravenous infusions.
9. Potassium chloride (KCl) is the preferred form; it enhances the reabsorption of potassium and chloride in exchange for sodium and bicarbonate. The average dose is 20-40 mEq BID to QID.
10. For maintenance when hypokalemia has been corrected or for prophylaxis, the average dose is 16-24 mEq daily.
11. Many different forms of potassium supplements are available. Potassium bicarbonate or potassium citrate are good choices for patients with metabolic acidosis.
12. Potassium supplements can cause GI distress and should be given with meals.
13. Hypomagnesemia should be treated in hypokalemic patients, because magnesium depletion impairs the ability to replace potassium losses.

14. If the patient is unable to take oral medications, IV replacement is indicated.
15. In patients with moderate to severe hypokalemia (less than 3 mEq/L) or if the patient is symptomatic, has ECG changes, or severe weakness, IV potassium should be given (20-40 mEq/hr). The serum potassium should be checked after infusing 60 mEq.
16. Potassium is never given IV push due to its effects on the vein and the heart.
17. When life-threatening dysrhythmias are present or paralysis occurs, patients should be admitted for cardiac monitoring and more aggressive replacement under close supervision (Lederer et al., 2005; Schaeffer & Wolford, 2005; Gennari, 2002; Smith, 2000).

EVIDENCE-BASED PRACTICE UPDATES

The following guidelines for potassium replacement in clinical practice have been provided by the National Council on Potassium in Clinical Practice (Cohn et al., 2000).

1. Dietary consumption of potassium-rich foods should be supplemented with potassium replacement therapy in patients with hypokalemia, because increasing dietary potassium intake is not completely effective in replacing the potassium loss.
2. Potassium replacement is recommended for individuals who are sensitive to sodium or who are unable or unwilling to reduce salt intake; it is especially effective in reducing blood pressure in such individuals.
3. Potassium replacement is recommended for individuals who are subject to nausea, vomiting, diarrhea, bulimia, or diuretic/laxative abuse.
4. Although laboratory measurement is convenient, it is not always an accurate indicator of total body potassium. Measurement of 24-hour urinary potassium excretion may be appropriate for patients at high risk.
5. An oral dose of 20 mEq/day of potassium generally is sufficient to prevent hypokalemia, and a dose of 40-100 mmol/day is sufficient for its treatment.
6. Maintenance of optimal potassium levels (at least 4 mEq/L) is critical in patients with cardiac arrhythmias, for whom routine potassium monitoring is obligatory.

TEACHING AND EDUCATION

1. Instruct the patient and family in the symptoms of hypokalemia or hyperkalemia, including palpitations or cardiac arrhythmias, muscle weakness, decreased control of diabetes, and polyuria.
2. Instruct the patient and family in the effects of medications, specifically, which of the patient's drugs can cause serum potassium abnormalities. For example, tell the patient to discontinue diuretics if nausea and vomiting or diarrhea occurs and to call the physician if such gastrointestinal losses persist. Depending on patient's underlying disease or diseases, sudden fluid losses can cause either hypokalemia or hyperkalemia if diuretics, potassium supplements, or antihypertensives are continued.
3. Instruct the patient and family about dietary intake. A high sodium intake tends to enhance renal potassium losses, therefore educate the patient and family about a low-sodium, high-potassium diet.
4. Instruct the patient and family about potassium supplements, which can irritate the GI tract and should be taken with food. The slow-release form should be taken with a full glass of water. Inform the patient and family of the potential side effects and encourage compliance (Lederer et al., 2005; Smith, 2000).

NURSING DIAGNOSES

1. **Decreased cardiac output** related to effect of hypokalemia on cardiac muscle

2. **Ineffective breathing pattern** related to severe hypokalemia (less than 2.0 mEq/L) which can cause ascending paralysis and eventual respiratory arrest
3. **Imbalanced nutrition: less than body requirements** related to low intake of potassium, diarrhea or laxative abuse leading to hypokalemia
4. **Deficient knowledge** related to potassium-rich foods and medications that may lead to hypokalemia
5. **Anxiety** related to severity of illness and hospitalization

EVALUATION AND DESIRED OUTCOMES

1. The potassium level will normalize and the underlying cause of the hypokalemia will resolve.
2. The conditions causing ECG abnormalities will resolve.
3. For severe hypokalemia, patients usually are monitored in the ICU or telemetry unit; the potassium level should be assessed every 3 to 6 hours until the outcome of stabilization.
4. Once the patient's condition has been stabilized, acid-base problems have resolved, and coexistent electrolyte problems have been corrected, the patient usually is moved to a regular unit or discharged with follow-up in 2 or 3 days to check serum potassium levels.
5. The patient should respond within 72 hours to oral potassium replacement. If an adequate response is not seen, check for other electrolyte abnormalities (e.g., magnesium deficiency) and correct them.
6. Once the patient is stable, to maintain stabilization, monitor potassium levels weekly for 1 to 3 weeks and then every 1 to 2 months. (Lederer et al., 2005; Smith, 2000).

DISCHARGE PLANNING AND FOLLOW UP CARE

- If the patient has no other medical conditions and the hypokalemia was the result of an acute episode (e.g., severe diarrhea), no follow-up care is needed.
- If the patient is likely to develop hypokalemia again, periodic monitoring of serum potassium levels is essential.
- In patients with tumors producing ectopic secretion of ACTH, severe symptoms may require the use of adrenal suppressant medications or, in rare cases, adrenalectomy (Casciato, 2004).

REVIEW QUESTIONS

QUESTIONS

1. **All of the following ECG changes are associated with hypokalemia** *except*:
   1. Depressed ST segment
   2. Elevated ST segment
   3. Flattened T wave
   4. Presence of a U wave

2. **All of the following are common causes of hypokalemia** *except*:
   1. Small cell lung cancer
   2. Thiazide diuretics
   3. Severe diarrhea
   4. Loop diuretics

3. **Ectopic secretion of ACTH is found in all of the following types of tumor** *except*:
   1. Small cell lung cancer
   2. Malignant thymoma
   3. Brain tumors
   4. Bronchial carcinoids

4. **A patient presents to the office with an incidental finding of a potassium level of 3.2 mEq/L. The ECG shows no changes. Which of the following options is the *most* appropriate course of action for this patient:**
   1. Admit the patient to the critical care unit for continuous cardiac monitoring.

2. Start calcium gluconate IV for cardiac protection.
3. Administer 20 mEq of potassium chloride IV for 3 hours, then recheck the level.
4. Discontinue the thiazide diuretic Start potassium chloride at 40 mEq PO daily. Recheck the potassium level in 2 days.

5. **All of the following foods are rich in potassium** *except*:
    1. Fresh fruit
    2. Dried fruit
    3. Milk
    4. Nuts

6. **Based on the following arterial blood gas (ABG) results in an adult, what is the cause of hypokalemia?**
    $ABG = pH = 7.30$, $PaCO_2 = 37$ mmHg, $PaO_2 = 85$ mmHg, $HCO_3 = 22$ mEq/L.
    1. Alkalosis
    2. Acidosis
    3. Decreased oxygen saturation
    4. Excess bicarbonate

7. **Based on the following complete blood count (CBC) results in an adult, what is the cause of pseudohypokalemia?**
    CBC =
    Hematocrit = 38%
    Hemoglobin = 14 g/dL
    Red blood cells = 5.1 million/mcL
    White blood cells = 21,000/mcL
    Platelets = 180,000/mcL
    1. Decreased percentage of red blood cells in a volume of whole blood
    2. Anemia
    3. Leukocytosis
    4. Thrombocytopenia

8. **The depletion of what electrolyte promotes the renal loss of potassium?**
    1. Chloride
    2. Magnesium
    3. Selenium
    4. Vitamin K

9. **Your patient has just been prescribed a potassium supplement to be taken orally twice a day. What intervention would be appropriate to educate the patient about to decrease the incidence of gastrointestinal distress?**
    1. Take both doses just prior to bedtime
    2. Take each dose 12 hours apart
    3. Take each dose with 60 mL of 2% milk
    4. Take each dose with meals

10. **Intravenous (IV) potassium should never be given by what method:**
    1. Mixed with D51/2NS
    2. Intravenous push
    3. Intravenous piggy back
    4. Mixed with 0.9% sodium chloride

ANSWERS

1. *Answer: 2*
   Rationale: An elevated ST segment is found in hyperkalemia.

2. *Answer: 1*
   Rationale: Hypokalemia caused by ectopic secretion of ACTH from a tumor is rare.

3. *Answer: 3*
   Rationale: Ectopic secretion of ACTH, causing hypokalemia, is not associated with brain tumors.

4. *Answer: 4*
   Rationale: A potassium level of 3.2 mEq/L is considered mild to moderate hypokalemia. It can be treated in the outpatient setting with medication adjustment and oral replacement of potassium.

5. *Answer: 3*
   Rationale: Fresh and dried fruit and nuts are rich in potassium, but milk is not.

6. *Answer: 2*
   Rationale: Acidosis, as the pH is below 7.35.

7. *Answer: 3*
   Rationale: Too many white blood cells increase the uptake of potassium.

8. *Answer: 1*
   Rationale: Chloride depletion alters the renal signals for potassium secretion and promotes potassium loss.

9. *Answer: 4*
Rationale: Taking potassium with meals helps decreased GI distress.

10. *Answer: 2*
Rationale: IV push causes severe venous damage and cardiac dysrhythmias.

REFERENCES

Casciato, D. A., (Ed.). Metabolic complications. In Carlson, H. E. *Manual of clinical oncology* (pp. 529-550). (5th ed.). Philadelphia: Lippincott Williams & Wilkins.

Cohn, J. N., Kowey, P. R., & Whelton, P. K., et al. (2000). New guidelines for potassium replacement in clinical practice: A contemporary review by the National Council on Potassium in Clinical Practice. *Archives of Internal Medicine, 160*(16):2429-2436.

Gennari, F. J. (2002). Disorders of potassium homeostasis: Hypokalemia and hyperkalemia. *Critical Care Clinics, 18*(2):273-288.

Hollander-Rodriguez, J. C., & Calvert, J. F. (2006). Hyperkalemia. *American Family Physician, 73*(2):283-290.

Lederer, E., Erbeck, K., & Ouseph, R. (2005). Hypokalemia. Retrieved June 27, 2007 from www.emedicine.com.

Schaefer, T. J., & Wolford, R. W. (2005). Disorders of potassium. *Emergency Medicine Clinics of North America, 23*(3):723-747.

Smith, W. J. (2000). Hypokalemia and Hyperkalemia. In D. Camp-Sorrell, *Clinical manual for the oncology advanced practice nurse* (pp. 1031-1042). Pittsburgh: Oncology Nursing Press.

HYPOMAGNESEMIA

LYLE STUART BAKER, Jr. • BRENDA K. SHELTON • MICHAEL I. AGUGO

PATHOPHYSIOLOGICAL MECHANISMS

Magnesium plays a fundamental role in many functions of the cell, including energy transfer, storage, and use; insulin release; protein, carbohydrate, and fat metabolism; maintenance of normal cell membrane function; and regulation of parathyroid hormone (PTH) secretion (Guerrero-Romero & Rodriguez-Moran, 2006; Tong & Rude, 2005; Topf & Murray, 2003; Rubeiz et al., 1993). It also has been linked to more than 300 enzymatic reactions. Approximately two thirds of magnesium stores are located in the bones, about one third is found in voluntary and involuntary muscles, and less than 1% is measurable in the extracellular space (Agraharkar & Fahlen, 2002; Dacey, 2001; Topf & Murray, 2003).

Plasma concentrations of magnesium are kept within a very narrow range and are regulated by adjustment in renal excretion, bone uptake, intestinal uptake, and soft tissue stores. Magnesium differs from other ions in two major respects: (1) it is not hormonally regulated, and (2) bone, as the principal storage site for magnesium, does not readily exchange with extracellular magnesium. This inability to mobilize magnesium stores means that in states of negative magnesium balance, initial losses come from the extracellular space, and equilibrium from bone stores does not begin for several weeks (Agraharkar & Fahlen, 2002).

The body contains an average of about 24 total grams of magnesium. Approximately 60% of magnesium is bound to protein, but it is the ionized, unbound magnesium that is ionically active (Topf & Murray, 2003). Despite this fact, ionized calcium levels have not proven to reliably reflect magnesium depletion, and no albumin correction factor has been defined (Topf & Murray, 2005; Dacey, 2001). Magnesium may be reported in mg/dL, mmol, or mEq/L. Plasma concentrations are usually reported in mEq/L, but replacement therapy is administered in units or grams.

The normal plasma magnesium concentration is 1.4 to 1.7 mEq/L (0.7 to 0.9 mmol, or 1.7 to 2.1 mg/dL) (Agraharkar & Fahlen, 2002). Hypomagnesemia is defined as a plasma level less than 1.4 mEq/L (0.7 mmol or 1.6 mg/dL). It is an accepted concept that plasma levels do not always indicate the body's true status of depletion, yet there are no established methods to define the body's total magnesium level (Topf & Murray, 2003; Dacey, 2001). Because so little magnesium is located extracellularly, plasma hypomagnesemia often indicates a more severe underlying cellular deficiency. Inability to readily recognize increases in plasma magnesium levels in response to replacement therapy may indicate this intracellular deficiency.

The average American diet contains approximately 360 mg (15 mmol) of magnesium; healthy individuals ingest 0.15 to 0.2 mmol/kg each day to maintain balance (Agraharkar & Fahlen, 2002). Magnesium is absorbed via the small intestine, and the amount absorbed depends on the amount ingested. When dietary ingestion is normal, approximately 30% to

40% is absorbed; when intake is low, approximately 80% is absorbed; if intake is increased (as with oral replacement therapy), only about 25% is absorbed.

The two major pathophysiologic mechanisms of hypomagnesemia are losses via the kidney or gastrointestinal tract. Because the exchange of stored and ionized active magnesium is a slow process, magnesium deficiency is apparent even with minimal losses. Uncommon disorders of metabolism cause a selective defect in magnesium absorption; these have been described as both an X-linked recessive trait and an autosomal recessive disorder linked to chromosome 9 (Chubanov et al., 2005; Schlingmann et al., 2005). There is a physiologic change in the TRPM6 gene that encodes proteins present in intestinal epithelia and kidney tubules that is similar to the receptor channels for magnesium and calcium (Schlingmann et al., 2005; Voets et al., 2004).

EPIDEMIOLOGY AND ETIOLOGY

Studies of the incidence of hypomagnesemia in the general population are sparse, but its prevalence is estimated to be 1.5% to 15% (Mouw, 2005; Topf & Murray, 2003). Dietary evaluations suggest that magnesium deficiency may be even more prevalent than estimated because of the effects of low dietary intake and the inability of standard testing measures to reflect true intracellular magnesium deficiency (Mouw, 2005; Topf & Murray, 2003). Hypomagnesemia occurs in approximately 12% of hospitalized patients, with the highest incidence in the critically ill (60% to 65%) (Agus, 2006a; Mouw, 2005; Tong & Rude, 2005; Topf & Murray, 2003). A proposed reason for this high incidence in the critically ill is the extent of oxidative stress and inflammation experienced by these patients (Guerrero-Romero & Rodriguez-Moran, 2006).

RISK PROFILE

- Reduced magnesium intake may be the etiology of hypomagnesemia in chronically malnourished individuals. Individuals who have an inadequate intake, an increased fat intake, or a poorly balanced diet that does not include adequate nuts, seeds, fish, or vegetables are more likely to become magnesium deficient. Water in some areas can supplement magnesium.
- **Gastrointestinal losses:** The upper gastrointestinal tract has higher levels of magnesium than the lower intestinal tract (15 mEq/L versus 1 mEq/L), therefore depletion of magnesium is more pronounced with small intestinal disorders such as small bowel obstruction, small bowel resection, or Crohn's disease (Agus, 2006a). The amount of small bowel resected may directly influence the severity of magnesium deficiency (Topf & Murray, 2003).
- Renal losses of magnesium occur as a result of primary or secondary defects in tubular reabsorption.
  - Magnesium deficiency may accompany inhibition of sodium reabsorption, because magnesium passively follows sodium transport (Topf & Murray, 2003).
  - Loop and thiazide diuretics inhibit net magnesium reabsorption (Topf & Murray, 2003).
  - Volume expansion leads to mild hypomagnesemia as a result of decreased passive transport.
  - An excessive alcohol intake has been linked to an approximate 30% incidence of hypomagnesemia as a result of alcohol-induced tubular dysfunction. This tubular abnormally is viewed as temporary and reverses after approximately 4 weeks of abstinence (Elisaf et al., 1995).

- Excess calcium competes with magnesium for reabsorption in the ascending loop of Henle, and higher levels of calcium lead to decreased magnesium reabsorption (Tong & Rude, 2005).
- Gitelman's syndrome is a autosomal recessive familial defect in the sodium-chloride transporter mechanism in the loop of Henle (also called the *thiazide-sensitive Na-Cl channel*). It is associated with concomitant hypocalciuria. A few case reports of this syndrome have been associated with a history of treatment with cisplatin (Agus, 2006a; Panichpisal et al., 2006).
- Bartter's syndrome is an X-linked genetic disorder of tubular reabsorption that causes hypocalciuria and hypomagnesemia (Agus, 2006a). The hypomagnesemia is less severe in this familial syndrome than in others (Topf & Murray, 2003).
- Manz syndrome is a rare disorder of absorption in the ascending loop of Henle that causes hypocalcemia and hypomagnesemia with polyuria, nystagmus, and tetany (Akhtar et al., 2006).
- Pancreatitis causes hypomagnesemia accompanied by hypocalcemia through the mechanism of saponification of magnesium and calcium in necrotic fat tissue (Agus, 2006a; Dacey, 2001).
- Hyperparathyroidism-induced hypocalcemia is often linked to concomitant hypomagnesemia. When this etiology is present, the hypocalcemia is refractory to calcium replacement therapy unless magnesium is also repleted (Topf & Murray, 2003).
- Diabetes mellitus, particular with uncontrolled hyperglycemia, causes excessive renal excretion of magnesium, resulting in an incidence of hypomagnesemia of approximately 25% to 40% in patients with diabetes mellitus of any etiology (Tong & Rude, 2005; Topf & Murray, 2003). It has been proposed that hypomagnesemia contributes to impaired glucose utilization and may be instrumental in the pathophysiology of complications of diabetes, such as nephropathy, vascular disease, and retinopathy (Sales & Pedrosa, 2006; Pham et al., 2005).
  - The risk of hypomagnesemia with diabetes mellitus is greater in type 2 diabetes (Pham et al., 2005).
  - Factors associated with an increased incidence of hypomagnesemia in patients with diabetes mellitus include high plasma triglycerides, waist circumference, and albuminuria (Corica et al., 2006). Glucosuria has also been associated with increased magnesium wasting.
  - Uncontrolled glucose levels and the metabolic syndrome are associated with a higher incidence of hypomagnesemia (Sales & Pedrosa, 2006; Corica et al., 2006).
- Postoperative hypomagnesemia may occur as a result of several distinctly different etiologic mechanisms (Agus, 2006a).
  - Chelation of circulating free fatty acids (especially after pancreatic and hepatobiliary surgery) causes decreased renal excretion (Topf & Murray, 2003).
  - Transfusion of citrate-rich blood products causes hypocalcemia and accompanying hypomagnesemia. This has been noted after traumatic injury and liver transplantation.
  - Postoperative parathyroidectomy patients have an induced "hungry bone syndrome" characterized by increased bone uptake of magnesium during bone remineralization, with plasma depletion (Dacey, 2001).
  - Postoperative bowel resection causes hypomagnesemia in approximately 20% of patients.
    - Variables that influence the incidence of this complication include the preoperative bowel cleansing regimen and the extent of bowel resection (Schwarz & Nevarez, 2005; Topf & Murray, 2003).
    - Inflammation of the bowel may exacerbate this problem in the immediate postoperative period.

- Nephrotoxins disrupt the loop of Henle and distal tubular reabsorption of magnesium (Table 30-1).* Some agents, such as the platinol antineoplastics, also alter gastrointestinal absorption of magnesium. With some drugs (e.g., cetuximab), the renal tubular injury resolves, as does the hypomagnesemia (Fakih et al., 2006). However, hypomagnesemia associated with cisplatin therapy has been reported as permanent (Bashir et al., 2006).
- **Transdermal losses:** Excessive sweating or massive burns cause loss of magnesium in as many as 40% of patients (Mouw, 2005; Topf & Murray, 2003; Dacey, 2001).
- Magnesium depletion has been associated with a number of other medical conditions, including acidosis, attention deficit disorder, elevated bilirubin levels, fibromyalgia, hemolysis, hyperglycemia, hypertension, migraine headaches, menopause, pre-eclampsia, stroke, and ulcerative colitis. Symptoms of these disorders may improve with magnesium repletion (Agus, 2006a; Mouw, 2005; Topf & Murray, 2003; Dacey, 2001).

PROGNOSIS

Patients with acute onset of hypomagnesemia from a clearly identifiable cause have an excellent prognosis for complete recovery from this condition. In conditions of chronic loss, correction of the disorder and its symptoms may be a continuous challenge, although death attributable solely to hypomagnesemia is rare. Despite this lack of evidence regarding the importance of magnesium contributory to death, studies of intensive care patients have shown that the mortality rate is two to three times higher among patients with hypomagnesemia (Topf & Murray, 2003; Rubeiz et al., 1993).

PROFESSIONAL ASSESSMENT CRITERIA (PAC)

1. The primary clinical manifestations of hypomagnesemia are neuromuscular in nature. Increased or hyperactive neuromuscular function is the predominant feature. This is manifested similarly to findings of hypocalcemia and hypokalemia. Common symptoms include:
   - Mood disturbances, such as apathy and depression (Agus, 2006c; Perrin et al., 2006).
   - Seizures (in more severe deficiency, defined as a plasma magnesium less than 1 mEq/L) (Dharnidharka & Carney, 2005; Dacey, 2001).
   - Aphasia (Dharnidharka & Carney, 2005).
   - Extrapyramidal symptoms (e.g., nystagmus, tremors).
   - Cortical blindness (reversible with magnesium replenishment) (Topf & Murray, 2003).
   - Tetany (prolonged, painful muscle contraction).
   - Respiratory muscle weakness, which can lead to shallow breathing, decreased respiratory effort, and hypercarbia.
   - Paresthesias
   - Increased skeletal muscle sensitivity to nerve stimulation, as evidenced by tetany in response to nerve pressure. Although these clinical findings are classic symptoms of hypocalcemia, they may be present with hypomagnesemia even without depleted calcium.

---

*Stohr et al., 2007; Thomson Healthcare, 2007; Fakih et al., 2006; Navaneethan et al., 2006; Aisa et al., 2005; Nawaz et al., 2005; Pearson & Woolsley, 2005; Schrag et al., 2005; Topf & Murray, 2003.

- Chvostek's sign: Facial muscle twitching in response to tapping the facial nerve on the side of the face.
- Trousseau's sign: Carpopedal spasm in response to pressure on the brachial nerve (pumping of the blood pressure cuff).
- Increased deep tendon reflexes.
2. Irritability of the conduction system in the heart also represents neuromuscular hyperactivity. Dysrhythmias of irritable foci are common (Bashir et al., 2006; Topf & Murray, 2003). Rhythm disturbances include:
  - Atrial rhythms: Atrial fibrillation, atrial flutter, atrial tachycardia, premature atrial beats.
    - Some data suggest that magnesium repletion aids in conversion of atrial arrhythmias to normal sinus rhythm (Topf & Murray, 2003).
    - Tachyarrhythmias associated with mitral valve prolapse are less prevalent when magnesium stores are normal (Topf & Murray, 2003).
  - Junctional rhythms: Junctional tachycardia, premature junctional beats.

Table 30-1	COMMON NEPHROTOXIC MEDICATIONS THAT CAUSE HYPOMAGNESEMIA	
Drug Category		**Examples of Agents**
Antibiotics		Amikacin
		Daptomycin
		Gentamycin
		Pentamidine
		Tobramycin
Antifungals		Amphotericin B
		Amphotericin lipid complex
		Itraconazole
Antineoplastics		Arsenic trioxide
		Busulfan
		Gallium nitrate
		Methotrexate
Antiretrovirals, nucleoside reverse transcriptase inhibitors		Didanosine
		Zalcitabine
Antiviral agents		Foscarnet
Biologics		Aldesleukin
		Sargramostim
Bisphosphonates		Ibandronate
		Pamidronate
		Zoledronic acid
Bowel stimulants		Docusate
		Glycerin
		Lactulose
		Sorbitol
Diuretics, loop type and thiazide type		Acetazolamide
		Amsacrine
		Clopamide
		Furosemide
		Hydrochlorothiazide
		Urea
Immunosuppressive agents		Cyclosporine
		Mycophenolic acid
		Tacrolimus

Continued

Table 30-1	COMMON NEPHROTOXIC MEDICATIONS THAT CAUSE HYPOMAGNESEMIA—cont'd	
Drug Category		**Examples of Agents**
Miscellaneous agents		Albuterol
		Amifostine
		Dextrose solution
		Glycine
		Ibutilide
		Lenalidomide
		Neseritide
		Vasopressin
Monoclonal antibody antineoplastic agents		Cetuximab
		Panitumumab
Opiates		Methadone
Platinols		Cisplatin
		Carboplatin

Data from Aisa, Y., Mori, T., & Nakazato, T., et al. (2005). Effects of immunosuppressive agents on magnesium metabolism after allogeneic hematopoietic stem cell transplantation. *Transplantation, 80*:1046-1050; Fakih, M. G., Wilding, G., & Lombardo, J. (2006). Cetuximab-induced hypomagnesemia in patients with colorectal cancer. *Clinical Colorectal Cancer, 6*(2):152-156; Navaneethan, S. D., Sankarasubbaiyan, S., & Gross, M. D., et al. (2006). Tacrolimus-associated hypomagnesemia in renal transplant recipients. *Transplant Proceedings, 38*(5):1320-1322; Nawaz, S. H., Zafar, M. N., & Naqvi, S. A., et al. (2005). Impact of cyclosporine immunosuppression on serum magnesium and its fractional excretion in renal transplant recipients. *Journal of the Pakistan Medical Association, 55*(3):98-100; Pearson, E. C., & Woosley, R. L. (2005). QT prolongation and torsades de pointes among methadone users: Reports to the FDA spontaneous reporting system. *Pharmacoepidemiology and Drug Safety, 14*(11):747-753; Schrag, D., Chung, K. Y., & Flombaum, C., et al. (2005). Cetuximab therapy and symptomatic hypomagnesemia. *Journal of the National Cancer Institute, 97*(16):1221-1224; Stohr, W., Paulides, M., & Bielack, S., et al. (2007). Nephrotoxicity of cisplatin and carboplatin in sarcoma patients: A report from the late effects surveillance system. *Pediatric Blood Cancer, 48*(2):140-147; Thomson Healthcare. (2007). Thomson micromedex healthcare series. Retrieved January 15, 2007, from http://www.thomsonhc.com; Topf, J. M., & Murray, P. T. (2003). Hypomagnesemia and hypermagnesemia. *Reviews in Endocrine and Metabolic Disorders, 4*:195-206.

- Ventricular rhythms: Ventricular tachycardia, ventricular fibrillation, premature ventricular beats, torsades de pointes.
  - These rhythms are less prevalent in patients with myocardial ischemia and normal magnesium (Topf & Murray, 2003).
3. The absence of adequate plasma magnesium alters membrane depolarization in the heart and causes changes in the conduction speed, creating classic ECG changes:
  - Prolonged PR interval
  - Prolonged QT interval
  - ST segment depression
  - T-wave inversions
  - Widening QRS complexes
  - Tall T waves
  - These depolarization changes can lead to the classic form of the life-threatening dysrhythmia of ventricular fibrillation called *torsades de pointes*. This "twisting of points" demonstrates an irritable electrical focus in the ventricle that becomes the focal point for electrical discharge in a sweeping circular fashion (Fig. 30.1).
4. Coronary vasospasm with chest pain and transient ischemic ECG changes has been attributed to hypomagnesemia (Agus, 2006c; Sedlacek et al., 2006). Magnesium hyperrepletion is an accepted treatment for vasospastic angina (Topf & Murray, 2003; Teragawa et al., 2000). Magnesium repletion has also been associated with reversal of ischemia, reduced dysrhythmias, and reduced infarct size (Topf & Murray, 2003).

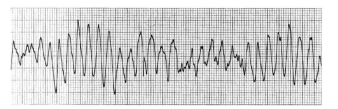

Fig. 30.1 • Torsades de pointes. *(From Phillips, R. E., & Feeney, M. D. [1990]. The* cardiac rhythms: A systematic approach to interpretation. *[3rd ed.]. Philadelphia: W. B. Saunders.)*

5. Magnesium is nature's own calcium channel blocker, and although hypertension is not a commonly reported clinical finding, patients with hypomagnesemia and hypertension often demonstrate significant reduction in blood pressure with magnesium replenishment (Topf & Murray, 2003).
6. Gastrointestinal distress (anorexia, nausea).
7. Respiratory suppression with carbon dioxide retention occurs as a result of weakness and inadequate contraction of respiratory muscles (Sedlacek et al., 2006).
8. Rare case reports of alopecia related to hypomagnesemia have been reported (Tataru & Nicoara, 2004).
9. Hypomagnesemia is reported to enhance platelet aggregation and hence hypercoagulability. Normalization of magnesium may reduce clotting risks (Dacey, 2001).
10. Reduced serum magnesium levels as part of an expanded chemistry panel are diagnostic for hypomagnesemia, but this does not reveal the etiology. The measured magnesium level reflects the total amount of serum magnesium bound to albumin and in a free ionized form. Approximately 70% of magnesium is "free" and unbound. Unlike with calcium, total and ionized magnesium levels do not clearly demonstrate clinical differences in symptomatology, and assessment of the ionized magnesium level is not required for an accurate measurement of magnesium levels in the body (Topf & Murray, 2003; Koch et al., 2002). When hyperreplacement therapy is used, ionized magnesium levels may more accurately reveal hypermagnesemia, and these determinations are recommended to prevent over-replacement (Escuela et al., 2005).
11. Urinary magnesium excretion for 24 hours or a random urine specimen and correction calculation can help differentiate between renal and gastrointestinal causes of hypomagnesemia. A 24-hour urine collection is done; this is followed by administration of a magnesium load of approximately 30 mmol of magnesium chloride over 24 hours. The 24-hour urine collection is repeated, and the excretion of magnesium is measured. A daily magnesium excretion level greater than 10 to 30 mg or a fractional excretion greater than 2% indicates renal wasting (Dacey, 2001). The formula for calculating the fractional excretion of magnesium (FeMg) is:

$$FeMg = \frac{\text{Urinary magnesium} \times \text{Plasma creatinine}}{(0.7 \times \text{Plasma Mg}) \times \text{Urinary creatinine}} \times 100$$

12. Unexplained hypokalemia or hypocalcemia may be the result of cellular magnesium depletion and is present in 10% to 40% of patients with these electrolytes disturbances (Topf & Murray, 2003). This may confirmed by low urinary magnesium excretion or reduced magnesium excretion in response to intravenous loading with magnesium (less than 80% over 24 hours), although no test has clear diagnostic utility (Topf & Murray, 2003; Hebert et al., 1997).

NURSING CARE AND TREATMENT

1. Primary treatment for hypomagnesemia is replenishment of the electrolyte magnesium. The route of administration depends on the severity of the deficit and the degree of symptoms.
2. In the absence of unintentional losses, the normal daily requirement for magnesium is 400 mg (NIH, 2005).
3. Magnesium uptake in cells can be enhanced by correction of metabolic variables that influence renal excretion, such as acidosis, hyperglycemia, elevated bilirubin levels, and hemolysis (Dacey, 2001).
4. Intravenous replacement therapy is provided with magnesium chloride (1 g = 9 mEq) or magnesium sulfate (1 g = 8 mEq) (Dacey, 2001).
   - In symptomatic hypocalcemic-hypomagnesemic-hypokalemic patients with tetany or dysrhythmias, up to 10 g of magnesium sulfate (80 mEq) is administered over 24 hours (Sedlacek et al., 2006).
     - The recommended hourly dose is 0.5-1 g given intravenously for the first 72 hours (Dacey, 2001).
     - In patients with renal insufficiency, magnesium should be replaced at 0.25 g/hr initially.
     - Ongoing intravenous replacement in a patient with normal renal function is 0.1-0.2 mEq/kg/day (Dacey, 2001).
   - Because the primary feedback mechanism for renal excretion of magnesium is the serum level as it passes through the loop of Henle, the more rapid the magnesium administration, the greater the renal loss. Up to 50% of infused magnesium is excreted in the urine (Agus, 2006b). For this reason, slow or constant infusion provides better repletion than bolus infusion. Often a combination of intravenous and oral replacement therapy is instituted.
5. Oral therapy:
   - Oral magnesium replacement is best achieved with a sustained-release form that permits slow absorption without sudden variations in blood levels.
   - Maintenance doses of magnesium replacement usually are uniform in the repletion plan, but the various forms of replacement require individualized dosing based on their magnesium content. The goal of therapy usually is 0.4 mEq/kg/day, although ongoing magnesium wasting may require alteration of this goal (Dacey, 2001).
   - Consider drug interactions with oral magnesium (UMCIM, 2006; Topf & Murray, 2003).
     - Quinolone antimicrobials have decreased absorption when administered with magnesium.
     - Concomitant magnesium administration increases the adverse effects of calcium channel blocking agents.
     - Concomitant magnesium administration increases the absorption of oral diabetic agents and may cause hypoglycemia.
     - Magnesium may decrease the effectiveness of levothyroxine.
     - Theophylline toxicity is enhanced by hypomagnesemia.
   - Magnesium chloride (Slow Mag) (1 g = 9 mEq)
   - Magnesium lactate (Mag-Tab SR) (84 mg = 7 mEq)
   - Magnesium oxide (1 g = 9 mEq)
   - Magnesium gluconate (500 mg = 2.4 mEq)
   - Liquid calcium and magnesium with zinc and vitamin D (www.netrtion.com)
   - The most common dose-limiting adverse effects of magnesium replacement therapy are weakness, fatigue, and diarrhea.

6. Correction of the underlying etiology of hypomagnesemia:
   - Discontinue diuretics or change to a potassium-sparing diuretic.
   - Change medication regimens to agents that do not deplete magnesium.
   - Control metabolic demands if they contribute to the hypomagnesemia.

EVIDENCE-BASED PRACTICE UPDATES

1. Low serum magnesium levels perpetuate renal loss of potassium. If potassium is replaced while the magnesium is still deficient, the kidneys will excrete potassium and levels will remain low. When possible, magnesium should be replenished before potassium (Agus, 2006b; Rubeiz et al., 1993).
2. Patients with diabetes mellitus and hypomagnesemia should have magnesium repletion, because normalization of magnesium may reduce diabetes-related long-term complications such as retinopathy, nephropathy, and vasculitis (Pham et al., 2005; Topf & Murray, 2003).
3. Oncology patients commonly present with atrial dysrhythmias and have many risk factors for hypomagnesemia, even if plasma levels are within the low normal range. One study of critically ill patients showed that magnesium repletion was more effective than amiodarone in the management of atrial dysrhythmias of the critically ill (Moran et al., 1995).

TEACHING AND EDUCATION

1. Teach the patient and family food sources of magnesium to enhance replenishment strategies (Table 30-2).

Table 30-2 ORAL SOURCES OF MAGNESIUM	
Food Category	**Food High in Magnesium**
Beans	Black beans
	Navy beans
	Soybeans
	White beans
Dairy	Canned condensed milk
	Low-fat yogurt
Fish	Halibut
	Tuna
Fruits	Prune juice
Grains	Barley, pearled, raw
	Bran, oat
	Buckwheat flour
	Cornmeal
	Oatmeal
Nuts and seeds	Almonds
	Brazil nuts
	Cashews
	Pine nuts
	Pumpkin seeds
Vegetables	Artichokes
	Spinach (canned)
	Tomato paste

Data from the National Institutes of Health, Office of Dietary Supplements. Foods high in magnesium. Retrieved January 9, 2007, from http://www.ods.od.nih.gov.

2. Discuss the signs and symptoms of worsening and severe hypomagnesemia.
3. Teach the patient how to take magnesium supplements for maximum absorption and minimal drug-drug interference.
4. Teach the patient about natural remedies for the diarrhea that can occur with magnesium replacement therapy, such as decreased dietary fiber, decreased fatty food intake, and increased intake of white and enriched breads and grains or bananas.
5. **Web sites for information:**
   http://www.emedicine.com/EMERG/topic274.htm An emedicine aticle by Nona P. Novello titled Hypomagnesemia. Retrieved September 19, 2007.
   http://www.emedicine.com/ped/topic1122.htm An emedicine article by Anastasios K. Konstantakos and Enrique Grisoni titled Hypomagnesemia. Retrieved September 19, 2007.
   http://www.fpnotebook.com/REN93.htm Family Practice Notebook. Retrieved September 19, 2007.
   http://www.fpnotebook.com/REN93.htm Cleveland Clinic, an algorithm for hypomagnesiemai in critical care. Retrieved September 19, 2007.

NURSING DIAGNOSES

1. **Decreased cardiac output** secondary to dysrhythmia related to hypotention and ECG changes of flat T wave, prominent U wave, and/or depressed ST segment
2. **Acute pain** related to muscle cramping
3. **Diarrhea** related to oral magnesium replacement therapy
4. **Activity intolerance** related to neuromuscular spasticity
5. **Imbalanced nutrition: less than body requirements** related to anorexia and nausea that occur with hypomagnesemia

EVALUATION AND DESIRED OUTCOMES

1. Plasma magnesium levels are within normal values. They are drawn routinely when patients are receiving therapies known to deplete magnesium or when other risk factors are present.
2. Urinary magnesium is within normal value range. When the etiology of the hypomagnesemia is unclear, measurement of the urinary magnesium level in response to a magnesium load can help determine whether the condition is renal or gastrointestinal in origin (Hebert et al., 1997).

DISCHARGE PLAN AND FOLLOW-UP CARE

- Make sure the patient knows which foods and fluids supplement body magnesium.
- Make sure the patient knows about specific food and drug interactions with magnesium supplements.
- Discuss possible lifestyle changes and long-term replacement therapy with patients who may have permanent hypomagnesemia from cisplatin-induced nephrotoxicity (Stohr et al., 2007).

REVIEW QUESTIONS

QUESTIONS

1. The primary mechanism of magnesium regulation is/are:
1. Hormonal feedback mechanisms
2. Hepatic blood flow
3. Renal tubular excretion
4. Intestinal absorption

2. Normal serum magnesium levels are:
1. 0.3 to 1.3 mEq/L
2. 1.3 to 2.3 mEq/L
3. 2.3 to 3.3 mEq/L
4. 3.5 to 5 mEq/L

3. Patients taking which of the following medications are at risk for hypomagnesemia:
1. Cyclosporine
2. Phenytoin
3. Glyburide
4. Ciprofloxacin

4. The diagnostic test *most* helpful for detecting hypomagnesemia is:
1. Ionized magnesium
2. Plasma magnesium
3. Urinary fraction of magnesium
4. Magnesium/calcium ratio

5. The *most* significant clinical manifestations of hypomagnesemia involve which organ system:
1. Neurologic system
2. Pulmonary system
3. Renal system
4. Hematologic system

6. The cardiac dysrhythmia *most* often associated with hypomagnesemia is:
1. Sinus bradycardia
2. Junctional rhythm
3. Heart block
4. Torsades de pointes

7. The optimal method of administering magnesium replacement is:
1. Dietary supplements
2. Oral magnesium
3. Intramuscular magnesium
4. Intravenous magnesium

8. A food that is high in magnesium is:
1. Baked beans
2. Salad greens
3. Oatmeal
4. Bananas

9. A patient undergoing magnesium replacement therapy complains of diarrhea. The best strategy to teach the patient for eradicating this symptom is:
1. Increase the fluid intake
2. Increase the fat intake
3. Divide the magnesium dose into more frequent but lower doses
4. Take over-the-counter antidiarrheal agents

10. When patients have refractory hypomagnesemia despite discontinuation of offending etiologies and replacement therapy, which of the following may be done:
1. Check for untreated hypokalemia and hypocalcemia.
2. Evaluate the urinary fraction of magnesium.
3. Check for hypoalbuminemia.
4. Check adrenal and thyroid function for hormonal influences on magnesium.

ANSWERS

1. *Answer: 3*
Rationale: Magnesium is an intracellular ion, and its primary storage site is the bones. The kidneys regulate the excretion or retention of magnesium based on blood levels, and in times of depletion, mobilization from the bones occurs over a prolonged period.

2. *Answer: 2*
Rationale: The normal serum magnesium level is between 1.3 and 2.3 mEq/L or 0.65-1.25 mmol/L.

3. *Answer: 1*
Rationale: Cyclosporine is known to cause hypomagnesemia. Although hypomagnesemia is associated with diabetes, it is not presumed to be related to the oral hypoglycemic medications. However, magnesium and these agents do interact in ways that affect absorption, as do ciprofloxacin and magnesium.

4. *Answer: 2*
Rationale: Although ionized magnesium levels are thought to show the actual amount of ionized, or active, magnesium, the levels are so small, given the fraction of extracellular magnesium, that plasma levels are more accurate and less prone to laboratory error.

5. *Answer: 1*
Rationale: Magnesium is essential for most metabolic functions in the body. The most important system that evidences changes in ATP and energy is the neuromuscular system, therefore it is the most important reflection of magnesium deficiency. Cardiac dysrhythmias occur not because of intrinsic cardiovascular abnormalities, but because of neuromuscular irritability.

6. *Answer: 4*
Rationale: Tachyarrhythmias reflect the effects of irritable foci rather than primary conduction pathway abnormalities. Because magnesium deficiency most affects neuromuscular activity, atrial, junctional, or ventricular tachycardia can occur. A specific type of ventricular tachycardia, called *torsades de pointes*, has been positively linked to magnesium deficiency to the extent that the American Heart Association recommends magnesium administration even with asymptomatic torsades de pointes.

7. *Answer: 2*
Rationale: Magnesium blood levels influence the percentage of reabsorption from the kidneys, therefore replacement therapy is best if continuous intake is implemented. Slow-release oral magnesium is recommended for most cases of hypomagnesemia unless gastrointestinal tract deficits are the cause of the deficiency.

8. *Answer: 3*
Rationale: Magnesium is highest in unrefined grains, chlorophyll segments of vegetables, and fish. Cooking often depletes the magnesium content of fish and vegetables but not of grains. Consequently, grains, nuts, and seeds are the most reliable sources of magnesium.

9. *Answer: 3*
Rationale: Diarrhea associated with magnesium replenishment is notoriously difficult to manage. If patients are taking immediate-release medications, a sustained-release product may be prescribed. Dividing the dose into more frequent but lower doses may also be helpful. Some individuals believe that the particular formulation of magnesium may influence the degree of diarrhea experienced, therefore changing the source of magnesium may be helpful. At times, oral and parenteral replacement may be combined to reduce the incidence of this adverse effect.

10. *Answer: 1*
Rationale: Plasma magnesium levels generally reflect active magnesium levels, and although some magnesium is bound to albumin, this does not usually affect measured levels. Magnesium is not regulated by any hormone, although it may be low with high levels of antidiuretic hormone. Low potassium and calcium affect renal absorption of magnesium and may cause refractory hypomagnesemia.

REFERENCES

Agraharkar, M., & Fahlen, M. (2002). Hyperchloremic acidosis. Retrieved November 26, 2007, from www.e-medicine.com/MED/topic1071.htm

Agus, Z. S. (2006a). Causes of hypomagnesemia. 2007 UpToDate. Retrieved January 2, 2007, from www.ut-dol.com/.

Agus, Z. S. (2006b). Diagnosis and treatment of hypomagnesemia. 2007 UpToDate. Retrieved January 2, 2007, from www.utdol.com/.

Agus, Z. S. (2006c). Signs and symptoms of magnesium depletion. 2007 UpToDate. Retrieved January 2, 2007, from www.utdol.com/.

Aisa, Y., Mori, T., & Nakazato, T., et al. (2005). Effects of immunosuppressive agents on magnesium metabolism after allogeneic hematopoietic stem cell transplantation. *Transplantation, 80*:1046-1050.

Akhtar, N., Hafeez, F., & Ahmad, T. M. (2006). A familial hypomagnesemia-hypercalciuria (Manz syndrome). *Jcpsp, Journal of the College of Physicians & Surgeons-Pakistan. 16*(6):428-430.

Bashir, H, Crom, D, & Metzger, M, et al. (2006). Cisplatin-induced hypomagnesemia and cardiac dysrhythmia. *Pediatric Blood Cancer, 49*:867-869.

Chubanov, V., Gudermann, T., & Schlingmann, K. P. (2005). Essential role of TRPM6 in epithelial magnesium transport and body magnesium homeostasis. *Pflugers Archives European Journal of Physiology, 451*(1):228-234.

Corica, F, Corsonello, A., & Ientile, R., et al. (2006). serum ionized magnesium levels in relation to metabolic syndrome in type 2 diabetic patients, *Journal of the American College of Nutrition, 25*(3):210-215.

Dacey, M. J. (2001). Endocrine and metabolic dysfunction in the critically ill. *Critical Care Clinics 17*(1):155-173.

Dharnidharka, V. R., & Carney, P. R. (2005). Isolated idiopathic hypomagnesemia presenting as aphasia and seizures. *Pediatric Neurology, 33*:61-65.

Elisaf, M., Merkouropoulos, M., & Tsianos, E. V., et al. (1995). Pathogenetic mechanisms of hypomagnesemia in alcoholic patients. *Journal Trace Elements in Medical Biology, 9*:210-214.

Escuela, M. P., Guerra, M., & Anon, J. M., et al. (2005). Total and ionized serum magnesium in critically ill patients. *Intensive Care Medicine, 31*:151-156.

Fakih, M. G., Wilding, G., & Lombardo, J. (2006). Cetuximab-induced hypomagnesemia in patients with colorectal cancer. *Clinical Colorectal Cancer, 6*(2):152-156.

Guerrero-Romero, F., & Rodriguez-Moran, M. (2006). Hypomagnesemia, oxidative stress, inflammation, and metabolic syndrome. *Diabetes/Metabolism Research and Reviews, 22*:471-476.

Hebert, P., Mehta, N., & Wang, J., et al. (1997). Functional magnesium deficiency in critically ill patients identified using a magnesium loading test. *Critical Care Medicine, 25*:749-755.

Koch, S. M., Warters, R. D., & Mehlhorn, U. (2002). The simultaneous measurement of ionized and total calcium and ionized and total magnesium in intensive care unit patients. *Journal of Critical Care, 17*(3):203-205.

Moran, J. L., Gallagher, J., & Peake, S. L., et al. (1995). Parenteral magnesium sulfate versus amiodarone in the therapy of atrial tachyarrhythmias: A prospective randomized study. *Critical Care Medicine, 23*:1816-1824.

Mouw, D. R. (2005). What are the causes of hypomagnesemia? *Family Practice, 54*(2):174-176.

National Institutes of Health, Office of Dietary Supplements (NIH). (2005). Foods high in magnesium. Retrieved January 9, 2007, from http://www.ods.od.nih.gov.

Navaneethan, S. D., Sankarasubbaiyan, S., & Gross, M. D., et al. (2006). Tacrolimus-associated hypomagnesemia in renal transplant recipients. *Transplant Proceedings, 38*(5):1320-1322.

Nawaz, S. H., Zafar, M. N., & Naqvi, S. A., et al. (2005). Impact of cyclosporine immunosuppression on serum magnesium and its fractional excretion in renal transplant recipients. *Journal of the Pakistan Medical Association, 55*(3):98-100.

Panichpisal, K., Angulo-Pernett, F., & Selhi, S., et al. (2006). Gitelman-like syndrome after cisplatin therapy: A case report and literature review. *BMC Nephrology, 7*:10-14.

Pearson, E. C., & Woosley, R. L. (2005). QT prolongation and torsades de pointes among methadone users: Reports to the FDA spontaneous reporting system. *Pharmacoepidemiology and Drug Safety, 14*(11):747-753.

Perrin, C., Fabre, C., & Raoul, J. L., et al. (2006). Behavioral disorders secondary to profound hypomagnesemia in a patient given cetuximab for metastatic colorectal cancer hypomagnesemia due to cetuximab treatment. *Acta Oncologica, 45*(8):1135-1136.

Pham, P. C., Pham, P. M., & Pham, P. A., et al. (2005). Lower serum magnesium levels are associated with a more rapid decline of renal function in patients with diabetes mellitus type 2. *Clinical Nephrology, 63*(6):429-436.

Rubeiz, G. J., Thill-Baharozian, M., & Hardit, D., et al. (1993). Association of hypomagnesemia and mortality in acutely ill medical patients. *Critical Care Medicine, 21*:203-209.

Sales, C. H., & Pedrosa, L. F. (2006). Magnesium and diabetes mellitus: Their relation. *Clinical Nutrition,* *25*(4):554-562.

Schlingmann, K. P., Sassen, M. C., & Weber, S., et al. (2005). Novel TRMP6 mutations in 21 families with primary hypomagnesemia and secondary hypocalcemia. *Journal of the American Society of Nephrology,* *16*(10):3061-3069.

Schrag, D., Chung, K. Y., & Flombaum, C., et al. (2005). Cetuximab therapy and symptomatic hypomagnesemia. *Journal of the National Cancer Institute, 97*(16):1221-1224.

Schwarz, R. E., & Nevarez, K. Z. (2005). Hypomagnesemia after major abdominal operations in cancer patients: Clinical implications. *Archives of Medical Research, 36:*36-41.

Sedlacek, M., Schoolwerth, A. C., & Remillard, B. D. (2006). Electrolyte disturbances in the intensive care unit. *Seminars in Dialysis, 19*(6):496-501.

Stohr, W., Paulides, M., & Bielack, S., et al. (2007). Nephrotoxicity of cisplatin and carboplatin in sarcoma patients: A report from the late effects surveillance system. *Pediatric Blood Cancer, 48*(2):140-147.

Tataru, A., & Nicoara, E. (2004). Idiopathic diffuse alopecias in young women correlated with hypomagnesemia. *Journal of the European Academy of Dermatology and Venereology, 18*(3):393-394.

Teragawa, H., Kato, M., & Yamagata, T., et al. (2000). The preventive effect of magnesium on coronary spasm in patients with vasospastic angina. *Chest, 118:*1690-1695.

Thomson Healthcare. (2007). Thomson micromedex healthcare series. Retrieved January 15, 2007, from http://www.thomsonhc.com.

Tong, G. M., & Rude, R. K. (2005). Magnesium deficiency in critical illness. *Journal of Intensive Care Medicine,* *20:*3-17.

Topf, J. M., & Murray, P. T. (2003). Hypomagnesemia and hypermagnesemia. *Reviews in Endocrine and Metabolic Disorders, 4:*195-206.

University of Maryland Center of Integrative Medicine (UMCIM). (2006). Integrated medicine: Research.. Retrieved January 14, 2007, from www.compmed.umm.edu.

Voets, T., Nillus, B., & Hoefs, S., et al. (2004). TRPM6 forms the Mg2+ influx channel involved in intestinal and renal Mg2+ absorption. *Journal of Biology and Chemistry, 279:*19-25.

HYPONATREMIA

CYNTHIA C. CHERNECKY • DEMICA N. JACKSON • ANGELA L. DANIEL

PATHOPHYSIOLOGICAL MECHANISMS

Hyponatremia is a disorder of hypo-osmolality in which the rate of sodium loss exceeds the rate of water loss (true hyponatremia). Another type of hyponatremia, *relative hyponatremia*, is a condition in which the rate of water intake exceeds the kidneys' ability to secrete free water and maximally dilute the urine. Hyponatremia is characterized by a low serum sodium level and a low serum osmolality. It is a very common electrolyte disorder (Palm et al., 2006; Siragy, 2006).

Hyponatremia occurs in patients with malignancies (Elejalde, 2004) and in those who are hospitalized and institutionalized. It is most frequently seen in elderly individuals. If the condition goes untreated or undiagnosed, many serious outcomes are possible. These consequences often are neurologic in nature and may include seizures, cerebral edema, apnea, coma, and death.

Hypotonic hyponatremia can be classified as euvolemic, hypervolemic, or hypovolemic based on an assessment of the serum sodium level, the serum and urine osmolality, and the body's fluid volume status.

Euvolemic hyponatremia occurs when the body retains too much electrolyte free water. This type of hyponatremia normally is related to impaired renal excretion in renal failure and the syndrome of inappropriate secretion of antidiuretic hormone (SIADH) (see Chapter 47).

Hypervolemic hyponatremia occurs with an increase in the extracellular fluid volume. It usually is accompanied by a disease process, such as heart failure.

Hypovolemic hyponatremia is related to a decrease in the extracellular volume as a result of renal sodium wasting, which leads to cerebral salt wasting (CSW), such as can occur in patients with subarachnoid hemorrhage. The CSW likely related is to decreased secretion of brain natriuretic peptide, with a resulting decrease in the secretion of aldosterone. If the condition goes untreated, cerebral edema occurs, with neurologic compromise and potential herniation of the brain. Hypovolemic hyponatremia also can be caused by conditions in which the body's need to replace intravascular volume outweighs the need to maintain appropriate serum and blood osmolality.

In all cases, the hyponatremia can lead to impaired cognitive function, a depressed level of consciousness, and convulsions.

In summary, hypotonic hyponatremia can be euvolemic (diuretic therapy, SIADH), hypervolemic (heart failure, cirrhosis, renal failure) or hypovolemic (CSW). It also can have the major clinical presentation of cerebral edema caused by water entering the brain.

A common cause of hyponatremia is hyperglycemia, which raises the plasma osmolality while sodium levels remain the same; this has the effect of lowering the plasma sodium concentration. Heart failure reduces the serum osmolality while raising the extracellular fluid volume, leading to hyponatremia.

Hormones are also involved with water balance regulation; these include antidiuretic hormone (ADH), atrial natriuretic peptide (ANP), brain natriuretic peptide (BNP) and c-type natriuretic peptide (CNP). ADH, also known as *arginine vasopressin* (AVP), is produced by the hypothalamic nuclei in response to increased plasma osmolality and decreased vascular volume. It acts on the distal tubules and collecting ducts of the nephrons to increase free water permeability and reabsorption of free water and promotes vasoconstriction. ANP is secreted mainly from the atria of the heart in response to atrial stretch caused by elevated intravascular volume or systolic heart failure. BNP is present in the brain and cardiac ventricles and is elevated in patients with cardiac hypertrophy or heart failure. C-type peptides promote shifting of fluid from the intravascular compartments to the extravascular compartments, thereby reducing blood pressure. As can easily be seen, if any of these hormone levels are altered, the resulting fluid volume changes can have serious consequences. In oncology patients, hyponatremia also can result from SIADH (see Chapter 47), which produces an overall euvolemic or mild hypervolemic state, and from CSW, which results in an overall hypovolemic state with compensatory tachycardia.

EPIDEMIOLOGY AND ETIOLOGY

Hyponatremia occurs in 1% to 2% of hospitalized patients (Offenstandt & Das, 2006) and in these cases is known as *hospital-acquired hyponatremia* (Moritz & Ayus, 2006). It is the second most common problem in oncology patients (Elejalde, 2004), and it occurs in 31.3% of institutionalized elderly individuals (Chen et al., 2006). Hyponatremia often is caused by overadministration of hypotonic intravenous fluids after surgery; this complicates the condition of 20% of all surgical patients (Achinger et al., 2006). Factors that contribute to hospital-acquired hyponatremia include administration of thiazide diuretics, administration of medications to stimulate ADH, surgery, and overadministration of hypotonic IV fluids (Hoorn et al., 2006). The average duration of an increased length of stay for hospital-acquired hyponatremia is 12 days; therefore it is clear that the condition has a serious impact on health care costs and the patient's quality of life (Hoorn et al., 2006).

RISK PROFILE

- Diseases and conditions associated with hyponatremia (Box 31-1).
- Drug classes and medications known to cause hyponatremia (Box 31-2).
- Chemotherapy medications known to cause hyponatremia (Box 31-3).
- Populations at risk for hyponatremia (Box 31-4).
- Surgery and treatments that increase the risk of hyponatremia (Box 31-5).

PROGNOSIS

In one study, pediatric oncology patients given hypotonic intravenous fluids were more likely to have hyponatremia with seizures (Duke et al., 2005). Symptomatic hyponatremia and hypoxia have high mortality rates (Kokko, 2006). The mortality rate for acute hyponatremia that develops in less than 48 hours is 50%. In symptomatic hyponatremia, when the serum sodium level is 120 to 130 mEq/L, the mortality rate is 15%. Hyponatremia in early phase ST elevation after an MI is a predictor of long-term mortality (Goldberg et al., 2006).

BOX 31-1	DISEASES AND CONDITIONS ASSOCIATED WITH HYPONATREMIA

- Acromegaly
- Anion gap, reduced
- Beer potomania syndrome
- Cancer: Brain, breast, colon, CNS lymphoma, Hodgkin's lymphoma, hypothalamic tumor, gastric, leukemia, lung (small cell), multiple myeloma (Sachs & Fredman, 2006), ovary, pancreas, pituitary tumor
- Cerebral salt wasting (CSW)
- Diabetes insipidus
- Diarrhea
- Gastroenteritis
- Gitelman's syndrome (Ogihara et al., 2004)
- Glucocorticoid deficiency
- Heart failure
- Hypercholesterolemia, severe (Inamoto et al., 2005)
- Hyperglycemia
- Hypothyroidism
- Malaria (Idro et al., 2006)
- Meningitis, bacterial
- Metabolic alkalosis (Sweetser et al., 2005)
- Mineralocorticoid deficiency
- Pertussis (Vaessen et al., 2006)
- Pituitary cyst
- Pre-eclampsia (Ravid et al., 2005)
- Prolactinoma
- Rathke's cleft cyst
- Renovascular hypertension
- Status epilepticus
- Subarachnoid hemorrhage
- Syndrome of inappropriate secretion of antidiuretic hormone (SIADH)
- Triple-A syndrome (Lam et al., 2006)
- Tuberculosis (TB) (Abal et al., 2005)

BOX 31-2	DRUG CLASSES AND MEDICATIONS KNOWN TO CAUSE HYPONATREMIA

- Antidepressants (trazodone, venlafaxine) (Egger et al., 2006)
- Antidiuretic hormones (desmopressin acetate [DDAVP])
- Antiepileptics/anticonvulsants (carbamazepine, mirtazapine, oxcarbazepine)
- Antifungals (Amphotericin B)
- Diuretics (bumetanide, furosemide)
- Hallucinogenics (Ecstasy [MDMA]) (Reingardiene, 2006)
- Herbals (weight reduction teas)
- Intravenous immunoglobulin (IVIG) (Nguyen et al., 2006)
- Monoamine anhydrase oxidase inhibitors (MAOIs)
- Neuroleptics
- Nonsteroidal antiinflammatory drugs (NSAIDs [Advil, ibuprofen, Motrin])
- Selective serotonin reuptake inhibitors (SSRIs [citalopram, fluoxetine, mirtazapine]) (Bavbek et al., 2006)
- Tricyclic antidepressants (amitriptyline, amoxapine, desipramine, doxepin, imipramine, nortriptyline, trimipramine)
- Urinary tract antispasmodic (tolterodine tartrate [Detrol]) (Juss et al., 2005)

| BOX 31-3 | CHEMOTHERAPY MEDICATIONS KNOWN TO CAUSE HYPONATREMIA |

- Cisplatin
- Cyclophosphamide (high dose)
- 5-FU
- Ifosfamide
- Methotrexate (intrathecal) (Diskin et al., 2006)
- Vinblastine
- Vincristine

Berghmans, T. (1996). Hyponatremia related to medical anticancer treatment (review). *Supportive Care in Cancer, 4(5)*:341-350.

PROFESSIONAL ASSESSMENT CRITERIA (PAC)

1. Serum sodium level less than 130 mEq/L.
2. **Serum osmolality:** Isotonicity and hypertonicity are seen in patients with hyperglycemia or with mannitol or sorbitol use. Hypotonicity (<280 mOsm/kg) is most commonly seen, and the nurse needs to determine whether the kidneys can eliminate urine by assessing and evaluating patient's glomerular filtration rates, urine outputs and serum creatinine levels.
3. Urine osmolality is low or high in the hypovolemic or hypervolemic state and high in the euvolemic state.
4. **Neurologic status:** Diminished deep tendon reflexes, confusion, and disorientation.
5. Assess the patient for high-risk treatments, surgeries, diagnoses, conditions, and medications, including chemotherapeutic drugs.
6. **Foods with diuretic properties:** Asparagus, artichoke, cabbage, foods that contain caffeine, corn, cucumbers, grapes, weight-loss herbal teas, spinach, and watermelon.
7. **Vital signs:** Hypovolemic hyponatremic patients often have an elevated temperature and a rapid, weak pulse. They may be tachypneic and have a lower systolic BP. Euvolemic hyponatremic patients often present with a temperature at or below baseline and the pulse, respirations, and BP are normal. Hypervolemic hyponatremic patients often have a temperature at or below normal, a rapid pulse, and an elevated BP. They may have tachypnea with dyspnea on exertion.
8. **Hallmark signs and symptoms:** Malaise, lethargy, weakness, muscle cramps, nausea. hyperreflexia, and muscle twitching. (See Box 31-6 for a list of early symptoms and Box 31-7 for a list of late symptoms.)
9. Assess laboratory values (Box 31-8).

| BOX 31-4 | POPULATIONS AT RISK FOR HYPONATREMIA |

- Elderly individuals
- Individuals who exercise for longer than 1 hour
- Infants (premature)
- Menstruant women
- Individuals with mental health problem (depression, schizophrenia)
- Pediatric patients
- Women as related to adverse drug effects(Grikiniene et al., 2004)

| BOX 31-5 | **SURGERY AND TREATMENTS THAT INCREASE THE RISK OF HYPONATREMIA** |

- Acoustic neuroma surgery
- Colonic enemas (Norlela et al., 2004)
- Colonoscopy with polyethylene glycol (PEG) preparation
- Neurosurgery (Frazer & Stieg, 2006)
- Transurethral prostatectomy (TURP)

| BOX 31-6 | **EARLY SIGNS AND SYMPTOMS OF HYPONATREMIA** |

- Decreased deep tendon reflexes
- Headache
- Irritability
- Lethargy
- Muscle cramps
- Nausea
- Vomiting

| BOX 31-7 | **LATE SIGNS AND SYMPTOMS OF HYPONATREMIA** |

- Anorexia
- Asterixis
- Bradycardia (if hypovolemic)
- Coma
- Coordination impairment
- Decreased cognitive function
- Dizziness
- Drowsiness
- Polydipsia
- Pupil dilation
- Respiratory insufficiency

| BOX 31-8 | **LABORATORY TESTS FOR HYPONATREMIA** |

- AAAS gene mutation (Lam et al., 2006)
- AVP (arginine vasopressin) 0.21-2.1 pg/mL
- $PO_2 < 50$ mm Hg (Arieff, 2006)
- Potassium, serum (high in hypovolemic state with adrenal metastasis and in hypervolemic state from renal dysfunction; normal in euvolemic state)
- Serum osmolality
- Thyroid hormone, serum (TSH, T_3, T_4)
- Serum sodium <130 mEq/L in hypovolemic, euvolemic, and hypervolemic states; values <125 mEq/L indicate severe hyponatremia)
- Urine osmolality: Low or high (>800 mOsm/kg H_2O) in hypovolemic state;, high in euvolemic state; and low (<100 mOsm/kg H_2O) or high (>300 mOsm/kg H_2O) in hypervolemic state
- Urine sodium: Low in hypovolemic state; high in euvolemic state; either high or low in hypervolemic state

10. Central venous pressure (CVP) is less than 2 mm Hg in hypovolemia; 2 to 6 mm Hg in euvolemia; and greater than 6 mm Hg in hypervolemia.

NURSING CARE AND TREATMENT

The following nursing interventions as presented are prioritized.

1. STAT serum electrolyte panel, creatinine, and AVP. After replacement therapy, the electrolyte panel can be evaluated each day × 48 hours.
2. Seizure precautions and supportive care for acute life-threatening conditions.
3. Vital signs and level of consciousness q2hr if acute. If patient is positive for signs of heart failure, assess q8hr for: rales, tachypnea, dyspnea, S3, tachycardia, jugular vein distension (JVD), peripheral edema, and bounding pulses.
4. Fluid restriction with renal failure or symptomatic hyponatremia. Fluid and sodium restriction for hypervolemic hyponatremia.
5. Hourly intake and output (more accurate with insertion of a urinary catheter).
6. IV normal saline with potassium and/or mineralocorticoids.
7. Placement of a vascular access device (VAD) for intravenous access and possible hemodynamic monitoring.
8. IV loop diuretics for hypervolemic hyponatremia.
9. AVP receptor antagonists:
   - Conivaptan 40-80 mg PO QD (Ghali et al., 2006)
   - Fludrocortisone 0.1 mg PO TID × 1 to 8 days (Wijdicks et al., 1988)
   - Oral urea (Berghmans et al., 2005).
10. Angiotensin-converting enzyme (ACE) for heart failure.
11. Thyroid hormone replacement if thyroid has been damaged by radiation or other factors.
12. Antidiarrheals and antiemetics as needed.
13. Weigh patient daily if acute.
    Box 31-9 presents a quick review of treatment strategies.

EVIDENCE-BASED PRACTICE UPDATES

1. Hyponatremia after initiation of chemotherapy is a warning signal of impending leukopenia and thrombocytopenia (Boku et al., 2001).
2. Hyponatremia is most likely to occur on day 8 of the chemotherapy nadir (Boku et al., 2001).
3. Patients with hyponatremia have a sixtyfold higher case fatality rate (Bennani et al., 2003).
4. Several nonpeptide vasopressin receptor antagonists have shown promise (Pham et al., 2006; Palm et al., 2006): VPA-985 (lixivaptan), YM-087 (conivaptan), OPC-41061 (tolvaptan), and SR-121463.
5. Mild hyponatremia contributes to an increased rate of falls (Decaux, 2006).
6. Overuse of NSAIDs can lead to severe hyponatremia (Wharam et al., 2006).

BOX 31-9	**TREATMENT FOR HYPONATREMIA**

- AVP (arginine vasopressin) receptor antagonists
- Conivaptan 40-80 mg PO QD (Ghali et al., 2006)
- Fludrocortisone 0.1 mg PO TID × 1 to 8 days (Wijdicks et al., 1988)
- Fluid replacement (hypertonic)
- Fluid restriction

TEACHING AND EDUCATION

1. Reduce or discontinue chemotherapy, because certain chemotherapeutic medications can induce kidney dysfunction and failure.
2. Obtain blood samples from the VAD and urine samples from the urinary catheter to track sodium levels.
3. Peripheral intravenous fluids may be necessary initially to begin fluid replacement.
4. Explain to the patient that fluid restriction is necessary to help the kidneys and heart function properly.
5. For patients with hypovolemic hyponatremia: Explain that dietary changes include eating foods that contain sodium.
6. Educate the patient and family to watch for signs of hyponatremia: Fatigue, weakness, confusion, muscle cramps, muscle twitching, nausea, vomiting, and convulsions or seizures.
7. **Web sites for information:**
   - Medline plus, US Library of Medicine and the National Institutes of Health http://www.nlm.nih.gov/medlineplus/ency/article/000394.htm
   - Mayo Clinic http://www.mayoclinic.com/health/low-blood-sodium/AN00621
   - Science Oxygen http://www.findarticles.com/p/articles/mi_m3225.is_10_69/ai_n6048503

NURSING DIAGNOSES

1. **Ineffective airway clearance** related to seizures or coma secondary to cerebral edema
2. **Acute confusion** related to cerebral edema and/or low serum sodium
3. **Deficient fluid volume** related to vomiting, diarrhea, increased urinary excretion, and decreased oral intake
4. **Excess fluid volume** related to infusion of hypotonic fluids, heart failure, liver metastasis, or oliguria secondary to chemotherapy
5. **Risk for injury** related to falls, motor deficits, and neurologic deficits from hyponatremia

EVALUATION AND DESIRED OUTCOMES

1. The serum sodium level will increase to greater than 120 mEq/L (greater than 120 mmol/L SI units) within 24 hours.
2. The serum sodium, urine sodium and osmolality, and serum potassium will return to normal levels within 48 hours.
3. Signs and symptoms of hyponatremia will be eliminated within 72 hours.
4. Chemotherapy will be resumed if appropriate.

DISCHARGE PLANNING AND FOLLOW-UP CARE

- Visit to physician's office in 1 week.
- Outpatient laboratory serum electrolytes and creatinine in 1 week.
- Continuation of dietary and fluid restrictions.
- Home visits for short-term enteral nutrition or IV fluids, intake and output, vital signs, and diuretic and other medication treatments.

REVIEW QUESTIONS

QUESTIONS

1. **Hyponatremia is primarily a disorder of:**
   1. Excess cerebrospinal fluid
   2. Lactic acidosis
   3. Hypo-osmolality
   4. Chloride depletion

2. **A primary nursing diagnosis for a patient with hyponatremia is:**
   1. Deficient fluid volume or excess fluid volume
   2. Ineffective coping
   3. Risk for infection
   4. Ampulla vater edema with insufficiency

3. **Patients at high risk for hospital-acquired hyponatremia are those who have:**
   1. Full-term babies
   2. Hyperoxygenation therapy
   3. Neurosurgery
   4. Low-dose corticosteroid therapy

4. **Hyponatremia is most common in people with which type of cancer:**
   1. Cervical cancer
   2. Small cell lung cancer
   3. Testicular cancer
   4. Malignant melanoma

5. **Which of the following is an early sign of hyponatremia:**
   1. Asterixis
   2. Pupil dilation
   3. Respiratory insufficiency
   4. Headache

6. **Which patient is at greatest risk for hyponatremia:**
   1. Child, age 14 years, post appendectomy, menstruant girl
   2. Elderly woman, postop neurosurgery, depressed
   3. Male, age 36 years, schizophrenic, exercises 20 minutes walking daily
   4. Male, age 6 months, pneumonia, receiving intravenous antibiotics

7. **Which intervention is the highest priority in a patient suspected of having hyponatremia:**
   1. Initiate seizure precautions
   2. Assess deep tendon reflexes
   3. Urinary catheter STAT
   4. Serum electrolytes STAT

8. **Eating foods that contain sodium is an appropriate intervention for a patient with:**
   1. Euvolemic hyponatremia
   2. Hypertonic chloremia
   3. Hypovolemic hyponatremia
   4. Hypervolemic hyponatremia

9. **A patient diagnosed with hyponatremia secondary to heart failure resulting from chemotherapy would primarily be taught about:**
   1. Alopecia
   2. Low-fat diet
   3. Symptoms of hypothyroidism
   4. Restriction of fluid intake

10. **Your patient is taking benazepril (Lotensin), furosemide (Lasix), trazodone (Desyrel), colonic irrigations, sildenafil citrate (Viagra), and vitamin E to try to cure his colon cancer. Which of these medications and treatments puts him at high risk for hyponatremia:**
    1. Benazepril and vitamin E
    2. Furosemide and trazodone
    3. Colonic irrigations and vitamin E
    4. Sildenafil citrate and benazepril

ANSWERS

1. *Answer: 3*
   Rationale: Hypo-osmolality occurs when the rate of sodium loss exceeds the rate of water loss (true hyponatremia) or when the rate of water intake exceeds the ability of the kidneys to excrete free water and maximally dilute urine (relative hyponatremia).

2. *Answer: 1*
   Rationale: Hypotonic hyponatremia is fluid volume excess, and fluid volume deficit is depletion of extracellular fluid.

3. *Answer: 3*
   Rationale: Patients who have neurosurgery are at risk as a result of

administration of intravenous fluids and cerebral edema.

4. *Answer: 2*
   Rationale: SCLC is a common cause of hyponatremia, along with breast cancer and multiple myeloma.

5. *Answer: 4*
   Rationale: Headache is an early sign of hyponatremia; the other signs listed are late signs.

6. *Answer: 2*
   Rationale: Older age, undergoing neurosurgery, depression, and female gender all are risk factors.

7. *Answer: 4*
   Rationale: A serum sodium level, which is part of an electrolyte panel, is essential for diagnosing hyponatremia.

8. *Answer: 3*
   Rationale: Patients with hypovolemic hyponatremia have a loss of sodium and water.

9. *Answer: 4*
   Rationale: Water and fluid restrictions are part of the dietary changes required to prevent excess water retention by the body.

10. *Answer: 2*
    Rationale: Diuretics (e.g., furosemide), antidepressants (e.g., trazodone), and colonic irrigations are known to increase the risk of hyponatremia.

REFERENCES

Abal, A. T., Jayakrishnan, B., & Parwer, S, et al. (2005). Demographic pattern and clinical characteristics of patients with smear-positive pulmonary tuberculosis in Kuwait. *Medical Principles and Practice, 14*(5):306-312.

Achinger, S. G., Moritz, M. L., & Ayus, J. C. (2006). Dysnatremias: Why are patients still dying? *Southern Medical Journal, 99*(4):353-362.

Arieff, A. I. (2006). Influence of hypoxia and sex on hyponatremic encephalopathy (review). *American Journal of Medicine, 119*(Suppl. 1):S59-S64.

Bavbek, N., Kargili, A., & Akcay, A., et al. (2006). Recurrent hyponatremia associated with citalopram and mirtazapine. *American Journal of Kidney Diseases, 48*(4):e61-e62.

Bennani, S. L., Abouqal, R., & Zeggwagh, A. A., et al. (2003). Incidence, causes and prognostic factors of hyponatremia in intensive care (French). *La Revue de Médecine Interne, 24*:224-229.

Berghmans, T. (1996). Hyponatremia related to medical anticancer treatment (review). *Supportive Care Cancer, 4*:341-350.

Berghmans, T, Meert, A., & Schulier, J. P. (2005). Correction of hyponatremia by urea in a patient with heart failure. *Acta Clinica Belgica, 60*(5):244-266.

Boku, N., Ohtsu, A., & Nagashima, F., et al. (2001). Retrospective study of hyponatremia in gastric cancer patients treated with a combination of chemotherapy of 5-fluorouracil and cisplatin: A possible warning sign of severe hematological toxicities? *Japanese Journal of Clinical Oncology, 31*(8):382-387.

Chen, L. K., Lin, M. H., & Hwang, S. J., et al. (2006). Hyponatremia among the institutionalized elderly in 2 long-term care facilities in Taipei. *Journal of the Chinese Medical Association, 69*(3):115-119.

Decaux, G. (2006). Is asymptomatic hyponatremia really asymptomatic? *American Journal of Medicine, 119*(Suppl. 1):S79-S82.

Diskin, C., Dansby, L. M., & Radcliff, L., et al. (2006). Recurrent hyponatremia after intrathecal methotrexate not related to antidiuretic hormone: Is a natriuretic peptide activated? *American Journal of the Medical Sciences, 331*(1):37-39.

Duke, T., Kinney, S., & Waters, K. (2005). Hyponatraemia and seizures in oncology patients associated with hypotonic intravenous fluids. *Journal of Paediatrics & Child Health, 41*(12):685-686.

Egger, C., Muehlbacher, M., & Nickel, M., et al. (2006). A case of recurrent hyponatremia induced by venlafaxine. *Journal of Clinical Psychopharmacology, 26*(4):439.

Elejalde, J. L. (2004). Metabolic emergencies in the oncology patient (review). *Anales del Sistema Sanitario de Narvarra, 27*(Suppl, 3):53-62.

Frazer, J. F., & Stieg, P. E. (2006). Hyponatremia in the neurosurgical patient: Epidemiology, pathophysiology, diagnosis, and management. *Neurosurgery, 59*(2):222-229.

Ghali, J. K., Koren, M. J., & Taylor, J. R., et al. (2006). Efficacy and safety of oral conivaptan: A V1A/V2 vasopressin receptor antagonist, assessed in a randomized, placebo-controlled trial in patients with euvolemic or hypervolemic hyponatremia. *Journal of Clinical Endocrinology & Metabolism, 91*(6):2145-2152.

Goldberg, A., Hammerman, H., & Petcherski, S., et al. (2006). Hyponatremia and long-term mortality in survivors of acute ST-elevation myocardial infarction. *Archives of Internal Medicine, 166*(7):781-786.

Grikiniene, J., Volbekas, V., & Stakisaitis, D. (2004). Gender differences of sodium metabolism and hyponatremia as an adverse drug effect (review). *Medicina (Kaunas, Lithuania), (Kaunas, Lithuania) 40*(10):935-942.

Hoorn, E. J., Lindemans, J., & Zietse, R. (2006). Development of severe hyponatremia in hospitalized patients: Treatment-related risk factors and inadequate management. *Nephrology Dialysis Transplantation, 21*(1):70-76.

Idro, R., Aketch, S., & Gwar, S., et al. (2006). Research priorities in the management of severe Plasmodium falciparum malaria in children (review). *Annals of Tropical Medicine & Parasitology, 100*(2):95-108.

Inamoto, Y., Teramoto, T., & Shirai, K., et al. (2005). Severe hypercholesterolemia associated with decreased hepatic triglyceride lipase activity and pseudohyponatremia in patients after allogeneic stem cell transplantation. *International Journal of Hematology, 82*(4):363-366.

Juss, J. K., Radhamma, A. K., & Forsyth, D. R. (2005). Tolterodine-induced hyponatremia. *Age & Ageing, 34*(5):524-525.

Kokko, J. P. (2006). Symptomatic hyponatremia with hypoxia in a medical emergency. *Kidney International, 69*(8):1319-1325.

Lam, Y. Y., Lo, I. F., & Shek, C. C., et al. (2006). Triple-A syndrome: The first Chinese patient with novel mutations in the AAAS gene. *Journal of Pediatric Endocrinology, 19*(5):765-770.

Moritz, M. L., & Ayus, J. C. (2006). Case 8-2006: A woman with Crohn's disease and altered mental status. *New England Journal of Medicine, 354*(26):2833-2834.

Nguyen, M. K., Rastogi, A., & Kurtz, I. (2006). True hyponatremia secondary to intravenous immunoglobulin. *Clinical and Experimental Nephrology, 10*(2):124-126.

Norlela, S., Izham, C., & Khalid, B. A. (2004). Colonic irrigation—induced hyponatremia. *Malaysian Journal of Pathology, 26*(2):117-118.

Offenstandt, G., & Das, V. (2006). Hyponatremia, hypernatremia: A physiological approach (review). *Minerva Anesthesiologica, 72*(6):353-356.

Ogihara, T., Katsuya, T., & Ishikawa, K., et al. (2004). Hypertension is a patient with Gitelman's syndrome. *Journal of Human Hypertension, 18*(9):677-679.

Palm, C., Pistrosch, F., & Herbrig, K, et al. (2006). Vasopressin antagonists as aquaretic agents for the treatment of hyponatremia (review). *American Journal of Medicine, 119*(Suppl. 1):S87-S92.

Pham, P. C., Pham, P. M., & Pham, P. T. (2006). Vasopressin excess and hyponatremia (review). *American Journal of Kidney Diseases, 47*(5):727-737.

Ravid, D., Massarwa, L. E., & Biron-Shental, T., et al. (2005). Hyponatremia in preeclampsia. *Journal of Maternal-Fetal & Neonatal Medicine, 18*(1):77-79.

Reingardiene, D. (2006). Ecstasy toxicity (review). *Medicina (Kaunas, Lithuania), 42*(6):519-523.

Sachs, J., & Fredman, B. (2006). The hyponatremia of multiple myeloma is true and not pseudohyponatremia. *Medical Hypotheses, 67*(4):839-840.

Siragy, H. M. (2006). Hyponatremia, fluid-electrolyte disorders, and the syndrome of inappropriate antidiuretic hormone secretion: Diagnosis and treatment options (review). *Endocrine Practice, 12*(4):446-457.

Sweetser, L. J., Douglas, J. A., & Riha, R. L., et al. (2005). Clinical presentation of metabolic alkalosis in an adult patient with cystic fibrosis. *Respirology, 10*(2):254-256.

Vaessen, S., Anthopoulou, A., & Bricteux, G. (2006). Clinical case of the month: Fatal pertussis infection in a 2 month old infant (French). *Revue Medicale de Liege, 61*(3):146-148.

Wharam, P. C., Speedy, D. B., & Noakes, T. D., et al. (2006). NSAID use increases the risk of developing hyponatremia during an Ironman triathlon. *Medicine & Science in Sports & Exercise, 38*(4):618-622.

Wijdicks, E. F., Vermeulen, M., & van Brummeleen, P., et al. (1988). The effect of fludrocortisone acetate on plasma volume and natriuresis in patients with aneurismal subarachnoid hemorrhage. *Clinical Neurologic Neurosurgery, 90*:209-214.

INCREASED INTRACRANIAL PRESSURE

KARA L. PENNE

PATHOPHYSIOLOGICAL MECHANISMS

Increased intracranial pressure (ICP) can be caused by numerous surgical and medical problems. The skull is a closed compartment, therefore an increase in volume can lead to symptoms of ICP. The skull contains the brain and interstitial fluid, intravascular blood, and cerebrospinal fluid (CSF). The Monro-Kellie hypothesis states that if one component increases in volume, another component must decrease in volume to maintain homeostasis (Goetz, 2003). The ICP is ever changing and is affected by several physiologic processes. A common cause of increased ICP is a malignant intracranial process. Malignant processes can increase pressure through displacement of brain tissue, obstruction of CSF flow, and increased vascularity associated with tumor growth (Fig. 32.1). Increased ICP often is an early sign of a progressive tumor, and increased ICP can quickly lead to life-threatening complications.

Increased ICP produces several warning symptoms, including papilledema, headaches, nausea and vomiting, vital sign changes, and neurologic dysfunction, depending on the location of the tumor and edema. Papilledema occurs secondary to tumor blockage of the CSF flow, which increases pressure around the optic nerve. Subsequently, venous blood outflow becomes impaired, which causes edema of the optic disk. Papilledema is almost always bilateral and does not affect vision. It may occur over several hours or several days, depending on the etiology (Greenberg et al., 1993).

Headache is another common presenting symptom of increased ICP. It usually is marked by an early morning onset of bilateral frontal or occipital pain. The pain is exacerbated by movements that increase ICP, such as lying down, bending over, coughing, and/or the Valsalva maneuver. The headache may be accompanied by projectile vomiting as a result of increased pressure on the vomiting center in the medulla oblongata. It is thought that headache pain occurs secondary to pressure exerted by the tumor on the large blood vessels and dura and on the cranial and cervical nerve fibers (Dalessio, 1978).

Patients may also develop Cushing's triad, a set of three clinical manifestations (i.e., bradycardia, systolic hypertension, and widening pulse pressure) caused by direct pressure and/or tumor invasion into the vasomotor center in the medulla. These signs, which may occur in response to intracranial hypertension or herniation syndrome, are a late finding of neurologic deterioration (Carlson, 2002). Other focal symptoms are possible and are directly related to the location of the tumor. These may include hemiparesis, aphasia, seizures, hemisensory loss, and/or personality changes.

Primary brain tumors account for only 1.3% of all cancers (ACS, 2006), but they often present with symptoms of increased ICP. Low-grade tumors grow slowly, therefore the intracranial pressure increases slowly, which may not always lead to symptom development. High-grade tumors, primarily glioblastoma multiforme, grow rapidly, leading to acute onset

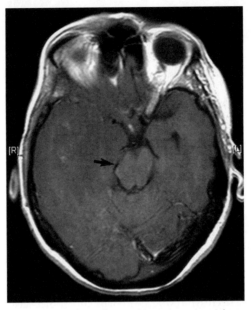

Fig. 32.1 • Subfalcine herniation *(arrow)* caused by progressive right temporal brain tumor.

of symptoms such as headache, hemiparesis, seizures, visual changes, and aphasia, depending on the tumor's location. Some tumors can cause acute blockage of CSF flow through the ventricles, resulting in a dramatic increase in ICP. Regardless of the cause, the increased pressure in the intracranial cavity can cause nerve cell damage and death.

The treatment for increased ICP includes procedures and pharmacologic approaches. Emergency placement of a ventriculostomy catheter through a burr hole is performed to reduce the ICP immediately by draining CSF fluid. This allows for close management and monitoring of CSF drainage. Surgical resection or debulking of malignant tissue can also alleviate ICP relatively quickly. Chemotherapy and/or radiation therapy is used to reduce the tumor burden, resulting in decreased ICP. These options are beneficial for patients who are not eligible for surgery because of the tumor's location or because of poor performance status.

Pharmacologic approaches to the management of ICP include osmotic diuretics, glucocorticoids, barbiturate therapy, and/or anticonvulsants. Mannitol, an osmotic diuretic, pulls fluid from the interstitial space into the vascular space. To prevent fluid overload in the vasculature, a loop diuretic may be administered (LeJeune & Howard-Fain, 2002). Glucocorticoids are most helpful for managing increased ICP secondary to intracranial or spinal cord malignancies (LeJeune, & Howard-Fain, 2002). Barbiturate therapy is used to lower cerebral blood flow and brain metabolism, which can lower the ICP; however, this may lead to hypotension, therefore caution should be used. Anticonvulsants are used to prevent seizure activity. It is critical that oncology nurses be alert for signs of increased ICP and its management so that emergency interventions can be initiated to reduce damage.

EPIDEMIOLOGY AND ETIOLOGY

Patients with cancer can develop increased ICP from primary brain tumors, brain metastases, hemorrhage, meningitis, head trauma, infarction, or abscess (Quinn & DeAngelis, 2000).

The onset can be acute or subacute. Cerebrovascular disease, specifically infarction and/or hemorrhage, is the most common etiology of neurologic symptoms in patients with cancer. One study found that 14.6% of 3426 patients with terminal cancer had cerebral hemorrhages or infarctions (Graus et al., 1985). Coagulation disorders, infection, cerebral metastases, and complications from cancer treatment are the most common causes of cerebrovascular disease in patients with cancer (Graus et al., 1985).

RISK PROFILE

- Cancer, especially primary gliomas, brain metastases, neuroblastomas, and leukemia. Primary cancers with an increased incidence of brain metastases include lung cancer, breast cancer, and melanoma
- Pediatric brain tumors, including cerebellar tumors, medulloblastoma, and ependymoma of the fourth ventricle
- Coagulation disorder, thrombocytopenia, or platelet dysfunction
- Bacterial or fungal infection, meningitis, or brain abscess
- Head trauma
- Previous whole brain or focal radiation therapy over 6000 cGy or radiosurgery
- Hydrocephalus

PROGNOSIS

The prognosis varies and can depend on whether the condition is rapidly diagnosed and treated. Compensatory mechanisms control the ICP, but these eventually fail. As the pressure increases, critical brain structures are compromised, including the brainstem. If left untreated, the increasing cerebral edema leads to ischemia, followed by coma and subsequently death. Treatment includes:
- Removal of the tumor
- Radiation therapy
- Shunt placement
- Chemotherapy

PROFESSIONAL ASSESSMENT CRITERIA (PAC)

1. Baseline neurologic exam, including:
   - **Orientation:** Person, place, and time.
   - **Level of consciousness (LOC):** Agitation, confusion, restlessness, lethargy.
   - **Muscle strength:** Hemiparesis, flexion, dorsiflexion, pronator drift, coordination.
   - **Vital signs:** Widened pulse pressure, irregular respirations, bradycardia secondary to pressure on the vasomotor centers of the medulla.
   - **Pupillary response:** Size and shape, equal and reactive to light.
2. Early signs and symptoms (Table 32-1):
   - Headaches
   - Nausea secondary to pressure on the medulla.
   - Projectile vomiting secondary to pressure on the vomiting center of the medulla.
   - Hemiparesis
   - Unilateral pupil dilation with slow reaction.
   - Visual disturbances, including blurred vision, diplopia, and decreased visual acuity.

Table 32-1 EARLY AND LATE SYMPTOMS OF INCREASED INTRACRANIAL PRESSURE	
Early Symptoms	**Late Symptoms**
Headaches	Change in the level of consciousness, including stupor and coma
Nausea	Worsening headache
Projectile vomiting	Abnormal motor functioning, including decorticate/decerebrate posturing
Hemiparesis	Cushing's triad (elevated BP, widening pulse pressure, and bradycardia)
Unilateral pupil dilation with slow reaction	Pupils dilated and fixed bilaterally
Visual disturbances, including blurred vision, diplopia, and decreased visual acuity	Papilledema

- Changes in LOC, including restlessness, agitation, and/or confusion.
3. Late signs and symptoms (see Table 32-1):
    - **Change in LOC:** Stupor, coma.
    - Worsening headache.
    - **Motor function:** Decorticate/decerebrate posturing.
    - **Cushing's triad:** Bradycardia, systolic hypertension, and widening pulse pressure.
    - Pupils dilated and fixed bilaterally.
    - **Papilledema:** An increase in the ICP leads to increased pressure on the optic nerve; this impairs the outflow of blood, causing edema of the optic disk.
4. Other signs and symptoms:
    - Memory loss
    - Decreased cognitive function
    - Personality changes
5. Head CT scan may demonstrate acute hemorrhage, hydrocephalus, or an acute mass with associated edema. CT scanning is a quick procedure that is helpful in emergency situations.
6. Magnetic resonance imaging (MRI) of the brain provides details of intracranial tumors and/or abscesses.
7. Magnetic resonance angiography (MRA) helps to assess for vascular abnormalities.
8. Positron emission tomography (PET) distinguishes radiation necrosis from tumor recurrence.
9. Single-photon emission computed tomography (SPECT) distinguishes infiltrating disease from solid tumors.
10. ICP monitoring shows an ICP greater than 30 mmHg.
11. Stereotactic biopsy may be done for tissue sampling to determine the pathology.
12. Craniotomy may be done for therapeutic debulking and to determine the pathology.

NURSING CARE AND TREATMENT

1. Perform and document a neurologic examination; assess for changes in level of consciousness.
2. **Positioning:** Elevate the head of the bed to 30 to 45 degrees to promote venous drainage. Avoid isometric muscle contractions, head extension, neck flexion, pressure on the abdomen, or Valsalva maneuver.
3. Perform intubation and hyperventilation to obtain a PCO_2 of 25 to 30 mm Hg. A low PCO_2 results in vasoconstriction, which causes a decrease in cerebral blood

volume and ICP. Hyperventilation is short acting, therefore additional therapy must be instituted (Colice, 1993).

4. Administer mannitol 20% to 25% solution at a dosage of 0.5-2 g/kg given IV over 20 to 30 minutes. Additional doses may be given if clinically indicated. Assess for rebound edema, because mannitol is a hyperosmotic agent that creates an osmotic gradient that pushes water from the brain across the blood-brain barrier into the bloodstream.

5. Dexamethasone, a glucocorticoid, is useful for reducing increased ICP secondary to brain metastases or infection in patients with cancer. It may be given IV or PO. The onset of action is several hours, and the effect lasts several days.

6. Monitor intake and output and urine specific gravity every hour.

7. Monitor for symptoms of hypovolemia (i.e., tachycardia, hypotension, serum osmolality greater than 300 mOsm/kg).

8. Treat fever with acetaminophen PRN and hypothermia blanket.

9. Institute seizure precautions, including padding, side rails up at all times. Administer prophylactic anticonvulsants.

10. Ensure patient's safety (e.g., raised side rails, assistive devices, and bed alarm).

11. Administer sedatives and/or paralyzing agents for severely increased ICP.

12. Monitor and maintain blood pressure with antihypertensives, vasopressors, and/or volume expanders.

13. Assess for and treat pain.

14. Provide regular passive range-of-motion exercises.

15. Ensure bowel regulation by administering stool softeners and laxatives to prevent constipation.

EVIDENCE-BASED PRACTICE UPDATES

1. Hyperbaric oxygen therapy has been shown to reduce cerebral edema, normalize the water content in the brain, and maintain an intact blood-brain barrier (Al-Waili et al., 2005).

2. Increased ICP secondary to pseudotumor cerebri has been associated with many medications, including vitamin A, isotretinoin, and other synthetic retinoic acid compounds; corticosteroid withdrawal; nalidixic acid; levonorgestrel; and tetracyclines (Friedman et al., 2004). Patients taking these medications should be monitored closely for this complication.

3. The results of a small study suggest that use of 23.4% hypertonic saline is a safe and effective treatment for elevated ICP in patients after traumatic brain injury (Ware et al., 2005).

TEACHING AND EDUCATION

1. Frequent neurologic exams provide information about the patient's current condition and the response to treatment.

2. Noxious stimuli should be limited, because they may lead to excitation of the patient, which may exacerbate intracranial pressure and lead to seizures.

3. Strict bowel regimens should be followed using stool softeners, because straining with bowel movements can further increase intracranial pressure.

4. A hypothermia blanket should be used for fevers. Fever increases the body's metabolism, which results in increased ICP.

5. Seizure precautions should be taken, because increased ICP can cause subsequent seizure activity.

NURSING DIAGNOSES

1. **Ineffective tissue perfusion (cerebral)** related to increased ICP
2. **Disturbed sensory perception** related to increased ICP and subsequent pressure on sensory control centers of the brain
3. **Disturbed thought processes** related to increased ICP
4. **Impaired verbal communication** related to increased ICP secondary to pressure on verbal centers of the brain
5. **Acute pain** (head and/or neck) related to increased ICP secondary to pressure on pain receptors in the brain

EVALUATION AND DESIRED OUTCOMES

1. The ICP will be normal within 24 hours.
2. Vital signs will be stable.
3. Neurologic status will return to baseline.
4. The patient's level of pain will be controlled.
5. The patient and family will be able to list the signs and symptoms of increased ICP and whom to call if they occurs.

DISCHARGE PLANNING AND FOLLOW-UP CARE

- Instruction for the patient and family in how to recognize the signs and symptoms of increased ICP and the health care provider to whom they should be reported.
- Acute or subacute inpatient rehabilitation for intensive physical therapy to regain any loss of function and/or strength.
- Home health nursing for assessment of the home environment for safety, provision of assistive devices, evaluation of the medication plan, and possible hospice referral.
- If the patient is homebound: Home health physical therapy for activity and assessment for need of assistive devices.
- Social services for identification of useful community services, financial assistance, and family support services.
- Close follow-up with physician or oncology nurse practitioner to evaluate for recurrence of increased ICP symptoms and management of any long-term deficits.

REVIEW QUESTIONS

QUESTIONS

1. **The normal range for intracranial pressure is:**
   1. 0 to 15 mm Hg
   2. 15 to 20 mm Hg
   3. 20 to 25 mm Hg
   4. 25 to 30 mm Hg

2. **Which of the following is *not* a possible cause of increased ICP:**
   1. Tumor
   2. Infection
   3. Hypovolemia
   4. Head trauma

3. **The symptom cluster for Cushing's triad includes:**
   1. Tachypnea, tachycardia, and hypotension
   2. Bradycardia, systolic hypertension, and widening pulse pressure
   3. Slow breathing, tachycardia, and hypertension
   4. Confusion, agitation, and intermittent somnolence

4. **A late sign of increased ICP is:**
   1. Mild headache
   2. Diplopia
   3. Bilateral dilation and fixation of the pupils
   4. Confusion

5. **You recently administered mannitol to Mr. P. for increased ICP. His serum osmolality is now 287 mmol/L. His wife asks you what that means. You respond with all of the following except:**
   1. "The mannitol has worked to improve your husband's ICP."
   2. "I need to notify the doctor, because he may need another dose."
   3. "The goal of mannitol therapy is a serum osmolality less than 300 mOsm/L, so it appears to be working."
   4. "The ICP has improved with the medication."

6. **The first priority in nursing interventions for a patient with increased ICP is:**
   1. Assess the vital signs
   2. Elevate the head of the bed to 90 degrees
   3. Perform a baseline neurologic exam
   4. Obtain blood for laboratory evaluation of electrolytes

7. **Hyperventilation is maintained until the PCO₂ is:**

   1. 15 to 20 mm Hg
   2. 20 to 25 mm Hg
   3. 25 to 30 mm Hg
   4. 30 to 35 mm Hg

8. **The cause of primary brain tumors is:**
   1. Chemical exposure
   2. Race
   3. Prior chemotherapy
   4. Unknown

9. **Patients and family members should be educated about safety at home, with emphasis placed on avoiding noxious stimuli, preventing constipation, and:**
   1. Administration of mannitol
   2. Neurologic evaluation
   3. Blood glucose levels
   4. Seizure precautions

10. **Medications used to treat increased ICP include all of the following except:**
    1. Mannitol
    2. Barbiturates
    3. Furosemide
    4. Dexamethasone

ANSWERS

1. *Answer: 1*
   Rationale: Normal ICP is 0 to 15 mm Hg. An ICP greater than 30 mm Hg requires immediate intervention, or permanent brain damage can occur.

2. *Answer: 3*
   Rationale: Hypovolemia is not a cause of increased ICP. Increased ICP can be caused by a primary brain tumor, brain metastases, infection, hemorrhage, infarction, and head trauma.

3. *Answer: 2*
   Rationale: Bradycardia, systolic hypertension, and widening pulse pressure are the components of Cushing's triad. These symptoms indicate rising ICP.

4. *Answer: 3*
   Rationale: Bilateral dilation and fixation of the pupils is a late sign of ICP and indicates pressure on the optic nerves. It also may indicate permanent damage.

5. *Answer: 2*
   Rationale: The goal of treatment with mannitol is a serum osmolality less than 300 mOsm/L. The serum osmolality requires close monitoring because of the potential rebound effect of ICP with the use of mannitol.

6. *Answer: 3*
   Rationale: A baseline neurologic exam is imperative so that the patient can be closely monitored for any subtle or dramatic changes that may indicate worsening ICP.

7. *Answer: 3*
   Rationale: The normal physiologic PCO₂ is 35 to 45 mm Hg. A low PCO₂ results in vasoconstriction, which causes a decrease

in cerebral blood volume and ICP. Hyperventilation is short acting, therefore additional therapy must be instituted (Colice, 1993).

8. *Answer: 4*
   Rationale: The cause of primary brain tumors is essentially unknown. Previous radiation therapy has been suggested as a possible cause.

9. *Answer: 4*
   Rationale: It is important that patients and family members understand seizure precautions. A person with increased ICP is at higher risk of having seizures. If the patient has a seizure, the person should be helped to the floor in a clear space, away from any furniture, and the head should be protected. Nothing should ever be put in the patient's mouth. If the seizure lasts longer than 3 to 4 minutes or if airway management is a concern, EMS should be called immediately.

10. *Answer: 3*
    Rationale: Furosemide is a loop diuretic that may worsen the ICP. Mannitol and dexamethasone are osmotic diuretics that draw fluid from the interstitial space into the intravascular space. Barbiturates are used to induce a coma, thereby limiting excitation that may worsen ICP (LeJeune & Howard-Fain, 2002).

REFERENCES

Al-Waili, N. S., Butler, G. J., & Beale, J., et al. (2005). Hyperbaric oxygen in the treatment of patients with cerebral stroke, brain trauma, and neurologic disease. *Advances in Therapy, 22*(6):659-678.

American Cancer Society (ACS) (2006). Brain tumors. Retrieved August 18, 2006, from http://www.cancer.org/docroot/CRI/CRI_2_3x.asp?dt=3.

Carlson, B. (2002). Neurologic clinical assessment. In L. Urden, K. Stacy, & M. Laugh (Eds.), *Thelan's critical care nursing: Diagnosis and management* (pp. 654-655). (4th ed.). St. Louis: Mosby.

Colice, G. L. (1993). How to ventilate patients when ICP elevation is a risk: Monitor pressure, consider hyperventilation therapy. *Journal of Critical Illness, 8:*1003-1020.

Dalessio, D. J. (1978). Mechanisms of headache. *Medical Clinics of North America, 62:*429-442.

Friedman, D. I., Gordon, L. K., & Egan, R. A., et al. (2004). Doxycycline and intracranial hypertension. *Neurology, 62*(12):2297-2299.

Goetz, C. G (2003). *Textbook of clinical neurology.* (2nd ed.). Chicago: Saunders.

Graus, F., Rogers, L. R., & Posner, J. B. (1985). Cerebrovascular complications in patients with cancer. *Medicine, 64:*16-35.

Greenberg, D. A, Aminoff, M. J., & Simon, R. P. (1993). Disturbances of vision. In *clinical neurology* (pp. 129-130). (2nd ed.). Standford, Connecticut: Appleton & Lange.

LeJeune, M., & Howard-Fain, T. (2002). Caring for patients with increased intracranial pressure. *Nursing2002, 32*(11):32cc1-32cc5.

Quinn, J. A., & DeAngelis, L. (2000). Neurologic emergencies in the cancer patient. *Seminars in Oncology, 27*(3):311-321.

Ware, M. L, Nemani, V. M., & Meeker, M., et al. (2005). Effects of 23.4% sodium chloride solution in reducing intracranial pressure in patients with traumatic brain injury: A preliminary study. *Neurosurgery, 57*(4):727-736.

LACTIC ACIDOSIS, TYPE B

CATHERINE SARGENT

PATHOPHYSIOLOGICAL MECHANISMS

Type B lactic acidosis is considered a rare metabolic oncologic emergency; if left untreated, it can be fatal. It generally is a complication seen with advanced disease; however, in some patients with cancer, it is the presenting symptom. Type B lactic acidosis was first described in 1963 by Huckabee. It was further delineated in 1976 by Cohen and Woods, who classified the disorder into three categories (Borron, 2005; Pignanelli & Budzinski-Braunscheidel, 1998) (Table 33-1). The onset of lactic acidosis can be either abrupt or insidious, depending on the cause.

Lactate Production

Approximately 1500 mmol of lactate are produced daily by various organs in the body. Lactate is the end product of anaerobic glycolysis. Serum lactate levels reflect the balance between production and elimination of lactate. The liver and kidneys are responsible for metabolizing and eliminating lactate (Moyle, 2002); about 70% to 90% of the body's lactate is metabolized by the liver, and 10% to 20% is eliminated by the kidneys.

The Cori cycle is the process by which lactic acid or lactate is recycled during anaerobic metabolism. When the energy needs of the body are greater than the oxygen supply, muscle cells and red blood cells produce adenosine triphosphate (ATP) through lactic acid fermentation. During anaerobic glycolysis, pyruvic acid is converted through gluconeogenesis into lactate, which is then converted into glucose for energy (Sharma, 2006). Some lactate is metabolized into CO_2 and water through the citric acid cycle and ultimately eliminated from the body. In normal circumstances, the Cori cycle allows the body to focus on the production of ATP while the liver handles lactate, thereby preventing lactic acidosis through the removal of lactate in the blood. Lactate is produced from pyruvic acid through a chemical reaction with the enzyme lactate dehydrogenase (LDH).

EPIDEMIOLOGY AND ETIOLOGY

Type A versus Type B Lactic Acidosis

Type A lactic acidosis occurs when the production of anaerobic lactic acid results in hypoxemia, or poor tissue perfusion. This deficit in oxygenation leads to difficulty generating ATP in the absence of oxygen (Moyle, 2002). Lactic acidosis induced by hypoxia is far more common than type B lactic acidosis. Etiologies of type A lactic acidosis include hypovolemic shock, sepsis, congestive heart failure, carbon monoxide poisoning, pheochromocytoma, and catecholamines (Sharma, 2006; Pignanelli & Budzinski-Braunscheidel, 1998). These etiologies can be subdivided into three primary causes: low PO_2 (pulmonary), poor delivery

Table 33-1	TYPES OF LACTIC ACIDOSIS	
Type	**Definition**	**Related Conditions**
Type A lactic acidosis (fast)	Poor tissue perfusion or oxygenation (hypoxia)	
	• Anaerobic muscle activity	Vigorous exercise, seizures
	• Tissue hypoperfusion	Sepsis, cardiogenic or hypovolemic shock, hypotension, myocardial infraction, acute heart failure, ischemic bowel, massive pulmonary emboli
	• Decreased tissue delivery or utilization	Hypoxemia, carbon monoxide poisoning
Type B lactic acidosis (slow)	Impaired lactate metabolism without evidence of inadequate tissue oxygenation (hypoxia)	
Type B1	Related to underlying disorder	Cancer (especially lymphomas, leukemia, and sarcoma), AIDS, sepsis, hepatic or renal failure, diabetes mellitus
Type B2	Associated with drugs and toxins	Antiretrovirals, acetaminophen, biguanide antihyperglycemics, cyanide, beta agonists, methanol, sorbitol, cocaine, parenteral nutrition, ethanol intoxication
Type B3	Related to congenital enzymatic defects of metabolism	Glucose-6-phosphatase deficiency (von Gierke's disease), pyruvate dehydrogenase deficiency, fructose-1,6-diphosphatase deficiency
Type D lactic acidosis (rare)	Bacterial overgrowth of gram-positive anaerobes	Jejunoileal bypass, small bowel resection, or other forms of short bowel syndrome and malabsorption

Data from Luft, F. C. (2001). Lactic acidosis: Update for critical care clinicians. *Journal of the American Society of Nephrology, 12*(Suppl 17): S15-S19; Moyle, G. (2002). Hyperlactatemia and lactic acidosis: Should routine screening be considered? *AIDS Read, 12*(8):344-348; and Sharma, S. (2006). Lactic acidosis. Retrieved May 29, 2006, from www.emedicine.com/med/topic1253.htm.

of oxygen (circulatory), or decreased oxygen-carrying capacity (as seen with hemoglobin disorders) (Luft, 2001).

Type B lactic acidosis occurs without hypoxia. It is considered to be the result of impaired lactate metabolism secondary to drugs, toxins, and/or disease processes. Type B lactic acidosis is characterized by a pH less than 7.35 and an arterial serum lactate level greater than 5 mEq/L (5 mmol/L in SI units) (Sharma, 2006). Arterial blood gas values in patients with type B lactic acidosis typically reflect a metabolic acidosis. The hallmark signs and symptoms of this rare oncologic emergency are changes in mental status and hyperventilation (Table 33-2).

Several theories have attempted to explain the etiology of type B lactic acidosis secondary to malignancy. Some propose that in patients with a large tumor burden, anaerobic glycolysis occurs as a result of decreased oxygenation in lactate-producing areas. Intrinsically, tumor cells have a higher rate of glycolysis than normal cells (DeKeulenaer et al., 2003). According to another theory, local tissue hypoxia and anaerobic metabolism occur as a result of microvascular aggregation of leukocytes and leukostasis, which result in

Table 33-2 SIGNS AND SYMPTOMS OF TYPE B LACTIC ACIDOSIS	
Early Signs and Symptoms	**Late Signs and Symptoms**
Nausea and vomiting	Shortness of breath
Abdominal pain	Tachypnea
Fatigue	Hyperventilation
Weight loss	Liver or renal failure
Enlarged liver	Clotting abnormalities
	Seizures
	Cardiac dysrhythmias
	Death

Data from Borron, S. (2005). Lactic acidosis. Retrieved May 11, 2005, from www.emedicine.com/emerg/topic291.htm; Pignanelli, A., & Budzinski-Braunscheidel, M. (1998). Lactic acidosis—type B. In C. Chernecky & B. Berger (Eds.), *Advanced and critical care oncology nursing* (pp. 384-397). Philadelphia: W. B. Saunders; and Vasseur, B. G., Kawanishi, H., & Shah, N., et al. (2002). Type B lactic acidosis: A rare complication of antiretroviral therapy after cardiac surgery. *Annuals of Thoracic Surgery, 74*(4):1251-1252.

the production of lactate. A third theory is that in patients with liver metastasis, lactate accumulates because the liver is unable to eliminate it. Finally, still others theorize that cancer cells themselves can produce lactate.

RISK PROFILE

- Sepsis: The exact mechanism of lactic acidosis in sepsis is not fully understood; however, it is thought to be related to increased lactate production during anaerobic and aerobic metabolism and decreased lactate clearance (Sharma, 2006).
- Liver dysfunction:
  - Alcohol intoxication
  - Hepatitis (B or C virus)
- Malignancies (e.g., leukemia; lymphoma; breast, colon, and lung cancer; and multiple myeloma) and AIDS. Type B lactic acidosis can occur with any malignancy.
- Cardiac or renal insufficiency
- Drug related:
  - Antiretrovirals (inhibit enzymes necessary for mitochondrial DNA synthesis) (Vasseur et al., 2002):
    - Stavudine (Mokrzycki et al., 2000).
    - Zidovudine
    - Didanosine
    - Lamivudine
    - Zalcitabine
    - Fialuridine
  - Biguanide antihyperglycemics (known to inhibit lactate metabolism)
    - Metformin (Glucophage)
    - Phenformin or buformin (off the market)
  - Other medications: Cyanide, beta agonists, methanol, epinephrine, salicylates, acetaminophen, cocaine, valproic acid, nitroprusside infusion, propofol, and 5-flourouracil
- Diabetic ketoacidosis
- Hyperglycemia greater than 300 mg/dL
- Intravenous radiographic contrast secondary to contrast-induced nephrotoxicity
- Pancreatitis

- Obesity
- Female gender (more often than males)
- Congenital disorders:
  - Glucose-6-phosphatase deficiency (von Gierke's disease)
  - Pyruvate dehydrogenase deficiency
  - Fructose-1,6-diphosphatatse deficiency
- Pediatric patients: Thiamine deficiency during TPN

PROGNOSIS

The prognosis for patients with type B lactic acidosis appears to be poor; the disorder is fatal in 56% to 75% of cases (Borron, 2005; Moyle, 2002). However, the severity of the acidosis can vary, and the prognosis depends on how rapidly it is identified and treated. Hyperlactemia secondary to antiretroviral therapy rarely is fatal, and it is effectively treated by discontinuing antiretroviral therapy and administering vitamins and antioxidants (Sharma, 2006). The higher the lactate level and the more acidotic the patient, the worse the prognosis. In patients with cancer, treatment should be directed at the underlying cause, not the acidosis. Cytoreduction therapy has been shown to reduce the acidosis as the tumor mass shrinks, which improves the prognosis. However, if the tumor mass recurs, the acidosis can recur, reducing survival.

PROFESSIONAL ASSESSMENT CRITERIA (PAC)

1. Vital signs:
   - Temperature: Normal unless infection or sepsis is present.
   - Pulse: Tachycardia.
   - Respirations: Tachypnea, dyspnea; may progress to compensatory hyperventilation, Kussmaul's breathing, and/or respiratory muscle fatigue.
   - Blood pressure: Hypotension (systolic blood pressure less than 90 mm Hg).
   - Pulse oximetry: May be normal.
2. Cancer:
   - Hematologic malignancies (leukemia).
   - Solid tumors with or without liver metastasis (breast, colon, lung cancers; lymphoma; multiple myeloma; sarcoma).
   - Advanced disease.
   - Previous episode of type B lactic acidosis secondary to cancer.
   - Recurrence of cancer.
3. Laboratory values:
   - Blood glucose: May be normal or elevated.
   - Serum lactate: Level greater than 5 mEq/L indicates hyperlactemia (NOTE: The blood specimen should be placed in ice before being sent to the laboratory.)
   - Blood urea nitrogen (BUN) and creatinine: Normal.
   - Urine for ketones.
   - Arterial blood gases (ABGs):
     - pH less than 7.35 indicates a metabolic acidosis.
     - PaO_2: Normal.
     - $PaCO_2$: Normal or decreased if lungs are compensating.
     - Bicarbonate: Low (less than 22 mEq/L).

- Anion gap: Increased,
4. Liver function tests:
   - Alkaline phosphatase: Increased.
   - Acid phosphatase: Increased.
   - Alanine aminotransferase (ALT) or serum glutamic pyruvic transaminase (SGPT): Increased.
   - Aspartate aminotransferase (AST) or serum glutamic oxaloacetic transaminase (SGOT): Increased.
   - Lactate dehydrogenase (LDH): Increased.
   - Aldolase: Increased.
   - Gamma glutamyl transpeptidase (GGTP): Increased.
   - 5′Nucleotidase: Increased.
   - Leucine aminopeptidase: Increased.
5. Strict intake and output.
6. **Neurologic status:** Changes in mental status, lethargy, confusion, disorientation, somnolence, coma, headache, mental dullness, disturbed perception, and/or loss of coordination.
7. **Other possible signs and symptoms:** Myalgia, hepatomegaly, and anxiety.
8. Cardiac monitoring for arrhythmias.
9. IV fluids to reduce hypovolemia.

NURSING CARE AND TREATMENT

1. Assess neurologic status hourly × 4, then every 4 hours.
2. Assess respiratory status hourly:
   - Check rate, rhythm, and depth.
   - Auscultate lung sounds.
   - Monitor for respiratory muscle fatigue.
   - Ensure continuous pulse oximetry.
3. Assess blood pressure, pulse, and temperature every hour × 4, then every 4 hours if stable.
4. Ensure IV access (ideally a central line, long-line catheter, or port) for chemotherapy, IV fluids, and/or blood transfusions.
5. Keep the head of the bed elevated at least 30 degrees.
6. Monitor intake and output hourly × 4, then every 4 hours.
7. Insert indwelling Foley catheter.
8. Initiate fall safety precautions with frequent monitoring.
9. Have suction setup available and ready in the room.
10. Have oxygen setup available and ready in the room.
11. Assess cardiovascular status to rule out type A lactic acidosis.
12. Obtain and send the following laboratory values:
    - STAT:
      - ABGs
      - Basic metabolic profile (BMP)
    - May be done on an emergent or nonemergent basis:
      - Liver function tests (LFTs)
      - Glucose levels
      - Blood cultures to rule out sepsis
      - Urine culture
      - Sputum culture
      - Toxicology screen for salicylates, methanol, ethanol, cocaine

- Chest x-ray film (CXR)
13. Thiamine level if patient is receiving TPN without thiamine.
14. Calculate anion gap:

$$\text{Anion gap} = (Na) - (Cl - HCO3^-) \text{ or } (Na + K) - (Cl + HCO3^-)$$

15. Administer IV sodium bicarbonate therapy (controversial).
16. Monitor for possible side effects of chemotherapy.

EVIDENCE-BASED PRACTICE UPDATES

1. Management of type B lactic acidosis primarily involves early recognition and removal of the causative factor and the use of supportive therapies.
2. Hemodialysis and antioxidants (e.g., riboflavin, thiamine, L-carnitine, coenzyme Q10, and vitamin C) all have been reported as possible treatments for type B lactic acidosis secondary to antiretroviral therapy (Vasseur et al., 2002).
3. Coexistence of metabolic alkalosis and lactic acidosis may result in an altered serum bicarbonate level.
4. Patients with an anion gap of 12 to 18 mEq/L have an almost fivefold greater chance of developing hyperlactemia than those with an anion gap less than 12 (for patients with an anion gap greater than 18, the risk increases to eightfold). It is believed that in some patients, the elevated lactate level indicates a shift in acid-base homeostasis (Moyle, 2002).

TEACHING AND EDUCATION

Teaching may be based on the condition of the patient, therefore education may need to be directed toward significant others.

Instruct significant others to monitor for changes in mental status or level of consciousness. *Rationale*: The brain is very sensitive to changes in the body's acid levels. When these levels are increased, a person can become confused, lethargic, or disoriented. If occurs, the person may not be able to perform normal activities such as bathing or eating.

Instruct significant others to monitor for changes in breathing and possible need for oxygen therapy. Instruct them in the use of a pulse oximeter if needed. *Rationale:* The level of acid in the body can affect how fast and how deeply a person breathes. One role your lungs play is to help regulate and change the amount of acid in the body. For example, the faster and deeper a person breathes, the more carbon dioxide is eliminated from the body, which helps reduce the level of acid. Oxygen therapy may be needed to help this process."

Discuss possible need for chemotherapy, surgery, or radiation. *Rationale*: By treating the underlying cause (cancer) with chemotherapy, the goal is to return your body to its normal, nonacidic state. As the acidic environment resolves, your breathing will return to normal, and you should not feel as sleepy or forgetful. If necessary, your physician may also recommend surgery or radiation.

Explain the need for an IV line, central line, or arterial line placement. *Rationale:* The IV line/arterial line allows the nurse to draw the blood samples needed to monitor the amount of lactate in the body and its effect, as well as provide fluids and administer chemotherapy or blood, if necessary.

Discuss possible need for mechanical ventilation with patient and significant others. *Rationale:* Increased lactate levels in the body can affect breathing. The respiratory muscles can become tired and weak. A ventilator can help support breathing until the person is strong enough to breathe without assistance.

Describe the signs and symptoms of type B lactic acidosis secondary to cancer. *Rationale:* It is important for you and your significant others to watch for signs and symptoms of increased acid levels in your body, because these can occur if your cancer worsens. You should look for changes in how you breathe, such as shortness of breath, difficulty breathing, or breathing too fast. You and your significant others also should be alert for any signs of confusion, disorientation, excessive sleepiness, and an inability to wake up. If you note any of these, you should call your doctor.

NURSING DIAGNOSIS

1. **Ineffective breathing pattern** related to respiratory compensation for metabolic acidosis
2. **Risk for injury** related to changes in mental status
3. **Impaired physical mobility** related to cognitive impairment, impaired coordination, and changes in metal status
4. **Acute confusion** related to cerebral lactic acidosis, which can result in increased intra-cranial pressure
5. **Imbalanced nutrition: less than body requirements** related to inability to eat secondary to changes in mental status and altered breathing pattern

EVALUATION AND DESIRED OUTCOMES

1. Acidosis will be corrected by treatment of the underlying disease, resulting in a decrease in tumor burden or remission.
2. Blood gas analysis will show a return to normal levels and a pH level of 7.35 to 7.45.
3. The serum lactate level will be less than 5 mEq/L.
4. The anion gap will be within normal limits (less than 12).
5. The patient's mental status will return to baseline.
6. Respiratory status will show lungs clear to auscultation and a respiratory rate of 12 to 20 breaths/min.
7. The patient and significant others will verbalize an understanding of the signs and symptoms of type B lactic acidosis.

DISCHARGE PLANNING AND FOLLOW-UP CARE

Based on the severity of the cancer and the patient's general health condition, the following may apply:

- Initiate a multidisciplinary discussion with the patient and significant others about the need for home care or possibly hospice care.
- If was surgery performed, educate the patient and significant others in how to manage the incisional wound at home.
- Educate the patient and significant others about the signs and symptoms of type B lactic acidosis and the side effects of chemotherapy and radiation therapy, if appropriate.
- Schedule appointments for outpatient laboratory work as indicated (e.g., ABGs, lactate levels).
- Arrange follow-up visit to the physician's office within 1 to 2 weeks after discharge.

REVIEW QUESTIONS

QUESTIONS

1. **Signs and symptoms of type B lactic acidosis secondary to malignancy include:**
   1. A pH greater than 7.35 and a respiratory rate of 12 breaths/min
   2. A low lactic acid level and confusion
   3. Lethargy and hyperventilation
   4. Hypoventilation and a high level of lactic acid

2. **Treatment for type B lactic acidosis related to malignancy should include:**
   1. Radiation therapy
   2. Chemotherapy
   3. Antibiotics
   4. Mechanical ventilation

3. **The primary nursing diagnosis for patients with type B lactic acidosis secondary to cancer is:**
   1. Deficient fluid volume
   2. Risk for infection
   3. Ineffective breathing pattern
   4. Acute confusion

4. **The hallmark signs and symptoms of type B lactic acidosis are:**
   1. Change in mental status, hyperventilation, and lethargy
   2. Hypoventilation, lethargy, and tachycardia
   3. Shortness of breath, pain, and wheezing
   4. Hypertension, hyperventilation, and confusion

5. **Type B lactic acidosis secondary to malignancy:**
   1. Occurs only in patients with metastasis
   2. Can occur with any malignancy
   3. More commonly occurs with solid tumors
   4. Occurs in patients with elevated BUN and creatinine levels

6. **Type A lactic acidosis due to hypoperfusion is the result of:**
   1. Diabetic ketoacidosis
   2. Liver failure
   3. Shock
   4. Exercise

7. **Lactate is:**
   1. The end product of anaerobic glycolysis
   2. An enzyme important for digestion
   3. A colony-stimulating factor produced by the kidneys
   4. A metabolic end product of angiogenesis

8. **An arterial line may be placed in a patient with lactic acidosis for the purpose of:**
   1. Instilling chemotherapy
   2. Administering intravenous (IV) fluids
   3. Obtaining frequent blood gas specimens
   4. Preventing blood clot formation

9. **Assessment of a patient with lactic acidosis associated with malignancy involves:**
   1. Monitoring intake and output daily
   2. Obtaining blood samples for serum sodium and potassium levels every 6 hours
   3. Obtaining a urine specimen for urine pH analysis every 4 hours
   4. Evaluating the patient's neurologic status every hour

10. **Type B lactic acidosis may be the result of:**
    1. Congestive heart failure
    2. Severe anemia
    3. Shock
    4. Malignancy

ANSWERS

1. *Answer: 3*
   Rationale: Changes in mental status occur secondary to a build up of acid in the brain; hyperventilation results as the lungs attempt to compensate for the metabolic acidosis.

2. *Answer: 2*
   Rationale: Treatment of the underlying cause (malignancy) with chemotherapy yields the best results for the patient.

3. *Answer: 3*
Rationale: The body tries to compensate for the metabolic acidosis by means of hyperventilation. As respiratory muscle fatigue occurs, the patient may require mechanical ventilation.

4. *Answer: 1*
Rationale: The classic signs and symptoms of type B lactic acidosis are a change in mental status, hyperventilation, and lethargy. Often, with type B lactic acidosis, the blood pressure is low and the patient does not complain of pain.

5. *Answer: 2*
Rationale: Type B lactic acidosis can occur with any malignancy; however, it is more common with hematologic malignancies.

6. *Answer: 3*
Rationale: The etiology of type A lactic acidosis is tissue hypoxia and hypoperfusion caused by shock. Hypoperfusion is not a cause of type B lactic acidosis.

7. *Answer: 1*
Rationale: Lactate is produced in the body by the skin, brain, muscles, and blood cells. It is the end product of anaerobic glycolysis.

8. *Answer: 3*
Rationale: An arterial line is placed to allow monitoring and to obtain blood gas and other arterial (not venous) blood samples for laboratory evaluation.

9. *Answer: 4*
Rationale: Assessment of the neurologic status is important in determining the patient's condition and the effectiveness of treatment.

10. *Answer: 4*
Rationale: Congestive heart failure, severe anemia, and shock result in tissue hypoxia or hypoperfusion, which are known causes of type A lactic acidosis. Type B lactic acidosis is not associated with perfusion problems. Malignancy is thought to cause an increase in lactate production.

REFERENCES

Borron, S. (2005). Lactic acidosis. Retrieved May 11, 2005, from www.emedicine.com/emerg/topic291.htm.

De Keulenaer, B., Van Outryve, S., & DeBacker, A., et al. (2003). Symptomatic lactic acidosis due to relapse of T-cell acute lymphoblastic leukaemia in the kidney. *Nephrology Dialysis Transplant, 18*(6):1214-1216.

Huckabee, W. E. (1963). Lactic acidosis. *American Journal of Cardiology, 12*:663-666.

Luft, F. C. (2001). Lactic acidosis update for critical care clinicians. *Journal of the American Society of Nephrology, 12*(Suppl. 17):S15-S19.

Mokrzycki, M., Harris, C., & May, H., et al. (2000). Lactic acidosis associated with stavudine administration: A report of five cases. *Clinical Infectious Disease, 30*:198-200.

Moyle, G. (2002). Hyperlactatemia and lactic acidosis: Should routine screening be considered? *AIDS Read, 12*(8):344-348.

Pignanelli, A., & Budzinski-Braunscheidel, M. (1998). Lactic acidosis—type B. In C. Chernecky & B. Berger (Eds.), *Advanced and critical care oncology nursing* (pp. 384-397). Philadelphia: W. B: Saunders.

Sharma, S. (2006). Lactic acidosis. Retrieved May 29, 2006, from www.emedicine.com/med/topic1253.htm.

Vasseur, B. G., Kawanishi, H., & Shah, N., et al. (2002). Type B lactic acidosis: A rare complication of antiretroviral therapy after cardiac surgery. *Annuals of Thoracic Surgery, 74*(4):1251-1252.

LAMBERT-EATON MYASTHENIC SYNDROME

DIONNE T. SAVAGE

PATHOPHYSIOLOGICAL MECHANISMS

Lambert-Eaton myasthenic syndrome (LEMS) is a rare, antibody-mediated autoimmune disorder. It can occur sporadically or as a paraneoplastic syndrome, most often associated with small cell carcinoma of the lung. The clinical presentation may be mistaken for myasthenia gravis, because the pathophysiologies of the two disorders have some similarities (Pascuzzi, 2002). Antibodies are directed against the voltage-gated calcium channels at the neuromuscular junction. The neuromuscular junction, or *synapse*, is the area where the nerve cells and the muscle fibers meet. Nerve cells regulate the function of the muscle fibers by controlling the frequency of the electrical signal, or *action potentials*, produced in the muscle fibers, resulting in a series of chemical events. These chemical events lead to muscle movement or contraction. At the neuromuscular junction, the nerve cell is known as the *presynaptic terminal* or *membrane*, where the action potential is initiated or produced, and the muscle fiber is known as the *postsynaptic terminal* or *membrane*, which receives the action potential.

Acetylcholine, a neurotransmitter, is released from the voltage-gated calcium channel of the presynaptic nerve at the neuromuscular junction. A *neurotransmitter* is a substance released from a presynaptic membrane that stimulates the action potential in the postsynaptic membrane. In LEMS the body produces antibodies that attack the presynaptic P/Q-type voltage-gated calcium channel (VGCC) of the neuromuscular junction. The antibodies bind to the particles that form the VGCC, causing clumping, which reduces the amount of calcium allowed to pass through the channels and also reduces the number of acetylcholine particles to be released. This attack on the VGCC, ultimately causes a decrease in acetylcholine. Anything that affects the production, release, and degradation of acetylcholine or its ability to bind to its receptor molecules on the postsynaptic membrane also affects the transmission of action potentials across the neuromuscular junction. This interferes with nerve impulses to the muscles. If the nerve impulses cannot get through to the muscle, the end result is proximal muscle weakness, hyporeflexia, and autonomic dysfunction.

EPIDEMIOLOGY AND ETIOLOGY

The incidence of LEMS is unknown, but 50% to 60% of these patients are diagnosed with non-small cell lung cancer. About 3% to 6% of patients with small cell lung cancer (SCLC) are diagnosed with LEMS. The median age of onset for LEMS is 60 years, although the disorder can occur in individuals anywhere from 7 to 80 years (Wirtz et al., 2002). If cancer has not been found in a patient presenting with LEMS, the patient should be screened for SCLC every 6 months, with chest imaging, for at least 2 years. In addition, evaluation for other autoimmune disorders, such as systemic lupus erythematosus and antibody-positive myasthenic gravis, should be considered (Pascuzzi, 2002).

If a patient is diagnosed with LEMS and a tumor is not found within the first 2 years after the onset of symptoms, cancer is unlikely; however, a latency period of 3 to 8 years has been reported (Scully et al., 1994).

RISK PROFILE

- Cancers: SCLC; breast, prostate, and laryngeal carcinomas; Non-Hodgkin's lymphoma; and leukemia.
- Paraneoplastic syndrome in middle-aged and elderly individuals.
- Autoimmune disorders: Systemic lupus erythematosus, thyroiditis, pernicious anemia, antibody-positive myasthenia gravis, rheumatoid arthritis, vitiligo, celiac disease, type 1 diabetes, and multiple sclerosis.
- Lifestyle: Smoking (which can lead to lung cancer).

PROGNOSIS

The survival rate depends on the underlying cancer and its response to treatment. LEMS can be resolved if the tumor successfully responds to the treatment. Little information is available on the prognosis for patients with LEMS who do not have a malignancy.

PROFESSIONAL ASSESSMENT CRITERIA (PAC)

1. Slowly progressive proximal leg and arm weakness, followed by generalized weakness, which is worse in the morning and tends to improve throughout the day. Difficulty climbing stairs or rising from a chair is noted.
2. Generalized fatigue after protracted exercise, with an increase in strength after mild exercise.
3. Waddling gait and impaired balance.
4. Dry mouth, related to the effects on the autonomic nervous system.
5. Difficulty chewing and swallowing.
6. Slurred speech and jaw and facial muscle weakness.
7. Constipation.
8. Vision changes: Blurred vision or diplopia.
9. Respirations: Decreased in rate and depth if the muscles of ventilation are affected. Cough associated with lung cancer or infection may be present.
10. Deep tendon reflexes may be decreased or absent.
11. Extremities: Numbness or paresthesias.
12. Impotence in males and postural hypotension.
13. Vaginal dryness.
14. Prolonged paralysis after the use of neuromuscular blocking agents during surgery.
15. Increased weakness after administration of aminoglycoside or fluoroquinolone antibiotics, magnesium channel blockers, and iodinated intravenous contrast agents.
16. Laboratory values:
    - Antibody assay: VGCC antibodies are found in 75% to 100% of patients with LEMS who have SCLC and in 50% to 90% of patients with LEMS alone.
17. CT scanning or MRI of the chest for SCLC.
18. Acetylcholine receptor antibodies.

19. Repetitive nerve stimulation studies: These studies confirm the LEMS diagnosis by demonstrating characteristic findings on electrodiagnostic studies.
20. Needle electromyography.
21. Single-fiber electromyography.
22. Bronchoscopy to detect SCLC.
23. Pain related to muscle stiffness.
24. Pulse oxygen for O_2 saturation related to SCLS.
25. ABGs: Acidosis, hypercapnia, hypoxia.

NURSING CARE AND TREATMENT

1. Asses ventilation status: Respiratory rate and depth may be decreased, and dyspnea or cough may be present. Administer oxygen therapy. Follow aspiration precautions. Respiratory failure is rarely the presenting symptom in LEMS patients, although it can develop later in the disease process (Eaton & Lambert, 1957). Administer decongestant PRN: guaifenesin or antitussive PRN: hydrocodone bitartrate (Hycodan/Robidone). Heliox treatment is a combination of helium and oxygen. Helium is a smaller, lighter molecule, which allows for oxygen delivery through smaller airways; this treatment works best for narrowed airways.
2. Assess mobility and balance: Provide safety measures to prevent falls.
3. Assess and document muscular strength.
4. Assess and document neurologic status.
5. Provide bowel function treatment for constipation.
6. Obtain and assess laboratory test and biopsy results.
7. Medications that may be ordered:
   - Pyridostigmine 30-60 mg PO q4-6h.
   - Guanidine hydrochloride 5-10 mg/kg/day PO to a maximum dose of 30 mg/kg/day in divided doses.
   - Aminopyridines 5-25 mg PO TID to QID.
   - Prednisone 60-80 mg/day PO until symptoms improve, then taper over weeks to months.
   - Azathioprine 50 mg/day, increased by 50 mg/day every 3 days to a total of 150-200 mg/day.
   - Cyclosporine 5-6 mg/kg/day divided into two doses q12hr initially, increased to produce blood levels of 100-150 ng/L until maximum response is achieved, then tapered.
   - IVIG 2 g/kg over 2-5 days.
   - Anxiolytics PRN.
8. Chemotherapy: Reduction of the cancer may reduce the autoimmune response and antibody production (Motomura et al., 2000).
9. Assess the patient's spirituality and support the patient in meeting spiritual needs.
10. Radiation to treat the underlining SCLC.
11. Referral to occupational therapy to evaluate and improve functional status.

EVIDENCE-BASED PRACTICE UPDATES

1. Younger patients who do not smoke, do not carry the autoimmune-prone HLA-B8DR3 haplotype, and do not have additional autoimmune diseases themselves or in first-degree family members, have the lowest risk. In one study, SCLC was detected during follow-up in 70% of patients with a history of smoking who did not have the HLA-B8DR3 haplotype (Wirtz et al., 2005).

2. 3,4-Diaminopyridine and IVIG have improved muscle strength scores and compound muscle action potential amplitudes in LEMS patients (Maddison & Newsom-Davis, 2003).

TEACHING AND EDUCATION

1. **Mobility:** Safety precautions must be enforced because of muscle weakness, which increases the risk of falls. Instruct the patient in the use of a walker or cane. The patient may need assistance with ambulation.
2. **Dyspnea:** Supplemental oxygen may be required to ease shortness of breath. Space activities to reduce oxygen consumption.
3. Dry mouth can be treated with frequent rinsing and artificial saliva.
4. **Nutrition:** A pureed diet and small, frequent meals may be necessary because of difficulty swallowing.
5. **Side of effects of chemotherapy and radiation:** Chemotherapy destroys rapidly dividing cells, such as cancer cells, and normal fast-growing cells, such as hair follicles, certain blood cells and the cells that line the mouth and gastrointestinal tract. A decrease in red blood cells may result in decreased energy, decreased white blood cells (with an increased risk of infection), and decreased platelets (with an increased risk of bleeding).
6. **Blood test:** Multiple blood samples are obtained to check for antibodies and to monitor the treatments' effects on the body.
7. Immunosuppression related to chemotherapy, radiation, and steroid therapy can make the patient more prone to infection; therefore good hand washing is imperative, and the patient should be advised to avoid people who are ill.
8. Good oral hygiene to prevent break down of mucosal lining or oral infections.

NURSING DIAGNOSES

1. **Impaired physical mobility** related to the onset of muscle weakness and impaired balance
2. **Activity intolerance** related to fatigue and muscle weakness
3. **Risk for injury** related to muscle weakness and impaired balance
4. **Ineffective coping** related to the diagnosis of cancer and LEMS
5. **Deficient knowledge** related to the cancer and treatments

EVALUATION AND DESIRED OUTCOMES

1. Weakness will decrease and mobility and performance status will increase.
2. Clinical response to cancer treatment will be seen.
3. O_2 saturation will be greater than 92%.
4. The patient will be able to maintain normal oral hygiene.
5. The patient and family will be able to verbalize the disease process and the treatment goals and plan.
6. The patient will have normal bowel function.
7. The patient's weight will be stable or the patient will be at an ideal body weight.

DISCHARGE PLANNING AND FOLLOW-UP CARE

- Home O_2 therapy referral.
- Physical therapy for evaluation of home safety and to provide muscle strengthening exercises and assistive devices for ambulation.

- Occupational therapy to maximize the patient's ability to perform ADLs and to provide assistive devices for ADLs.
- Home health nurse to evaluate the patient's response to treatment and medications.
- Assistive devices for ambulation.
- Follow-up laboratory work if s/p chemotherapy: CBC, CMP.
- Instruct the patient to notify the physician or nurse practitioner if he or she develops a fever higher than 100.5° F, shortness of breath, or exacerbation of muscle weakness and fatigue.
- Ensure that a follow-up appointment is scheduled with the physician or nurse practitioner.

REVIEW QUESTIONS

QUESTIONS

1. **The initial symptom of LEMS is:**
   1. Gait disturbance
   2. Shortness of breath
   3. Decreased appetite
   4. Pain

2. **The percentage of patients diagnosed with SCLC who have LEMS is:**
   1. 10% to 20%
   2. 50% to 60%
   3. 3% to 6%
   4. 80%

3. **All of the following treatments are helpful in managing LEMS associated with SCLC *except:***
   1. Chemotherapy
   2. Surgery
   3. Radiation
   4. IVIG

4. **In the pathophysiology of LEMS, the neurotransmitter that is inhibited is:**
   1. Sodium
   2. Potassium
   3. Chloride
   4. Acetylcholine

5. **One of the procedures done to diagnose LEMS is repetitive nerve stimulation. Which of the following results indicates a diagnosis of LEMS:**
   1. Greater than 400% facilitation
   2. Positive deep tendon reflexes
   3. Decreased neuromuscular jitter
   4. Stable motor unit action potential

6. **Ms. Salmond is a 55-year-old African American woman who has smoked since she was 17. She has just been** diagnosed with SCLC and LEMS. The greatest risk factor for SCLC is:
   1. Smoking
   2. African American race
   3. Female gender
   4. Age

7. **LEMS is a disorder of the:**
   1. Neuromuscular junction
   2. Nervous system only
   3. Muscle fibers only
   4. Deep tendon reflexes

8. **The median age of onset for LEMS is:**
   1. 30 to 40
   2. 50 to 60
   3. 40 to 50
   4. 70 to 80

9. **Mr. Miller has been diagnosed with SCLC, and he completed his first chemotherapy treatment 2 weeks ago. He informs you that he is only brushing his teeth in the morning, when he gets up, because he has noticed some bleeding when he brushes. Your best response to his statement is:**
   1. "Continue to brush once a day, because your platelets are low and you don't want to cause increased bleeding."
   2. "You really only need to brush a couple of times a week."
   3. "Maybe you should get a softer tooth brush and rinse your mouth several times a day to keep your mouth moist."
   4. "Don't worry about brushing your teeth. It's not important while you are getting chemotherapy."

10. **Michael has LEMS, but he does not have an underlying malignancy. It has been 2 years since his diagnosis, and he is experiencing chronic SOB with increased activity. He cannot understand why he is having this problem, because he does not have lung cancer. The likely reason for his SOB is:**
    1. Muscle weakness
    2. IVIG treatment for his chronic disease
    3. Asthma
    4. Pulmonary fibrosis

ANSWERS

1. *Answer: 1*
   Rationale: Patients with LEMS typically present with slowly progressive proximal leg weakness that results in an altered gait.

2. *Answer: 3*
   Rationale: About 3% to 6% of patients with SCLC are diagnosed with LEMS, a rare paraneoplastic syndrome. About 60% of patients diagnosed with LEMS have SCLC.

3. *Answer: 2*
   Rationale: Surgery does not treat the symptoms of LEMS as effectively as systemic treatment for cancer, such as chemotherapy.

4. *Answer: 4*
   Rationale: The antibodies bind to the receptors of the presynaptic nerve membrane, leading to a decrease in acetylcholine.

5. *Answer: 1*
   Rationale: Repetitive nerve stimulation facilitation greater than 400% indicates a positive diagnosis of LEMS. The other reactions are the opposite of what they would be with LEMS.

6. *Answer: 1*
   Rationale: Smoking is the greatest risk factor for SCLC. The disease does not have a predilection for any particular race or gender. Although the patient is middle aged, age alone is not a risk factor.

7. *Answer: 1*
   Rationale: LEMS is a disorder of the neuromuscular junction, which includes the nerve and muscle fibers that affect the deep tendon reflexes.

8. *Answer: 2*
   Rationale: The median age of onset is 50 to 60 years.

9. *Answer: 3*
   Rationale: It is important to teach the patient good oral hygiene to reduce the risk of infection.

10. *Answer: 1*
    Rationale: LEMS is characterized by proximal muscle weakness that can slowly progress to involve the muscles of ventilation. Respiratory failure is rare with LEMS, but it can occur with progressive chronic disease.

REFERENCES

Eaton, L., & Lambert, E. (1957). Electromyography and electric stimulation of nerves in diseases of motor units: Observations on myasthenic syndrome associated with malignancy. *Journal of the American Medical Association, 163*:1117-1124.

Maddison, P., & Newsom-Davis, J. (2003). Treatment for Lambert-Eaton myasthenic syndrome. Cochrane Database of Systematic Reviews 2003, Issue 2. Art. No.: CD00379. DOI:10.1002114651858. CD003279.pub2.

Motomura, M., Hamasaki, S., & Nakane, S., et al. (2000). Apheresis treatment in Lambert-Eaton myasthenic syndrome. *Therapeutic Apheresis, 4*:287-290.

Pascuzzi, R. (2002). Myasthenic gravis and Lambert-Eaton syndrome. *Therapeutic Apheresis, 6*:57-68.

Scully, R. E., Mark, D. J., & McNeely, S. F., et al. (1994). Case records of the Massachusetts General Hospital: Case 32. *New England Journal of Medicine, 331*(8):528-535.

Wirtz, P. W., Wilcox, N., & van der Slik, A. R., et al. (2005). HLA and smoking in prediction and prognosis of small cell lung cancer in autoimmune Lambert-Eaton myasthenic syndrome. *Journal of Neuroimmunology, 159*:230-237.

Wirtz, P. W., Smallegange, T. M., & Wintzen, A. R., et al. (2002). Differences in clinical features between the Lambert-Eaton myasthenic syndrome with and without cancer: An analysis of 227 published cases. *Clinical Neurology and Neurosurgery, 104*:359-363.

MALNUTRITION AND CACHEXIA

KATHY G. KRAVITS • MARCIA GRANT

Malnutrition and cachexia continue to complicate the course of disease and treatment in patients with cancer. Agreement exists in the literature and among clinicians that malnutrition is a common problem. However, a predictable and measurable definition of malnutrition has yet to be established (Corish & Kennedy, 2000). Elia (2001) has suggested that cancer-related malnutrition be defined as "a state of nutrition in which a deficiency or excess (or imbalance) of energy, protein, and other nutrients causes measurable adverse effects on tissue/body form, function, and clinical outcome."

Primary cachexia, also known as *primary anorexia/cachexia*, is a specific syndrome characterized by protein breakdown and/or increased energy expenditure, resulting in anorexia, emaciation, loss of muscle tissue, weakness, and fatigue (Strasser & Bruera, 2002). Cachexia frequently does not respond to nutritional supplements or an increased food intake (Mantovani et al., 2003; Van Halteren et al., 2003). Researchers' understanding of the pathophysiology of these complications is still evolving. Supportive nutrition interventions consisting of assessment, treatment, and monitoring of the patient's nutritional status are an expanding area of study to delineate the outcomes for patients with cancer (Ottery, 1995).

PATHOPHYSIOLOGY

Primary Anorexia/Cachexia

Primary anorexia/cachexia syndrome is a metabolic imbalance associated with the chronic inflammatory response generated by the patient's body (the host) as a result of exposure to malignant cells (Strasser & Bruera, 2002). This imbalance causes an alteration in glucose metabolism, muscle protein synthesis, proteolysis of muscle proteins, and decreased lipogenesis (Van Halteren et al., 2003). Increased energy expenditure in relation to lean body mass is a consequence of this imbalance. The patient often presents with loss of appetite, early satiety, chronic nausea, muscle wasting, loss of fat, overall weight loss, and fatigue (Strasser, 2002).

Proinflammatory cytokines, which are small proteins that can be produced by any cell in the body, play a significant role in the host's response (Dinarello, 2000). Examples of cytokines commonly associated with primary anorexia/cachexia syndrome are tumor necrosis factor (TNF) and interleukins 1 and 6 (IL-1, IL-6) (Van Halteren et al., 2003). The research suggests that TNF mediates the loss of muscle proteins by causing fragmentation of muscle DNA, which results in muscle cell death (apoptosis) (Carbo et al., 2002). IL-1 appears to support TNF by enhancing TNF's ability to kill targeted cells (Dinarello, 2000). IL-6 also seems to support TNF and has been implicated in the development of anorexia and the breakdown of fats and proteins (Van Halteren et al., 2003).

Malignant cells not only act as a trigger for the host's inflammatory response, they also contribute glycoprotein molecules that appear to accelerate muscle breakdown and

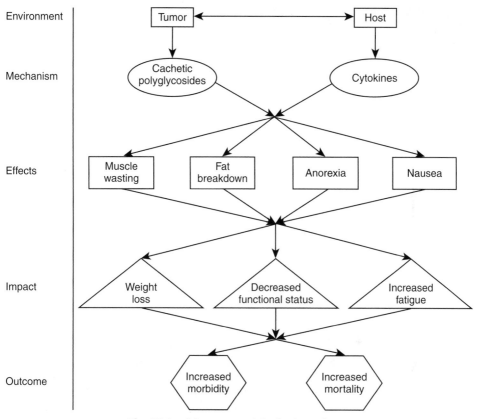

Fig. 35.1 • Primary anorexia/cachexia syndrome.

metabolism (Strasser, 2004). Examples of tumor-generated glycoprotein molecules are proteolysis-inducing factor (PIF) and lipid-mobilizing factor (LMF). PIF contributes to muscle protein breakdown, and LMF contributes to the breakdown of fat. Both substances are detectable in the blood and correlate with weight loss (Fig. 35.1) (Strasser & Bruera, 2002).

Secondary Anorexia/Cachexia

Secondary anorexia/cachexia is a constellation of conditions that can co-occur with primary anorexia/cachexia. The presence of secondary anorexia/cachexia with primary anorexia/cachexia complicates the presentation, assessment, and management of both syndromes (Strasser, 2002).

The conditions that make up secondary anorexia/cachexia are grouped into three major categories: starvation/malnutrition, loss of muscle mass, and other catabolic states. Multiple etiologies are responsible for the changes associated with each category and the pathophysiology depends on the etiology of the co-morbid conditions involved (Strasser, 2002).

Starvation/malnutrition occurs as a result of decreased oral intake, alteration in gastro-intestinal absorption, and/or loss of protein-rich body fluids (Strasser & Bruera, 2002). Examples of commonly encountered contributing factors to starvation and malnutrition in

Table 35-1	METABOLIC ALTERATIONS IN PRIMARY ANOREXIA/CACHEXIA VERSUS STARVATION	
	ALTERATION	
Characteristic	**Primary Anorexia/Cachexia**	**Starvation**
Glucose turnover	↑	↓
Ketone bodies	↓	↑
Acute phase protein synthesis	↑	↔
Muscle protein synthesis	↓	↓
Proteolysis of muscle proteins	↑↑	↑
Lipogenesis	↓	↓
Lipolysis	↑	↑↑
Energy expenditure/lean body mass	↑	↓

Data adapted from Strasser, F. (2002). Eating-related disorders in patients with advanced cancer. *Supportive Care in Cancer*. Retrieved August 23, 2002, from http://www.springerlink.com/content/rtqcauvgdprlyged/fulltext.pdf.

the oncology patient include stomatitis, taste alteration and food aversions, xerostomia, dysphagia, nausea, vomiting, constipation, diarrhea, bowel obstruction, ascites, nephrotic syndrome, pain, dyspnea, depression, and cognitive impairment (Strasser & Bruera, 2002). This is not an all-inclusive list. The significance is that all these conditions contribute to a disruption in the intake of nutrients that, if severe enough, results in significant weight loss and malnutrition.

Loss of muscle mass is another category of secondary anorexia/cachexia. Circumstances associated with loss of muscle mass not previously discussed include prolonged immobility and deconditioning, growth hormone deficiency, aging, and muscle wasting (Strasser & Bruera, 2002). These conditions tend to be found in aging and ill people.

Catabolism is the breakdown of tissue. Catabolic states that may contribute to secondary anorexia/cachexia include infections, treatment with proinflammatory cytokines, chronic heart failure, renal failure, liver failure, diabetes mellitus, and hyperthyroidism (Strasser & Bruera, 2002).

The mechanisms of action of primary anorexia/cachexia and secondary anorexia/cachexia are different. In simple starvation and malnutrition, a form of secondary anorexia/cachexia, oral intake is either voluntarily or involuntarily withheld, depriving the body of needed calories and nutrients. This form of starvation emphasizes fat breakdown and limited protein breakdown, and generally is associated with a reduction in energy expenditure (Strasser, 2002).

The enhanced catabolic state of primary anorexia/cachexia promotes increased breakdown of muscle proteins and fats (Strasser, 2002). The most significant difference between these two syndromes from a management perspective is that increased intake of nutrients does not improve primary anorexia/cachexia (Strasser, 2002). Table 35-1 compares and contrasts the changes associated with primary anorexia/cachexia and simple starvation.

EPIDEMIOLOGY AND ETIOLOGY

Epidemiology

Nutritional problems are the most common secondary diagnosis for patients with cancer. The incidence varies, depending on the disease's stage, location, and treatment. Cachexia occurs in 24% of patients in the early stages of advanced cancer and in 80% of patients with cancer in the terminal stages. It is the cause of death in 20% of patients with terminal-stage cancer (Mantovani et al., 2003; Van Halteren et al., 2003; Strasser & Bruera, 2002).

The location of the cancer influences the occurrence of cachexia. Patients with pancreatic cancer commonly present with a history of digestive disturbance and weight loss (Ottery, 1996a). Patients with esophageal cancer complain of difficulty swallowing and a resulting loss of appetite and weight (Woodtli & Van Ort, 1993). Many patients with head and neck cancer undergoing radiation therapy are at risk for anorexia, loss of weight, and the beginning stages of malnutrition and cachexia (Woodtli & Van Ort, 1991).

Treatment approaches also affect the occurrence of malnutrition and cachexia. Patients receiving cytotoxic chemotherapy experience varying digestive symptoms, such as nausea, vomiting, stomatitis, and diarrhea; all of these, when uncontrolled, lead to anorexia, loss of weight, and eventually cachexia (Grant & Kravits, 2000).

Patients undergoing surgery are on restricted intake before and after the surgical procedure. If the surgery involves the mouth, neck, esophagus, and other areas of the gastrointestinal track, limited intake and disrupted absorption may occur, leading to anorexia/cachexia. Surgical procedures support and promote catabolism. As a result of increased catabolism coupled with a stress-related increase in metabolic requirements, surgical patients are susceptible to loss of weight and eventually cachexia (Strasser & Bruera, 2002).

Patients undergoing radiation therapy experience symptoms at the local site of therapy. This could mean a loss of appetite, difficulty swallowing, and lack of digestion and absorption, all of which may lead to anorexia and cachexia (Woodtli & Van Ort, 1993). The more toxic the chemotherapy, the more extensive the surgery, and the larger the radiation field, the more likely the patient is to be vulnerable to anorexia/cachexia.

Etiology

Evidence suggests that the presence of malignant cells in the host stimulates a chronic inflammatory response fueled by cytokines. This creates an imbalance between increased energy needs and the body's diminished ability to process nutrients to meet those needs. A likely clinical effect of this imbalance is the development of malnutrition with significant risk of progression to anorexia/cachexia (Strasser, 2002).

Etiologies of primary anorexia/cachexia include metabolic abnormalities produced by the relationship of the tumor and host tissues, resulting in a decreased intake of nutrients and increased energy requirements (Strasser, 2002). Secondary anorexia/cachexia is caused by starvation/malnutrition (impaired oral intake and/or impaired gastrointestinal absorption), other catabolic states (chronic infections, poorly controlled diabetes), and loss of muscle mass (prolonged bed rest) (Strasser & Bruera, 2002).

Secondary etiologies are associated with cancers that occur in the gastrointestinal tract, causing direct interference with food intake, digestion, and absorption, and with responses to cancer treatments, such as chemotherapy and radiation therapy. For patients with oral, esophageal, or stomach cancer, early loss of oral intake leads to anorexia/cachexia, followed by weight loss. For patients with cancer of the pancreas, digestive difficulties, including pain, may be the presenting symptom. Co-morbidities, especially if uncontrolled, may lead to anorexia/cachexia. For example, acute infections can increase the catabolic state. Organ failures (heart, lungs, kidneys), poorly controlled diabetes, and hyperthyroidism can lead to secondary anorexia/cachexia in patients with cancer. In addition, with bed rest, a lack of activity ensues, and muscle wasting begins (Strasser & Bruera, 2002).

RISK PROFILE

- Patients with specific cancers:
  - Cancer of the head and neck
  - Cancer of the esophagus, stomach, and small intestine
  - Cancer of the pancreas
- Patients in specific cancer stages:
  - Recurrent disease
  - Advanced or terminal cancer
- Patients undergoing specific cancer therapies:
  - Patients undergoing radical surgical procedures or surgery, especially those involving the head, neck, and gastrointestinal system.
  - Patients undergoing radiation therapy that includes the gastrointestinal tract within the treatment field.
  - Patients experiencing chemotherapy-associated side effects of nausea, vomiting, diarrhea, and pain, especially of the mouth and gastrointestinal tract.
  - Patients undergoing hematopoietic cell transplantation.
- Patients with cancer who have uncontrolled or poorly controlled co-morbidities (e.g., heart disease, renal disease, diabetes).
- Patients with cancer who are on bed rest or are bedridden.
- Patients with cancer who are experiencing psychological or spiritual crises.

PROGNOSIS

The presence of primary anorexia/cachexia has been associated with alterations in functioning, increased symptoms, intolerance for treatment, and impaired clinical outcome (Strasser & Bruera, 2002). Primary anorexia/cachexia has been commonly associated with a loss of 10% or more of the prediagnosis weight within the previous 6 months. Additional research has demonstrated that weight loss alone is not the best predicator of the impact of cachexia. Factors such as weight loss, a decreased food intake, and the presence of an inflammatory response, as measured by the C-reactive protein level, may be useful for assessing the impact of cachexia on outcome (Fearon et al., 2006).

PROFESSIONAL ASSESSMENT CRITERIA (PAC)

Primary anorexia/cachexia is a complex syndrome that may be affected by the presence of co-occurring conditions, including therapies such as chemotherapy, radiation therapy, and surgery. A comprehensive assessment that includes both subjective and objective data is essential for the formulation of an appropriate plan of care. The assessment should be initiated at the first patient contact, and the patient should be reassessed at regularly scheduled intervals throughout treatment. Proactive planning and symptom management helps minimize the impact of changes in nutritional status.

Areas of focus that facilitate the formulation of a comprehensive nutritional profile include the involuntary weight loss history, history of nutritional intake, perceptions of body image, subjective global assessment, symptom distress measures, laboratory values, anthropometric measurements, quality of life measures, and diagnostic tests. Referral to appropriate health care professionals for evaluation of specialized aspects of the patient's presentation is useful.

Involuntary Weight Loss History

Regular measurement of weight and height is a fundamental component of the assessment. The body mass index (BMI), which is calculated from height and weight measurements, provides an objective measure of chronic protein-energy status (Elia, 2001). Loss of 10% or more of the body weight within 6 months indicates the presence of cachexia and may be associated with a reduced tolerance for treatment and a worsening prognosis (Strasser, 2002). Patient and caregiver reports of subjective experiences of weight loss (e.g., clothes that no longer fit, an awareness of being thinner) should be incorporated into the weight loss history and, when present, should increase the clinician's sensitivity to the probability that significant weight loss has already occurred.

History of Nutritional Intake

The history of nutritional intake may be obtained in a number of ways, including interviews using open-ended questions. A dietary journal kept by the patient, with input by the caregiver, for a minimum of 3 days, including at least one weekend day, provides a wealth of data and may be revealing to the patient as well as the clinician. Types of foods, food portions, and food preferences should be recorded. It also is useful to ask the patient to note food aversions, taste changes, and aroma sensitivities in the journal entries (Grant & Kravits, 2000).

Perceptions of Body Image

Documentation of the patient's impression of her or his appearance, as measured with a visual analog scale, is valuable (Strasser, 2002).

Patient-Generated Subjective Global Assessment

Because of the variability of definitions, measures, and thresholds for action, developing consistently applied criteria for diagnosing malnutrition and cachexia has been difficult (Corish & Kennedy, 2000). The Patient Generated Subjective Global Assessment was created to provide a systematic methodology for collecting clinical nutritional assessment data, including weight loss history, intake history, symptom distress levels, functional status and evidence of fat loss, muscle wasting, and edema in the oncology patient (Fig. 35.2) (Ottery, 1996b).

Symptom Distress Measures

Anorexia, nausea, vomiting fatigue and pain (symptom distress) should be measured using a visual analog scale (Strasser & Bruera, 2002).

Laboratory Values

The serum albumin, serum transferrin, C-reactive protein, and retinol-binding protein measurements can be used to assess nutritional status (Fearon et al., 2006). They are decreased with malnutrition and cachexia (Brown, 2002). It is important to note that alterations in serum protein levels may be seen with chronic infection, inflammation, and other medical conditions (Corish & Kennedy, 2000).

Medical History	SGA Rating		
1. Weight change	**A**	**B**	**C**
A. Clothing size _____ No change _____ Change			
B. Overall weight loss in _____ past month _____ 6 months _____ 1 year			
C. % Loss of usual weight _____ <5% _____ 5-10% _____ >10%			
D. Change in past 2 weeks _____ Increase (gain)			
_____ No change (stabilization)			
_____ Decrease (continued loss)			
2. Dietary intake			
A. Reduction _____ Yes _____ No			
_____ Unintentional _____ Intentional			
B. Overall change _____ No change _____ Change			
_____ Increase _____ Decrease			
C. Duration _____ Weeks _____ Months			
D. Diet change _____ Suboptimal solids (i.e., 75%, 50%, 25% intake)			
_____ Full liquid diet			
_____ Hypocaloric fluids			
_____ NPO (starvation)			
3. Gastrointestinal symptoms (persisting daily for >2 weeks)			
_____ None _____ Diarrhea _____ Dysphagia/odynaphagia			
_____ Nausea _____ Vomiting _____ Anorexia			
4. Functional impairment			
A. Overall impairment _____ None _____ Mild _____ Severe			
B. Duration _____ Days _____ Weeks _____ Months			
C. Type _____ Ambulatory (Walking or wheelchair)			
_____ Bedridden			
Physical Examination			
5. Muscle wasting _____ Bicep _____ Tricep _____ Quadricep			
_____ Deltoid _____ Temple			
6. Subcutaneous fat loss _____ Tricep _____ Chest _____ Eyes			
_____ Perioral _____ Intraosseous _____ Palmar			
7. Edema _____ Hands _____ Sacral _____ Lower extremity			

A=Well nourished; B=Mild/moderate under nutrition; C=Severe under nutrition

Fig. 35.2 • Subjective global assessment. *(From Ottery, F. D. [1996]. Definition of standardized nutritional assessment and interventional pathways in oncology.* Nutrition, *12[1 Suppl.]:S15-S19.)*

Anthropometric Measurements

The midarm muscle circumference, triceps skin fold thickness, and subscapular skin fold thickness are examples of measurements that can be used to assess changes in the body mass index (Elia, 2001). However, their accuracy has not been established definitively. These measurements may be most useful when taken multiple times in the same patient, which allows the findings to be tracked and trended over the course of the illness (Corish & Kennedy, 2000).

Quality of Life Measures

Quality of life measures may clarify the context of the patient's experience. Areas of exploration can include the patient's level of knowledge about the disease and its treatment, the integrity of the patient's social support system, and the patient's family history, orientation on existential issues, and coping styles.

NURSING CARE AND TREATMENT

1. Assess nutritional status:
   - Evaluation for anorexia and food intake.
   - Periodic laboratory assessments, including plasma protein analysis, urinary creatinine, electrolytes, and minerals.
   - Periodic anthropometric tests, including body weight, skin fold thickness, midarm circumference, and body mass index.
   - 24-Hour dietary analysis.
   - Intake and output.
   - Height and weight.
2. Treat symptoms that interfere with food intake, digestion, and absorption:
   - Nausea, vomiting, stomatitis, diarrhea
   - Unrelieved pain
3. Provide oral care before and after meals.
4. Provide an environment conducive to eating (e.g., clear out bedpans, reduce odors).
5. Provide small, frequent meals high in calories and protein.
6. Provide for culturally appropriate foods.
7. Assist patient to eat as needed.
8. Limit procedures, treatments and psychological upsets before mealtimes.
9. Provide range of motion and exercise for patients who are bedridden.
10. Help patient to exercise to reduce fatigue, maintain muscle mass, and increase appetite,
11. Specialized nutritional support (enteral and parenteral nutrition) should be considered for patients undergoing hematopoietic cell transplantation, for malnourished patients undergoing radiation or chemotherapy, and for patients prone to ingestion or absorption problems.
12. Administer pharmacologic agents (Table 35-2).
13. Reassess patient's nutritional status after intervening.

EVIDENCE-BASED PRACTICE UPDATES

1. Oral nutritional supplements are more effective than dietary advice in improving body weight and energy intake in people with illness-related malnutrition (Baldwin et al., 2001).

Table 35-2	POSSIBLE MECHANISMS OF ACTION OF ESTABLISHED AND EMERGING PHARMACOLOGIC AGENTS IN THE MANAGEMENT OF CACHEXIA	
Possible Mechanism	**Agent**	
Central nervous system effects	Metoclopramide	
	Corticosteroids	
	Progestational agents	
	Cannabinoids	
	Thalidomide	
Modulation of immune response/reduction of inflammation	Corticosteroids	
	Progestational agents	
	Polyunsaturated fatty acids	
	Thalidomide	
	Melatonin	
	NSAIDs	
	ATP	
Anabolic effect	Growth hormone/insulin growth factor-1	
	Androgenic anabolic agents	
	Beta-2 adrenergic agents	
	ATP	
Stimulation of gastrointestinal motility/increase in gastric emptying	Metoclopramide	

From Bruera, E. D., & Sweeney, C., (2004). Pharmacological interventions in cachexia and anorexia. In D. Doyle, G. Hanks, and N.I. Cherny (Eds.), *Oxford textbook of palliative medicine* (p. 556). (3rd Ed.). Oxford: Oxford University Press.

2. Patients who have undergone bone marrow transplantation who are given parenteral nutrition with additional glutamine are likely to have a reduced rate of infection and to leave the hospital earlier (Murray & Pindoria, 2002).
3. In a review of trials aimed at improving the quality of life of patients with lung cancer, one trial of nutritional interventions found positive effects for increasing energy intake but no improvement in quality of life (Sola et al., 2004).
4. An examination of the role of nutritional factors in survival after the diagnosis of breast cancer identified recommendations for healthy weight control with an emphasis on exercise to preserve or increase lean muscle mass and a diet that includes nutrient-rich vegetables (Rock & Demark-Wahnefried, 2002).
5. Research focused on increasing food intake using supplements, counseling, and pharmacologic agents led to an increased food intake but did not improve body composition, nutritional status, tumor response to therapy, survival, or quality of life (Brown, 2002).

TEACHING AND EDUCATION

Oral care: *Rationale*: Good oral hygiene will help maintain your appetite and prevent or help heal any mouth sores.

Medications: *Rationale*: Management of symptoms such as nausea, vomiting, diarrhea, and pain require the administration of medications in a timely manner. Keeping a medication schedule and following the times for each medication are essential to managing the symptoms.

Meals: *Rationale*: Keep meals simple, including carbohydrates and protein. Eat half of your daily calories at breakfast, and divide the other half between lunch and dinner. Small meals and high-calorie, between meal snacks are recommended. Avoid uncomfortable procedures before mealtime.

Nutritional status: *Rationale*: You may be asked to evaluate your appetite daily on a 10-point scale, with 1 being little or no appetite and 10 being an excellent appetite. Use the same time for evaluation each day. Also, weigh yourself daily, at the same time each day wearing approximately the same amount of clothing.

Diet: *Rationale*: Consult a dietician to obtain recipes and meal recommendations. A dietician can also analyze your 24-hour food intake and help you plan your diet.

Enteral and parenteral nutrition: *Rationale*: Meet with the enteral/parenteral nutrition nurse to learn how to perform daily care and keep records of your intake.

NURSING DIAGNOSES

The following are some of the nursing diagnoses most commonly associated with primary and secondary anorexia/cachexia in patients with cancer (Courtens & Abu-Saad, 1998; Woodtli & Van Ort, 1993; MacAvoy & Moritz, 1992; Woodtli & Van Ort, 1991):

1. **Imbalanced nutrition: less than body requirements** related to reduced intake
2. **Risk for infection** related to nutritional deficit
3. **Impaired tissue integrity** related to nutritional deficit
4. **Impaired swallowing** related to disease progression and/or treatment related side-effects
5. **Deficient fluid volume** related to reduced intake

These diagnoses fall under the functional health pattern of nutritional-metabolic. The characteristics associated with the nursing diagnoses include taste aversion, bloating, decreased appetite, early satiety, constipation, nausea, fatigue, decreased intake, decreased weight, and weeping, blistered skin.

EVALUATION AND DESIRED OUTCOMES

1. The patient will have no weight loss during debilitating procedures.
2. Normal levels of blood proteins, glucose, and minerals will be maintained.
3. The patient will be able to complete the whole radiation and chemotherapy cycle.
4. Symptoms affecting nutritional status will be kept in control.
5. Infections will be minimized,
6. Fluid balance will be maintained.
7. Any surgical wounds will heal cleanly without indications of infection.

DISCHARGE PLANNING AND FOLLOW UP CARE

- A patient with primary and/or secondary anorexia/cachexia will need the following:
- Ongoing assessment and reassessment of symptom pattern and progression.
- Sufficient nutrient sources to meet energy requirements, preferably in forms that may be taken orally. Enteral and parenteral supplements should be available if the patient is unable to tolerate oral intake.
- Physical care provided by family support systems and/or professional caregivers.
- Education related to the importance of nutritional intake, monitoring of nutritional intake and weight, and other individualized features of care.
- End of life cachexia: Requires the support of professionals prepared to provide care in all domains of life experience.
- Access to educational resources.

- Recommendations for professional consultation as needed.
- Mobilization of social systems, including family, friends, and formal, nonrelated support groups to provide emotional support and to reduce feelings of isolation.
- Assistance with processing of existential issues and spiritual practice.

REVIEW QUESTIONS

QUESTIONS

1. **According to Ottery, a standardized nutritional assessment for patients with cancer should include:**
   1. History of weight loss, food intake, disease stage, and current medications.
   2. History of weight loss, food intake, disease stage, and treatment status.
   3. History of weight loss, food intake, functional capacity, and symptom distress.
   4. History of weight loss, food intake, functional capacity, and current medications.

2. **Anorexia/cachexia of cancer occurs primarily as a result of:**
   1. Loss of desire for food
   2. Taste aversions
   3. Inability to absorb nutrients
   4. A metabolic imbalance

3. **Examples of proinflammatory cytokines include:**
   1. IL-4, IL-10, and TNF
   2. IL-6, TNF, and IL-1
   3. IL-6, TNF, and IL-10
   4. IL-4, IL-1, and IL-10

4. **Secondary anorexia/cachexia of cancer can complicate the presentation of primary anorexia/ cachexia of cancer. The condition or conditions that contribute to secondary anorexia/cachexia include:**
   1. Chronic infection
   2. Stomatitis
   3. Immobility
   4. All of the above

5. **The incidence of cancer-related cachexia at the end of life is approximately:**
   1. 80%
   2. 20%
   3. 30%
   4. 40%

6. **Cancers commonly associated with an increased risk of secondary anorexia/ cachexia include all of the following *except*:**
   1. Head and neck cancer
   2. Esophageal cancer
   3. Sarcoma
   4. Pancreatic cancer

7. **Loss of 10% or more of the body weight within the previous 6 months is associated with:**
   1. No increased risk of cachexia
   2. An increased risk of cachexia
   3. An increased tolerance for chemotherapy
   4. An increased tolerance for radiation therapy

8. **Laboratory values that may be useful in assessing malnutrition include:**
   1. Serum albumin
   2. Serum transferrin
   3. Retinol-binding protein
   4. All of the above

9. **Examples of interventions that can mitigate the effects of anorexia/ cachexia include:**
   1. Perform oral care before and after meals.
   2. Serve large meals at regularly scheduled intervals,
   3. Limit snacks,
   4. Minimize exercise and range of motion.

10. **One of the nursing diagnoses most commonly identified with anorexia/ cachexia is:**
   1. Deficient diversional activity
   2. Ineffective role performance
   3. Imbalanced nutrition: less than body requirements
   4. Altered self-concept

ANSWERS

1. *Answer: 3*
Rationale: Functional capacity and symptom distress are included in Ottery's nutritional assessment.

2. *Answer: 4*
Rationale: The loss of appetite and weight loss in primary cachexia are due to a metabolic imbalance.

3. *Answer: 3*
Rationale: IL-6, TNF, and IL-10 are the main proinflammatory cytokines known to be related to cachexia.

4. *Answer: 4*
Rationale: Secondary anorexia/cachexia is related to an inability to obtain adequate nutrients for a variety of physiologic reasons.

5. *Answer: 1*
Rationale: About 80% of patients with advanced cancer have cachexia near the end of life.

6. *Answer: 3*
Rationale: Sarcoma is associated with secondary anorexia/cachexia. Head and neck cancer, esophageal cancer, and pancreatic cancer affect the ability to swallow or the appetite, leading to weight loss.

7. *Answer: 2*
Rationale: Loss of 10% or more of the body weight is associated with an increased risk of cachexia. In general, weight loss reduces tolerance for chemotherapy and radiation therapy, depending on the specific chemotherapeutic agent or the location of the irradiation.

8. *Answer: 4*
Rationale: All of the laboratory values listed reflect nutritional status.

9. *Answer: 1*
Rationale: Oral care may help moisten the mucosa, aiding swallowing and helping to improve taste. Large meals are discouraged, because the sight of large quantities of food may be overwhelming to a patient without an appetite. Frequent snacks are encouraged, because small amounts of food may be better tolerated than large quantities. Exercise may help increase appetite, bowel regularity, a sense of well-being, and digestion.

10. *Answer: 3*
Rationale: The most specific and appropriate nursing diagnosis for patients with anorexia/cachexia is imbalanced nutrition: less than body requirements.

REFERENCES

Baldwin, C., Parsons, T., & Logan, S. (2001). Dietary advice for illness-related malnutrition in adults. *Cochrane Database of Systematic Reviews*, (2):CD002008. Retrieved August 4, 2006, from http://www.medscape.com/viewarticle/485966.

Brown, J. K. (2002). A systematic review of the evidence on symptom management of cancer-related anorexia and cachexia. *Oncology Nursing Forum*, 29(3):517-532.

Bruera, E. D., & Sweeney, C. (2004). Pharmacological interventions in cachexia and anorexia. In D. Doyle, G. Hanks, & N. I. Cherny (Eds.), *Oxford textbook of palliative medicine* (p 556) (3rd ed.). Oxford: Oxford University Press.

Carbo, N., Busquets, S., & van Royen, M., et al. (2002). TNF-alpha is involved in activating DNA fragmentation in skeletal muscle. *Journal of Cancer*, 86(6):1012-1016.

Corish, C. A., & Kennedy, N. P. (2000). Protein-energy undernutrition in hospital in-patients. *British Journal of Nutrition* 83(6):575-591.

Courtens, A. M., & Abu-Saad, H. H. (1998). Nursing diagnoses in patients with leukemia. *Nursing Diagnosis* 9(2):49-61.

Dinarello, C. A. (2000). Proinflammatory cytokines. *Chest*, 118(2):503-508.

Elia, M. (2001). The Malnutrition Advisory Group concensus guidelines for the detection and management of malnutrition in the community. *Nutrition Bulletin*, 26(1):81-83.

Fearon, K. C., Voss, A. C., & Hustead, D. S. (2006). Definition of cancer cachexia: Effect of weight loss, reduced food intake, and systemic inflammation on functional status and prognosis. *American Journal of Clinical Nutrition, 83*(6):1345-1350.

Grant, M., & Kravits, K. (2000). Symptoms and their impact on nutrition. *Seminars in Oncology Nursing, 16*(2):113-121.

MacAvoy, S., & Moritz, D. (1992). Nursing diagnoses in an oncology population. *Cancer Nursing, 15*(4):264-270.

Mantovani, G., Maccio, A., & Madeddu, C., et al. (2003). Cancer-related cachexia and oxidative stress: Beyond current therapeutic options. *Expert Review of Anticancer Therapy, 3*(3):381-392.

Murray, S. M., & Pindoria, S. (2002). Nutrition support for bone marrow transplant patients. *Cochrane Database of Systematic Reviews* (2):CD002920. Retrieved August 4, 2006, from http://www.medscape.com/viewarticle/486309.

Ottery, F. D. (1995). Supportive nutrition to prevent cachexia and improve quality of life. *Seminars in Oncology, 22*(2 Suppl. 3):98-111.

Ottery, F. (1996a). Supportive nutritional management of the patient with pancreatic cancer. *Oncology (Williston Park), 10*(9 Suppl):26-32.

Ottery, F. D. (1996b). Definition of standardized nutritional assessment and interventional pathways in oncology. *Nutrition, 12*(1 Suppl):S15-S19.

Rock, C. L., & Demark-Wahnefried, W. (2002). Nutrition and survival after the diagnosis of breast cancer: A review of the evidence. *Journal of Clinical Oncology, 20*(15):3302-3316.

Sola, I., Thompson, E., & Subirana, M., et al. (2004). Non-invasive interventions for improving well-being and quality of life in patients with lung cancer. *Cochrane Database of Systematic Reviews* (4):CD004282. Retrieved August 4, 2006, from http://www.medscape.com/viewarticle/502113.

Strasser, F. (2002). Eating-related disorders in patients with advanced cancer. *Supportive Care in Cancer.* Retrieved August 23, 2002, from http://www.springerlink.com/content/rtqcauvgdprlyged/fulltext.pdf.

Strasser, F. (2004). Nutrition in palliative medicine. In D. Doyle, G. Hanks, & N. I. Cherny (Eds.), *Oxford textbook of palliative medicine* (pp. 526-528). (3rd ed.). Oxford: Oxford University Press.

Strasser, F., & Bruera, E. D. (2002). Update on anorexia and cachexia. *Hematology and Oncology Clinics of North America, 16*(3):589-617.

Van Halteren, H. K., Bongaerts, G. P., & Wagener, D. J. (2003). Cancer cachexia: What is known about its etiology and what should be the current treatment approach? *Anticancer Research, 23*(6D):5111-5116.

Woodtli, M. A., & Van Ort, S. (1991). Nursing diagnoses and functional health patterns in patients receiving external radiation therapy: Cancer of the head and neck. *Nursing Diagnosis, 2*(4):171-180.

Woodtli, M. A., & Van Ort, S. (1993). Nursing diagnoses and functional health patterns in patients receiving external radiation therapy: Cancer of the digestive organs. *Nursing Diagnosis, 4*(1):15-25.

PAIN MANAGEMENT: NOCICEPTIVE AND NEUROPATHIC

CHRISTINE MIASKOWSKI

PATHOPHYSIOLOGICAL MECHANISMS

From a mechanistic perspective, cancer pain can be classified as *nociceptive* or *neuropathic* in origin. Nociceptive pain results from activity in neural pathways caused by tissue damage. Examples of nociceptive pain include postoperative pain, pain from bone metastasis, or pain associated with an intestinal obstruction. In contrast, neuropathic pain results from injury to nerves in the peripheral or central nervous system. In patients with cancer, neuropathic pain can result from tumor-related compression of neural tissue or injury to the nervous system from radiation, chemotherapy, or infection (Nicholson, 2006; Miaskowski, 2004).

EPIDEMIOLOGY AND ETIOLOGY

Unrelieved pain is one of the problems that patients with cancer fear most. Both adults and children can experience acute or chronic pain associated with cancer and its treatment. Epidemiologic studies suggest that 20% to 75% of adults with cancer report pain at the time of diagnosis, that 17% to 57% of patients undergoing active treatment experience pain, and that 23% to 100% of patients with advanced disease report moderate to severe pain (Goudas et al., 2005; Miaskowski et al., 2005). In addition, 23% to 90% of patients with cancer experience episodic breakthrough pain (BTP), a transitory exacerbation of pain superimposed on a background of persistent yet tolerable and generally adequately controlled pain (Svendsen et al., 2005; Caraceni & Portenoy, 1999; Portenoy et al., 1999). Because cancer has become a chronic illness, cancer survivors may experience pain as a result of their cancer or cancer treatment or from other chronic medical conditions unrelated to their cancer.

RISK PROFILE

- Cancer:
  - **Nociceptive pain:** Breast, gastrointestinal, kidney, lung, ovarian, and prostate cancer and multiple myeloma.
  - **Neuropathic pain:** Myeloma; metastasis to the base of the skull; brachial plexopathy from breast cancer, lung cancer, or lymphoma; cervical plexopathy from head and neck tumors; and lumbosacral plexopathy from colorectal and renal cancer, sarcoma, and lymphoma.

- Cancer treatments
  - **Nociceptive pain:** Surgery, administration of stomatotoxic chemotherapy (e.g., methotrexate, 5-fluorouracil, doxorubicin, bleomycin), infectious processes in soft tissues, radiation-induced desquamation, extravasation of chemotherapy (e.g., actinomycin D, doxorubicin, mitomycin C), intraperitoneal chemotherapy, intestinal obstruction, hepatic metastasis, abdominal radiation (diarrhea), and pelvic irradiation (cystitis).
  - **Neuropathic pain:** Surgical procedures that damage peripheral nerves (e.g., limb amputation, breast cancer surgery, nephrectomy, head and neck resection, thoracotomy), herpes zoster infection, radiation damage to peripheral nerves, and neurotoxic chemotherapy (e.g., vinca alkaloids, platinum compounds, taxanes, thalidomide).

PROGNOSIS

1. Ninety percent of all cancer pain can be managed effectively through noninvasive pharmacologic and nonpharmacologic interventions (Miaskowski et al., 2005).
2. Unrelieved cancer pain has a negative impact on a patient's mood, functional status, and quality of life (Paul et al., 2005; Rustøen et al., 2005; Miaskowski et al., 1997; Glover et al., 1995).

PROFESSIONAL ASSESSMENT CRITERIA (PAC)

1. Screen all patients for pain at every visit.
2. Perform a *comprehensive* pain assessment that includes:
   - A detailed history to determine the presence of persistent and breakthrough pain (BTP)
   - A psychosocial assessment
   - A physical examination
   - A diagnostic evaluation to determine whether the patient has a common cancer pain syndrome (e.g., spinal cord compression, postherpetic neuralgia)
3. Persistent pain is described as constant pain that lasts for long periods (Miaskowski et al., 2005). The assessment of *persistent pain* should include the following information:
   - Onset and temporal pattern
   - Location
   - Description
   - Intensity
   - Aggravating and relieving factors
   - Previous and current pharmacologic treatments and their effectiveness
   - Effects of pain on function
4. BTP is described as sudden, severe flare-ups of pain that come and go. These flare-ups are called breakthrough pain because the pain "breaks through" the treatment for persistent pain (Miaskowski et al., 2005). The assessment of *BTP* should include the following information:
   - Presence of BTP
   - Frequency and duration of the episodes of BTP
   - Intensity of the BTP
   - Occurrence of BTP (e.g., spontaneous, with movement)
   - Previous and current pharmacologic and nonpharmacologic treatments and their effectiveness

Table 36-1	DIFFERENCES IN THE CHARACTERISTICS OF NOCICEPTIVE AND NEUROPATHIC PAIN	
Characteristic	**Nociceptive Pain**	**Neuropathic Pain**
Mechanism	Tissue injury	Nerve injury
Description	Aching, throbbing, sharp, gnawing, dull, pressurelike	Burning, tingling, numbing, shooting, electrical, jolting
Location	Usually localized over the site of tissue injury	Usually localized to the site of neuronal injury; may radiate
Severity	Use a 0 (no pain) to 10 (worst pain imaginable) numeric rating scale to assess the severity of average and worst pain.	Use a 0 (no pain) to 10 (worst pain imaginable) numeric rating scale to assess the severity of average and worst pain.
Aggravating factors	May include movement, activity, work, increased stress.	May include clothing rubbing against the site, water or wind hitting the site, or movement.
Relieving factors	May include the application of heat or cold, massage, and splinting of the affected site.	May include gentle rubbing of the affected site.
Additional signs and symptoms	Muscle spasms, diaphoresis, distention, feeling of fullness, nausea, and vomiting	Allodynia; atrophy; hair loss; hyperalgesia; loss of reflexes; loss of normal sensations; dysesthesias; smooth, fine skin
Psychological symptoms	Depression, anxiety, fear	Depression, anxiety, fear

5. The differences between chronic nociceptive and neuropathic pain are summarized in Table 36-1.
6. The physical examination should focus on the site of the pain.
   - Consider common pain problems associated with cancer and cancer treatment.
   - Perform a focused neurologic examination related to the site of the pain (e.g., for back and neck pain, focus on motor and sensory function in the upper and lower extremities, as well as the function of the rectal and urinary sphincters).
7. Diagnostic tests should be done to evaluate for recurrence or progression of disease and/ or tissue injury caused by cancer treatment.
   - Pain should be treated to facilitate completion of the diagnostic tests.
8. Assess the patient for the most common cancer pain syndromes (i.e., bone metastasis; epidural spinal cord compression; cervical, brachial, or lumbar plexopathy; peripheral neuropathy; postherpetic neuralgia).
9. Perform ongoing reassessments of pain to evaluate the effectiveness of the pain management plan.
   - Have the patient or family complete a pain management diary and have them bring it to each clinic visit. The diary recordings of pain intensity and medication intake facilitate evaluation of the effectiveness of the pain management plan, allow for evaluation of the patient's level of adherence to the analgesic regimen, and guide revisions of the pain management plan.

NURSING CARE AND TREATMENT

1. Perform a comprehensive pain assessment and facilitate the diagnostic workup to determine the cause of the pain.

2. Establish patent intravenous access if the worst pain is uncontrolled and the patient rates it as 7 or higher (based on a numeric rating scale on which 0 is no pain and 10 is the worst pain imaginable).
3. Treat a worst pain intensity score of 7 or higher as a **pain emergency**. The patient should be titrated on oral or intravenous opioids until the worst pain score drops to 4 (Miaskowski et al., 2005).
4. Position the patient to enhance comfort.
5. Initial treatment of cancer pain should be based on the severity of the pain that the patient reports.
6. Adjust the dosage of analgesic medications to achieve pain relief with acceptable side effects.
7. Monitor for and prophylactically treat analgesic side effects:
   • **Nonopioid analgesics:** Gastric distress, bleeding, renal failure, central nervous system toxicity, hepatotoxicity (acetaminophen).
   • **Opioid analgesics:** Constipation, sedation, nausea, pruritus, urinary retention, respiratory depression (rare with patients on chronic opioids).
   • **Co-analgesics:** Monitor for side effects that are specific to each class of co-analgesic.
8. Use relaxation exercises to reduce pain and anxiety.
9. Refer the patient to the pain management service if severe pain persists.

EVIDENCE-BASED PRACTICE UPDATES

1. For patients with chronic cancer pain, administer a long-acting opioid analgesic on an around-the-clock basis, along with an immediate-release opioid to be used on an as-needed basis for BTP, once the patient's pain intensity and dosage have been stabilized (Miaskowski et al., 2005).
2. For nociceptive pain, use adequate doses of nonopioid and opioid analgesics, either alone or in combination, depending on the severity of the patient's pain.
   • Table 36-2 lists the most common nonopioid analgesics and the recommended dosing regimens.
   • Table 36-3 lists the most common opioid analgesics and the recommended dosing regimens.
3. Neuropathic pain associated with cancer and cancer treatment is usually managed with co-analgesics (e.g., anticonvulsants, antidepressants). Most of the studies on the use of these drugs to manage neuropathic pain were done with patients who had diabetic neuropathy or postherpetic neuralgia. These medications need to be administered in the appropriate dose, titrated to effect or tolerable side effects, and given an adequate trial. Until the co-analgesic becomes effective, patients may require a short-acting opioid analgesic for pain management (Miaskowski et al., 2005; Dworkin et al., 2003).

Table 36-2 NONOPIOID ANALGESICS

Nonopioid Analgesic	Usual 24-Hour Dose Range	Usual Daily Dose	
		Dosage	Frequency
Acetaminophen	2-4 g	325-650 mg	Every 4 hours
		650 mg-1 g	Daily
Aspirin	2.4-6 g	600-1500 mg	Daily
Ibuprofen	1.2-3.2 g (pain)	200-400 mg	Daily
Naproxen sodium	550-1100 mg	275-550 mg	Twice daily

Table 36-3 OPIOID ANALGESICS

| Opioid Analgesic | Usual starting dose for moderate to severe cancer pain in adults weighing >50 kg | |
	Oral	Parenteral
Morphine	15-30 mg every 3-4 hours	10 mg every 3-4 hours
Morphine, controlled-release formulations		
MS Contin	15-30 mg every 12 hours	N/A
Oramorph SR	15-30 mg every 12 hours	N/A
Kadian	20 mg every 24 hours	N/A
Avinza	30 mg every 24 hours	N/A
Hydromorphone	4-8 mg every 3-4 hours	1.5 mg every 3-4 hours
Oxycodone	10-30 mg every 4 hours	N/A
Oxycodone, controlled-release formulation	10 mg every 12 hours	N/A
Transdermal fentanyl	25 mcg/hr patch every 72 hours	N/A

4. Patients with certain types of cancer pain or with refractory pain that is inadequately controlled with opioid analgesics may benefit from local anesthetic nerve blocks or neurolytic blocks (Miaskowski et al., 2005).
   - Local anesthetic nerve blocks may be used to provide immediate but temporary relief for regional pain problems that originate in a nerve or muscle (e.g., pain associated with acute herpes zoster infection).
   - Neurolytic nerve blocks have a role in the management of refractory, persistent cancer pain that is often incapacitating (e.g., celiac plexus block for pain associated with pancreatic cancer).
5. Radiation therapy may be used to palliate pain associated with bone metastasis or spinal cord compression.
6. Surgical procedures may be performed to debulk tumors or to relieve obstructions caused by tumors. Orthopedic procedures may be used to treat the pain associated with pathologic fractures.

TEACHING AND EDUCATION

Effective pain management: *Rationale:* It is extremely important to keep your pain under control Unrelieved pain can result in sleep disturbance, depression, anxiety, decreased mobility, and decreased enjoyment of life.

Management of persistent pain and BTP: *Rationale:* Approximately 90% of your persistent pain can be relieved by taking your pain medication on a regular schedule. If you have episodes of BTP, these can be managed with short-acting analgesic medications that you take when you need them.

Management of side effects: *Rationale:* Side effects occur with pain medicines. Some of these side effects will decrease over time, as long as the dose of the pain medicine remains the same. Your body will become used to the pain medicine, and the side effects of sedation and nausea will decrease. If they become intolerable, you can receive medicine to treat them.

Management of constipation: *Rationale:* Constipation is the one side effect that continues for the entire time you take your pain medication. It is important that you drink fluids and eat a diet high in fiber. In addition, you need to take a stool softener and a laxative to prevent constipation. The dose of the stool softener and the laxative will need to be adjusted until your normal bowel pattern returns.

Ongoing reassessment of pain: *Rationale:* At each follow-up visit, you will be asked about your pain management. It is a good idea to keep a daily diary about your pain and pain management. Each day, record in the diary your average pain, your worst pain, and the doses of pain medication that you took that day. Record any other thoughts or notes you want to share with your doctor or nurse at the next visit. If the pain medicine is not working, call the doctor's office and have the pain medicine changed.

Development of tolerance: *Rationale:* Sometimes your body gets used to the pain medicine. This effect is called tolerance. Tolerance is not a problem, because the amount of pain medicine can be changed to keep your pain under control.

Development of addiction: *Rationale:* You will not "get hooked" or become addicted to the pain medicine. You need to take your pain medicine to treat your pain, just as you would take antibiotics to treat an infection.

NURSING DIAGNOSES

1. **Acute pain** related to diagnostic procedures, surgery, stomatotoxic chemotherapy, skin desquamation from radiation therapy
2. **Chronic pain** related to specific nociceptive etiology, specific neuropathic etiologies
3. **Constipation** related to intake of opioid analgesics, intake of tricyclic antidepressants
4. **Sleep deprivation** related to chronic pain
5. **Hopelessness** related to chronic pain

EVALUATION AND DESIRED OUTCOMES

1. Persistent pain and BTP will be controlled.
2. Bowel elimination pattern will return to normal.
3. The patient will be free of side effects from the analgesic regimen.
4. The patient will use nonpharmacologic strategies on a routine basis.
5. The patient will engage in activities as tolerated.
6. The patient will report any new complaints of pain promptly.
7. The patient will adhere to the pain management plan.

DISCHARGE PLANNING AND FOLLOW-UP CARE

- Escalate the dose of pain medication as tolerance develops.
- Monitor for changes in pain intensity. If pain intensity increases, evaluate the patient for the development of tolerance or disease progression.
- Evaluate the effectiveness of the pain management plan weekly.
- Provide ongoing education to alleviate fears about the development of psychological addiction.

- Anticipate that the patient may need referrals and make them as appropriate:
  - To a pain specialist when pain is not controlled by conventional means and more specialized pain management strategies are required (e.g., celiac plexus block).
  - To hospice care during the terminal phases of the illness to manage escalating doses of pain medication and additional symptoms of the disease and treatment.
  - For psychological counseling and support to manage some of the psychosocial issues associated with a chronic illness and chronic pain.
  - For education and skills training for the patient and family in pain assessment and how to communicate with health care professionals about unrelieved pain.

REVIEW QUESTIONS

QUESTIONS

1. The percentage of oncology patients who will have pain while receiving treatment for their cancer is:
   1. 10%
   2. 20%
   3. 50%
   4. 100%

2. The type of cancer pain that results from tissue damage is called:
   1. Nociceptive pain
   2. Chronic pain
   3. Neuropathic pain
   4. Idiopathic pain

3. The most common cause of nociceptive pain in patients with cancer is:
   1. Oral mucositis
   2. Herpes zoster infection
   3. Bone metastasis
   4. Limb amputation

4. All of the following chemotherapy agents can cause neuropathic pain *except:*
   1. Adriamycin
   2. Cisplatin
   3. Taxol
   4. Vincristine

5. One of the most troublesome side effects of opioid analgesics that needs to be anticipated and treated prophylactically is:
   1. Pruritus
   2. Respiratory depression
   3. Dry mouth
   4. Constipation

6. A comprehensive pain assessment should include all of the following *except:*
   1. A detailed pain history
   2. A psychosocial evaluation
   3. Physical examination
   4. Psychiatric evaluation

7. To manage persistent cancer pain effectively, analgesic medications should be given:
   1. On a regular schedule
   2. On an as-needed basis
   3. Only when the pain becomes severe
   4. Only for a limited time

8. The teaching plan for a patient with cancer pain should include all of the following information *except:*
   1. An explanation of tolerance
   2. How to keep a pain management diary
   3. The use of a pain rating scale
   4. How to manage respiratory depression

9. Neuropathic pain has all of the following characteristics *except:*
   1. Allodynia
   2. Hyperesthesias
   3. Numbness and tingling
   4. Pressurelike sensation

10. Patients with neuropathic pain will most likely be placed on which of the following analgesic medications:
    1. Acetaminophen
    2. Codeine
    3. Anticonvulsant
    4. Morphine

ANSWERS

1. *Answer: 3*
   Rationale: Approximately 50% of oncology patients who undergo active treatment for their cancer report pain.

2. *Answer: 1*
   Rationale: Nociceptive pain is the result of tissue injury.

3. *Answer: 3*
   Rationale: The most common cause of nociceptive pain in patients with cancer is pain from bone metastasis.

4. *Answer: 1*
   Rationale: The vinca alkaloids, taxanes, and platinum compounds can cause neuropathic pain.

5. *Answer: 4*
   Rationale: Constipation is the only opioid-induced side effect for which tolerance does not develop.

6. *Answer: 4*
   Rationale: A comprehensive pain assessment focuses on establishing the cause of the pain and the impact of the pain on the patient's functional status and quality of life, not on psychiatric disorders.

7. *Answer: 1*
   Rationale: Persistent pain, which is chronic in nature, requires that analgesics be given on a regular schedule to maintain a therapeutic blood level of the pain medicine.

8. *Answer: 4*
   Rationale: Respiratory depression is not a significant problem in patients taking opioid analgesics to manage chronic cancer pain.

9. *Answer: 4*
   Rationale: A pressurelike sensation is more characteristic of nociceptive pain.

10. *Answer: 3*
    Rationale: Co-analgesics (e.g., anticonvulsants, antidepressants) are the most common treatments used to manage neuropathic pain.

REFERENCES

Caraceni, A., & Portenoy, R. K. (1999). An international survey of cancer pain characteristics and syndromes. IASP Task Force on Cancer Pain, International Association for the Study of Pain. *Pain, 82*(3):263-274.

Dworkin, R. H., Backonja, M., & Rowbotham, M. C., et al. (2003). Advances in neuropathic pain: Diagnosis, mechanisms, and treatment recommendations. *Archives of Neurology, 60*(11):1524-1534.

Glover, J., Dibble, S. L., & Dodd, M. J., et al. (1995). Mood states of oncology outpatients: Does pain make a difference? *Journal of Pain Symptom Management, 10*(2):120-128.

Goudas, L. C., Bloch, R., & Gialeli-Goudas, M., et al. (2005). The epidemiology of cancer pain. *Cancer Investigation, 23*(2):182-190.

Miaskowski, C. (2004). Recent advances in understanding pain mechanisms provide future directions for pain management. *Oncology Nursing Forum, 31*(4 Suppl.):25-35.

Miaskowski, C., Cleary, J., & Burney, R., et al. (2005). *Guideline for the management of cancer pain in adults and children.* (Vol. 3) Glenview, IL: American Pain Society.

Miaskowski, C., Zimmer, E. F., & Barrett, K. M., et al. (1997). Differences in patients' and family caregivers' perceptions of the pain experience influence patient and caregiver outcomes. *Pain, 72*(1–2):217-226.

Nicholson, B. (2006). Differential diagnosis: Nociceptive and neuropathic pain. *American Journal of Managed Care, 12*(9 Suppl.):S256-S262.

Paul, S. M., Zelman, D. C., & Smith, M., et al. (2005). Categorizing the severity of cancer pain: Further exploration of the establishment of cutpoints. *Pain, 113*(1–2):37-44.

Portenoy, R. K., Payne, D., & Jacobsen, P. (1999). Breakthrough pain: Characteristics and impact in patients with cancer pain. *Pain, 81*(1–2):129-134.

Rustøen, T., Moum, T., & Padilla, G., et al. (2005). Predictors of quality of life in oncology outpatients with pain from bone metastasis. *Journal of Pain Symptom Management, 30*(3):234-242.

Svendsen, K. B., Andersen, S., & Arnason, S., et al. (2005). Breakthrough pain in malignant and non-malignant diseases: A review of prevalence, characteristics and mechanisms. *European Journal of Pain, 9*(2):195-206.

PATHOLOGIC FRACTURES

CYNTHIA C. CHERNECKY

PATHOPHYSIOLOGICAL MECHANISMS

Normal bone activity includes osteoclasts that wear away bone and osteoblasts that build up new bone. A pathologic fracture in a person with cancer is a fracture that occurs in a bone because it is weakened by primary or metastatic disease, sometimes as a consequence of minimal trauma. Other diseases and conditions that involve pathologic fractures include Paget's disease, fibrous dysplasia, tuberculosis, osteoporosis, pyogenic osteomyelitis, osteoid osteoma, gout, Gorham's disease, fibrous dysplasia, and benign bone cysts. The most common condition associated with noncancerous pathologic fractures is osteoporosis.

Bone metastases are a common cause of morbidity in cancer patients (Rubens, 1998). Pathologic factures impair ambulation and can cause spinal cord compression and severe neurologic impairment. Pathologic fractures rarely heal if left untreated.

When tumor cells become lodged adjacent to bone, the cells of the bone produce growth factors and angiogenic factors that support tumor growth. Some tumor cells stimulate osteoclasts and, along with the tumor cells' response to the calcium in the extracellular fluid of the bone, cause osteolytic lesions (holes in the bone) and thus destruction of the bone itself. Some tumors cause mineral release from the bone, which wears away, resulting in a matrix resorption that leaves holes in the bone. Some tumors release osteoclastic-stimulating factors that cause bone weakness. Tumor cells can also secrete chemicals that cause the build up of abnormal bone, called *osteosclerotic bone*.

Repair of bone is a unique form of healing involving two processes—intramembranous ossification and endochondral ossification—both of which contribute to successful repair. Intramembranous ossification begins in the mesenchyme, where an ingrowth of capillaries aids in the differentiation of mesenchymal cells into osteoblasts, which lay down the organic matrix of bone. This results in the formation of an early callus. In endochondral ossification, bone formation occurs in the primary and secondary centers of the bone, creating a stabilization process that is seen in displaced bones or unstable bones, such as fractured ribs. Table 37-1 presents the specific stages of fracture repair.

Pain is a primary symptom of bone metastasis. It is caused by tumor enlargement, perilesional edema, increased intraosseous pressure, or weakness from bone loss. Direct pressure stimulates the release of pain mediators, such as prostaglandins, bradykinins, and histamine. Tumor invasion causes activation of mechanoreceptors and nociceptors, which leads to the development of pain.

Clinically I have found that patients are extremely accurate about feeling bone metastasis and pinpointing its site, even before its presence is confirmed by diagnostic tests.

EPIDEMIOLOGY AND ETIOLOGY

Bone is the third most common site for metastasis after the lungs and liver. The incidence of pathologic fracture is approximately 2%. Up to 70% of newly diagnosed patients with

Table 37-1 STAGES OF FRACTURE REPAIR

Stage	Time Frame	Characteristics
Inflammation	Begins after the initial injury and lasts until cartilage and bone begin to form a few days to several months later	Swelling and pain
Soft callus	Begins when pain and swelling decrease; may last 3 weeks to months	Bone fragments are united by fibrocartilage or fiberbone, and a soft callus forms. This is the point of clinical stability.
Hard callus	Begins after a soft callus forms and lasts 3 to 6 months after fracture	After the soft callus is initially stable, it is converted to bone. This corresponds to clinical and radiologic union.
Remodeling	Begins after clinical and radiologic union and may last years	Bone structure, including the medullary canal, is restored to normal. Primary cortical healing is an extremely slow process, estimated to progress 1 mm every 3 weeks.

Data from Connolly, J. (1995). Fractures and dislocations: Closed management. Philadelphia: W. B. Saunders.

cancer develop bone metastasis, and of these approximately 20% develop a pathologic fracture that requires surgical intervention (Wedin, 2001; Townsend et al., 1994). Interventions to treat bone metastases include radiotherapy (Hartsell et al., 2005), radio-isotopes, surgery, hormone therapy, chemotherapy (Struthers et al., 1998), and bisphosphonates (Table 37-2).

Prevention of pathologic fractures is superior to treatment after the fracture occurs. In general, breast cancer metastases that are purely lytic are more likely to fracture than those that are blastic or mixed; 18.5% of pathologic fractures from breast cancer occur in the humerus (Flemming & Beales, 1986). After reconstruction of the humerus, fracture occurs as a complication in about 40% of these patients, with a mean bone union time of 12 months (Rose et al., 2005). Blastic lesions in the proximal femur have a high rate of fracture. Pathologic fractures are associated with a significant increase in the risk of death, especially for pateints' with breast cancer and multiple myeloma (Saad et al., 2007).

RISK PROFILE

Risk factors include the type of cancer, type of treatment, size of the lesion, location of the lesion, whether the lesion is lytic or blastic, symptoms associated with the lesion, environmental safety, and co-morbidities (e.g., diabetes, malnutrition, alcoholism). Overall the common metastatic sites are the femur and then the humerus. Other sites are the tibia and the ulna, and vertebral compression also is common.

Table 37-2 BISPHOSPHONATES

Generic Name	Trade Name	Uses	Reference
Clodronic acid	Clodronate	Breast, prostate cancers	Gulley & Dahut, 2005
Ibandronate sodium	Boniva	Postmenopausal osteoporosis	Coleman, 2005
Pamidronate disodium	Aredia	Breast, myeloma cancers and hypercalcemia	Coleman, 2005
Zoledronic acid	Zometa	Breast, myeloma, prostate, lung, and solid tumor cancers	Kohno et al., 2005; Hirsh et al., 2004

- Cancer types include primary bone cancers (Ewing's, malignant fibrous histiocytoma, osteosarcoma) and metastatic cancers of the breast, prostate, lung, thyroid, renal cell, bowel, pancreas, rectum, and ovary, myeloma, lymphoma and, in rare cases, vulvar cancer (Marcocci et al., 1989).
- In patients with breast cancer, a metastatic lesion 2.5 cm or larger in the femoral cortex or anywhere in the body that is accompanied by pain requires fixation and treatment to prevent fractures (Parrish & Murray, 1970; Snell & Beals, 1964).
- Treatment of prostate cancer with androgen deprivation therapy (Malcolm et al., 2007), LHRH agonists, orchiectomy, and/or radiation therapy increases the fracture rate by 9% (Townsend et al, 1997).
- Lytic lesions a have a higher fracture incidence (Mirels, 2003), because they reduce both the strength and stiffness of the bone. Lung cancer metastasis is typically a lytic lesion in bones below the elbow and knee. Because patient survival is short, these painful lesions usually are treated with radiation or surgery.
- Thyroid cancer has a long survival time, and these patients require lifetime follow-up for possible fractures.
- Renal cell metastasis to bone occurs in about 25% to 50% of patients.
- Radiation therapy to the bone increases the risk of fracture by up to 41%. This is theorized to be due to failure of reossification or to softening of the bone.
- Women over 55 years of age with sarcoma who have radiation doses of 60 Gy or higher have an increased risk of pathologic fractures (Holt et al., 2005).
- In patients with sarcoma, more than 50% of fractures occur in the distal femur and 25% in the proximal femur (Ebeid et al., 2005).
- Unsafe environments, such as clutter, throw rugs, loose edges on floors, uneven floors, and icy pavements, can lead to fractures. Children with bone metastasis are vulnerable to fractures associated with falls while running or playing.

PROGNOSIS

The prognosis depends on the underlying disease process. The quality of the bone proximal and distal to the fracture site must be adequate to support fixation. Internal fixation with postoperative radiation has been found to afford the best prognosis (Perez et al., 1972). Complete pathologic fracture and soft tissue metastasis are negative prognostic variables for 1-year survival in patients with breast cancer, with 11% requiring reoperation for repair of pathologic fractures (Wedin, 2001). The 5-year event-free survival rate is 60% in patients with nonmetastatic extremity osteosarcoma, but it drops to 17% with recurrence (Bacci et al., 2006). Predictors of survival for patients who undergo surgery for treatment of bone metastasis include the diagnosis, clinical estimation of survival, hemoglobin count, number of visceral metastases, and ECOG performance score (Nathan et al., 2005). Administration of zoledronic acid (Zometa) prolonged the median survival time in patients with lung cancer and other solid tumor by 2.5 months (Hirsh et al., 2004).

PROFESSIONAL ASSESSMENT CRITERIA (PAC)

1. Assess the patient for pain history: Dull, aching, steady pain that increases during the daytime or sharp pain with swelling, redness, and reduced range of motion. Pain develops gradually over weeks to months and becomes progressively more severe.

2. Hallmark symptoms include sharp pain initially, then dull pain that increases with movement, as well as limited range of motion.
3. Assess the wound site (if applicable): Color, temperature, sensation distal to area, ability to bear weight; also patient anxiety, apprehension.
4. Assess vital signs for indicators of pain: Increased heart rate, blood pressure, and respiratory rate. Fever indicates an inflammatory process or tumor growth.
5. Rib fractures lead to restricted breathing (assess respiratory rate and excursion) and pain (assess severity on a 1 to 10 scale).
6. Assess patient's mobility and ability to perform ADLs.
7. Assess serum calcium levels for an increase that indicates bone disease.
8. Assess the patient for depression.
9. Assess total Gy of radiation received; if 60 Gy or greater, the patient is at increased risk for pathologic fractures.

NURSING CARE AND TREATMENT

1. Immobilize the limb and avoid lifting or movement of the affected area.
2. Initiate pain control (e.g., large doses of corticosteroids [dexamethasone 20-100 mg IV for epidural tumor]; analgesics; radiation; chemotherapy; nerve blocks; radiopharmaceutical agents; bisphosphonates [see Table 37-2]; calcitonin; surgical intervention for fixation of fracture site). Reassess pain every 1 to 2 hours.
3. Diagnostics: Bone scan to detect bone metastasis and to assess overall extent of disease except in myeloma, renal cell, and thyroid cancers, for which skeletal x-ray films are used. Note that bone scans do not provide detail of the structural lesion in the bone. PET scans are very sensitive to metastatic diseases and are often used as comparison studies throughout the patient's life. MRI (superior to myelography) (Kent & Larson, 1988) is superior in detecting epidural tumors and has great accuracy for differentiating pathologic fractures from stress fractures (Fayad et al., 2005). CT scans are often prescribed, especially before a biopsy.
4. Initiate treatment:
   • Pamidronate for patients with multiple myeloma.
   • Zoledronic acid (Zometa), a bisphosphonate that is a potent inhibitor of osteoclast-mediated bone resorption, to reduce the risk of bone complications (Kohno et al., 2004; Saad et al., 2004; Rosen et al., 2001) in patients with breast cancer, prostate cancer (Saad et al., 2006), myeloma, lung cancer, and other solid tumors. May cause osteonecrosis of the jaw (Lipton, 2007).
   • Radioisotopes (e.g., strontium-89 and samarium-153) in patients with prostate metastasis.
5. Orthopedic, pain management, physical therapy, and palliative care consults as needed.
6. Ensure that the patient has a caregiver.

EVIDENCE-BASED PRACTICE UPDATES

1. Limb salvage management in sarcoma is possible in some cases with the use of reconstructive modalities such as joint fusion and rotationplasty (Ebeid et al., 2005).
2. Patients with osteosarcoma who have a pathologic fracture and who undergo limb salvage are at no greater risk of recurrence or death than those who undergo amputation (Scully et al., 2002).
3. Patients with pathologic fractures of the humerus who had cemented nailing rather than endoprosthetic reconstruction had better shoulder motion, hand positioning, lifting

ability, and emotional acceptance. Pain alleviation and dexterity were comparable in the two groups (Bickels et al., 2005).

4. Single-fraction radiotherapy of 8 Gy works as well as fractionated regimens in controlling pain from pathologic fractures (Jeremic, 2001). However, an 8 Gy delivery has a higher rate of retreatment, although less toxicity, than a 30 Gy delivery (Hartsell et al., 2005).

5. HIV-positive patients taking Tenofovir have increased pathologic fractures through its effects on phosphorus balance and vitamin D metabolism (Brim et al., 2007).

TEACHING AND EDUCATION

Ambulation: *Rationale:* Standing up, bearing weight, and walking will increase the blood supply to the fractured area and promote healing.

Safety: *Rationale:* It is necessary to prevent further fractures through careful body movement and avoiding environmental hazards that can increase the risk of falls.

Signs and symptoms: *Rationale:* Bone disease usually starts with a dull, aching type discomfort or pain and gets worse as time goes on. Tell your health care provider if you have any aches.

Web sites for information:
- Novartis Oncology, Novartis Pharma AG: www.zometa.com
- National Center for Biotechnology Information: www.ncbi.nlm.nih.gov
- Elsevier, Inc.: www.linkinghub.elsevier.com/retrieve/pii/S0020138303002407

NURSING DIAGNOSES

1. **Acute pain** related to actual fracture or destruction of bone from malignant disease
2. **Impaired physical mobility** related to instability of bone, healing process, and/or depression
3. **Ineffective coping** related to change in activity, hormonal manipulation, diagnosis, stress related to treatment(s)
4. **Risk for infection** related to surgical and/or medical interventions for cancer treatment, including transfusions
5. **Risk for injury** related to increased risk of falls as a result of bone instability and environmental hazards

EVALUATION AND DESIRED OUTCOMES

1. The patient will be able to ambulate.
2. The patient will be able to participate in activities of daily living.
3. The patient will be able to reduce the use of analgesics as the fracture heals.
4. The severity of the patient's pain will be decreased.
5. The patient will be able to name potential new sites for fracture and associated symptoms.

DISCHARGE PLAN AND FOLLOW-UP CARE

- Ensure that the patient has a caregiver.
- Home health care for progressive weight bearing, wound care, and mental health management.

- Surgical and medical follow-up 2 weeks after discharge.
- Follow-up diagnostics to monitor for bone regeneration and possible metastasis.

REVIEW QUESTIONS

QUESTIONS

1. **Pathologic fractures occur commonly in which type of cancer:**
   1. Gallbladder cancer
   2. Glioblastoma brain tumor
   3. Parotid tumor cancer
   4. Breast cancer

2. **Bone weakness in pathologic fractures is caused by:**
   1. Osteoclasts
   2. Osteoblasts
   3. Mitochondrial engulfment
   4. Hypernatremia

3. **Which of the following processes would indicate bone healing:**
   1. Internal toenail matrix formation
   2. Callus formation
   3. Pancytopenia
   4. Hypomagnesemia

4. **Which of the following statements leads you to believe that your patient, who has breast cancer, may have a pathologic fracture:**
   1. "I've got a sharp pain in my belly, knifelike."
   2. "My pain gets better as the day goes on and I move more."
   3. "My pain stings, and then my arm goes numb for a while."
   4. "My pain is dull and achy and has gotten worse since 3 days ago."

5. **Which condition would inhibit healing of a pathologic fracture:**
   1. Anemia
   2. Gastroesophageal reflux disease (GERD) that responds to treatment
   3. Hypertension of 148/92
   4. Hypercholesterolemia

6. **What types of lesions have a higher fracture incidence:**
   1. Melanoma lesions
   2. Blastic lesions
   3. Lytic lesions
   4. Eczema-type lesions

7. **Your patient may have an epidural tumor. The best test to substantiate this diagnosis is a:**
   1. Bone scan
   2. Serum calcium
   3. CT scan without contrast
   4. MRI study

8. **Which of the following radioisotopes is used to treat bone metastasis in patients with prostate cancer:**
   1. Samarium-153
   2. Cesium-121
   3. Iridium-128
   4. Cobalt 152

9. **Which of the following patients is at greatest risk for a pathologic fracture:**
   1. Breast cancer, stage I, lumpectomy
   2. Prostate cancer, white male, age 57, TURP surgery
   3. Osteosarcoma, total Gy 70, combination chemotherapy, age 58
   4. Lung cancer, metastatic lesion left rib, 0.05 cm in size

10. **With which of the following cancers might you recommend limb salvage:**
    1. Liver cancer
    2. Astrocytoma
    3. Osteosarcoma
    4. Lung cancer

ANSWERS

1. *Answer: 4*
   Rationale: Fractures are most common in breast, lung, and prostate cancers and lymphomas.

2. *Answer: 1*
   Rationale: Osteoclasts wear away bone, thereby causing fractures. Osteoblasts build up bone.

3. *Answer: 2*
Rationale: Both soft and then hard callus formation are stages of fracture repair.

4. *Answer: 4*
Rationale: Dull, achy pain that increases over time is a sign of a pathologic fracture.

5. *Answer: 1*
Rationale: Anemia reduces the number of red cells to the fracture area that can help heal bone.

6. *Answer: 3*
Rationale: Lytic lesions have the highest fracture incidence because they reduce both the strength and the stiffness of the bone.

7. *Answer: 4*
Rationale: MRI is superior for detecting epidural tumors, because it reveals the structure and placement of bone and soft tissue.

8. *Answer: 1*
Rationale: Samarium-153 and strontium-89 are the radioisotopes used to treat bone metastasis from prostate cancer.

9. *Answer: 3*
Rationale: Of the patients described, the patient with osteosarcoma who was treated with a total Gy greater than 60 is at greatest risk. The risk of fracture is increased for a patient with breast cancer who has a femoral lesion larger than 2.5 cm and for a patient with prostate cancer who is treated with LHRH agonists, orchiectomy, or radiation. Lung cancer metastasis is too small for fracture compared to other choices.

10. *Answer: 3*
Rationale: Bone cancer of an extremity (e.g., osteosarcoma) may allow the limb to be saved through limb salvage surgery.

REFERENCES

Bacci, G., Longhi, A., & Versari, M., et al. (2006). Prognostic factors for osteosarcoma of the extremity treated with neoadjuvant chemotherapy: 15-Year experience in 789 patients treated at a single institution. *Cancer, 106*(5):1154-1161.

Bickels, J., Kollender, Y., & Wittig, J. C., et al. (2005). Function after resection of humeral metastases: Analysis of 59 consecutive patients. *Clinical Orthopaedics & Related Research, 437*:201-208.

Brim, N. M., Cu-Uvin, S., & Hu, S. L., et al. (2007). Bone disease and pathologic fractures in a patient with tenofovir-induced Fanconi syndrome. *AIDS Reader 17*(6):322-328.

Coleman, R. E. (2005). Bisphosphonates in breast cancer. *Annals of Oncology, 16*(5):687-695.

Ebeid, W., Amin, S., & Abdelmegid, A. (2005). Limb salvage management of pathologic fractures of primary malignant bone tumors. *Cancer Control, 12*(1):57-61.

Fayad, L. M., Kawamoto, S., & Kamel, I. R., et al. (2005). Distinction of long bone stress fractures from pathologic fractures on cross-sectional imaging: How successful are we? *American Journal of Roentgenology, 185*(4):915-924.

Flemming, J. E., & Beales, R. K. (1986). Pathologic fracture of the humerus. *Clinical Orthopaedics and Related Research, 203*:258-260.

Gulley, J., & Dahut, W. L. (2005). Clodronate in the prevention and treatment of skeletal metastasis. *Expert Review of Anticancer Therapy, 5*(2):221-230.

Hartsell, W. F., Scott, C. B., & Bruner, D. W., et al. (2005). Randomized trial of short- versus long-course radiotherapy for palliation of painful bone metastases. *Journal of the National Cancer Institute, 97*(11):798-804.

Hirsh, V., Tchekmedyian, N. S., & Rosen, L. S., et al. (2004). Clinical benefits of zoledronic acid in patients with lung cancer and other solid tumors: Analysis based on history of skeletal complications. *Clinical Lung Cancer, 6*(3):170-174.

Holt, G. E., Griffin, A. M., & Pintilie, M., et al. (2005). Fractures following radiotherapy and limb-salvage surgery for lower extremity soft-tissue sarcomas: A comparison of high-dose and low-dose radiotherapy. *Journal of Bone and Joint Surgery Am, 87*(2):315-319.

Jeremic, B. (2001). Single fraction external beam radiation therapy in the treatment of localized metastatic bone pain: A review. *Journal of Pain and Symptom Management, 22*(6):1048-1058.

Kent, D. L., & Larson, E. B. (1988). Magnetic resonance imaging of the brain and spine: Is clinical efficacy established after the first decade? *Annals of Internal Medicine, 108*(3):402-424.

Kohno, N., Aogi, K., & Minami, H., et al. (2004). A randomized, double blind, placebo-controlled, phase III trial of zoledronic acid in the prevention of skeletal complications in Japanese women with bone metastases from breast cancer. Presented at the American Society of Clinical Oncology 2004 Annual Meeting (ASCO); June 5-6, Abstract 668.

Kohno, N., Aogi, K., & Minami, H., et al. (2005). Zoledronic acid significantly reduces skeletal complications compared with placebo in Japanese women with bone metastases from breast cancer: A randomized, placebo-controlled trial. *Journal of Clinical Oncology, 23*(15):3314-3321.

Lipton, A. (2007). Efficacy and safety of intravenous bisphosphanates in patients with bone metastases caused by metastatic breast cancer. *Clinical Breast Cancer, 7*(Suppl 1):S14-S20.

Malcolm, J. B., Derweesh, I. H., & Kincade, M. C., et al. (2007). Osteoporosis and fractures after androgen deprivation initiation for prostate cancer. *Canadian Journal of Urology 14*(3):3551-3559.

Marcocci, C., Pacini, F., & Elisei, R., et al. (1989). Clinical and biologic behavior of bone metastases from differentiated thyroid carcinoma. *Surgery 106*(6):960-966.

Mirel, H. (2003). Metastatic disease in long bones: A proposed scoring system for diagnosing impending pathologic fractures. *Clinical Orthopaedics and Related Research, 415*(Suppl.):S4-S13.

Nathan, S. S., Healey, J. H., & Mellano, D., et al. (2005). Survival in patients operated on for pathologic fracture: Implications for end-of-life orthopedic care. *Journal of Clinical Oncology, 23*(25):6072-6082.

Parrish, F. F., & Murray, J. A. (1970). Surgical treatment for secondary neoplastic fractures. A retrospective study of ninety-six patients. *Journal of Bone & Joint Surgery - American Volume 52*(4):665-686.

Perez, C. A., Bradfield, J. S., & Morgan, H. C. (1972). Management of pathologic fractures. *Cancer, 29*(3):684-693.

Rose, P. S., Shin, A. Y., & Bishop, A. T., et al. (2005). Vascularized free fibula transfer for oncologic reconstruction of the humerus. *Clinical Orthopaedics and Related Research, 438*:80-84.

Rosen, L. S., Gordon, D., & Kaminski, M., et al. (2001). Zoledronic acid versus pamidronate in the treatment of skeletal metastases in patients with breast cancer or osteolytic lesions of multiple myeloma: A phase III, double-blind, comparative trial. *Cancer Journal, 7*(5):377-387.

Rubens, R. D. (1998). Bone metastases: The clinical problem. *European Journal of Cancer, 34*(2):210-213.

Saad, F., Gleason, D. M., & Murray, R., et al. (2004). Long-term efficacy of zoledronic acid for the prevention of skeletal complications in patients with metastatic hormone-refractory prostate cancer. *Journal of the National Cancer Institute, 96*(11):879-882.

Saad, F., Lipton, A., & Cook, R., et al. (2007). Pathologic fractures correlate with reduced survival inpatients with malignant bone disease. *Cancer 110*(8):1860-1867.

Saad, F., McKiernan, J., & Eastham, J. H. (2006). Rationale for zoledronic acid therapy in men with hormone-sensitive prostate cancer with or without bone metastasis. *Urologic Oncology, 24*(1):4-12.

Scully, S. P., Ghert, M. A., & Zurakowski, D., et al. (2002). Pathologic fracture in osteosarcoma: Prognostic importance and treatment implications. *Journal of Bone and Joint Surgery Am, 84A*(1):49-57.

Snell, W., & Beals, R. K. (1964). Femoral metastases and fractures from breast cancer. *Surgery, Gynecology & Obstetrics, 119*:22-24.

Struthers, C., Mayer, D., & Fisher, G. (1998). Nursing management of the patient with bone metastases. *Seminars in Oncology Nursing, 14*(3):199-209.

Townsend, M. F., Sanders, W. H., & Northway, R. O., et al. (1997). Bone fractures associated with luteinizing hormone-releasing hormone agonists used in the treatment of prostate carcinoma. *Cancer, 79*(3):545-550.

Townsend, P. W., Rosenthal, H. G., & Smalley, S. R., et al. (1994). Impact of postoperative radiation therapy and other perioperative factors on outcomes after orthopedic stabilization of impending or pathologic fractures due to metastatic disease. *Journal of Clinical Oncology, 12*(11):2345-2350.

Wedin, R. (2001). Surgical treatment for pathologic fracture. *Acta Orthopaedica Scandinavica Supplementum, 72*(302):1-29.

Pleural Effusions: Malignant

DIANE G. COPE

PATHOPHYSIOLOGICAL MECHANISMS

Malignant pleural effusions are collections of excess body fluid in the pleural space. The pleural space is located between the visceral and parietal pleura. Normally, fluid is shifted from the parietal pleural surface to the pleural surface, over the intrapleural space, and then reabsorbed through the visceral pleura. The pleural space contains 0.13 mL of pleural fluid (composed of hypoproteinemic plasma) per kilogram of body mass (about 7 mL per lung). This fluid reduces friction between the lung and the chest wall.

Approximately 100 to 200 mL of fluid moves across the pleural space daily (Noppen et al., 2000). A balance between the osmotic and hydrostatic pressures governs the secretion and reabsorption of pleural fluid. Pleural fluid develops in the pleural membrane vessels and is reabsorbed by pleural lymphatics (which absorb protein) and capillaries (which absorb fluids). An increase in the amount of fluid moving into the pleural space can result from increased permeability of the endothelial tissue and increased microvascular pressure. A decrease in the amount of fluid exiting the pleural space can result from cytokine-mediated lymphatic constriction; damage to the lymphatics caused by medications, radiation, surgery, malignancy; or increased systemic venous pressure (Spiea & Brahmer, 2004).

Specifically, malignant pleural effusions can develop as a result of increased fluid production or obstruction of pleural lymphatic drainage. Pulmonary neoplasms can cause obstruction by direct pleural invasion or through seeding and deposits of malignant cells, which alter capillary permeability (Schrump & Nguyen, 2001). A decrease in the amount of fluid exiting the pleural space can be caused by cytokinine-mediated lymphatic constriction (infection or tumor); damage to lymphatics from chemotherapy, radiation, or surgery; or invasion of the lymphatics by malignancy.

The development of a malignant pleural effusion indicates a grave prognosis. The condition is associated with distressing symptoms such as dyspnea, chest pain, pleuritic chest pain, cough, orthopnea, hemoptysis, fever, and dysphagia. Nurses can manage symptoms and provide supportive care to patients and their caregivers.

EPIDEMIOLOGY AND ETIOLOGY

The incidence of malignant pleural effusion is about 40% to 50% in patients with cancer (Schrump & Nguyen, 2001; Walker & Casciato, 2001). An estimated 200,000 to 250,000 new cases of malignant pleural effusions are diagnosed annually as a result of the

Table 38-1	MALIGNANT NEOPLASMS ASSOCIATED WITH PLEURAL EFFUSION*	
Cause	Number	Percentage
Total malignant effusions	1283	100
Lung cancer	450	35
Breast cancer	246	20
Lymphomas and leukemia	256	20
Unknown primary (adenocarcinoma)	154	12
Unknown primary (all types)	95	7
Reproductive tract	70	5
Gastrointestinal tract	90	7
Genitourinary tract	66	5
All other	39	3

From Abeloff, M. D., Armitage, J. O., & Niederhuber, J. E., et al. (Eds.). (2004). *Clinical oncology*. (3rd ed.). New York: Churchill Livingstone.
*Includes causes of malignant effusion each less than 1%: Endocrine, head and neck cancer; mesothelioma; soft tissue sarcoma; bone cancer; and myeloma.

increasing incidence of breast and lung cancer (Light, 2002). Approximately 75% of malignant pleural effusions are caused by lung and breast cancers and lymphomas (Table 38-1) (Shuey & Payne, 2005).

RISK PROFILE

- Lung and breast cancer, lymphomas, leukemia, and adenocarcinoma of unknown primary cause.
- Cancers resistant to chemotherapy.
- Advanced cancer.

PROGNOSIS

Upon diagnosis of malignant pleural effusion, 54% of patients die within 1 month, and 84% die within 3 months (Schrump & Nguyen, 2001). Survival time is also related to the underlying tumor histology. Patients with lung or gastric carcinomas may survive only months; those with ovarian cancer may survive 9 months; and those with breast cancer may survive a year or longer (Schrump & Nguyen, 2001).

PROFESSIONAL ASSESSMENT CRITERIA (PAC)

1. Dry, nonproductive cough; chest discomfort near the involved lung; pleuritic pain; dyspnea on exertion; and increased fatigue.
2. Decreased or absent breath sounds, crackles at the superior border of the effusion.
3. Decreased chest expansion during inspiration.
4. Absence of fremitus.
5. Dullness on percussion over involved lung.
6. Hypertension
7. Tachypnea
8. Tachycardia

9. Cyanosis or decreased oxygen saturation.
10. Chest x-ray films (posteroanterior, lateral, and decubitus) showing an opaque shadow in the involved lung and costophrenic angle blunting, with possible mediastinal shift if a large pleural effusion is present.
11. CT scan is helpful for evaluating masses, nodules, and pleural-based thickening.
12. Thoracentesis with pleural fluid analysis may be done for diagnosis and treatment planning.
    • Transudative fluid: Strawlike color; results from altered hydrostatic/colloid forces; low protein, low cellular content; usually a non-inflammatory process.
    • Exudative fluid: Pusslike color; formed by active secretion, inflammation, or leakage; increased cellular or protein content. Fluid is considered exudative if:
        • The ratio of pleural to serum protein is greater than 0.5.
        • The LDH level is greater than 2/3 of the upper limit for the serum reference range.
        • The ratio of protein to serum LDH is greater than 0.6.
    • Fluid analysis results with regard to malignancy may include the following studies:
        • pH: Less than 7.3.
        • Cell count: Hypercellular, predominantly lymphocytes and monocytes.
        • Albumin gradient (serum albumin minus pleural albumin): Less than 1.2 g/dL.
        • Cholesterol: Elevated with exudative fluid.
        • Glucose and tumor markers may be evaluated, although these results have not been found to be useful clinically.

NURSING CARE AND TREATMENT

1. **Vital signs:** Assess for hypertension, tachycardia, tachypnea, chest discomfort, or fever.
2. Obtain and interpret O_2 saturation values.
3. Administer oxygen as needed.
4. Assess for nonproductive cough.
5. Obtain pleural fluid analysis and review results.
6. Obtain and review the results of a chest x-ray film, CT scan of the chest.
7. Weigh the patient daily.
8. Administer morphine sulfate for dyspnea and chest discomfort as ordered.
9. Provide small frequent meals with high calories.
10. **Activity**: Have the patient conserve energy by spacing and limiting activity; provide assistance with ambulation.
11. Educate the patient and family about the disease process; explain the etiologies of malignant pleural effusion and anticipated treatment plans, such as thoracentesis, possible pleurodesis, and supportive care.

EVIDENCE-BASED PRACTICE UPDATES

1. Vascular endothelial growth factor (VEGF) is believed to be a major contributor to the development of pleural effusions (Grove & Lee, 2002). VEGF is a cytokine that facilitates endothelial vasodilation and increases the permeability of the mesothelium.
2. Thoracoscopic pleurodesis, using talc as the sclerosing agent, has proved to be the most effective means of preventing recurrence of pleural effusions (Shaw & Agarwal, 2004).
3. In one study, intrapleural catheterization (e.g., the Denver Pleurx System) provided symptomatic benefit for 91% of patients with trapped lung or multiloculated effusions (Pollak, 2002).

TEACHING AND EDUCATION

Dyspnea: *Rationale*: You may need oxygen to ease your breathing.

Activity: *Rationale*: You need to conserve energy and limit or space out your activities to reduce the shortness of breath.

Nutrition: *Rationale*: Eat small, high-calorie meals.

Tests and procedures: *Rationale*: You may need additional chest x-ray films to assess for fluid in your lungs. If the fluid has returned and you are short of breath, the fluid may be removed through a needle inserted into the pleural space. Sometimes the fluid is left in the lung because it tends to reaccumulate, and frequent taps may pose a risk of infection or complications.

Web sites for information:
- American Thoracic Society: www.thoracic.org
- Lung Cancer: www.lungcancer.org
- American Cancer Society: www.cancer.org
- Oncology Nursing Society: www.ons.org

NURSING DIAGNOSES

1. **Ineffective tissue perfusion** related to decreased oxygen saturation
2. **Imbalanced nutrition: less than body requirements** related to early satiety, anorexia, and fatigue
3. **Activity intolerance** related to dyspnea and fatigue
4. **Risk for caregiver role strain** related to patient's physical assistance needs and increased symptoms
5. **Ineffective coping** related to progression of disease

EVALUATION AND DESIRED OUTCOMES

1. Pain will be absent or tolerable.
2. Dyspnea will be absent or not distressing.
3. Cough will be absent or not distressing.
4. Fatigue will be absent or not distressing.
5. O_2 saturation will be greater than 92%.

DISCHARGE PLAN AND FOLLOW-UP CARE

- Home oxygen as prescribed.
- Caregiver or family member to assist with patient care, meal preparation, and household maintenance.
- Home health nursing or hospice care for assessment of pulmonary status, symptom management, and medication evaluation.
- Instruct patient and family to notify health care provider if the patient experiences increased shortness of breath and/or increased nonproductive cough.
- Follow-up visit with nurse practitioner or physician.
- Repeat chest x-ray film for increasing shortness of breath.

REVIEW QUESTIONS

QUESTIONS

1. Malignant pleural effusions are most frequently related to:
   1. Lung cancer
   2. Colon cancer
   3. Leukemia
   4. Breast cancer

2. An early presenting symptom of pleural effusion is:
   1. Nausea
   2. Fever
   3. Shortness of breath
   4. Weight gain

3. Mr. K. is a 66-year-old male who was diagnosed with stage III non-small cell lung cancer. He received chemotherapy and radiation to the chest and completed treatment 8 months ago. He presents to your clinic with complaints of increasing shortness of breath, right-sided chest discomfort, and cough. You suspect a pleural effusion. You anticipate assessment findings that correlate with pleural effusion, including:
   1. Hypotension and fever
   2. Brachypnea and bradycardia
   3. Oxygen saturation less than 96%
   4. Decreased breath sounds in the right lower lobe

4. Mr. K. is sent for a chest x-ray film. A chest x-ray film confirming a pleural effusion would reveal:
   1. Fibrotic streaking
   2. Costophrenic angle blunting
   3. Cardiomegaly
   4. Water bottle–shaped pericardium

5. Mr. K. has a thoracentesis for pleural fluid analysis and symptom management. Mrs. K. asks you what caused the fluid in his lung. After reviewing the report on the pleural fluid analysis, you tell Mrs. K. the results suggest that the fluid is most likely malignant. Your statement is based on the knowledge that malignant pleural fluid has the following characteristic:
   1. Clear, light yellow color
   2. High pH (greater than 7.3)
   3. Elevated cell count
   4. Elevated LDH

6. Mr. K. remains short of breath after the thoracentesis. Your nursing care should include:
   1. Elevate the head of the bed to reduce pressure on the chest
   2. Measure the O_2 saturation and administer oxygen
   3. Administer morphine sulfate
   4. All of the above

7. Mrs. K. voices concern about being able to care for Mr. K. at home. To assist Mrs. K., you would recommend:
   1. Nursing home placement
   2. Physical therapy
   3. Referral to home care nursing or home hospice care
   4. Occupational therapy

8. Mr. and Mrs. K. decide to go home with hospice care. Mrs. K. should be instructed to notify the home care or hospice nurse if Mr. K. experiences:
   1. Hemoptysis
   2. Increasing shortness of breath
   3. Loss of appetite
   4. Distressing symptoms

9. Discharge instructions for Mr. K. would include:
   1. Use oxygen only at night.
   2. Prepare low-calorie meals if weight gain occurs.
   3. Encourage Mr. K. to perform activities of daily living.
   4. The rationale for using morphine sulfate for dyspnea.

10. The hospice nurse visits and finds Mr. K. sitting in a chair, holding his right ribs. The nurse's assessment is: BP 160/100, temperature 98.7, pulse 120, shallow respirations 22,

decreased tactile fremitus and decreased breath sounds in the right lung. The appropriate nursing action would be:
1. Reposition Mr. K. with pillows
2. Administer oxygen, 2 to 4 L/nasal cannula
3. Administer morphine sulfate
4. All of the above

ANSWERS

1. *Answer: 1*
   Rationale: Lung cancer is the malignancy most frequently associated with pleural effusions.

2. *Answer: 3*
   Rationale: Early presenting symptoms of pleural effusion are shortness of breath, nonproductive cough, chest discomfort near the involved lung, and fatigue.

3. *Answer: 4*
   Rationale: A sign of pleural effusion is decreased breath sounds or crackles during auscultation of the lungs.

4. *Answer: 2*
   Rationale: Chest x-ray findings consistent with pleural effusion are costophrenic angle blunting and an opaque shadow in the involved lung. A water bottle–shaped pericardium is associated with pericardial effusion.

5. *Answer: 4*
   Rationale: Pleural fluid analysis results indicative of a malignancy may include cloudy, bloody, or purulent color; low pH (less than 7.3); elevated LDH, and low glucose level. An elevated cell count is not diagnostic.

6. *Answer: 4*
   Rationale: Patients experiencing shortness of breath after removal of pleural fluid may require repositioning, oxygen, and pain and dyspnea medication management.

7. *Answer: 3*
   Rationale: A referral to home nursing care or hospice helps in the further assessment of home needs and discharge planning. Home hospice is indicated if Mr K.'s prognosis is likely less than 6 months.

8. *Answer: 4*
   Rationale: The hospice nurse needs to reassess Mr. K.'s condition and provide symptom management if his symptoms change or worsen.

9. *Answer: 4*
   Rationale: Patients using morphine for dyspnea need to be taught the rationale for its use, the drug's side effects, and safety issues.

10. *Answer: 4*
    Rationale: The nurse's assessment findings suggest increasing pleural effusion, which should be treated symptomatically.

REFERENCES

Grove, C. S., & Lee, Y. C. (2002). Vascular endothelial growth factor: The key mediator in pleural effusion formation. *Current Opinions in Pulmonary Medicine, 8*:294-301.

Light, R. W. (2002). Pleural effusion. *New England Journal of Medicine, 25*:1971-1977.

Niedrehuber, et al. (Eds.), *Clinical oncology* (pp. 1179-1212). New York: Churchill Livingstone.

Noppen, N., DeWaele, M. R., & Li, R., et al.,(2000). Volume and cellular content of normal pleural fluid in humans examined by pleural lavage. *American Journal of Respiratory Critical Care Medicine, 162*, pp. 1023-1026.

Pollak, J. S. (2002). Malignant pleural effusions: Treatment with tunneled long-term drainage catheter. *Circulation Opinion in Pulmonary Medicine, 8*, pp. 302-307.

Schrump, D. S., & Nguyen, D. M. (2001). Malignant pleural and pericardial effusions. In V. T. DeVita, S. Hellman, & S. A. Rosenberg (Eds.), *Cancer: Principles and practice of oncology* (pp. (6th ed.). Philadelphia: Lippincott Williams & Wilkins.

Shaw, P., & Agarwal, R. (2004). Pleurodesis for malignant pleural effusions. *Cochrane Database of Systematic Reviews*, 1:CD002916. Retrieved: May 1, 2007 from www.cochrane.org/reviews/-18K.

Shuey, K., & Payne, Y. (2005). Malignant pleural effusion. *Clinical Journal of Oncology Nursing, 9*:529-532.

Walker, D. L., & Casciato, D. A. (2001). Malignant effusions. In C. M. Haskell (Ed.) *Cancer treatment* (pp. (5th ed.). Philadelphia: W. B. Saunders.

PULMONARY FIBROSIS

CYNTHIA C. CHERNECKY

PATHOPHYSIOLOGICAL MECHANISMS

Pulmonary fibrosis (PF) is a pathologic term for excessive connective tissue in the lungs that hampers lung recoil and lung deflation during expiration. The disorder is more commonly referred to as *interstitial pulmonary fibrosis, fibrosing alveolitis, interstitial pneumonitis,* and *Hamman-Rich syndrome,* although it has many more names (Table 39-1).

Although no clear mechanisms have been validated to explain pulmonary fibrosis in humans, we do know that in mice it involves the loss of E prostanoid receptors for prostaglandin 2 (EP2) on fibroblasts (Moore et al., 2005). The current understanding is that excessive connective tissue results from bodily tissue repair mechanisms associated with a variety of types of injury to the lungs. With injury, the inflammatory response and coagulation cascade are activated; this results in an increase in fibroblasts, myofibroblasts, inflammatory cells, and collagen deposits in the lungs, which twist the lung alveoli and capillaries out of shape. The air sacs (alveoli) fill with fluid (alveolitis), the lung capillaries become inflamed (vasculitis), and ultimately, scarring of the lung tissue (fibrosis) occurs. The end result is restrictive lung disease with loss of lung elasticity, sometimes called *stiff lungs.* Increased tissue resistance reduces the internal diameter of the pulmonary vascular bed, which increases the work of respiration. The lack of lung recoil and elasticity makes deflation of the lungs difficult, and compensation, through an increase in the work of breathing, must occur to achieve oxygenation. The overall results of diminished recoil include increased work of breathing, destruction of alveoli and pulmonary vessels, hypoxemia, pulmonary hypertension, and finally, cor pulmonale and heart failure. Pulmonary fibrosis can have a devastating effect on quality of life and can be fatal. The nurse's main role includes early detection of fibrosis to minimize its severity, efficient treatment to increase or maintain the patient's quality of life, and/or effective end of life care. Current research is focusing on finding treatments to eliminate or diminish the fibrosis.

EPIDEMIOLOGY AND ETIOLOGY

The incidence of pulmonary fibrosis is about 5% to 15% in the general population (Chisam & Douglas, 2002). It increases with increased doses of radiation therapy to the lung fields, increases in the volume of lung irradiated, and use of concomitant chemotherapy. Moderate or severe radiation pneumonitis occurs in 2% to 9% of patients treated with radiation and chemotherapy. Pulmonary fibrosis can take months or years to develop. Diffuse pulmonary fibrosis has several causes (Table 39-2), unlike idiopathic pulmonary fibrosis (IPF), the cause of which is unknown.

Table 39-1	OTHER NAMES AND CAUSES OF PULMONARY FIBROSIS
Name	**Examples of Causes***
Acute interstitial pneumonitis	Polymyositis, dermatomyositis, psoriasis
Chronic diffuse fibrosing pneumonitis	Albinism, SARS, congenital misalignment lung vessels
Chronic diffuse sclerosing pneumonitis	Hemangioma
Chronic interstitial pneumonia	MPO-ANCA vasculitis, smoking, mesalamine drug use, heroin use, coal worker, EBV, acute lung injury, traction bronchiectasis, plaster worker, nontuberculosis Mycobacterium bronchiolitis (hot tub lung)
Cryptogenic fibrosing alveolitis	HTLV-1 virus, systemic sclerosis, antiphospholipid antibody syndrome, metal exposure, hepatitis C virus
Diffuse idiopathic interstitial fibrosis	Sarcoidosis, viral infection
Diffuse idiopathic pulmonary fibrosis	Bone marrow dysfunction, ARDS, systemic sclerosis, bronchiolitis obliterans
Diffuse infiltrative pulmonary disease	Sarcoidosis, autoimmune disease
Desquamative interstitial pneumonitis	Dermatomyositis, ABCA3 mutation, smoking, asbestosis
Familial pulmonary fibrosis	Familial idiopathic fibrosis
Fibrosing alveolitis	Rheumatoid arthritis (RA), Jo-1 autoimmune disease, EBV, atrial myxoma, d-penicillamine therapy, systemic sclerosis, Wegener's granulomatosis, nickel dust exposure, zinc oxide inhalation, scleroderma
Hamman-Rich disease or syndrome	Dermatomyositis, polymyositis, ARDS, pseudoinfluenza, goldsmith work
Honeycomb lung	Lung cancer, connective tissue disease
Honey lung	Lung cancer, connective tissue disease
Idiopathic fibrosing alveolitis	Connective tissue disease, systemic sclerosis, pulmonary arterial hypertension, sarcoidosis, lung cancer
Idiopathic interstitial fibrosis of lung syndrome	Polymyositis, dermatomyositis, smoking
Interstitial pneumonitis	HIV mismatch, post BMT, CMV infection, sirolimus medication, smoking, ABCA-3 mutation, polymyositis, dermatomyositis
Interstitial pulmonary fibrosis	Systemic sclerosis, asbestosis, Jo-1 autoimmune disease, chronic paraquat intoxication, ammonia gas inhalation, atrial myxoma, ARDS
Shrinking lung	SLE, traction bronchiectasis, autoimmune diseases, systemic sclerosis, Sjögren's syndrome
Stiff lung	Atrial-septal defect
Usual interstitial pneumonitis (UIP)	Smoking, surfactant protein C mutation, antiphospholipid antibody syndrome, Erdheim-Chester disease, varicella pneumonia, dermatomyositis, polymyositis

*Other than radiation and chemotherapy.

RISK PROFILE

- Radiation therapy to the lung fields within the past 2 years, usually for treatment of lung cancer, breast cancer, lymphoma, cancer of the larynx, and thymoma.
- Chemotherapy, single or combination (Table 39-3).
- Chronic allograft rejection (Dosanjh, 2007)
- **Biologic response modifiers:** Interferon alpha or interferon gamma1b (Antoniou et al., 2003).
- **Medications:** Amiodarone (Cordarone), nitrofurantoin (Furadantin, Macrobid, Macrodantin) used for UTIs.

Table 39-2	CAUSES OF DIFFUSE PULMONARY FIBROSIS
Category	**Specific Causes**
Occupational dust inhalation	Asbestos, beryllium, coal, cotton, detergent, gold, grain, iron, lead, malt, maple bark, moldy hay, mushrooms, paprika, plutonium (Newman et al., 2005), silica from and/or rock, sugar cane, talc (Honda et al., 2002), zinc
Noxious gas inhalation	Chlorine, metals, nitrogen oxide, sulfur
Drug sensitivities	Amiodarone (Cordarone), busulfan (Myleran), interferon alpha or gamma 1b, nitrofurantoin (Furadantin, Macrobid, Macrodantin), phenytoin (Dilantin)
Radiation therapy to lung fields	Radiation for treatment of cancers (breast, head and neck, lung, Hodgkin's lymphoma)
Pneumonia or infection	Bird breeder's lung, chronic bacterial pneumonia, hepatitis C infection (Aisa et al., 2001), viral pneumonia
Diseases	AIDS, amyloidosis, ARDS, arthritis, bagassosis, diabetes mellitus (Zisman et al., 2005), diffuse alveolar hemorrhage syndrome, eosinophilic granuloma, familial pulmonary fibrosis (FPF), GERD (Zisman et al., 2005), Hermansky Pudlak syndrome, polymyositis (Aisa et al., 2001), sarcoidosis, scleroderma, Sjögren's syndrome, systemic lupus erythematosus, systemic sclerosis (Leandro & Isenberg, 2001), tuberculosis
Smoking, heavy	Cigarettes (Zisman et al., 2005), marijuana
Poisoning	Herbicide (paraquat) (Hong et al., 2005), orthophenylphenol (OPP) used in fungicides and antibacterial agents (Cheng et al., 2005)

- High-dose chemotherapy and/or radiation therapy, especially in patients who have undergone bone marrow transplantation (BMT).
- *Lifestyle*: Smoking (Grubstein et al, 2005; Zisman et al., 2005), marijuana (Phan et al, 2005), inhalation of dusts or gases, drug sensitivities, poisoning, and diseases or conditions that cause fibrosis (see Table 39-1).

Table 39-3	CHEMOTHERAPEUTIC AGENTS ASSOCIATED WITH PULMONARY FIBROSIS
Generic Name	**Trade Name**
Bleomycin	Blenoxane
Busulfan	Myleran
Carmustine	BCNU
Cetuximab	Erbitux
Cyclophosphamide	Cytoxan
Dactinomycin	Actinomycin D, Cosmegen
Docetaxel	Taxotere
Doxorubicin	Adriamycin
Gefitinib	Iressa
Gemcitabine	Gemzar
Irinotecan	Camptosar
Lomustine	CCNU
Methotrexate	Folex
Mitomycin	Mutamycin
Oxaliplatin	Eloxatin
Paclitaxel	Taxol
Vincristine	Oncovin

- Females may be at higher risk as a result of female sex hormones, as shown by laboratory research on mice (Gharaee-Kermani et al., 2005).
- Genetic factors: Individuals with the interleukin-1 receptor antagonist gene (+2018) allele 2 and tumor necrosis factor–alpha gene (−308) allele 2 (Satoh et al., 2002), transfection of the Sflt-1 gene attenuated PF (Hamada et al., 2005), and telomerase RNA component (TERC) gene mutation have an increased risk of developing PF (Marrone et al., 2007). Expression of the H2-EA gene protects against bleomycin-induced PF in mice (Du et al., 2004).
- Other risk factors include increased serum levels of sialyl Lewis X-i antigen (greater than 50 units/mL) (Satoh et al., 2002); YKL-40 growth factor (Nordenbaek et al., 2005); pulmonary and activation–regulated chemokine (PARC) (Kodera et al., 2005); and CYFRA-21 (Suzuki et al., 1996). An increased serum level of CA 19-9 reflects progression of PF (Totani et al., 2005).

PROGNOSIS

The 5-year survival rate is 90% if the patient is young and has minimal fibrosis; it is 25% if the patient is older and has severe fibrosis. The mortality rate is estimated to be 1% to 2%.

PROFESSIONAL ASSESSMENT CRITERIA (PAC)

1. **Classic symptoms:** Dyspnea on exertion (DOE) and/or nonproductive cough (Chernecky & Sarna, 2000). Typical symptoms of drug-induced fibrosis: Dyspnea, nonproductive cough, and tachycardia.
2. History of chemotherapy (see Table 39-3), interferon alpha or interferon gamma1b, radiation therapy to the lungs, and/or BMT.
3. **History of comorbidities:** Smoking, inhalation of dusts or gases, drug sensitivities, poisoning, pneumonia, collagen disease.
4. Finger clubbing
5. Decreased breath sounds or crackles during auscultation of the lungs.
6. Decreased chest expansion during expiration on excursion assessment.
7. Hypoxemia (PaO_2 less than 92%).
8. Hypotension
9. Tachypnea
10. **Chest x-ray film (*CXR*):** Diffuse infiltrates (Fig. 39.1), haziness around the hilar region, honeycomb or mottled lung appearance, elevation of hemidiaphragm, or pneumothorax. With pulmonary hypertension: Enlarged pulmonary artery and right atrium and ventricle.
11. **Pulmonary function tests:** Decreased total lung capacity (TLC), diffusion capacity (DLCO), forced vital capacity (FVC) and residual volume (RV).
12. Tachycardia and prominent S2.
13. Anxiety, restlessness.
14. **Labs:** Total WBC count may be elevated; pH indicates acidosis (Chernecky & Berger, 2004).
15. **Electrocardiogram (*ECG*):** May show PVC, V-tach, or V-flutter.
16. **Hemodynamic monitoring:** Increased pulmonary hypertension. Increased PA pressures with variable pulmonary artery occlusion pressure (PAOP); or, PAWP/PAOP may be normal but pulmonary end diastolic pressure (PAD) is increased.

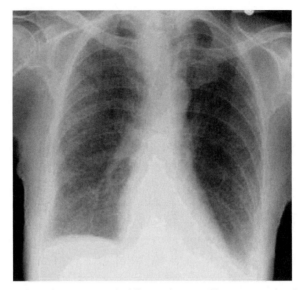

Fig. 39.1 • Chest x-ray film of a patient with diffuse pulmonary fibrosis. Note the shadows at the lung base and the diffuse ground-glass appearance.

17. **MRI:** Low signal intensity and low contrast enhancement compared to alveolitis. CT scan of the chest (Fig. 39.2): Ground-glass opacity, decreased lung volume, pleural thickening, honeycomb or mottled lung fields, pneumothorax, pneumomediastinum.

18. **Lung biopsy:** Fibrosis, positive stain for TGF-1 or TGF-B1 or increased osteonectin expression (Siddiq et al., 2004); broncholavage shows increased hyaluronan.

19. **Lung perfusion scan, FDG-PET scan or 3-D SPECT scan:** Underperfusion and/or poor alveolar subunit function.

20. **Cardiac catheterization:** High pulmonary vascular resistance.

21. **Cor pulmonale and heart failure:** ECG (Chernecky et al., 2006) and CVP changes, cough, peripheral edema, jugular vein distension (JVD), nausea, anorexia, polyuria at night, weight gain, acidosis, hepatomegaly, ascites, positive hepatojugular (HJ) reflex.

NURSING CARE AND TREATMENT

1. Hold chemotherapy, radiation therapy, and interferon alpha.
2. Elevate the head of the bed to high Fowler's position.
3. **Vital signs:** Assess for hypotension, tachycardia, tachypnea, chest pain, or fever (for pulmonary infection).
4. Obtain O_2 saturation reading (signs of hypoxia include restlessness, dyspnea, anxiety, and cyanosis), PFTs (decreased DLCO), ABGs (acidosis, hypercapnia, hypoxia).
5. Administer oxygen to treat hypoxia and high-dose corticosteroids (over 100 mg/day or 1 mg/kg) for inflammation.
6. Maintain venous access with an 18 or 20-gauge peripheral IV (in adults) or a venous access device (VAD).
7. Measure dyspnea on a 0 to 10 scale, with 0 being no dyspnea and 10 being severe dyspnea. Note whether dyspnea occurs at rest or with exertion.

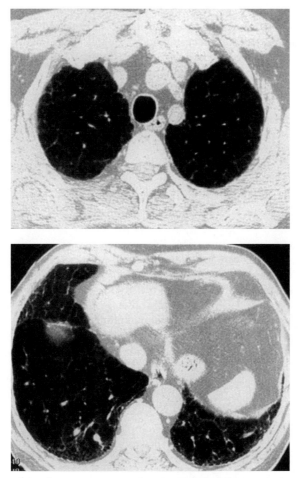

Fig. 39.2 • CT scans of the chest in a patient with pulmonary fibrosis. Note the honeycomb appearance.

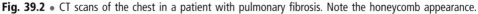

8. Assess for nonproductive cough.
9. Auscultate the lung fields for crackles and adventitious breath sounds; also assess for decreased chest expansion.
10. Obtain and assess laboratory test and biopsy results: WBC total, electrolytes, lung biopsy.
11. Obtain and assess chest x-ray film, CT/MRI of the chest for infiltrates, pleural thickening, pneumothorax, mottled or honey comb appearance.
12. **Assess for right-side heart failure/cor pulmonale:** Dependent peripheral edema, fatigue, nausea, anorexia, weight gain, hepatomegaly, JVD, systolic or diastolic murmur, prominent S2, polyuria at night, ascites.
13. Intake and output (I&O) q2-8hr.
14. Weigh patient daily and compare result to previous days; retention of 450 mL of fluid equals 1 pound of weight gain.
15. **Hemodynamic monitoring** (Hodges et al., 2005): Note that pulmonary hypertension can predispose a person to PA rupture when a PA catheter is placed for hemodynamic

monitoring. Pulmonary hypertension causes increased PA pressures with variable PAOP, or PAWP/PAOP may be normal but PAD is increased.

16. Administer calcium channel blockers (e.g., verapamil HCl [Calan] or diltiazem [Dilacor XR]), and a vasodilator (e.g., isosorbide dinitrate [Isordil]) to treat pulmonary hypertension.

17. Administer ACE inhibitors of Ngiotensin II receptor blockers to protect the lungs form radiationinduced fibrosis (Molteni et al., 2007).

18. Anticipate administration of digitalis for cardiac dysfunction; furosemide or hydro-chlorothiazide (HCTZ) for diuresis; and antibiotics (e.g., azithromycin [Zithromax] or levofloxacin [Levaquin]) for infection.

19. Administer by inhalation: Nitric oxide 10-20 ppm plus oral sildenafil (Viagra) 50 mg daily (which enhances the effect of nitric oxide) to reduce pulmonary vascular resistance (Ghofrani et al., 2002).

20. Administer decongestant and cough suppressant or narcotic antitussive (e.g., guaifenesin [Hytuss, Tussin]) or hydroiodone bitartrate-homatropine methylbromide (Hycodan).

21. Administer low-dose morphine sulfate for anxiety and dyspnea.

22. Use relaxation techniques (e.g., guided imagery, music therapy) to reduce anxiety.

23. Anticipate administration of ginkgo biloba extract 1 g three times per day for 3 months, because this may be useful in reducing the occurrence of PF (He et al., 2005).

24. Anticipate anticoagulant therapy in addition to prednisolone, because this increases survival in patients with idiopathic PF (Kubo et al., 2005).

25. **Diet:** Small, frequent high-calorie meals; fluid and sodium restriction for cor pulmonale.

26. **Activity:** Bed rest with bathroom privileges as tolerated.

27. Assess spirituality of patient and support patient in meeting spiritual needs (Albaugh, 2003).

28. Referral to clinical nurse specialist, dietician, home health nurse, hospice, social worker, and/or respiratory therapist as appropriate.

EVIDENCE-BASED PRACTICE UPDATES

1. Patients who have a proteinase activated–receptor 1 (PAR-1) deficiency have increased pulmonary fibrosis after bleomycin chemotherapy (Howell et al., 2005).

2. Administration of platelet-derived growth factor (PDGF) receptor tyrosine kinase inhibitors (RTKIs) reduces pulmonary fibrosis in patients receiving radiation therapy to the lungs (Abdollahi et al., 2005; Tada et al., 2003). The administration of monoclonal anti-CD40L antibody (MR1) (Adawi et al., 1998), Houttuynia cordata extract (Ng et al., 2007), Hu-qi-yin (Zhou et al., 2007) and alpha-lipoic acid (Liu et al., 2007) protects against bleomycin induced PF in mice.

3. For patients with IPF, single lung transplantation is superior to bilateral lung transplantation (Meyer et al., 2005), and low-concentration inhaled carbon monoxide (CO) suppresses bleomycin-induced lung fibrosis in mice (Zhou et al., 2005).

4. Overexpression of platelet-derived growth factor receptors (PDGFRs) causes radiation-induced PF in rats (Tada et al., 2003).

5. Administration of follistatin in bleomycin-treated rats attenuated lung fibrosis (Aoki et al., 2005), as do mesna (El-Medany et al., 2005); imatinib (Aono et al., 2005); CXCL11, an angiostatic chemokine (Burdick et al., 2005); and the Chinese herb combination known as Feitai (Gong et al., 2005).

6. Chrondroitin sulfate proteoglycans digestive enzyme, chondroitinase ABC (ChABC) alleviates bleomycin induced pulmonary fibrosis (Kai et al., 2007).

TEACHING AND EDUCATION

Discontinuation of chemotherapy, radiation therapy, and interferon alpha: *Rationale*: These types of therapies can cause further lung inflammation and make it harder for you to breathe.

Dyspnea: *Rationale*: Oxygen may be necessary to make you less short of breath and to help your heart pump more easily. You should keep your activity level to a minimum.

Anxiety: *Rationale*: When you are short of breath, you sometimes feel anxious and restless, which puts you in a cycle of more anxiety and more shortness of breath. To break this cycle, try using guided imagery, watching TV, listening to music, or taking medication, if necessary.

Nutrition: *Rationale*: Eat small, high-calorie meals. You may have to restrict liquids and salt.

Tests and procedures: *Rationale*: You may need x-rays or scans of your chest made by a special machine. Also, a tube may need to be placed in your artery, similar to an IV being placed in your vein, although this tube is longer. The tube is attached to a machine that helps us make sure your heart and lungs are working well.

New or increased symptoms: *Rationale*: High pressure can develop in your lungs and heart. It is important to tell your nurse or physician if you are more short of breath, have swelling in your ankles, feet, or hands, feel faint, have chest pain, or feel as if your heart is beating unevenly.

Prevention of infections in the lungs: Be sure to get influenza and pneumococcal vaccines, avoid people with coughs, colds, or the flu, and wash your hands often (especially after touching someone or a commonly used item, such as a door handle, and after toileting). Call the nurse or physician immediately if you have a fever over 100.5° F (38° C) or if you are coughing up red, yellow, green, or brown phlegm.

Pulmonary rehabilitation: Your health care practitioner may prescribe pulmonary rehabilitation for you. This type of program can benefit people with PF, because it includes exercise and air circulation and oxygen therapies.

Web sites for information:
- American Lung Association: www.lungusa.org (telephone: 1-800-LUNGSUSA)
- Mayo Clinic: www.mayoclinic.com
- American Cancer Society: www.cancer.org
- Cleveland Clinic Foundation: www.chemocare.com
- American Thoracic Society: www.ajrccm.atsjournals.org/cgi/content/full/161/2/646

NURSING DIAGNOSES

1. **Ineffective tissue perfusion** related to lung fibrosis, hypoxia, and/or anxiety
2. **Decreased cardiac output** related to increased pulmonary vascular resistance
3. **Activity intolerance** related to dyspnea, fever, and/or anxiety
4. **Risk for infection** related to immunosuppressive therapy (chemo, radiation, interferon, steroids), fever and/or pulmonary edema resulting from loss of lung elasticity

5. **Imbalanced nutrition: less than body requirements** related to fatigue, fever, dyspnea, hypoxia, cor pulmonale, and/or chest pain

EVALUATION AND DESIRED OUTCOMES

1. The patient will rate dyspnea, cough, fatigue, and anxiety each as less than 3 on a 0 to 10 scale (assess for improvement and medicate accordingly).
2. O_2 saturation will be greater than 92%.
3. The patient will have no adventitious lung sounds or congestion, pneumonia, productive cough, peripheral edema, or jugular vein distention.
4. WBCs, electrolytes, ECG, hemodynamic monitoring values, and diagnostic tests of CXR/ CT/MRI will be within normal limits.
5. The patient will have no nausea or anorexia. The patient will not gain more than 1 pound/week, or his or her weight will remain stable.

DISCHARGE PLANNING AND FOLLOW-UP CARE

- Home oxygen via tube or mask as prescribed.
- Caregiver to assist with meal preparation, ADLs, and household maintenance (laundry, shopping, housework).
- Home health nursing visits for assessment of pulmonary and cardiac status, medication evaluation, and antianxiety interventions for 1 to 2 months.
- Follow-up visit to physician's office 1 to 2 weeks after discharge. Discuss pulmonary rehabilitation program as an option.
- Follow-up chest x-ray film, PFTs, and/or ABGs every 2 to 3 months.
- Call the health care provider immediately for the following: fever higher than 100.5° F (38° C), coughing up blood or blood-tinged mucus, unusual swelling of the hands or feet, weight gain of more than 3 pounds in 1 week, heart palpitations, chest discomfort, increased shortness of breath, or skin rash.

REVIEW QUESTIONS

QUESTIONS

1. **An early symptom of pulmonary fibrosis is:**
   1. Vomiting
   2. Confusion
   3. Dyspnea
   4. Seizures

2. **Excessive connective tissue in the lungs associated with pulmonary fibrosis is caused by:**
   1. Hyperoxygenation
   2. Inflammatory response
   3. Heart failure
   4. Gastrointestinal bleeding

3. **Mrs. Enron had lung cancer 8 months ago and was treated with chemotherapy and radiation therapy** to the lungs. On her clinic visit, she complains of nausea and polyuria at night. Upon taking her vital signs, you note a prominent S2. Which condition might these symptoms indicate:
   1. Kidney failure
   2. Liver failure
   3. Pancreatitis
   4. Cor pulmonale

4. **Your patient, who has pulmonary fibrosis, complains of shortness of breath. The most immediate nursing intervention you can provide to help relieve this complaint is:**
   1. Administer oxygen at 5 L by mask.
   2. Raise the head of the bed to high Fowler's position.

3. Place the bed in Trendelenburg position.
4. Administer haloperidol (Haldol) 5 mg orally now.

5. **Which of the following results from a pulmonary function test (PFT) would indicate pulmonary fibrosis:**
    1. Decreased total lung capacity (TLC)
    2. Increased diffusion capacity (DLCO)
    3. Increased forced vital capacity (FVC)
    4. Hyponatremia

6. **You are assessing the chest x-ray film of a person you believe may have pulmonary fibrosis. Which description of the chest x-ray film would indicate PF:**
    1. Bite wing appearance
    2. Glasslike appearance
    3. Mottled appearance
    4. Granulomatous appearance

7. **Your patient has been placed on corticosteroids as part of his treatment for pulmonary fibrosis. The main area of teaching in which you need to instruct your patient is:**
    1. Infection
    2. Hypoglycemia
    3. Peripheral neuropathy
    4. Diarrhea

8. **Mr. Johanson is a 56-year-old male who is receiving doxorubicin and cyclophosphamide as part of his chemotherapy regimen for lung cancer. He has been a farmer all his life. He does all the work himself, including feeding the horses hay and cleaning their stables, welding his farm equipment when it breaks, preparing the soil with manure, and dusting his crops with herbicides. He loves to fish and take walks when he has some time to do so. His wife is very supportive, although she wishes her husband would stop smoking cigarettes, which he has done since he was 15 years old. From this information, which factors place Mr. Johanson at risk for pulmonary fibrosis:**
    1. Chemotherapy, history of working with hay, and welding
    2. Fishing, smoking, and being married

3. Crop dusting, walking, and shoveling manure
4. Smoking, eating fish, and being outdoors receiving ultraviolet radiation

9. **Mrs. Wolinski, who has a history of lung cancer, is in the physician's office waiting room. She has come for her 2-month postlobectomy office visit. After being shown to the examination room, she complains of dyspnea. You notice that she now appears anxious. Your immediate nursing assessment should be to:**
    1. Take her temperature
    2. Measure her blood pressure
    3. Obtain a pulse oximetry reading
    4. Perform a finger stick for determination of her glucose level

10. **You are the home health nurse visiting Mrs. Wallace, who has been diagnosed with cor pulmonale. She states that she cannot cook because of her dyspnea, and she wants to know whether her prepackaged frozen dinners or canned food from the grocery store are okay to eat. Your best response is:**
    1. "I don't see why not; food is food. You eat whatever you want."
    2. "As long as you do not eat foods too high in potassium, you should be fine."
    3. "As long as they contain protein and carbohydrates and some fiber you should be okay, so go ahead and eat them."
    4. "With your condition, it's important not to drink too many liquids and not to take in a lot of sodium. Frozen and canned foods are not a good choice because they contain large amounts of sodium."

ANSWERS

1. *Answer: 3*
   Rationale: Dyspnea, particularly on exertion, and nonproductive cough are early symptoms of pulmonary fibrosis.

2. *Answer: 2*
Rationale: Excessive connective tissue is caused by an inflammatory response with an increase in fibroblasts, myofibroblasts, and inflammatory cells.

3. *Answer: 4*
Rationale: The symptoms of cor pulmonale include fatigue, nausea, vomiting, prominent S2, peripheral edema, hepatomegaly, JVD, and ascites. These may occur months to years after treatment with chemotherapy and/or radiation to the lungs.

4. *Answer: 2*
Rationale: High Fowler's position increases the breathing capacity of the lungs.

5. *Answer: 1*
Rationale: PF, or stiff lungs, is associated with a decrease in PFT values, including TLC, DLCO, FVC, and RV.

6. *Answer: 3*
Rationale: A mottled or honeycomb appearance is a classic description of a CXR showing pulmonary fibrosis.

7. *Answer: 1*
Rationale: Steroids can suppress the immune system, putting the patient at risk for infection.

8. *Answer: 1*
Rationale: Chemotherapy, moldy hay, and metal dust can contribute to pulmonary fibrosis, as can smoking and using the herbicide paraquat.

9. *Answer: 3*
Rationale: Dyspnea and anxiety are signs of hypoxia.

10. *Answer: 4*
Rationale: Cor pulmonale is failure of the right ventricle. To reduce stress on cardiac output, the patient should limit her fluid intake, and to prevent edema, she should restrict her salt intake.

REFERENCES

Abdollahi, A., Li, M., & Ping, G., et al. (2005). Inhibition of platelet-derived growth factor signaling attenuates pulmonary fibrosis. *Journal of Experimental Medicine, 201*(6):925-935.

Adawi, A., Zhang, Y., & Baggs, R., et al. (1998). Blockade of CD40-CD40 ligand interactions protects against radiation-induced pulmonary inflammation and fibrosis. *Clinical Immunology and Immunopathology, 89*(3):222-230.

Aisa, Y., Yokomori, H., & Kashiwagi, K., et al. (2001). Polymyositis, pulmonary fibrosis and malignant lymphoma associated with hepatitis C virus infection. *Internal Medicine, 40*(11):1109-1112.

Albaugh, J. A. (2003). Spirituality and life-threatening illness: A phenomenologic study. *Oncology Nursing Forum, 30*(4):593-598.

Antoniou, K. M., Ferdoutsis, E., & Bouros, D. (2003). Interferons and their application in the diseases of the lung. *Chest, 123*(1):209-216.

Aoki, F., Kurabayashi, M., & Hasegawa, Y., et al. (2005). Attenuation of bleomycin-induced pulmonary fibrosis by follistatin. *American Journal of Respiratory and Critical Care Medicine, 172*(6):713-720.

Aono, Y., Nishioka, Y., & Inayama, M., et al. (2005). Imatinib as a novel antifibrotic agent in bleomycin-induced pulmonary fibrosis in mice. *American Journal of Respiratory and Critical Care Medicine, 171*(11):1279-1285.

Burdick, M. D., Murray, L. A., & Keane, M. P., et al. (2005). CXCL11 attenuates bleomycin-induced pulmonary fibrosis via inhibition of vascular remodeling. *American Journal of Respiratory and Critical Care Medicine, 171*(3):261-268.

Cheng, S. L., Wang, H. C., & Yang, P. C. (2005). Acute respiratory distress syndrome and lung fibrosis after ingestion of a high dose of ortho-phenylphenol. *Journal of the Formosan Medical Association, 104*(8):585-587.

Chernecky, C., & Berger, B (2004). *Laboratory tests and diagnostic procedures.* Philadelphia: W. B. Saunders.

Chernecky, C., Garrett, K., & Hodges, B., et al. (2006). *ECGs and the heart.* (2nd ed.). St. Louis: Mosby.

Chernecky, C., & Sarna, L. (2000). Pulmonary toxicities of cancer therapy. *Critical Care Nursing Clinics of North America, 12*(3):281-295.

Chisam, M., & Douglas, R. (2002). Radiation pneumonitis. Retrieved May 26, 2007, pp. 1-7. www.emedicine.com/radio/topic590.

Dosanjh, A. (2007). Pirfenidone: a novel potential therapeutic agent in the management of chronic allograft rejection. *Transplantation Proceedings* 39(7):2153-2156.

Du, M., Irani, R. A., & Stivers, D. N., et al. (2004). H2-Ea deficiency is a risk factor for bleomycin-induced lung fibrosis in mice. *Cancer Research, 64*(19):6835-6839.

El-Medany, A., Hagar, H. H., & Moursi, M., et al. (2005). Attenuation of bleomycin-induced lung fibrosis in rats by mesna. *European Journal of Pharmacology, 509*(1):61-70.

Gharaee-Kermani, M., Hatano, K., & Nozaki, Y., et al. (2005). Gender-based differences in bleomycin-induced pulmonary fibrosis. *American Journal of Pathology, 166*(6):1593-1606.

Ghofrani, H. A., Wiedemann, R., & Rose, F., et al. (2002). Sildenafil for treatment of lung fibrosis and pulmonary hypertension: A randomized controlled trial. *Lancet, 360*(9337):895-900.

Gong, L. K., Li, X. H., & Wang, H., et al. (2005). Effect of Feitai on bleomycin-induced pulmonary fibrosis in rats. *Journal of Ethnopharmacology, 96*(3):537-544.

Grubstein, A., Bendayan, D., & Schactman, I, et al. (2005). Concomitant upper-lobe bullous emphysema, lower-lobe interstitial fibrosis and pulmonary hypertension in heavy smokers: Report of eight cases and review of the literature. *Respiratory Medicine, 99*(8):948-954.

Hamada, N., Kuwano, K., & Yamada, M., et al. (2005). Anti-vascular endothelial growth factor gene therapy attenuates lung injury and fibrosis in mice. *Journal of Immunology, 175*(2):1224-1231.

He, M., Zhang, X. M., & Yuan, H. Q. (2005). Clinical study of treatment of pulmonary interstitial fibrosis with ginkgo extract (Chinese). *Journal of Integrated Traditional and Western Medicine 25*(3):222-224.

Hodges, B., Garrett, K., & Chernecky, C., et al. (2005). *Hemodynamic monitoring*. St. Louis: Mosby.

Honda, Y., Beall, C., & Delzell, E., et al. (2002). Mortality among workers at a talc mining and milling facility. *Annals of Occupational Hygiene, 46*(7):575-585.

Hong, S. Y., Gil, H. W., & Yang, J. O., et al. (2005). Clinical implications of the ethane in exhaled breath of patients with acute paraquat intoxication. *Chest, 128*(3):1506-1510.

Howell, D. C., Johns, R. H., & Lasky, J. A., et al. (2005). Absence of proteinase-activated receptor-1 signaling affords protection from bleomycin-induced lung inflammation and fibrosis. *American Journal of Pathology, 166*(5):1353-1365.

Kai, Y., Yoneyama, H., & Koyama, J., et al. (2007). Treatment with chondroitinase ABC alleviates bleomycin-induced pulmonary fibrosis. *Medical Molecular Morphology 40*(3):128-140.

Kodera, M., Hasegawa, M., & Komura, K., et al. (2005). Serum pulmonary and activation-regulated chemokine/CCL18 levels in patients with systemic sclerosis: A sensitive indicator of active pulmonary fibrosis. *Arthritis and Rheumatism, 52*(9):2889-2896.

Kubo, H., Nakayama, K., & Yanai, M., et al. (2005). Anticoagulant therapy for idiopathic pulmonary fibrosis. *Chest, 128*(3):1475-1482.

Leandro, M. J., & Isenberg, D. A. (2001). Rheumatic diseases and malignancy: Is there an association? *Scandinavian Journal of Rheumatology, 30*(4):185-188.

Liu, R., Ahmed, K. M., & Nantajit, D., et al. (2007). Therapeutic effects of alpha-lipoic acid on bleomycin-induced pulmonary fibrosis in rats. *International Journal of Molecular Medicine 19*(6):8658-8673.

Marrone, A., Sokhal, P., & Walne, A., et al. (2007). Functional characterization of novel telomerase RNA (TERC) mutations in patients with diverse clinical and pathological presentations. *Haematologica,, 92*(8):1013-1020.

Meyer, D. M., Edwards, L. B., & Torres, F., et al. (2005). Impact of recipient age and procedure type on survival after lung transplantation for pulmonary fibrosis. *Annals of Thoracic Surgery 79*(3):950-957; discussion 957–958.

Molteni, A., Wolfe, L. F., & Ward, W. F., et al. (2007). Effect of an angiotensin II receptor blocker and two angiotensin converting enzyme inhibitors on transforming growth factor-beta (TGF-beta) and alpha-actomyosin (alpha SMA), important mediators of radiation-induced pneumopathy and lung fibrosis. *Current Pharmaceutical Design 13*(13):1307-1316.

Moore, B. B., Ballinger, M. N., & White, E. S., et al. (2005). Bleomycin-induced E prostanoid receptor changes alter fibroblast responses to prostaglandin E2. *Journal of Immunology, 174*(9):5644-5649.

Newman, L. S., Mroz, M. M., & Ruttenber, A. J. (2005). Lung fibrosis in plutonium workers. *Radiation Research, 164*(2):123-131.

Ng, L. T., Yen, F. L., Liao, C. W., & Lin, C. C. (2007). Protective effect of Houttuynia cordata extract on bleomycin-induced pulmonary fibrosis in rats. *American Journal of Chinese Medicine 35*(3):465-475.

Nordenbaek, C., Johansen, J. S., & Halberg, P., et al. (2005). High serum levels of YKL-40 in patients with systemic sclerosis are associated with pulmonary involvement. *Scandinavian Journal of Rheumatology, 34*(4):293-297.

Phan, T. D., Lau, K. K., & Li, X. (2005). Lung bullae and pulmonary fibrosis associated with marijuana smoking. *Australasian Radiology, 49*(5):411-414.

Satoh, H., Ishikawa, H., & Yamashita, Y. T., et al. (2002). Serum sialyl Lewis X-I antigen in lung adenocarcinoma and idiopathic pulmonary fibrosis. *Thorax, 57*(3):263-266.

Siddiq, F., Sarkar, F. H., & Wali, A., et al. (2004). Increased osteonectin expression is associated with malignant transformation and tumor associated fibrosis in the lung. *Lung Cancer, 45*(2):197-205.

Suzuki, A., Masuda, T., & Koito, N., et al. (1996). Studies of serum markers inpatients with interstitial pneumonia/pulmonary fibrosis complicated with collagen diseases: Clinical evaluation of CYFRA21-1 (Japanese). *Ryumachi, 36*(6):837-843.

Tada, H., Ogushi, F., & Tani, K., et al. (2003). Increased binding and chemotactic capacities of PDGF-BB on fibroblasts in radiation pneumonitis. *Radiation Research, 159*(6):805-811.

Totani, Y., Saito, Y., & Miyachi, H., et al. (2005). Clinical characterization of CA19-9 in patients with interstitial pneumonia showing pathological nonspecific interstitial pneumonia pattern (Japanese). *Nihon Kokyuki Gakkai Zasshi, 43*(2):77-83.

Zhou, X. M., Zhang, G. C., Li, J. X., & Hou, J. (2007). Inhibitory effects of Hu-qi-yin on the bleomycin-induced pulmonary fibrosis in rats. *Journal of Ethnopharmacology 111*(2):252-264.

Zhou, Z., Song, R., & Fattman, C. L., et al. (2005). Carbon monoxide suppresses bleomycin-induced lung fibrosis. *American Journal of Pathology, 166*(1):27-37.

Zisman, D. A., Keane, M. P., & Belperio, J. A., et al. (2005). Pulmonary fibrosis. *Methods in Molecular Medicine, 117:3-44.*

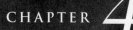

SEIZURES

MARY P. LOVELY

PATHOPHYSIOLOGICAL MECHANISMS

The brain controls how the body moves by sending electrical signals. Seizures occur when the normal signals from the brain are changed. These signals are caused by hyperactivity of an action potential, an impulse that moves from one cell to the next and passes along information. In the normal physiology of an action potential, thousands of cells that emit excitatory transmitters (acetylcholine and glutamate) and inhibitory transmitters (gaba aminobutyric acid [GABA]) converge on one cell. Excitatory neurotransmitters cause sodium to rush into a cell, and inhibitory neurotransmitters cause chloride to enter. Summation of the conversion of the excitatory and inhibitory neurons then takes place. If the excitatory neurons prevail, sodium enters the cell and potassium leaves the cell, resulting in an action potential. In this way, a signal is sent down the axon to the next cell (Armstrong et al., 2003).

A seizure occurs as a result of an imbalance characterized by more excitatory or less inhibitory activation in the central nervous system. Calcium causes an increase in excitatory neurotransmitter release, resulting in sodium entering the cell and potassium leaving. A long plateau of depolarization follows, causing numerous action potentials, then a period of hyperpolarization occurs as a result of GABA and chloride entering the cell. The hyperpolarization is soon replaced by depolarization, which increases in amplitude (Schaller & Ruegg, 2003). The cell then begins to fire repeatedly and produces sustained membrane depolarization, causing seizure activity.

Seizures usually start in one area of the brain, where the imbalance of cell activation occurs; this area is called the *epileptogenic focus*. If sufficient activation occurs to recruit surrounding neurons, the seizure propagates and activates other parts of the brain (Hickey, 2003). This results in a generalized seizure.

The preictal phase is the interval before the actual seizure. The patient is alert and oriented, without altered consciousness. The ictal phase is the initiation of seizure activity. The patient may experience activity consistent with the area of cerebral involvement. For example, if a tumor is located in the right frontal motor area of the brain, the patient will have arm or leg jerking on the left side. The postictal phase is the period after the seizure, during which the patient may be tired, confused, or disoriented (Fisher et. al., 2004).

Epilepsy is a condition marked by recurrent, unprovoked seizures caused by biochemical, anatomic, and physiologic changes (Jacobs & Shafer, 2000). Management of this condition usually requires daily medication to prevent seizures.

Many types of seizures have been described (Table 40-1) (Krouwer et al., 2000). The seizures commonly seen in patients with cancer or primary brain tumors are simple focal, complex partial, and generalized tonic-clonic seizures (Keles & Berger, 2000).

A simple focal seizure is *localized*, or generated from a specific part of the brain. It may involve a sensory function such as a funny smell, a strange feeling, visual changes,

Table 40-1	TYPES OF SEIZURES	
Seizure Type	**Description**	**Variations**
Simple partial seizure	Consciousness not impaired; usually unilateral hemispheric involvement	With motor symptoms With somatosensory symptoms With autonomic symptoms With psychic symptoms
Complex partial seizure	Impairment of consciousness; frequently bilateral hemispheric involvement	Begins as simple partial seizure and progresses to impairment of consciousness With no other features With features as in simple partial seizures With automatisms (aberration of behavior, such as lip smacking, fidgeting with the hands) With impairment of consciousness at onset Partial seizures secondarily generalized
Generalized seizure (convulsive or nonconvulsive)	Consciousness always impaired, frequently as first manifestation Bilateral motor manifestations	Absence seizures Myoclonic seizures Clonic seizures Tonic seizures

a sensation in the stomach, or a feeling of impending doom. A motor seizure may produce hand, leg, or mouth twitching. The patient does not lose consciousness. It may happen rarely or several times a day. A focal seizure can progress to the whole side of the body and become a generalized tonic-clonic seizure (Lovely, 2004).

A complex partial seizure occurs when the epileptic focus is in the temporal or frontal temporal lobe. The patient may have an initial feeling (aura or preictal phase) of an upset stomach or a funny smell. Consciousness is not lost, but the patient may lose track of the environment. Although the person may seem to be acting purposefully, he or she may have no control of behavior. For example, repetitive actions, known as *automatisms*, may happen, such as buttoning and unbuttoning a shirt, lip smacking, or hand wringing. These seizures may continue for only minutes or may last for days.

A generalized tonic-clonic seizure, informally known as a *grand mal seizure*, occurs if the chemical imbalance spreads into both sides of the brain. A patient may have an initial feeling that a seizure is imminent, such as a sensation or a focal seizure. Subsequently, a patient shows excessive movement of the arms and legs (tonic-clonic movements) with possible bowel and bladder incontinence (ictal phase). This type of seizure usually lasts about 1 to 2 minutes. After the seizure, during the postictal phase, the patient is quite tired and may want to sleep for hours.

Status epilepticus is a generalized tonic-clonic seizure that lasts longer than 5 minutes, or the occurrence of two or more seizures in succession without recovery. In rare cases, patients can experience continuous seizures, most often in the hospital setting. Detection requires electroencephalographic testing. Status epilepticus is a medical emergency (Victor et al., 2001). Left untreated, it may cause massive activation of the "stress" response of the sympathetic nervous system, resulting in elevated blood pressure and serum glucose. During prolonged seizures, the homeostatic mechanisms fail, and profound abnormalities result, including hypoxia, hypoglycemia, hypotension, and acidemia, with the potential to cause cortical nerve damage (Armstrong et al., 2003).

The nurse's role in seizure disorders includes managing seizures when they occur, administering the appropriate medication to prevent further seizures, and providing the patient and family with education and counseling to help them work toward self-esteem and a good quality of life. Medical research has focused on a new generation of antiepileptic medications that stops seizures with fewer side effects. Nursing research has opened the doors to an understanding of how individuals can live with seizures and the stigma of epilepsy.

EPIDEMIOLOGY AND ETIOLOGY

In patients with cancer, seizures may be caused by a structural lesion in the brain (e.g., direct tumor involvement), vascular events, or central nervous system infections.

Seizures are known to originate from the disrupted normal tissue around the tumor rather than from the tumor itself. They also may be a result of treatment of a tumor (e.g., surgery, chemotherapy). Cranial radiation rarely causes seizures. However, focal radiation necrosis (i.e., dead tissue due to the radiation) can behave like an expanding intracerebral mass and cause seizures (Bromfield, 2004).

Seizures also may be caused by cerebrovascular disorders, such as hemorrhage or thrombosis. In addition, some medications may cause seizures, including certain chemotherapeutic drugs, antiemetics (phenothiazines), and allergy and cold products that contain diphenhydramine, which is thought to make patients with underlying neurologic damage more prone to having seizures. Metabolic abnormalities, such as hepatic failure, electrolyte abnormalities, hypoxia, and hyperglycemia, also are a cause of seizures (Armstrong et al., 2003).

RISK PROFILE

- Tumors involving the frontal, frontal parietal, and frontal temporal lobes are associated with the occurrence of seizures more often than are tumors in other parts of the brain (Liigant et al., 2001).
- Seizures are more common in patients 30 to 50 years of age (Liigant, 2001).
- Seizures are the presenting feature of intracranial tumors in 30% to 90% of patients (Keles & Berger, 2000).
- Patients with low-grade gliomas have a higher incidence of seizures than patients with higher grade gliomas (Hildebrand et al., 2005).
- Patients with metastatic brain tumors have a 35% risk of seizures, and nearly 25% occur as the first sign of neurologic dysfunction in patients with a pre-existing diagnosis of cancer (Beaumont & Whittle, 2000).
- With regard to the worst aspects of having epilepsy, stigma was rated second, after the unpredictability of the next seizure's occurrence (Fisher et al., 2000).

PROGNOSIS

Seizures induced by tumors usually are controlled with antiepileptic medication. In most cases, seizures do not cause death. Several episodes of status epilepticus may result in systemic and neurologic deterioration and a morbidity and mortality rate of 20% (Hickey, 2003). Adult onset epilepsy is associated with a poor quality of life because of mood changes and the adverse effects of antiepileptic medications. Coping measures help improve quality of life (Szalflarski et al., 2006).

PROFESSIONAL ASSESSMENT CRITERIA (PAC)

1. **Description of seizure:** Preictal, ictal, and postictal; also timing.
2. History of previous seizure disorder.
3. Description of triggering factors (e.g., hot showers, flashing lights, fatigue, drinking alcohol).
4. **History of co-morbidities:** Cerebrovascular disease, renal disease, cancer, brain tumors or metastasis.
5. **History of medications:** High-dose narcotics, meperidine, phenothiazine antiemetics, products with diphenhydramine, chemotherapy, compliance with antiepileptic medication, toxic levels of antiepileptics.
6. **Neurologic examination:** Executive thinking, memory, movement, sensation, balance, and coordination.
7. **Neuroimaging:** CT scan or MRI with and without contrast may show structural changes related to the cause of the seizures.
8. **Labs:** Hepatic and renal dysfunction, electrolyte imbalance (hyponatremia, hypomagnesemia, hypocalcemia or hypercalcemia, hyperglycemia, hyperphosphatemia).
9. **Electroencephalogram:** To localize a seizure focus or determine whether seizure activity is ongoing.

NURSING CARE AND TREATMENT

1. Simple focal seizure:
   - Time and observe the seizure activity.
   - Document the date, time, and description.
   - Note whether movement or sensation extended to another part of the body.
2. Complex partial seizure:
   - Observe the behavior and protect the patient from harm.
   - Keep a calm manner to lessen the patient's agitation and the family's anxiety.
   - Do not restrain the patient; instead, guide the movements to prevent harm.
   - Stay with the patient until consciousness is fully regained.
   - Gently reassure and reorient the patient.
   - Document the date and time of the seizure and the activities before, during, and after it.
3. Tonic-clonic generalized seizure (Fig. 40.1):
   - Assess the patient's level of consciousness.
   - Protect the patient from self-harm during the ictal phase.
   - Place a pillow, towel, or something soft under the patient's head.
   - Provide privacy.
   - Remove eyeglasses and loosen constraining clothing.
   - Do not force anything into the patient's mouth.
   - Time the seizure and observe actions and behaviors.
   - After the seizure, observe the patient's level of consciousness.
   - Turn the patient onto his or her side; do not give liquids because of the high risk of choking.
   - Allow the patient to sleep, then reorient the patient upon awakening.
   - The patient may bite his or her tongue; if this happens, examine the mouth to prevent the patient from swallowing blood.

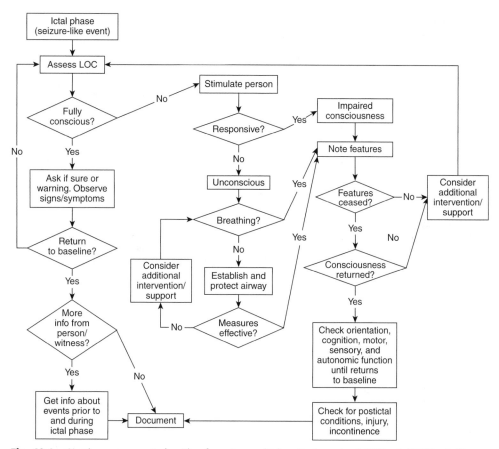

Fig. 40.1 • Nursing assessment algorithm for seizures. (Fisher, R., Long, L., & White, I. [2004]. *Guide to care of the patient with seizures.* American Association of Neuroscience Nurses. Retrieved May 10, 2006, from http://www.aann.org.)

- Document the date and time of the seizure and the activities before, during, and after it.
4. Status epilepticus:
   - Evaluate airway, breathing, and circulation.
   - Rapidly determine and treat for hypoglycemia and hypoxia to prevent further seizures.
   - Give initial injection of diazepam or lorazepam. Additional antiepileptic drugs (e.g., fosphenytoin, phenytoin, and phenobarbital) may be required to prevent more seizures (Table 40-2).
5. Give antiepileptic medication as prescribed. Begin with one drug and titrate the dosage to achieve appropriate blood concentration levels (see Table 40-2). Drugs approved for monotherapy include phenytoin, carbamazepine, valproate, phenobarbital, and topiramate. If this drug does not control the seizures, changing to another antiepileptic drug may be considered. A combination of two drugs may be needed to control the seizures. Finding the most suitable combination for seizure control and minimum side effects may take several attempts.
6. Monitor blood levels of antiepileptic medications.

Table 40-2	COMMONLY USED ANTIEPILEPTIC DRUGS		
Drug/Daily Dose	**Therapeutic Blood Levels**	**Toxicities**	**Monitoring**
Phenytoin (Dilantin) 300-500 mg Fosphenytoin (Cerebyx) IV	10-20 mcg/mL	Drowsiness, lethargy, confusion, slurred speech, irritability, rash, constipation, dizziness, nausea Long-term effects include gingival hyperplasia	Initial blood work: Liver function, CBC, and platelet counts; repeat CBC and platelet counts 2 weeks after maintenance dose is given to establish level Uses P450 enzyme system
Carbamazepine (Tegretol or Carbatrol, a timed-release form) 600-1200 mg	4-12 mcg/mL	Drowsiness, dizziness, nausea, vomiting, visual abnormalities, dry mouth, tongue irritation, headache, water retention, increased sweating, constipation/diarrhea Rare blood dyscrasias	Initial blood work: Liver function, CBC, and platelet counts; blood tests repeated frequently during the first 3 months of therapy and at monthly intervals thereafter for 2-3 years Uses P450 enzyme system
Valproate (Depakote) 1000-3000 mg	50-100 mcg/mL	Abdominal/stomach pain, loss of appetite, changes in menstrual period, diarrhea, hair loss, indigestion, nausea, trembling in arms/hands, weight gain, drowsiness Hepatotoxicity may occur in the first 6 months	Initial blood work: CBC, platelet count before and 2 weeks after therapy begins, then 2 weeks after the maintenance dose is given Take with food May accentuate hepatotoxicity associated with chemotherapy or tumor-induced hepatic function Does not use P450 enzyme system
Phenobarbital 60-200 mg	10-30 mcg/mL	Drowsiness, sedation, dizziness, irritability, mood changes, mental/cognitive slowing, joint aches	Liver function tests, CBC, and platelet counts done before therapy and periodically during therapy Uses P450 enzyme pathway
Gabapentin (Neurontin) 900-3600 mg	None	Fatigue, dizziness, ataxia, nystagmus	Cautionary measures to be taken if renal impairment Does not use P450 enzyme system
Lamotrigine (Lamictal) 100-400 mg	None	Headache, dizziness, nausea, vision disturbances, rash, fatigue; rash is more common when given with valproate	Distributed in breast milk Breast-feeding not recommended Phenobarbital, phenytoin, carbamazepine, and valproate decrease lamotrigine concentration Does not use P450 enzyme system
Levetiracetam (Keppra) 1000-3000 mg	None	Somnolence, ataxia, incoordination, behavior changes, decreased hemoglobin	Use cautiously with impaired renal function Does not use the P450 enzyme pathway

Table 40-2	COMMONLY USED ANTIEPILEPTIC DRUGS		
Drug/Daily Dose	Therapeutic Blood Levels	Toxicities	Monitoring
Topiramate (Topamax) 400 mg	None	Dizziness, nausea/vomiting, hepatotoxicity, SIADH, bone marrow suppression, rash, somnolence	Use cautiously with hepatic impairment Does not use the P450 enzyme pathway
Diazepam (Valium) 2-10 mg Status: 5-10 mg IV Lorazepam (Ativan) 1 mg Status: 4 mg IV	None	Drowsiness, dizziness, nausea, respiratory depression	Short-term use for control of refractory seizures Monitor closely for respiratory depression

7. Monitor for seizure control and for tolerance and side effects of medications. Common side effects are fatigue, drowsiness, incoordination, and nystagmus (i.e., rapid vertical eye movements).

8. Keep a list of all drugs the patient is taking to evaluate for interactions (Patsalos et al., 2002). Enzyme-induced antiepileptic drugs use the P450 pathway in the liver for breakdown. These antiepileptic medications are known to alter the metabolism of some chemotherapy agents and other drugs that use this same pathway for metabolism (see Table 40-2) (Patsalos et al., 2002). Some anticancer agents that use this pathway include temozolomide, irinotecan, etoposide, cyclophosphamide, and paclitaxel. Many other drugs interact with antiepileptic medications, including the commonly used corticosteroids and dexamethasone.

9. Surgical removal of brain tissue is performed for uncontrolled seizures if an epileptogenic focus is identified through extended electroencephalographic testing.

10. Vagus nerve stimulation is approved as adjunctive therapy for patients with partial onset seizures that are refractory to antiepileptic medications.

11. For patients at the end of life, seizures may be best treated with rectal antiepileptic drugs (Krouwer et al., 2000). The two drugs that have shown good rectal absorption are carbamazepine and valproic acid. For status epilepticus, diazepam or lorazepam rectal gel may be given. Phenobarbital, given rectally, by mouth, or intravenously, may also be given at the end of life to reduce seizures and agitation (Stirling et al., 1999).

EVIDENCE-BASED PRACTICE UPDATES

1. Antiepileptic medications that involve the P450-induced liver enzyme must be monitored carefully, because the drug levels alter dramatically (Armstrong et al., 2003). For this reason, many clinical trials specify that patients be placed on non-enzyme-induced antiepileptic drugs (NEIADs) before joining the trial study.

2. Guidelines established by the Academy of Neurology state that the use of anticonvulsants in patients who have not had a seizure should be discouraged (Glantz et al., 2000).

3. Prophylactic anticonvulsants are not likely to be effective or useful in patients with brain tumors who have not had a seizure (Forsyth et al., 2003).

4. Routine use of antiepileptic prophylaxis in patients with brain tumors undergoing neurosurgical procedures remains the prevailing practice pattern among members of the American Association of Neurosurgeons (Siomin et al., 2005).

5. Adolescents with epilepsy showed significantly higher levels of depression and social anxiety and higher numbers of obsessive symptoms than adolescents without epilepsy. High seizure frequency was significantly associated with low self-esteem. Tonic-clonic seizures were associated with higher levels of depression. Low levels of epilepsy knowledge were associated lower self-esteem and high levels of social anxiety (Baker et al., 2005).

TEACHING AND EDUCATION

Preventive medications: *Rationale:* It is important that you understand how and when to take your antiepileptic medication and how to manage its side effects. Talk with your doctor about drug interactions. The best way to prevent seizures is to take the medication properly.

Seizure triggers: *Rationale:* Seizures can be triggered by stress; fatigue; bright, flashing lights; or something that is particular to you. Determine the specific factors that may trigger your seizures and then eliminate them or avoid them as much as possible.

Safety: *Rationale:* You and your family members should be trained in appropriate first aid measures and home medication intervention if required. If you have an indication that a seizure is commencing, put yourself in a safe environment. Wear an identification bracelet to alert others that you have seizures. Take a shower rather than a tub bath to eliminate the risk of drowning.

Documentation of seizures: *Rationale:* You or a family member should keep a journal noting when a seizure occurs, how long it lasts, and what happened before, during, and after the seizure.

End of life seizures: *Rationale:* Develop a plan for medications in the home if seizures are possible. Learn the method of giving seizure medication rectally. If a seizure that lasts longer than 15 minutes occurs at the end of life, rectal diazepam in gel form is highly effective. Adults may be treated with one of three doses, based on the person's weight: 10 mg (28-50 kg); 15 mg (51-75 kg); or 20 mg (76-111 kg) (Krouwer et al., 2000). In the case of a witnessed seizure in the home, diazepam rectal gel should be administered to prevent progression of a single seizure into a cluster of seizures or status epilepticus.

Lifestyle alterations: *Rationale:* Maintain a healthy diet, engage in regular exercise, and restrict alcohol consumption. Avoid identified trigger situations. Regular sleep patterns on a consistent schedule are important.

Emergencies: *Rationale:* Call for emergency services if a seizure:
- Lasts longer than 5 minutes.
- Occurs in water and causes potential cardiac and pulmonary symptoms.
- Causes injury.
- Occurs in a patient with a history of diabetes, and the patient is unable to check his or her blood glucose level.

- Occurs in a patient who is pregnant.
- Occurs repeatedly without a return to consciousness.
- Occurs for the first time with no history of epilepsy.

Living with the stigma of epilepsy: *Rationale*: Contact the Epilepsy Foundation of America for help with emotional and psychological stress related to having seizures or living with a person who has seizures.

Limitations due to epilepsy: *Rationale*: Be aware of driving restrictions related to seizures. Each state has different rules. (Epilepsy Foundation, 2003). Be aware of triggers that cause seizures and limit exposure to them.

Web sites for information:
- Epilepsy Foundation: www.epilepsyfoundation.org
- National Brain Tumor Foundation: www.braintumor.org
- American Brain Tumor Association: www.abta.org
- The Epilepsy Development Project: www.epilepsy.com

Other Web sites that are sponsored by pharmaceutical companies can be quite informative. They can be found by using an Internet search engine to search for "epilepsy sites."

NURSING DIAGNOSES

1. **Risk for injury** related to trauma during a seizure
2. **Noncompliance** related to not taking antiepileptic medication as prescribed
3. **Fatigue** related to side effects of antiepileptic medications
4. **Disturbed thought processes** related to several bouts of status epilepticus
5. **Situational low self-esteem** related to having seizures in public

EVALUATION AND DESIRED OUTCOMES

1. The patient will not be harmed during a seizure.
2. The patient and family will understand when and how the patient should take the antiepileptic medications, and they also will know their side effects.
3. The patient and family will understand what to do if a seizure occurs.
4. The patient will remain seizure free.
5. The patient and family will have a plan if seizures occur at the end of life.

DISCHARGE PLANNING AND FOLLOW-UP CARE

- Instruction sheet on first aid for a seizure to be given to the patient and family.
- Medication sheet with prescribed dosage and side effects to be given to the patient and family.
- Follow-up visit with physician or nurse practitioner 1 to 2 weeks for monitoring of seizure activity and antiepileptic medication blood levels and side effects.
- Call health care provider immediately if:
- A seizure lasts longer than 5 minutes, or if one, two, or more seizures occur in a row.
- A skin rash occurs, because it may indicate an autoimmune response to the seizure medication that could be fatal.

REVIEW QUESTIONS

QUESTIONS

1. The diagnostic test or tests done when a person has a first seizure is/are:
   1. Chest x-ray film
   2. MRI or CT scan with and without contrast and blood work
   3. Electroencephalogram
   4. Visual field tests

2. Mrs. H. is taking phenytoin (Dilantin) for her seizure management. She has fatigue, poor balance, and her phenytoin blood levels are 25 mcg/mL. What could be happening, and what should the nurse do:
   1. She does not have enough phenytoin in her system; the nurse should instruct her to talk with her doctor about adjusting her dosage.
   2. These are clear signs that her tumor has returned; the nurse should instruct her to consult her physician.
   3. She is toxic on the phenytoin; the nurse should instruct her to contact her doctor about reducing the dosage.
   4. The nurse should inform her that these are just side effect of living with a brain tumor.

3. Mrs. M. has a history of seizures, and she usually is well controlled with her medications. She has just had a generalized tonic-clonic seizure. It stopped, but she then had two more seizures. Which action is not appropriate:
   1. Have someone call 911 immediately, because this is a medical emergency.
   2. Stay with her and keep her from harming herself.
   3. Roll her on her side if possible to reduce the risk of aspirating secretions.
   4. Stick something in her mouth.

4. The best alternative method of giving medications for seizure control at the end of life is:
   1. Rectal medications
   2. IV medications
   3. Sublingual medications
   4. Crushed pills

5. Mrs. G. had a seizure as the presenting sign of her glioblastoma. Concurrent with her radiation therapy, she is taking temozolomide and phenytoin. She developed fatigue and severe effects from the temozolomide. The logical cause of the change is:
   1. She has not been taking the phenytoin.
   2. An interaction between the two medications has raised the level of phenytoin, because they use the same P450 enzyme system.
   3. She had developed liver disease.
   4. She is very sensitive to drugs.

6. Mr. M. is attending a lecture. All at once, the presenter begins to look off into space, smack his lips, and wring his hands. He is showing signs of which type of seizure:
   1. Tonic-clonic generalized seizure
   2. Simple focal seizure
   3. Complex partial seizure
   4. Absence seizure

7. Mrs. N.'s chemotherapy has made her very nauseated and prone to vomiting. When she arrives in the emergency department, she appears dehydrated, and she proceeds to have a generalized tonic-clonic seizure. A logical cause of her seizure would be:
   1. She has a new brain metastasis.
   2. She has an electrolyte imbalance.
   3. She forgot to take her medications.
   4. She fell and suffered a head injury.

8. Mr. G., an 18-year-old boy, has a history of seizures that are moderately controlled. He tells you that the worst part of having seizures is that he is embarrassed when they occur. If he has a seizure, which

of the following might be a very important part of the management process:
1. Make sure he does not hurt himself.
2. Provide privacy and speak softly when he wakes up.
3. Ask him if he takes his medication properly.
4. Call an ambulance immediately.

9. An alternative method for managing seizures, besides medication, is:
   1. Deep brain stimulation
   2. Surgery
   3. Colonics
   4. Taking herbs

10. Mr. L. has been very tired because he is undergoing chemotherapy and has an active home life. He finds that when life gets hectic, he has more simple focal seizures. Which of the following do you think may be causing these seizures:
    1. Not taking his medications
    2. Worrying too much
    3. Fatigue
    4. Walking

ANSWERS

1. *Answer: 2*
   Rationale: The two most common causes of seizure in patients with cancer are structural changes and changes in hemodynamics.

2. *Answer: 3*
   Rationale: Adequate phenytoin levels are 10 to 20 mcg/mL. Fatigue and poor balance are symptoms of toxicity, and the nurse should instruct the patient to call her doctor about reducing the dosage.

3. *Answer: 4*
   Rationale: Sticking an object in her mouth may cause trauma. The airway usually stays patent.

4. *Answer: 1*
   Rationale: Most medications are well absorbed rectally. The patient runs no risk

of aspiration. IV routes may be considered if the patient has IV access, but IV medications are more costly and difficult for the family to administer.

5. *Answer: 2*
   Rationale: Phenytoin alters the level of temozolomide, causing possible toxic side effects.

6. *Answer: 3*
   Rationale: In a complex partial seizure, the person remains conscious but is not totally present. Common movements associated with this seizure type are lip smacking and hand wringing.

7. *Answer: 2*
   Rationale: The vomiting was caused by an electrolyte imbalance, which resulted from dehydration. A CT scan probably would be done to make sure the tumor has not grown. The patient would be given intravenous antiepileptic medication, and her electrolytes would be balanced.

8. *Answer: 2*
   Rationale: Adolescent patients often become depressed about having seizures and have low self-esteem. It is best to provide them with privacy during a seizure and to be accepting of the condition. Speaking softly puts the person at ease.

9. *Answer: 2*
   Rationale: Surgery may be done to remove the seizure focus, thereby reducing or eliminating the seizures.

10. *Answer: 3*
    Rationale: Knowing what triggers a seizure is very important to the management of this disorder. Reducing his fatigue by simplifying his surroundings may reduce the patient's seizures.

ACKNOWLEDGMENT

The author thanks Harriet Patterson, MPH, at the National Brain Tumor Foundation for her efforts in editing this chapter.

REFERENCES

Armstrong, T. S., Kanusky, J. T., & Gilbert, M. R. (2003). Seize the moment to learn about epilepsy in people with cancer. *Clinical Journal of Oncology Nursing, 7*(2):163-169.

Baker, G., Spector, S., & McGrath, Y., et al. (2005). Impact of epilepsy in adolescence: A UK controlled study. *Epilepsy and Behavior, 6:*556-562.

Beaumont, A., & Whittle, I. R. (2000). The pathogenesis of tumor epilepsy. *Acta Neurochirurgica (Wein), 142*(1):1-15.

Bromfield, E. (2004). Epilepsy in patients with brain tumors and other cancers. *Review of Neurological Diseases, 1*(Suppl 1):527-533.

Epilepsy Foundation. (2003). Driver licensing and reporting requirements. Retrieved May 10, 2006, from www.epilepsyfoundation.org/answerplace/legal/transit/drivelaw/drivers.cfm.

Fisher, R., Long, L., & White, I. (2004). *Guide to care of the patient with seizures.* American Association of Neuroscience Nurses. Retrieved May 10, 2006, from http://www.aann.org.

Fisher, R. S., Vickrey, B. G., & Gibson, P., et al. (2000). The impact of epilepsy from the patient's perspective. II. Views about therapy and health care. *Epilepsy Research, 41:*53-61.

Forsyth, P. A., Weaver, S., & Fulton, D., et al. (2003). Prophylactic anticonvulsants in patients with brain tumor. *Canadian Journal of Neurological Sciences, 30*(2):106-112.

Glantz, M. J., Cole, B. F., & Forsyth, P. A., et al. (2000). Practice parameter: Anticonvulsant prophylaxis in patients with newly diagnosed brain tumors. Report of the Quality Standards Subcommittee of the American Academy of Neurology. *Neurology, 54:*1886-1893.

Hickey, J. (2003). Seizures and epilepsy. In J. Hickey (Ed.), *The clinical practice of neurological and neurosurgical nursing* (pp. 619-640). Philadelphia: Lippincott Williams & Wilkins.

Hildebrand, J., Lecaille, C. L., & Perennes, J., et al. (2005). Epileptic seizures during follow-up of patients treated for primary brain tumor. *Neurology, 65*(2):212-215.

Jacobs, M. P., & Shafer, P. O. (2000). Care versus cure of epilepsy: The paradigm shift. *Clinical Nursing Practice in Epilepsy, 3*(1):1-7.

Keles, M., & Berger, M. (2000). Seizures associated with brain tumors. In M. Berstein & M. Berger (Eds.), *Neuro-oncology: The essentials* (pp. 473-477). New York: Thieme.

Krouwer, H. G. K., Pallagi, J., & Graves, N. M. (2000). Management of seizures in brain tumor patients at the end of life. *Journal of Palliative Medicine, 3*(4):465-475.

Liigant, A., Haldie, S., & Oun, A., et al. (2001). Seizure disorders in patients with brain tumors. *European Neurology, 45:*46-51.

Lovely, M. P. (2004). Symptom management of brain tumor patients. *Seminars in Oncology Nursing, 20*(4):273-283.

Patsalos, P., Froscher, W., & Pasani, F., et al. (2002). The importance of drug interactions in epilepsy therapy. *Epilepsia, 43*(4):365-385.

Schaller, B., & Ruegg, S. (2003). Brain tumor and seizures: Pathophysiology and its implications for treatment revisited. *Epilepsia, 44*(9):1223-1232.

Siomin, V., Angelov, L., & Liang, L., et al. (2005). Results of a survey of neurosurgical practice patterns regarding the use of anti-epilepsy drugs in patients with brain tumors. *Journal of Neuro-Oncology, 74:*211-215.

Stirling, L. C., Kurowska, A., & Tookman, A. (1999). The use of phenobarbitone in the management of agitation and seizures at the end of life. *Journal of Pain and Symptom Management, 17*(5):363-368.

Szalflarski, M., Meckler, J. M., & Privitera, M. D., et al. (2006). Quality of life in medication resistant epilepsy: The effects of patient's age at seizure onset, and disease duration. *Epilepsy Behavior, 8*(3):547-551.

Victor, M., Robber, A. H., & Adams, R. D. (2001). *Principles of neurology.* (7th ed.). New York: McGraw-Hill.

Sepsis and Septic Shock

KATHY A. SHANE

PATHOPHYSIOLOGICAL MECHANISMS

Healthy individuals with an intact immune system are able to mount a normal immune response to a microbe exposure, preventing colonization of the host. Patients with cancer are at a significantly increased risk for infection because their immune response is impaired as a result of the malignant process and its treatment. As a complication in patients with cancer, infection frequently leads to sepsis and prolongs hospitalization.

The pathophysiologic progression of infection to sepsis to multiorgan dysfunction syndrome (MODS) is a continuum of an inflammatory response to a microbial invasion that becomes increasingly pathologic as organ dysfunction progresses. In 1992, the American College of Chest Physicians and the Society of Critical Care Medicine Consensus Panel defined the various stages of sepsis.

Infection

Infection is an inflammatory response to the presence of microbes; invasion of normally sterile host tissue by these organisms is characteristic. Infection is the most significant complication of cancer therapy and a major cause of sepsis.

A presumed or known site of infection is indicated by one of the following:

- Purulent sputum or respiratory sample, or a chest x-ray film showing new infiltrates not explained by a noninfectious process.
- Spillage of bowel contents noted during an operation.
- Radiographic or physical exam evidence of an infected collection.
- WBCs in a normally sterile body fluid.
- Positive blood culture.
- Physical exam or x-ray film evidence of infected mechanical hardware.

Bacteremia

Bacteremia is the presence of viable bacteria in the blood. The most prevalent organisms in cancer are coagulase-negative staphylococci, viridans group streptococci, *Staphylococcus aureus*, *Escherichia coli*, and *Pseudomonas aeruginosa*. Predisposing factors for nosocomial bacteremias (within 48 hours), in order of occurrence, are the presence of a central venous access device (VAD), peripheral VAD, or urinary catheter; administration of total parenteral nutrition (TPN); intensive care unit (ICU) stay; ventilator support; presence of an arterial line; and dialysis. No significant seasonal or geographic patterns of bacteremia are apparent in the oncology population (Wisplinghoff et al., 2003).

Systemic Inflammatory Response Syndrome

Systemic inflammatory response syndrome (SIRS) is a nonspecific inflammatory process that may follow a variety of clinical insults, including trauma, infection, burns, pancreatitis, ischemia, hemorrhagic shock, or immune-mediated diseases, The inflammatory reaction exceeds local mechanisms of containment, and inflammatory mediators invade the bloodstream, causing systemic disturbances.

Evidence of a systemic inflammatory response includes at least two or more of the following:

- Fever or hypothermia: Core body temperature of 38° C or higher or 36° C or lower.
- Tachypnea: Respiratory rate of 20 breaths/min or higher, or the need for mechanical ventilation for an acute process.
- Tachycardia: HR of 90 beats/min or higher, unless the patient has a pre-existing tachycardia.
- WBCs: WBC count of 12,000 cells/mm^3 or higher, or 4000 cells/mm^3 or lower, or greater than 10% bands on differential.

Sepsis

Sepsis is a systemic response to infection or SIRS. It is an autodestructive process of malignant intravascular inflammation that permits extension of the normal pathophysiologic response to infection.

Severe Sepsis (Septic Shock)

Severe sepsis, or *septic shock*, is sepsis with hypotension (systolic BP less than 90 mm Hg or a reduction of 40 mm Hg from baseline) despite adequate fluid resuscitation. Vasoactive mediators and nitric oxide cause vasodilation and increase vascular permeability, which results in widespread interstitial edema. Changes in both systolic and diastolic function by myocardial depressant substances result in perfusion abnormalities, as evidenced by acidosis, oliguria, and obtundation. Patients with pre-existing cardiac disease are unable to increase cardiac output appropriately, and venous return is diminished. All these events result in profound hypotension.

Multiorgan Dysfunction Syndrome

Multiorgan dysfunction syndrome is the presence of altered organ function in a patient who is acutely ill such that homeostasis cannot be maintained without intervention. Primary MODS is the direct result of a well-defined insult in which dysfunction occurs early and can be directly attributed to the insult itself. Secondary MODS develops as a consequence of a host response and is identified within the context of SIRS.

Sepsis-induced organ failure is indicated by one of the following criteria:

- Cardiovascular dysfunction: Mean arterial pressure (MAP) equal to or less than 60 mm Hg; need for vasopressors to maintain this blood pressure despite adequate intravascular volume (CVP greater than 8 cm H$_2$O or PAOP greater than 12 torr) or after an adequate fluid challenge.
- Respiratory organ failure: PaO$_2$/FiO$_2$ ratio less then 250 in the absence of pneumonia or less than 200 with pneumonia.
- Renal dysfunction: Urine output less than 0.5 mL/kg for 1 hour despite adequate intravascular volume or after an adequate fluid challenge.

- Hematologic dysfunction: Thrombocytopenia, with 80,000 platelets/mm^3, a 50% drop in the previous 3 days, or an INR greater than 1.2 that cannot be explained by liver disease or concomitant warfarin use.
- Unexplained metabolic acidosis: pH less than 7.3 and plasma lactate greater than 1.5 times the upper limit of normal for the lab.

Bacteria are the pathogens most commonly associated with sepsis, but fungi, viruses, and parasites may also be the culprits, particularly in patients with prolonged immunosuppression. The outer membrane components of both gram-negative bacteria (endotoxin, lipid A, lipopolysaccharide) and gram-positive bacteria (peptidoglycan) initiate the pathophysiology of sepsis by binding to the CD14 toll-like receptors on the surface of monocytes. This sends a signal to the cell, leading to the production of proinflammatory cytokines (TNF alpha and IL-1). These cytokines have a toxic effect on tissues and also activate phospholipase, which leads to further tissue damage. Cytokines promote nitric oxide production, tissue infiltration by neutrophils, generation of oxygen free radicals, and increased concentrations of platelet-activating factor. IL-1 and TNF also have direct effects on the endothelial surface of cells; as a result of these inflammatory cytokines, tissue factor, which is the first step in the extrinsic pathway of coagulation, is activated. Tissue factor leads to the production of thrombin, which also is a proinflammatory substance. Thrombin results in fibrin clots in the microvasculature, leading to decreased tissue perfusion. IL-1 and TNF alpha also lead to the production of plasminogen activator inhibitor-1, a potent inhibitor of fibrinolysis.

Proinflammatory cytokines also disrupt the body's modulators of coagulation and inflammation, activated protein C and antithrombin. Activated protein C has direct antiinflammatory properties, such as inhibiting production of proinflammatory cytokines and inhibiting leukocyte adhesion and neutrophil accumulation. Although neutrophils are essential for the eradication of pathogens, excessive release of oxidants and proteases by neutrophils is also believed to be responsible for injury to organs, particularly the lungs.

Antithrombin inhibits thrombin production at multiple steps in the coagulation cascade. Binding of antithrombin to the surface of endothelial cells leads to the production of the antiinflammatory molecule prostacyclin. This accounts for the fact that sepsis initially is characterized by increases in inflammatory mediators but, as the sepsis persists, a shift occurs toward an antiinflammatory immunosuppressive state.

Apoptotic cell death may trigger sepsis-induced anergy, a state of nonresponsiveness to an antigen, and cytokine release. A potential mechanism of lymphocyte apoptosis may be stress-induced endogenous release of glucocorticoids. Large numbers of lymphocytes and gastrointestinal epithelial cells die by apoptosis during sepsis. A second wave of bacterial multiplication (known as the *second hit*) occurs in late sepsis, 4 to 5 days after the initial insult, that is related to this immune dysfunction and intestinal translocation of bacteria. Autopsy studies in people who died of sepsis have shown a profound apoptosis-induced loss of cells of the adaptive immune system (i.e., B cells, CD4 T cells, and follicular dendritic cells), cells that should have proliferated during life-threatening infection. These cells are responsible for antibody production, macrophage activation, and antigen presentation.

This vicious cycle of inflammation and coagulation, if unchecked, leads to cardiovascular insufficiency. TNF exerts a myocardial-depressant effect, as well as promoting vasodilation and capillary leakage (LaRosa, 2002). Additional organ systems fail as a result of poor perfusion. Autopsy studies reveal a discordance between histologic findings and the degree of organ dysfunction. It is speculated that organ dysfunction in sepsis is due to "cell stunning," or hibernation, rather than cellular necrosis. This explains why patients who survive sepsis with associated organ dysfunction can return to baseline function. (Hotchkiss & Karl, 2003).

EPIDEMIOLOGY AND ETIOLOGY

Nosocomial bacteremias are the thirteenth leading cause of death in the United States, with approximately 250,000 cases reported annually; this represents a 78% increase in the past two decades. Of these patients with bacteremias, 10% have an underlying malignancy. Gram-positive organisms account for 60% to 75% of bacteremias in patients with cancer, and gram-negative organisms for 14% to 22%; 30% to 35% of bacteremic patients are neutropenic.

In 2004, critical care and infectious disease experts representing 11 international organizations developed management guidelines for severe sepsis and septic shock for practical use by the bedside clinician. This was an international effort to increase awareness and improve the outcome in severe sepsis. A set of core changes extracted from these guidelines have been incorporated into a package of key elements or goals that, when introduced into clinical practice, have a high likelihood of reducing mortality from severe sepsis. The package is referred to as the *sepsis bundle* (Levy et al., 2004). Areas addressed in the sepsis bundle include initial resuscitation, diagnosis, antibiotic therapy, source control, fluid therapy, vasopressors, inotropic therapy, steroids, recombinant human activated protein C (Xigris), blood product administration, mechanical ventilation of sepsis-induced acute lung injury with sedation, analgesia, and neuromuscular blockade guidelines, glucose control, renal replacement therapy, DVT prophylaxis, stress ulcer prophylaxis, consideration for limitation of support, and pediatric considerations (Dellinger et al., 2004).

According to Cross and Opal (2003), "Given the likelihood that many processes in the complex pathophysiology of sepsis are simultaneously activated, it is unlikely that therapy directed at one of them will dramatically improve survival; rather, a combination of therapies directed at many arms of the septic process, much like the strategy used for cancer and HIV, is required."

RISK PROFILE

The exact process that occurs after an infectious insult is still the subject of many studies.
- **Cancers:** Patients with hematologic malignancies, acute and chronic leukemias (especially in pediatric patients), lymphomas, Hodgkin's disease, and multiple myeloma have an increased risk of infection. The solid tumor malignancies most frequently associated with infection include lung and bronchus cancers (most common) and colon, esophageal, gastric, head and neck, lung, melanoma, and ovarian cancers.
- **Conditions:** An absolute neutrophil count of $500/mm^3$, prolonged neutropenia, marrow-suppressive chemotherapy regimens, radiation therapy, gastrointestinal surgery, loss of mucosal or skin integrity, foreign bodies (e.g., VADs, stents, or catheters), poor nutritional status, poor performance status, the very young or elderly, and the existence of co-morbidities (e.g., collagen vascular diseases; diabetes; and respiratory, cardiac, or renal diseases), particularly if treatment includes glucocorticosteroids (Lyman, et al., 2005; Khan & Wingard, 2001).
- **Environment:** Neutropenic patients are more susceptible to pathogens in the air, water, food, and animals.
- **Chemotherapy medications:** Antineoplastics associated with moderate (grade III) neutropenic toxicity include 5-fluorouracil (greater than 500 mg/m^2), arsenic trioxide, BCNU, bleomycin, cisplatin (greater than 100 mg/m^2), dacarbazine, doxorubicin (greater than 50 mg/m^2), gemcitabine, ifosfamide (greater than 1 g/m^2), Gleevec (greater than 400 mg/day), lomustine, mechlorethamine, melphalan, procarbazine, vinblastine, and vincristine. Antineoplastics associated with severe (grade IV) neutropenic toxicity include 6-mercaptopurine, 6-thioguanine, Campath, busulfan, chlorambucil, cyclophosphamide, cytarabine, daunorubicin, docetaxel, epirubicin, etoposide (greater than

200 mg/m^2), fludarabine, Mylotarg, hydroxyurea, idarubicin, irinotecan, mitoxantrone, paclitaxel, topotecan, ATRA, and vinorelbine.

• **Other medications:** Other medications that may cause mild neutropenia include acetaminophen, allopurinol, amiodarone, aminophylline, amoxicillin, ace inhibitors, cephalosporins, cimetidine, clindamycin, Dilantin, Bactrim, Flagyl, ganciclovir, gentamicin, haloperidol, HCTZ, ibuprofen, Keppra, NNRTIs, nifedipine, nitrofurantoin, norfloxacin, omeprazole, Phenergan, ranitidine, rifampin, Ritalin, Sinemet, spironolactone, sulfonylurea derivatives, Tegretol, valproate. Combinations of any of these medications may have a synergistic effect on the bone marrow.

• **Elderly patients:** Many patients have multiple risk factors that exponentially increase their risk for the development of sepsis. The elderly, in particular, have poorer outcomes because of an increased incidence of hematologic malignancies, a higher degree of co-morbidity, and excessive toxicity and complications related to treatment (Norgaard et al., 2005).

PROGNOSIS

The mortality rate for patients with bacteremia who are neutropenic is 30% to 36%. According to Donowitz and colleagues (2001), "Infection in the neutropenic patient has remained a major challenge for over three decades."

Sepsis is the major cause of mortality worldwide. In the United States, the incidence of severe sepsis is approximately 800,000 cases per year, with a mortality rate ranging from 30% to 50%, depending on the population studied. Sepsis among all patient populations is increasing by an average of 16% per year in the United States, accounting for more than $15 billion in health care costs annually. Severe sepsis is a costly complication of cancer treatment, resulting in approximately 5% of cancer hospitalizations and 8% to 10% of cancer deaths per year at a cost exceeding $3.5 billion annually. Patients with cancer are nearly four times as likely to be hospitalized with severe sepsis than patients without cancer, and patients with hematologic malignancies are 15 times more likely to develop severe sepsis than the general population.

PROFESSIONAL ASSESSMENT CRITERIA (PAC)

1. According to Cohen and colleagues (2004), obtaining a precise bacteriologic diagnosis is paramount for the success of therapeutic strategy during sepsis (see the following table).
2. The admission test for a neutropenic fever should include a comprehensive chemistry panel, CBC with diff, coags, source control by appropriate cultures (peripheral blood and VAD samples, urine, sputum, and wound drainage), and CXR and other radiographic procedures as indicated for source identification.
3. If sepsis is suspected, d-dimer and fibrinogen, lactate, troponin, and ABG tests should be added.
   A cortisol stimulation test is indicated for any patient with refractory hypotension (Manglik et al., 2003).
4. Other possible procedures include a right upper quadrant (RUQ) ultrasound to rule out cholecystitis, transduced bladder pressure for detection of abdominal compartment syndrome, pan-CT scanning as indicated, and LP if neurologic symptoms persist (Cohen et al., 2004).
5. The procalcitonin value is superior to the C-reactive protein finding for diagnosing the severity of sepsis and its outcome.

6. Neopterin is useful in the diagnosis of viral infection.
7. An endotoxin assay in combination with CRP, PCT, or neopterin may aid the diagnosis of gram-negative bacterial infection (Mitaka, 2005).
8. The most common sources of neutropenic fever should be evaluated; this includes inspection of any catheter, VAD, or drainage site; evaluation for mucositis, a common risk factor for bacterial and fungal infections, including oral and perineal inspection (Khan & Wingard, 2001); and targeted H & P for pharyngitis, gastroenteritis, cellulitis, DVT, and respiratory infection (Perrone et al., 2004).

Localized Infection	Sepsis (Generalized Infection)	Septic Shock	MODS
Vital Signs/Labs			
Fever, chills, malaise, BP may be slightly ↑ + Cultures, ↑ ESR, procalcitonin < 1.5 ng/mL, ↑ thyroid hormones	Fever, BP ↓ ↑ Lactate, ↑ C-reactive protein, ↓ phosphate, procalcitonin 30-150 ng/mL, ↓ thyroid hormones, ↓ Mg	Fever or hypothermia, BP ↓↓ ↑↑ Lactate, ↑ anion gap, ↓ cortisol, ↓albumin, ↑ serum and urine myoglobin, procalcitonin > 150 ng/mL, ↑ troponin, ↑ alk phos	Loss of thermal regulation ↓ Calcium
Neurologic Findings			
Headache, meningismus, photophobia (meningitis, encephalitis)	Intellectual impairment, anxiety, agitation	Confusion, obtundation, tremors	Coma, seizures
Respiratory Findings			
Cough, rales, infiltrates, pleuritic chest pain, DOE (pneumonia) Adenopathy, headache, nasal discharge, sore throat (sinusitis, pharyngitis)	↓ PaO$_2$, requiring supplemental oxygen, ↓ PaCO$_2$, tachypnea, shortness of breath	Hypoxia, hypercarbia, effusions, atelectasis, respiratory acidosis, pulmonary capillary leakage; ventilatory support usually required	Apnea, vent-dependent, refractory hypoxia, PEEP, ↑ FiO$_2$ requirement (ARDS)
Cardiovascular Findings			
Tachycardia, regurgitant murmur (endocarditis)	Tachycardia, peripheral edema secondary to capillary leakage, hyperdynamic state: ↑ CO and EF, ↓ SVR	Dysrhythmias, fluid refractory hypotension, vasopressors necessary to support BP, sluggish CRTs	Vasopressor refractory hypotension, need for multiple agents to support BP, ↓ EF, anasarca
Gastrointestinal/Hepatic Findings			
Abdominal pain, diarrhea, nausea, vomiting, ↑ amylase and lipase (mucositis, enteritis, pancreatitis, cholecystitis)	Gastroparesis, ↓ bowel sounds, intolerance of enteral intake, abdominal distention, ↑bilirubin	Ileus, stress ulcer, translocation of gut bacteria, mesenteric ischemia (second hit) ↑ LFTs (shock liver)	GI bleeding, ascites, stasis cholecystitis, bowel perforation, LFTs may return to normal, ↑↑ bilirubin, ↑ coags (liver failure)
Renal Findings			
Dysuria, cloudy urine, CVA tenderness (UTI)	Oliguria or high-output ATN, ↓HCO$_3^-$, ↑ BUN and creatinine, proteinuria, ↑ K	Anuria, ↓↓ HCO$_3^-$ (ARF, Metabolic acidosis)	Dialysis dependent ARF, refractory acidosis

Localized Infection	Sepsis (Generalized Infection)	Septic Shock	MODS
Dermatologic/Musculoskeletal Findings			
Erythema, induration, edema, local tenderness, pus (unless neutropenic) (cellulitis) Diaphoretic	Flushed, hot Myalgias	Petechiae, purpura; skin may be cold, clammy, mottled, jaundiced (rhabdomyolysis)	Diminished skin integrity; tissue necrosis; cool, clammy; pallor; cyanotic Muscle weakness
Hematologic Findings			
↑ WBC with left shift (unless neutropenic)	↑ Platelets, ↑ fibrinogen Xigris may be beneficial	+ D-dimer, ↓ fibrinogen ↑ DVT risk (DIC)	Bleeding from puncture sights, Relative pancytopenia
Endocrine Findings			
↓ or ↑ in blood sugar	Labile blood sugar, may require exogenous insulin	Stress-induced adrenal insufficiency may require exogenous steroids; hyperglycemia may require insulin drip (shock pancreas)	Refractory glucose control despite insulin drip (necrotizing pancreatitis)

NURSING CARE AND TREATMENT

1. **Surgery:** Serves as a component of source control through abscess drainage, wound débridement, exploratory lap for suspected bowel perforation, bronchial stent placement to relieve postobstructive pneumonia, removal of tunneled or implanted VADs, and removal of infected hardware (Marshall et al., 2004).

2. **Chemotherapy:** Indicated if tumor burden reduction is necessary to relieve obstruction of anatomic passageways (i.e., biliary tract, bronchial tree, bowel obstruction with potential perforation).

3. **Radiation:** As for chemotherapy.

4. **Medications:** According to Sepkowitz (2005), "Local patterns of microbiological findings and drug susceptibility, as well as general assistance from national guidelines, are the most important determinants in the selection of empirical therapy for fever in immunocompromised patients." However, studies agree that broad-spectrum antibiotics should be started immediately in sepsis and re-evaluated at 48 to 72 hours if a source of infection has not been identified (Sepkowitz, 2005; Bochud et al., 2004). Gea-Banacloche and colleagues (2004) have said, "Immunosuppressed patients, by definition, are susceptible to a wider spectrum of infectious agents and thus require a broader spectrum of antimicrobial regimen when they present with sepsis."

   The use of antifungals and antivirals remains a challenge, but they should be administered as indicated, particularly in immunosuppressed patients (Gea-Banacloche et al., 2004). Invasive mold infections in general, and *Aspergillus* in particular, are increasing, and the number of patients at risk for them continues to grow. (DiNubile et al., 2005; Richardson, 2005). New agents in the antifungal arsenal include broad triazole agents, (e.g., voriconazole) and the echinocandins (e.g., caspofungin) (Rubin & Somani, 2004). Growth factors, such as G-CSF or GM-CSF, may shorten periods of neutropenia and may be a necessary adjunct in the treatment of sepsis (Ozer et al., 2000).

Immediate fluid resuscitation to maintain the CVP greater than 8 cm H_2O, the MAP greater than 60 mmHg, the UO greater than 0.5 mL/kg., and the SVO_2 saturation greater than 70% (Rhodes & Bennett, 2004; Vincent & Gerlach, 2004) is essential to prevent hypoperfusion states. Administration of packed cells to maintain the Hgb greater than 7 g/dL may be done to supplement crystalloid resuscitation (Zimmerman, 2004). Vasopressors (Levo-phed is the preferred agent in adult sepsis) should be used after sufficient fluid resuscitation; dobutamine is the preferred inotropic agent, but it should not be used to increase cardiac output above physiologic levels (Beale et al., 2004; Hollenberg et al., 2004). Dopamine is recommended in pediatric sepsis with therapeutic endpoints of CRT greater than or equal to 2 seconds, normal pulses with no differential between peripheral and central, warm extremities, UO greater than or equal to 1 mL/kg/hr, and decreased lactate.

Up to 60% of patients admitted for septic shock have relative adrenal insufficiency, as evidenced by refractory hypotension, and might benefit from stress steroid bolusing after adrenal function tests are completed (Keh & Sprung, 2004). Xigris, in controlled settings, has shown promise if initiated early in the course of sepsis (Cross & Opal, 2003; Pastores et al., 2002). Tight glucose control (i.e., maintaining the blood glucose level at 80 to 110 mg/dL) has been shown to improve survival in critically ill patients. Insulin should be given as needed, either by continuous infusion or sliding scale, to achieve this goal (Cariou et al., 2004; Van den Berghe et al., 2003). Proton pump inhibitors or H_2-receptor blockers are indicated for stress ulcer prevention. Low-molecular-weight heparin and graduated compression stockings or intermittent compression devices for DVT prophylaxis are also indicated for patients with severe sepsis (Trzeciak & Dellinger, 2004). Granulocyte transfusions, particularly patients with documented candidemia, have been associated with improved survival rates (Safdar et al., 2004).

5. **Other:** Ventilatory support using low tidal volume, permissive hypercapnia, and sedation protocols is a new trend in the management of respiratory failure. Renal replacement therapy as needed by means of continuous venovenous hemofiltration or intermittent hemodialysis is indicated to correct fluid and electrolyte derangements and acid-base imbalances in patients with acute renal failure.

- Nutritional support should not be overlooked in these critically ill patients. When possible, the enteral route is preferred, but many patients do not tolerate tube feedings because of gastroparesis and ileus, therefore parenteral alimentation may be required.
- Surveillance cultures, prophylactic antibiotics, and VAD salvage by guidewire and antibiotic lock therapy have been studied in various oncology patient trials, with mixed reviews (Cullen et al.,2005; Van de Wetering et al., 2005; Donowitz et al., 2001).

EVIDENCE-BASED PRACTICE UPDATES

"The unmet challenge in sepsis research is not the identification of therapeutic targets, but the development of sensible, robust, and validated methods of stratifying patients, analogous to those that currently guide the use of adjuvant therapy in oncology" (Macias et al., 2005; Marshall et al., 2004; Benoit et al., 2003; Larché et al., 2003; Marshall et al., 2003). The Acute Physiology, Age, and Chronic Health Evaluation (APACHE) scale roughly attempts this but more accurately predicts mortality in the critically ill. The Theoretical Predisposition, Nature of Acute Insult, Host Response, and Baseline Degree of Organ Dysfunction (PIRO) model attempts to stratify septic patients. The Sequential Organ Failure Assessment (SOFA) score has proven to have predictive value for survival in general ICU populations (Cornet et al., 2005). The Monoclonal Anti-TNF: A Randomized Controlled Sepsis (MONARCS) trial sought to determine whether adequate antibiotic therapy in suspected sepsis was associated with a decreased mortality rate

(MacArthur et al., 2004; Marshall et al., 2001). Other trials that have attempted to meet this challenge with regard to appropriate timing of Xigris administration include the Protein C Worldwide Evaluation in Severe Sepsis (PROWESS) trial, the Alfa-Activated Drotrecogin Recombinant in the Treatment of Severe Sepsis (ADDRESS) trial (Abraham et al., 2005), and the Extended Evaluation of Human Activated Protein C in the United States (ENHANCE US) trial.

Another challenge is overcoming the reluctance to offer critical care management to patients with cancer, an attitude found in many institutions. Studies have shown that careful selection of patients and early intervention can result in improved survival among this patient population (Soares et al., 2005; Williams et al., 2004; Benoit et al., 2003; Maschmeyer et al., 2003).

Specific updates include the following:

1. Glutamine injected into rats with sepsis-enhanced heat shock protein increased lung function and improved survival (Singleton et al., 2005).
2. Endocan, a circulating proteoglycan, is increased (greater than 6.8 ng/mL) in individuals with severe sepsis and septic shock (Scherpereel et al., 2006).
3. An antiinflammatory state of the gut is induced in rats fed an immune-enhancing diet of L-arginine, fish oil, and RNA fragments; this helps control sepsis (Hurt et al., 2006).
4. Procalcitonin (PCT) and C-reactive protein (CRP) plasma levels are useful markers for sepsis. PCT increases early on and differentiates infective from noninfective causes of inflammation (Spapen et al., 2006).
5. An increase has been seen in the antimicrobial resistance of *Acinetobacter baumannii* and *Klebsiella pneumoniae* to amikacin, ciprofloxacin, imipenem, and piperacillin/tazobactam (Falagas et al, 2006).

TEACHING AND EDUCATION

1. Oncology patients in general should be instructed in the signs of infection and the need for *immediate* intervention, particularly during periods of neutropenia.
2. Emergency departments should provide rapid triage of patients with a neutropenic fever to prevent sepsis (Nirenberg et al., 2004). The national standard for neutropenic fever is appropriate cultures with administration of antibiotics within 1 to 2 hours of the onset of fever.
3. Patients discharged with indwelling VADs should be instructed in the signs and symptoms of line infection, (e.g., chills and fever with catheter flushing, redness or drainage at the insertion site). If further treatment is not indicated, VADs should be removed as soon as they are no longer needed.
4. **Web sites for information:** Sepsis.com defines pathophysiology, management, and the clinical consequences of sepsis: http://sepsis.com/index.jsp.

NURSING DIAGNOSES

The nursing diagnoses will differ, depending on the stage of infectious insult in the sepsis continuum. The following are some of the common diagnoses for this patient population.

1. **Deficient fluid volume** related to capillary permeability secondary to generalized inflammatory response
2. **Ineffective tissue perfusion** related to hypotension secondary to generalized inflammatory response and infection
3. **Risk for infection** related to infectious exo or endotoxins

4. **Impaired gas exchange** related to capillary leakage, and acute lung injury secondary to hypoperfusion and infection.
5. **Risk for impaired liver function** related to acute liver hypoperfusion.

EVALUATION AND DESIRED OUTCOMES

1. As mentioned previously, acuity scales can predict survival rates as septic shock and MODS progresses.
2. Identification of sepsis in its earliest stages and prevention of shock are the keys to improved survival; rapid intervention by patients, caregivers, and health care professionals is required to accomplish these goals.
3. Patient and caregiver education, as previously outlined, is essential.
4. Institutions with standing protocols, order sets, and stock antibiotics for neutropenic fever can achieve the goal of fever workup and antibiotic delivery within 1 hour of entry to the health care arena.

DISCHARGE PLANNING AND FOLLOW-UP CARE

- Some studies suggest that "oral antibiotics in conjunction with early hospital discharge for patients who remain stable after a 24-hour period of inpatient monitoring offers a feasible and cost-effective alternative to conventional management of low-risk neutropenic fever" and may reduce the risk of virulent hospital-acquired infections (Innes et al., 2003).
- Patients who have survived a septic event must be followed carefully, particularly if further treatment cycles are planned. The need for dose reduction for future cycles must be considered to prevent prolonged neutropenic periods.

REVIEW QUESTIONS

QUESTIONS

1. A nonspecific inflammatory process best describes:
   1. Bacteremia
   2. Sepsis
   3. SIRS
   4. MODS

2. The solid tumor malignancies most commonly associated with infection include all of the following *except:*
   1. Lung and bronchus cancer
   2. Colorectal cancer
   3. Ovarian cancer
   4. Astrocytoma

3. All of the following chemotherapeutic agents are associated with grade I neutropenia toxicity *except:*
   1. Interleukin-2
   2. Busulfan
   3. Cytarabine
   4. Idarubicin

4. The most common source of infection in an oncology patient who is neutropenic is:
   1. Mucositis
   2. Venous access device
   3. Cholestasis
   4. Urinary tract infection

5. **Rapid intervention (within the first hour of admission) for a patient presenting with sepsis includes all of the following *except:***
   1. Identifying the source through appropriate cultures
   2. Aggressive fluid resuscitation
   3. Establishing a central line
   4. Administering broad-spectrum antibiotics

6. **The Surviving Sepsis Campaign addressed all of the following in the "sepsis bundle" *except:***
   1. DVT prophylaxis
   2. Nutritional support
   3. Glucose control
   4. Steroid administration

7. **Indications of *sepsis-induced* organ failure include all of the following *except:***
   1. Unexplained metabolic acidosis (pH less than 7.3)
   2. Thrombocytopenia (less than 80,000 platelets/mm^3 or a 50% drop over 3 days)
   3. Mean arterial pressure less than or equal to 60 mm Hg with vasopressors after adequate fluid resuscitation
   4. Blood glucose control requiring an insulin drip in a nondiabetic patient

8. **Which of the following statements about sepsis is *false*:**
   1. Sepsis is the major cause of mortality worldwide.
   2. The mortality rate for sepsis in the United States is 30% to 50%.
   3. Sepsis among all patient populations is slowly declining as a result of improved antibiotic and supportive therapy.
   4. Cancer patients are four times as likely to be hospitalized with sepsis than the general population.

9. **Which of the following patients has the greatest risk of developing sepsis:**
   1. A 40-year-old, otherwise healthy man with a new diagnosis of lung cancer by routine CXR.
   2. A 25-year-old man with an absolute neutrophil count of 0.75 or 750/

mm^3 6 days after chemotherapy for Hodgkin's disease.
   3. A 50-year-old woman with chronic myelocytic leukemia with a WBC count of 40,000/mm^3.
   4. A 38-year-old woman with newly diagnosed acute leukemia with a WBC count of 3000/mm^3.

10. **Which of the following statements about the pathophysiology of sepsis is *false*:**
   1. The outer membrane components of gram-negative and gram-positive bacteria initiate the septic process by binding to the surface of monocytes.
   2. Cytokines have a toxic effect on tissues and disrupt the body's modulators of coagulation and inflammation.
   3. Neutrophils are essential for the eradication of pathogens, and neutrophil accumulation at the site of infection prevents tissue damage in that organ.
   4. A second wave of bacterial multiplication occurs in late sepsis that is related to immune dysfunction and intestinal translocation of bacteria.

ANSWERS

1. *Answer: 3*
   Rationale: SIRS is a nonspecific inflammatory process that may follow a variety of clinical insults. The inflammatory reaction exceeds local mechanisms of containment.

2. *Answer: 4*
   Rationale: Lung and bronchial cancer are the most common solid malignancies associated with infection, followed by cancers of the gastrointestinal tract. Brain tumors generally are not complicated by an infectious process.

3. *Answer: 1*
   Rationale: Interleukin-2 (IL-2) is a biologic response modifier that activates the immune system. The most common complications of IL-2 therapy are fever, agitation, and capillary leakage syndrome. The other agents are very myelosuppressive and are

frequently used in the treatment of hematologic malignancies.

4. *Answer: 2*
   Rationale: Venous access devices, particularly central VADs, are the most common source of infection in oncology patients who are neutropenic. For this reason, patients require education in signs of infection and in the care of these devices. VADs should be removed when they are no longer needed for active cancer treatment.

5. *Answer: 3*
   Rationale: Large-bore peripheral access is an effective means of achieving fluid resuscitation and administering IV antibiotics. Antibiotics should be administered after the results of appropriate cultures have been obtained.

6. *Answer: 2*
   Rationale: The sepsis bundle included guidelines for initial resuscitation, diagnosis, antibiotic therapy, source control, fluid therapy, vasopressors, inotropic support, steroids, Rha protein C, blood product administration, mechanical ventilation, glucose control, renal replacement therapy, DVT prophylaxis, stress ulcer prophylaxis, pediatric considerations, and consideration for limitation of support. It did not make recommendations for nutritional support.

7. *Answer: 4*
   Rationale: Tight glycemic control has been shown to improve survival in critically ill patients. It is not uncommon for patients to require an insulin drip to achieve this goal without evidence of pancreatic shock or failure. Additional indications of sepsis-induced organ failure include a paO_2/FiO_2 ratio less than 250 without pneumonia (less than 200 with pneumonia); a urine output less than 0.5 mL/kg for 1 hour after adequate fluid resuscitation; and an INR greater than 1.2 without liver disease or warfarin use.

8. *Answer: 3*
   Rationale: Sepsis among all patient populations is *increasing* by an average of 16% per year in the United States, with approximately 800,000 cases per year.

9. *Answer: 2*
   Rationale: Severe neutropenia is the single greatest risk for the development of sepsis in the oncology population. A normal absolute neutrophil count is 1.5 to 8.0 or 1,500 to 8,000/mm³. Patients with hematologic malignancies, which this patient also has, have an increased risk because of the effect on immune function. Lung cancer is the solid tumor malignancy with the highest rate of sepsis, but this patient is asymptomatic.

10. *Answer: 3*
    Rationale: Although neutrophils are essential for the eradication of pathogens, excessive release of oxidants and proteases by neutrophils is also believed to be responsible for injury to organs, particularly the lungs.

REFERENCES

Abraham, E., Laterre, P. F., & Garg, R., et al. (2005). Drotrecogin alfa (activated) for adults with severe sepsis and a low risk of death. *New England Journal of Medicine, 353*:1332-1341.

Beale, R. J., Hollenberg, S. M., & Vincent, J. L., et al. (2004). Vasopressor and inotropic support in septic shock: An evidence-based review. *Critical Care Medicine, 32*(11):S455-S465.

Benoit, D. D., Vandewoude, K. H., & Decruyenaere, J. M., et al. (2003). Outcome and early prognostic indicators in patients with a hematologic malignancy admitted to the intensive care unit for a life-threatening complication. *Critical Care Medicine, 1*:320-321.

Bochud, P. Y., Bontne, M., & Marchetti, O., et al. (2004). Antimicrobial therapy for patients with severe sepsis and septic shock: An evidence-based review. *Critical Care Medicine, 32*(11):S495-S512.

Cariou, A., Vinsonneau, C., & Dhainaut, J. F. (2004). Adjunctive therapies in sepsis: An evidence-based review. *Critical Care Medicine, 32*(11):S562-S570.

Cohen, J., Brun-Buisson, C., & Torres, A., et al. (2004). Diagnosis of infection in sepsis: An evidence-based review. *Critical Care Medicine, 32*(11):S466-S494.

Cornet, A. D., Issa, A. I., & van de Loosdrecht, A. A., et al. (2005). Sequential organ failure predicts mortality of patients with a haematological malignancy needing intensive care. *European Journal of Haematology,* 74:511-516.

Cross, A. S., & Opal, S. M. (2003). A new paradigm for the treatment of sepsis: Is it time to consider combination Therapy? *Annals of Internal Medicine, 138*:502-505.

Cullen, M., Steven, N., & Billingham, L., et al. (2005). Antibacterial prophylaxis after chemotherapy for solid tumors and lymphomas. *New England Journal of Medicine, 353*(10):988-998.

Dellinger, R. P., Darlet, J. M., & Masur, H., et al. (2004). Surviving sepsis campaign guidelines for management of severe sepsis and septic shock. *Critical Care Medicine, 32*(3):858-873.

DiNubile, M. J., Hille, D., & Sable, C. A., et al. (2005). Invasive candidiasis in cancer patients: Observations from a randomized trial. *Journal of Infection, 50*(5):443-449.

Donowitz, G. R., Maki, D. G., & Crnich, C. J, et al. (2001). Infections in the neutropenic patient: New views of an old problem. *Hematology, 1*:113-139.

Falagas, M. E., Kasiakou, S. K., & Nikita, D., et al. (2006). Secular trends of antimicrobial resistance of blood isolates in a newly found Greek hospital. *BMC Infectious Diseases, 6*:99.

Gea-Banacloche, J. C., Opal, S. M., & Jorgenson, J., et al. (2004). Sepsis associated with immunosuppressive medications: An evidence-based review. *Critical Care Medicine, 32*(11):S578-S590.

Hollenberg, S. M., Ahrens, T. S., & Annane, D., et al. (2004). Practice parameters for hemodynamic support of sepsis in adult patients: 2004 Update. *Critical Care Medicine, 32*(9):1928-1948.

Hotchkiss, R. S., & Karl, I. E. (2003). The pathophysiology and treatment of sepsis. *New England Journal of Medicine, 348*(2):138-150.

Hurt, R. T., Matheson, P. J., & Mays, M. P., et al. (2006). Immune-enhancing diet and cytokine expression during chronic sepsis: An immune-enhancing diet containing L-arginine, fish oil, and RNA fragments promotes intestinal cytokine expression during chronic sepsis in rats. *Journal of Gastrointestinal Surgery, 10*(1):46-53.

Innes, H. E., Smith, D. B., & O'Reilly, S. M., et al. (2003). Oral antibiotics with early hospital discharge compared with in-patient intravenous antibiotics for low-risk febrile neutropenia in patients with cancer: A prospective randomized controlled single centre study. *British Journal of Cancer, 89*:43-49.

Keh, D., & Sprung, C. L. (2004). Use of corticosteroid therapy in patients with sepsis and septic shock: An evidence-based review. *Critical Care Medicine, 32*(11):S527-S533.

Khan, S. A., & Wingard, J. R. (2001). Infection and mucosal injury in cancer treatment. *Journal of the National Cancer Institute Monographs, 29*:31-36.

Larché, J., Azoulay, É., & Fieux, F., et al. (2003). Improved survival of critically ill cancer patients with septic shock. *Intensive Care Medicine, 29*(10):1688-1695.

Larosa, S. P. (2002). Sepsis: Menu of new approaches replaces one therapy for all. *Cleveland Clinic Journal of Medicine, 69*(1):65-73.

Levy, M. M., Pronovost, P. J., & Dellinger, R. P., et al. (2004). Sepsis change bundles: Converting guidelines into meaningful change in behavior and clinical outcome. *Critical Care Medicine, 32*(11):S595-S597.

Lyman, G. H., Lyman, C. H., & Agboola, O. (2005). Risk models for predicting chemotherapy-induced neutropenia. *Oncologist, 10*(6):427-437.

MacArthur, R. D., Miller, M., & Albertson, T., et al. (2004). Adequacy of early empiric antibiotic treatment and survival in severe sepsis: Experience form the MONARCS trial. *Clinical Infectious Diseases, 38*(2):284-288.

Macias, W. L., Nelson, D. R., & Williams, M., et al. (2005). Lack of evidence for qualitative treatment by disease severity interactions in clinical studies of severe sepsis. *Critical Care, 9*:R607-R622.

Manglik, S., Flores, E., & Lubarsky, L., et al. (2003). Glucocorticoid insufficiency in patients who present to the hospital with severe sepsis: A prospective clinical trial. *Critical Care Medicine, 31*:1668-1675.

Marshall, J. C., Maier, R. V., & Jimenez, M., et al. (2004). Source control in the management of severe sepsis and septic shock: An evidence-based review. *Critical Care Medicine, 32*(11):S513-S526.

Marshall, J. C., Penacek, E. A., & Tech, L., et al. (2001). Modeling organ dysfunction as a risk factor, outcome, and measure of biologic effect of sepsis: Results of the MONARCS trial. *Critical Care Medicine, 28*:A46.

Marshall, J. C., Vincent, J. L., & Fink, P. M., et al. (2003). Measures, markers, and mediators: Toward a staging system for clinical sepsis. A report of the Fifth Toronto Sepsis Roundtable, Toronto, Ontario, Canada, October 25-26, 2000. *Critical Care Medicine, 31*(5):1560-1567.

Maschmeyer, G., Bertschat, F. L., & Moesta, K. T., et al. (2003). Outcome analysis of 189 consecutive cancer patients referred to the intensive care unit as emergencies during a 2-year period. *European Journal of Cancer, 39*(6):783-792.

Mitaka, C. (2005). Clinical laboratory differentiation of infectious versus non-infectious systemic inflammatory response syndrome. *Clinica Chimica Acta, 351*:17-29.

Nirenberg, A., Mulhearn, L., & Lin, S., et al. (2004). Emergency department waiting times for patients with cancer with febrile neutropenia: A pilot study. *Oncology Nursing Forum, 31*(4):711-715.

Norgaard, M., Larsson, H., & Pedersen, G., et al. (2005). Short-term mortality of bactaeremia in elderly patients with haematological malignancies. *British Journal of Haematology, 132*:25-31.

Ozer, H., Armitage, J. O., & Bennett, C. L., et al. (2000). 2000 Update of recommendations for the use of hematopoietic colony-stimulating factors: Evidence-based, clinical practice guidelines. *Journal of Clinical Oncology, 18*(20):3558-3585.

Pastores, S. M., Papadopoulos, E., & van den Brink, M., et al. (2002). Septic shock and multiple organ failure after hematopoietic stem cell transplantation: Treatment with recombinant human activated protein C. *Bone Marrow Transplantation, 30*:131-134.

Perrone, J., Hollander, J. E., & Datner, E. M. (2004). Emergency department evaluation of patients with fever and chemotherapy-induced neutropenia. *Journal of Emergency Medicine, 27*(2):115-119.

Rhodes, A., & Bennett, D. (2004). Early goal-directed therapy: An evidence-based review. *Critical Care Medicine, 32*(11):S448-S450.

Richardson, M. D. (2005). Changing patterns and trends in systemic fungal infections. *Journal of Antimicrobial Chemotherapy, 56*:S1, 5-11.

Rubin, Z. A., & Somani, J. (2004). New options for the treatment of invasive fungal infections. *Seminars in Oncology, 2*:91-98.

Safdar, A., Hanna, H. A., & Boktour, M., et al. (2004). Impact of high-dose granulocyte transfusions in patients with cancer with candidemia. *Cancer, 101*(12):2859-2865.

Scherpereel, A., Depontieu, F., & Grigoriu, B., et al. (2006). Endocan, a new endothelial marker in human sepsis. *Critical Care Medicine, 34*(2):532-537.

Sepkowitz, K. A. (2005). Treatment of patients with hematologic neoplasm, fever, and neutropenia. *Clinical Infectious Diseases, 40*(Suppl. 4):S253-S256.

Singleton, K. D., Serkova, N., & Beckey, V. E., et al. (2005). Glutamine attenuates lung injury and improves survival after sepsis: Role of enhanced heat shock protein expression. *Critical Care Medicine, 33*(6):1206-1213.

Soares, M., Salluh, J. I. F., & Spector, N., et al. (2005). Characteristics and outcomes of cancer patients requiring mechanical ventilatory support for longer than 24 hours. *Critical Care Medicine, 33*(3):520-526.

Spapen, H. D., Hachimi-Idrissi, S., & Corne, L., et al. (2006). Diagnostic markers of sepsis in the emergency department. *Acta Clinica Belgica, 61*(3):138-142.

Trzeciak, S., & Dellinger, R. P. (2004). Other supportive therapies in sepsis: An evidence-based review. *Critical Care Medicine, 32*(11):S571-S577.

Van de Wetering, M. D., de Witte, M. A., & Kremer, L. C. M., et al. (2005). Efficacy of oral prophylactic antibiotics in neutropenic febrile oncology patients: A systemic review of randomized controlled trials. *European Journal of Cancer, 41*(10):1372-1382.

Van den Berghe, G., Wbuters, P. J., & Bouillon, R., et al. (2003). Outcome benefit of intensive insulin therapy in the critically ill: Insulin dose versus glycemic control. *Critical Care Medicine, 31*:359-366.

Vincent, J. L., & Gerlach, H. (2004). Fluid resuscitation in severe sepsis and septic shock: An evidence-based review. *Critical Care Medicine, 32*(11):S451-S454.

Williams, M. D., Braun, L. A., & Cooper, L. M., et al. (2004). Hospitalized cancer patients with severe sepsis: Analysis of incidence, mortality, and associated costs of care. *Critical Care Forum, 8*(5):1-15.

Wisplinghoff, H., Seifert, H., & Wenzel, R. P., et al. (2003). Current trends in the epidemiology of nosocomial bloodstream infections in patients with hematological malignancies and solid neoplasms in hospitals in the United States. *Clinical Infectious Diseases, 36*:1103-1110.

Zimmerman, J. L. (2004). Use of blood products in sepsis: An evidence-based review. *Critical Care Medicine, 32*(11):S542-S546.

Sinusoid Occlusive Syndrome

PATRICIA C. BUCHSEL

PATHOPHYSIOLOGICAL MECHANISMS

Sinusoid occlusive syndrome (SOS) is increasingly replacing the term *venulo-occlusive disease* (VOD), because current research suggests that the initial target of this syndrome is primarily the liver sinusoids rather than the venule sinusoids (Kumar et al. 2003; DeLeve et al., 2002). This chapter uses SOS to reflect current language.

SOS was first reported to be linked to the use of Senecio tea in South Africa (Willmot & Robertson, 1920). Other studies described epidemics of VOD associated with the ingestion of plants that contained pyrrolizidine alkaloids (Datta et al., 1978; Tandon et al., 1976). The term *VOD* subsequently made its way into the scientific literature until recent research determined otherwise.

SOS was first described in Western culture in 1979 in recipients of bone marrow transplants (BMTs) (Berk et al., 1979; Jacobs et al., 1979). SOS also can occur in other settings (although it is rare), such as in patients receiving chemotherapy after high-dose radiation therapy (Fajardo & Colby, 1980), individuals who have ingested alkaloid toxins, and recipients of liver transplants (Sebagh et al., 1999).

Management of a patient with hepatic SOS continues to be the subject of intensive research. Until such time that successful modalities emerge, supportive care remains the first-line treatment. Prophylactic and treatment measures have been disappointing, but clinical research continues to focus on eliminating or diminishing the effects of SOS. Surprisingly, 70% of SCT recipients with SOS spontaneously overcome this disorder (Kumar et al., 2003), which emphasizes the need for intense supportive care until the disease resolves

Oncology nurses practicing in this setting carry many responsibilities in symptom management to support the recipient through numerous symptoms of SOS. In addition to reducing the physical discomforts of this syndrome, advanced nurse practitioners need to attend to the psychologic needs of patients who are great risk for morbidity and mortality. Those practicing in clinical trials for prevention and treatment of SOS can disseminate the results of ongoing research and nursing-sensitive outcomes (Kapustay & Buchsel, 2000). This chapter discusses the pathophysiology, risk factors, and medical management and nursing care for SOS in the SCT setting.

The histologic changes in the liver of the SCT recipient are caused by a number of events that make the liver vulnerable to the insults of co-morbidities before and during treatment. The pathophysiology of SOS is complex and remains somewhat unclear, but research in the rat model has contributed to new understanding of the histologic changes in the liver affected by SOS. Study rats given pyrrolizidine manifested the initial symptoms of SOS. Damage to the liver endothelium appeared to initiate a cascade of events that led to the loss of the endothelial cell fenestrations and the appearance of gaps in the lining, which were followed by extravasation of red cells into the space of Disse. This was followed by obstructions caused by engorged hepatocytes and red blood cells, leading to coagulation in the liver sinusoids. These obstructions are thought to result in the classic symptoms of water retention, weight gain, elevation of serum bilirubin, and painful hepatomegaly.

In summary, SOS manifests during the first 2 week after SCT. The classic signs and symptoms of SOS are weight gain, ascites, and pain in the upper right quadrant of the abdomen. Supportive care until the disease resolves, usually within several weeks, remains the gold standard of treatment. Current research is aimed at preventive and treatment measures, but no new agents or combinations of agents have as yet been accepted worldwide as curative measures.

EPIDEMIOLOGY AND ETIOLOGY

SOS is a specific treatment complication that can lead to substantial morbidity and treatment-related mortality. It develops in individuals who have a mutation in the gene encoding the PML nuclear body protein Sp110. Hepatic SOS is frequently linked to high-dose chemotherapy and total body irradiation in recipients of hematopoietic SCT; long-term use of azathioprine after organ transplantation; the use of other chemotherapeutic agents (e.g., oxaliplatin and CBV therapy [cyclophosphamide, VP-16, high-dose BCNU]) in the treatment of lymphoma; and the use of the Chinese herbal Gymura segetum. Although it occurs in patients treated with oxaliplatin, it is not associated with an increased risk of perioperative death. The incidence of hepatic SOS ranges from 0 to 70% (Helmy, 2006) and is decreasing. Disease risk is higher in patients with malignancies, hepatitis C virus infection, those who present late, when norethisterone is used to prevent menstruation, and when broad-spectrum antibiotics and antifungals are used during and after the conditioning therapy. Patients who undergo the transjugular intrahepatic portosystemic shunt (TIPS) procedure have a higher risk of developing SOS, because shunt dysfunction occurs in 50% of patients within 1 year. The prognosis varies, depending on the etiology and severity of the disease and on associated conditions. Patients who receive liver transplants have an average 5-year disease-free survival rate of 50% to 95% if the procedure was done at a specialized transplant center. Death most often is caused by renal or cardiopulmonary failure.

RISK PROFILE

The results of most large, well-conducted research studies agree on the primary risk factors, incidence, and morbidity and mortality rates for STC recipients who develop SOS. These studies include a multicenter study (N = 1653) from 73 SCT centers (Carreras et al., 1998); a cohort study of 355 patients (McDonald et al., 1993); and an extensive review of more than 32 studies (Kumar et al., 2003). The findings of other significant studies are consistent with those of these studies (Schoch et al., 2005; El-Sayed et al., 2004; Gooley et al., 2005; Bearman, 1995). Risk factors include the following:
- Pretransplant elevation in the serum aspartate aminotransferase (AST)
- Decreased albumin levels, decreased pseudocholinesterase
- Cirrhosis
- Metastatic liver disease
- Pretransplant hepatotoxic drug therapy (i.e., acyclovir, amphotericins, vancomycin, cyclophosphamide) (De Jonge et al., 2006)
- Karnovsky scores less than 90%
- Previous radiation therapy to the abdomen

- Advanced age
- Previous STC transplantation
- Allogenic STC versus autologous
- Previous therapy with gemtuzumab
- Viral hepatitis C
- Use of cyclophosphamide, busulfan, or total body irradiation in conditioning regimens for SCT
- Administration of methotrexate for GVHD
- Possible cytomegalovirus (CMV) infection

PROGNOSIS

SOS is proportional to the extent of liver damage. The incidence of SOS ranges from 20% to 70%, depending on the diagnostic criteria used, the population studied, and the conditioning protocol. Patients with SOS usually succumb to multisystem organ failure and die of other causes, most commonly renal failure, pulmonary compromise requiring mechanical ventilation, cardiac failure, and bacteremia. Late complications of SOS are rare (Kumar et al., 2003).

PROFESSIONAL ASSESSMENT CRITERIA (PAC)

SOS typically occurs within the first 2 weeks after SCT. The classic symptoms are hepatomegaly, right upper quadrant pain, jaundice, and ascites. Computed tomography (CT) scans show periportal edema and small diameter of the right hepatic vein (less than 0.27 cm) (Ertuck et al., 2006). SCT recipients manifest numerous overlapping symptoms caused or mimicked by myriad complications of transplantation, especially in the early stages of SCT. For example, the clinical symptoms and laboratory findings for acute liver (GVHD) or fungal infections are similar (Kapustay & Buchsel, 2000).

Three recognized scales for diagnosing SOS are similar and are accepted by researchers in the worldwide community of transplant medicine. These are the Seattle Criteria, the Baltimore Criteria, and the Modified Seattle Criteria (Kumar et al., 2003).

1. As mentioned, the classic initial symptoms are manifested within the first 2 weeks of SCT. Symptoms are often overlooked early in SCT because of the administration of high volumes of intravenous fluids. Such symptoms include the following:
   - Pain (upper right abdominal pain caused by enlarged liver and ascetics).
   - Tender, enlarged liver (narcotics may be required for pain, which may be severe enough to require opioids).
   - Asymptomatic weight gain thought to be due to water and salt retention by the kidneys (ascites may not be relieved by diuretics).
   - Serum total bilirubin concentration greater than 2 mg/dL.
   - Jaundice related to liver dysfunction.
   - Renal dysfunction (occurs frequently, and 50% of cases require hemodialysis).
   - Thrombocytopenia (may be due to increased consumption of platelets in the liver sinusoids and increased splenic sequestration related to portal hypertension).
   - Coagulation factor deficiencies and prolonged prothrombin time.
   - Encephalopathy

2. The initial diagnosis of SOS is made primarily on the basis of the classic symptoms. Other diagnostic approaches include the following:
   - Transjugular biopsies, rather than percutaneous needle biopsies, are done because of the high risk of thrombocytopenia and abnormal coagulopathies. Histopathology may reveal hepatic venular occlusion, sinusoidal fibrosis, phlebosclerosis, hepatocyte necrosis, and luminal narrowing of the hepatic venules.
   - Ultrasound scanning has not been a useful tool in the STC setting, but it is useful for making a differential diagnosis regarding disorders that mimic SOS, such as hepatomegaly, ascites, and hepatic vein dilation.
   - Doppler findings of portal hypertension can be useful.
   - Magnetic resonance imaging (MRI) may support ultrasound findings, but it is not useful for diagnosing SOS.
3. Pretransplantation assessment:
   - History of risk factors for morbidity and mortality related to SCT.
   - History of co-morbidities, particularly hepatitis C infection.
4. Assessment during stem cell transplantation:
   - Right upper quadrant pain.
   - Increased abdominal girth.
   - Weight gain, fluid retention.
   - Thrombocytopenia with increased platelet requirements.
   - Jaundice
   - Psychological distress
   - Renal dysfunction secondary to intraperitoneal pressure.
   - Hepatic encephalopathy secondary to liver inability to metabolize waste products and the metabolites of drugs (i.e., confusion, lethargy, disorientation).
   - Anxiety, depression, fear of dying.
   - Lung biopsy shows fibrosis, positive staining for TGF-1 or TGF-B1 or increased osteonectin expression (Murase et al., 1995).
   - Broncholavage shows increased hyaluronan.

NURSING CARE AND TREATMENT

1. Maintain fluid and electrolyte balance, strict I & O; daily weights; measure abdominal girth, estimate insensible losses
2. Assess and manage pain using a recognized pain scale.
3. Postural blood pressure and heart rate; assess for peripheral edema.
4. Limit sodium intake; minimize fluids to prevent fluid from entering interstitial spaces, particularly pulmonary fluid; monitor serum sodium levels.
5. Auscultate lung fields for crackles and adventitious breath sounds; assess for decreased chest expansion secondary to possible pulmonary distress.
6. Assess for bleeding after liver biopsies; monitor complete blood count (CBC).
7. Anticipate that confounding symptoms of liver graft versus host disease may obscure diagnosis of SOS.
8. Administer medications specific for SOS (e.g., anticoagulants) if ordered.
9. Use relaxation techniques (e.g., imagery or music therapy) to reduce anxiety.
10. Ensure patient safety, especially for those with encephalopathy.
11. Assess spirituality of patient and support patient in meeting spiritual needs.
12. Prophylactic and treatment measures with ursodiol (UDCA), defibrotide, and low-dose heparin have centered on anticoagulant therapy but have had mixed results in clinical trials (Negrin, 2006; Essel et al., 1998; Strausser & McDonald, 1999; Bearman et al., 1997). The use of type plasminogen activator (tPA) to treat SOS appeared

promising in case studies and small trials, but larger trials determined that these patients typically have thrombocytopenia. tPA heightens bleeding, which prevents its use in a patient at significant risk for bleeding. At that time, further study was halted (Bearman et al., 1997). Other approaches have met with negative or inconsistent results. These include the use of high-dose methylprednisolone (Khoury et al., 2000); transjugular intrahepatic portosystemic shunts (Azoulay et al., 2000), and orthoptic liver transplantation (Dowlati et al., 1995). Defibrotide, initially found to have positive results in compassionate use studies, was further investigated by Richardson and colleagues (2002) in a multiinstitutional study (N = 88). No adverse events related to the treatment were noted, and SOS resolved in 36% of high-risk patients studied. More recently this agent has been tested as a prophylactic agent in combination with low-dose heparin in an historically controlled study (N = 52) (Chalandon et al., 2004). None of the patients in the treatment arm developed SOS or adverse effects related to this therapy. The researchers encourage further study in randomized controlled trials.

13. Immediate nursing interventions:
    - Twice daily weights on same scale.
    - Measure abdominal girth every shift.
    - Strict intake and output measurement.
    - Monitor serum electrolytes, liver function enzymes, bilirubin, coagulation studies, and complete blood counts.
    - Assess pain with standardized pain scale used by institution.
    - Assess for level of consciousness.
    - Assess for all classic signs and symptoms of SOS per institutional protocol.
    - Offer emotional support to patient and family.
14. Anticipated physician prescriptions and interventions:
    - Possible anticoagulant therapy.
    - Possible diuretic therapy.
    - Possible new agents being studied in clinical trials.
15. Ongoing nursing assessment, monitoring, and interventions:
    - Level of consciousness.
    - Pain
    - Nutrition
    - Shortness of breath, tachypnea due to effusions, diminished breath sounds, and/or crackles.
    - Psychological assessments (SOS carries a high level of morbidity and morality).
    - Interact with family with respite care and emotional support.
    - Assess for possibility of concomitant liver graft versus host disease.
    - Bleeding

EVIDENCE-BASED PRACTICE UPDATES

Few advances have been made in the prevention and treatment of SOS. Evidenced-based practice includes identification of risk factors before SCT, knowledge of the cardinal presenting symptoms of SOS, and exquisite assessment and symptom management throughout the SCT process. Supportive care remains the standard approach for treating SCT with SOS (Kumar et al., 2003).

1. Transjugular intrahepatic portosystemic shunts are beneficial for some patients with refractory disease (Schoppmeyer et al., 2006).
2. Mutations in PML nuclear body protein Sp110 have been seen in VOD (Roscioli et al., 2006).

3. The incidence of VOD in children after hematopoietic stem cell transplantation is 11% (Cesaro et al., 2005), and this rate increases if the child's regimen includes busulfan.

TEACHING AND EDUCATION

Pretransplantation evaluation: *Rationale:* You will be asked if you have a history of liver disease such as hepatitis, alcoholism, or other insults to the liver. Some the laboratory tests you will have, such as your liver function tests, may show that you have some liver damage. If there are concerns, your SCT transplant team will order more tests for you. Most patients who go on to SCT and experience SOS respond spontaneously. You may be given some medications for SOS that have been studied in clinical trials.

Management of ascites: *Rationale:* You will be placed on a low-salt diet and receive concentrated fluids to reduce bodily fluids and ascites. Your abdominal girth and weight will be measured daily to determine the status of the ascites.

Comfort: *Rationale:* You will be made as comfortable as possible during your STC. You will be evaluated for painful conditions and given medication or other comfort measures, such as body positioning. Be sure to report any discomfort as soon as possible; don't be hesitant or ashamed.

Nutritional support: *Rationale:* You may need nutrition by IV to maintain your nutritional needs.

Coping: *Rationale:* You and your family will receive as much information as possible about the course of SOS so that you feel informed. This information will help you cope during this time.

Anticipated patient and family questions and possible answers:

When does SOS occur, and how long will it last? *Rationale:* SOS occurs within the first 2 weeks after your STC. The signs and symptoms are weight gain, changes in your liver function tests, swelling in your abdomen, possible pain, nausea and vomiting, jaundice, and loss of appetite. SOS has to run its course, which can be 1 to 2 weeks. Mild symptoms could continue after you are discharged from the hospital. You will be evaluated frequently and given supportive care.

What are my chances of survival if I have SOS? *Rationale:* This is an important question to ask your physician. SOS can be mild or severe. Watching for symptoms of SOS and receiving supportive care are important treatment measures. Managing SOS through relief of swelling, pain management, nutritional support, and fluid and salt restrictions, as well as treatments by your physician, are part of supportive care.

When I recover from SOS, can it recur? *Rationale:* Generally SOS occurs in the first several weeks after BMT. Once your liver has recovered, SOS will not return. You may have other liver problems, such as chronic GVHD, that will be monitored and treated.

NURSING DIAGNOSES

1. **Excess fluid volume** related to abdominal ascites
2. **Acute pain** related to right upper quadrant tenderness

3. **Imbalance nutrition: less than body requirements** related to nausea, vomiting, and anorexia
4. **Disturbed body image** related to jaundice and edema
5. **Risk for deficient fluid volume** related to thrombocytopenia

EVALUATION AND DESIRED OUTCOMES

1. Fluid volume will return to baseline.
2. Weight and abdominal girth will return to baseline.
3. Nausea, vomiting, and anorexia will diminish with medication or appropriate nutritional support.
4. Jaundice will resolve.
5. Pain will be diminished by analgesics and comfort measures.
6. The lungs will remain clear on auscultation.
7. The patient and family will understand all support care measures.
8. The patient and family will obtain emotional support throughout the course of the syndrome, especially if the hepatic SOS progresses to a severe or potentially fatal state.

DISCHARGE PLANNING AND FOLLOW-UP CARE

The patient will need the following:
• Ongoing assessment of liver function tests.
• Short-term nutritional support to prevent weight loss and to normalize fluids and electrolytes.
• Referrals to support groups near home.
  Important phone numbers and ways to contact the health care team.
• Follow-up transplant care, including weekly or more frequent visits to the referring care physician for 3 months and then annual visits to the transplant physician and weekly laboratory tests to assess healing. The tests will include liver function tests, electrolytes, CBC, and other tests if problems such as graft versus host disease are a factor.

REVIEW QUESTIONS

QUESTIONS

1. **Hepatic SOS is a complication associated with SCT. This syndrome is best described as:**
   1. Similar to hepatitis B.
   2. An autoimmune dysfunction of the liver as a result of the preparative regimen for SCT.
   3. Liver damage characterized by extensive damage to the sinusoidal cells, resulting in widespread damage to the sinusoidal epithelial lining.
   4. Similar to chronic graft versus host disease.

2. **A risk factor associated with the development of SOS is/are:**
   1. Multiple pregnancies
   2. Frequent red blood cell transfusions
   3. Aged donors
   4. Hepatitis C

3. **The initial signs of SOS are most often evidenced by:**
   1. Computed tomography (CT) scans, liver biopsy, and jaundice.
   2. Hepatomegaly, sudden weight gain, and hyperbilirubinemia greater than 2 mg/dL.
   3. Liver biopsy, weight loss, and hair loss.
   4. Presence of liver graft versus host disease.

4. **A drug that has had some success in the treatment of SOS is:**
   1. Busulfan
   2. Low-dose heparin
   3. Amphotericin B
   4. Aspirin

5. **The optimal time to evaluate an SCT patient for the possible occurrence of SOS is:**
   1. At the time of the 3 day, 72 hour,post-transplantation evaluation
   2. At the start of conditioning regimens
   3. Approximately 5 to 10 days after SCT
   4. During the pretransplantation evaluation

6. **The initial symptoms of SOS manifest:**
   1. 70 to 80 days after SCT
   2. 1 year after SCT
   3. Approximately 10 to 12 days after SCT
   4. In an unpredictable sequence

7. **Which of the following is an accepted diagnostic criteria scale for SOS:**
   1. Karnofsky score
   2. Baltimore Criteria
   3. International Stem Cell Transplant Group
   4. Emory Cancer Center Criteria Tool

8. **Your SCT patient asks you whether he can expect SOS as a long-term adverse effect of SCT. You tell him:**
   1. "Long-term SOS manifests itself 100 days after SCT."
   2. "SOS is not a long-term complication of SCT."
   3. "If you have SOS as a long-term effect, you may need a liver transplant."
   4. "If you have symptoms of jaundice, nausea and vomiting a year after SCT, you likely have SOS."

9. **You are caring for an SCT recipient who complains of severe right upper quadrant pain associated with SOS. You tell him:**
   1. "You can't have pain medications, because your liver is damaged."
   2. "You can have acetaminophen, but you can't have an opioid."
   3. "Your pain is not caused by SOS but by skin GVHD."
   4. "I can give you something to ease your pain. How would you rate your pain on a scale of 0 to 10?"

10. **Which of the following tests is used to confirm a diagnosis of SOS:**
    1. Hepatitis C
    2. Fasting blood sugar
    3. Transjugular liver biopsy
    4. Doppler studies

ANSWERS

1. *Answer: 3*
   Rationale: The exact cause of SOS is unclear. Hepatic SOS appears to result from release of tumor necrosis factor, which in turn triggers coagulation and consequent obstruction of hepatic sinusoids and venules.

2. *Answer: 4*
   Rationale: A history of hepatitis C has been implicated in the development of SOS. Although the reason is unclear, major research studies have documented hepatitis C as a risk factor.

3. *Answer: 2*
   Rationale: These are the classic symptoms of SOS. CT scans are not useful for diagnosis, liver biopsies are performed after symptoms occur, and liver GVHD, although it may mimic GVHD, does not indicate SOS.

4. *Answer: 2*
   Rationale: Low-dose heparin interferes with the clotting cascade and may lessen SOS. Busulfan is used in conditioning regimens for SCT. Amphotericin is an antifungal agent and is not appropriate for SOS treatment. Aspirin is contraindicated in SCT recipients because it would put the patient at risk for bleeding.

5. *Answer: 4*
   Rationale: The risk of SOS is determined when the patient is evaluated for SCT. Patients with significant risk factors may not meet the criteria for SCT.

6. *Answer: 3*
    Rationale: SOS manifests itself in a predictable manner and occurs within the first 2 weeks after SCT. Only rarely is SOS a long-term complication of SCT.

7. *Answer: 2*
    Rationale: The Baltimore Criteria is an accepted scale. The Karnofsky scale measures patient performance status. The International Stem Cell Transplant Group and the Emory Cancer Center Criteria Tool do not exist.

8. *Answer: 2*
    Rationale: SOS manifests itself approximately 10 to 12 days after SCT. It is not a long-term complication. The occurrence of jaundice, nausea, and vomiting as long-term complications of SCT can have several causes. Liver transplants are not the first-line treatment for VOD.

9. *Answer: 4*
    Rationale: Right upper quadrant pain is a common adverse effect of VOD. Pain management with appropriate analgesics (acetaminophen, opioids) is warranted. Pain associated with skin GVHD is localized to the affected areas.

10. *Answer: 3*
    Rationale: A transjugular liver biopsy is the most reliable test for SOS. A positive hepatitis C test is not indicative of SOS but is a possible risk factor. Abdominal CT scans are not reliable for diagnosing SOS.

REFERENCES

Azoulay, D., Castaing, D., & Lemoine, A., et al. (2000). Transjugular intrahepatic portosystemic shunt (TIPS) for severe veno-occlusive disease of the liver following bone marrow transplantation. *Bone Marrow Transplantation, 25*:987-992.

Bearman, S. I. (1995). The syndrome of hepatic veno-occlusive disease after marrow transplantation. *Blood, 85*:3005-3020.

Bearman, S. I., Lee, J. L., & Baron, A. E., et al. (1997). Treatment of hepatic veno-occlusive disease with recombinant human tissue plasminogen activator and heparin in 42 marrow transplant patients. *Blood, 89*:1501-1506.

Berk, P. D., Popper, H., & Krueger, G. R., et al. (1979). Veno-occlusive disease of the liver after bone marrow transplantation: Possible association with graft versus host disease. *Annals of Internal Medicine, 90*:158-164.

Carreras, E., Bertz, H., & Arcese, W., et al. (1998). Incidence and outcome of hepatic veno-occlusive disease after blood or marrow transplantation: A prospective cohort study of the European Group for Blood and Marrow Transplantation, European Group for Blood and Marrow Transplantation Chronic Leukemia Working Party. *Blood, 9*:3599-3604.

Cesaro, S., Pillon, M., & Talenti, E., et al. (2005). A prospective survey on incidence, risk factors and therapy of hepatic veno-occlusive disease in children after hematopoietic stem cell transplantation. *Haematologica, 90*(10):1396-1404.

Chalandon, Y., Roosnek, E., & Mermillod, B., et al. (2004). Prevention of veno-occlusive disease with defribtide after allogeneic stem cell transplantation. *Biology of Blood and Marrow Transplantation, 10*:347-354.

Datta, D. V., Khuroo, M. S., & Mattocks, A. R., et al. (1978). Herbal medicines and veno-occlusive disease in India. *Postgraduate Medicine Journal, 54*:511-515.

De Jonge, M. E., Huitema, A. D., & Beijnen, J. H., et al. (2006). High exposures to bioactivated cyclophosphamide are related to the occurrence of veno-occlusive disease of the liver following high-dose chemotherapy. *British Journal of Cancer, 94*(9):1226-1230.

DeLeve, I. D., Schulman, H. M., & McDonald, G. M. (2002). Toxic injury to hepatic sinusoids: Sinusoidal obstructive syndrome (veno-occlusive disease). *Seminars in Liver Disease, 22:*27-41.

Dowlati, A., Honore, P., & Damas, P., et al. (1995). Hepatic rejection after orthotopic liver transplantation for hepatic veno-occlusive disease or graft versus host disease. *Transplantation, 60:*106-109.

El-Sayed, M. H., El-Haddad, A., & Fahmy, O. A., et al. (2004). Liver disease is a major cause of mortality following allogeneic bone-marrow transplantation. *European Journal of Gastroenterology and Hepatology, 16:*1347-1354.

Erturk, S. M., Mortele, K. J., & Binkert, C. A., et al. (2006). CT features of hepatic veno-occlusive disease and hepatic graft-versus-host disease in patients after hematopoietic stem cell transplant. *American Journal of Roentgenology, 186*(6):1497-1501.

Essel, J. H., Schroeder, M. T., & Harman, G. S., et al. (1998). Ursodiol prophylaxis against hepatic complications of allogeneic bone marrow transplantation. *Annals of Internal Medicine, 112:*975-981.

Fajardo, L. F., & Colby, T. V. (1980). Pathogenesis of veno-occlusive disease. *Archives of Pathology Laboratory Medicine, 104:*584-588.

Gooley, T. A., Rajvanshi, P., & Schoch, G., et al. (2005). Serum bilirubin levels and mortality after myeloablative allogenic hematopoietic cell transplantation. *Hepatology, 41:*345-352.

Helmy, A. (2006). Review article: updates in the pathogenesis and therapy of hepatic sinusoidal obstruction syndrome. *Alimentary Pharmacology & Therapeutics 23*(1):11-25.

Jacobs, P., Miller, J. L., & Uys, C. J. (1979). Fatal veno-occlusive disease after chemotherapy, whole body irradiation and bone marrow transplantation for refractory acute leukemia. *South African Medical Journal. Suid-Afrikaanse Tydskrif Vir Geneeskunde. 55*(1):5-10.

Kapustay, P. M., & Buchsel, P. C. (2000). Process, complications, and management of peripheral stem cell transplantation. In P. C. Buchsel, & P. M. Kapustay (Eds), *Stem cell transplantation: A clinical textbook* (pp. 5.3-5.28). Pittsburgh: Oncology Nursing Press.

Khoury, H., Adkins, D., & Brown, R., et al. (2000). Does early treatment with high-dose methylprednisolone alter the course of hepatic regimen-related toxicity? *Bone Marrow Transplantation, 25:*737-743.

Kumar, S., DeLeve, L. D., & Kamath, P. S., et al. (2003). Hepatic veno-occlusive disease (sinusoidal obstruction syndrome) after hematopoietic stem cell transplantation. *Mayo Clinic Proceedings, 78:*589-598.

McDonald, G. B., Hinds, M., & Fisher, L. B. (1993). Veno-occlusive disease of the liver and multiorgan failure after bone marrow transplantation: A cohort study of solid tumors and lymphomas. *Annals of Internal Medicine, 118:*255.

Murase, T., Anscher, M. S., & Petros, W. P., et al. (1995). Changes in plasma transforming growth factor beta in response to high-dose chemotherapy for stage II breast cancer: Possible implications for prevention of hepatic veno-occlusive disease and pulmonary drug toxicity. *Bone Marrow Transplantation, 15:*173-178.

Negrin, R. S., & Bonis, P. A. L. (2006). Pathogenesis and clinical features of hepatic veno-occlusive disease following hematopoietic cell transplantation. Retrieved September 7, 2006, from http://www.utdol.com/utd/content/topic.do?topickey=hcell_tr/4965&type=a&selectedtitle=2~17.

Richardson, P. G., Murakami, C., & Jin, Z., et al. (2002). Multi-institutional use of defibrotide in 88 patients after stem cell transplantation with severe veno-occlusive disease and multisystem organ failure: response without significant toxicity in a high-risk population and factors predictive of outcome. *Blood. 100*(13):4337-4343.

Roscioli, T., Cliffe, S. T., & Bloch, D. B., et al. (2006). Mutations in the gene encoding the PML nuclear body protein Sp110 are associated with immunodeficiency and hepatic veno-occlusive disease. *Nature Genetics, 38*(6):620-622.

Schoch, C., Kern, W., & Kohlmann, A., et al. (2005). Acute myeloid leukemia with a complex aberrant karyotype is a distinct biological entity characterized by genomic imbalances and a specific gene expression profile. *Genes, Chromosomes, & Cancer. 43*(3):227-238.

Schoppmeyer, K., Lange, T., & Wittekind, C., et al. (2006). TIPS for veno-occlusive disease following stem cell transplantation. *Zeitschrift fur Gastroenterologie, 44*(6):483-486.

Sebagh, M., Debette, M., & Samuel, D., et al. (1999). "Silent" presentation of veno-occlusive disease after liver transplantation as part of the process of cellular rejection with endothelial predilection. *Hepatology, 30:*1144-1150.

Strasser, S. I., & McDonald, G. B. (1999). Gastrointestinal and hepatic complications. In E. D. Thomas, K. G. Blume, & S. J. Forman (Eds), *Hematopoietic cell transplantation* (pp. 627-658). (2nd ed.). Malden, MA: Blackwell Science.

Tandon, B. N., Tandon, H. D., & Tandon, R. K, et al. (1976). An epidemic of venule occlusive disease in central India. *Lancet, 2:*271-272.

Willmot, F. C., & Robertson, G. W. (1920). Senecio disease, or cirrhosis of the liver due to Senecio poisoning. *Lancet, 2:*848-849.

Spinal Cord Compression

CHRISTINE MIASKOWSKI

PATHOPHYSIOLOGICAL MECHANISMS

Spinal cord compression (SCC) is an oncologic emergency that requires prompt diagnosis and treatment. Delays in diagnosis result in loss of mobility, loss of bladder function, and decreased survival. Therefore a recent onset of back pain in a patient with cancer should suggest a diagnosis of SCC until it is ruled out (Prasad & Schiff, 2005; Abrahm, 2004).

SCC is a compression of the thecal sac by a tumor in the epidural space, at the level of either the spinal cord or the cauda equina (Abrahm, 2004). Most cancers cause SCC as a result of metastatic disease to the vertebral column. The spinal cord can be compressed as a result of direct extension from a metastatic lesion in the vertebral body. In addition, frank bone collapse can occur, adding to the compression. Some patients, particularly those with lymphoma or retroperitoneal tumors, may develop SCC from tumors that grow through the intravertebral foramen and compress the spinal cord without involving the vertebrae (Prasad & Schiff, 2005; Abrahm, 2004; Gabriel & Schiff, 2004; Schiff, 2003).

Injury to the spinal cord from direct extension of a tumor or metastatic disease occurs as a result of ischemia and edema. In response to tissue injury and hypoxia, prostaglandins and vascular endothelial growth factors are released. The release of these inflammatory substances results in increased vascular permeability and vasogenic edema. Subsequent edema and hypoxia results in neuronal injury, ischemia, and infarction. Once the spinal cord infarcts, neurologic damage is permanent (Prasad & Schiff, 2005; Abrahm, 2004; Gabriel & Schiff, 2004; Schiff, 2003).

EPIDEMIOLOGY AND ETIOLOGY

SCC occurs in 2.5% to 5% of adult patients with terminal cancer. However, the cumulative incidence of SCC in adults declines with age. The prevalence of SCC in children ranges from 4% to 5.5%. The prevalence of SCC varies with the site of the cancer; 15% to 20% of cases are seen in patients with prostate, breast, and lung cancers. About 5% to 10% of cases occur in patients with non-Hodgkin's lymphoma, multiple myeloma, or renal cancer (Abrahm, 2004; Klimo & Schmidt, 2004).

RISK PROFILE

- Cancers of the breast, prostate, lung, kidney, and thyroid; non-Hodgkin's lymphoma, myeloma, sarcoma, lymphoma, leukemia, neuroblastoma, chordoma, neurofibroma, meningioma, glioma, epidermoid, and gastrointestinal cancers; rare in retinoblastoma (Chang et al., 2006).
- Cancer treatment that leads to lytic lesions in the vertebrae; development of a granulomatous mass from intrathecal morphine (Miele et al., 2006).

Table 43-1	MEDIAN SURVIVAL AFTER SCC
Cancer Diagnosis	**Median Survival (Months)**
Lymphoma	6.7
Multiple myeloma	6.4
Breast cancer	5
Prostate cancer	4
Lung cancer	1.5

Modified from Abrahm, J. L. (2004). Assessment and treatment of patients with malignant spinal cord compression. *Journal of Supportive Oncology*, 2(5):377-388, 391.

PROGNOSIS

Patients with SCC that is localized to a single site have a better prognosis. Median survival according to tumor type is shown in Table 43-1. A positive correlation exists between preoperative motor status and treatment outcomes. For example, 75% to 100% of patients who are ambulatory at the time of diagnosis are ambulatory after treatment. In contrast, only 14% to 35% of paraparetic and 15% of paralyzed patients regain useful function after treatment for SCC. Loss of sphincter control at the time of diagnosis is associated with a poor prognosis (Schiff, 2003).

PROFESSIONAL ASSESSMENT CRITERIA (PAC)

1. General pain assessment parameters include onset, description, location, severity, aggravating and relieving factors, previous treatments and effectiveness, and associated symptoms. Pain is the most frequent initial symptom of SCC. At the time of diagnosis, 83% to 95% of patients have had pain for a median of 8 weeks.
   - Pain is usually localized to the involved spinal segment.
   - Characteristics of the localized pain include a gradual onset (usually) and an increase in pain with movement, coughing, sneezing, or the Valsalva maneuver.
   - Pain may be worse after a period of lying down.
   - Pain can be radicular in nature.
   - Vertebral tenderness can occur over the site of SCC.
   - Neck flexion often produces pain of a local or radicular nature at the site of the lesion.
2. Weakness occurs in 60% to 85% of patients at the time of diagnosis.
   - Approximately two thirds of patients are not ambulatory at the time of diagnosis.
   - Weakness is most severe with thoracic SCC.
   - The pretreatment neurologic status is the most important predictor of function after treatment for SCC.
3. Motor examination includes an evaluation of muscle strength, muscle tone, motor deficits (e.g., ataxia), coordination, abnormal muscle movements, and deep tendon reflexes.
   - Both the upper and lower extremities must be evaluated.
   - Damage to the corticospinal tracts usually results in spasticity, spastic paralysis, hyperreflexia, and a positive Babinski's reflex.

- Damage to the lower motor neurons usually results in hypotonicity, flaccid paralysis, hyporeflexia, and muscular atrophy.
- Any weakness associated with back pain in a patient with cancer requires an evaluation for SCC.

4. Sensory changes occur in 40% to 90% of cases of spinal cord compression. Patients may be less aware of sensory changes than weakness or motor deficits.
   - Assessment should include evaluation of light touch, temperature, pinprick, position, and vibration.
   - Sensory deficits result from pressure on the spinothalamic tracts (STTs). Initial involvement of the anterior STT results in the loss of light touch. Involvement of the lateral STT results in the loss of pain and temperature. Lesions in the posterior columns cause changes in proprioception.

5. Bowel and bladder dysfunction are late signs of SCC. About 50% of patients are catheter dependent at the time of diagnosis.
   - An evaluation of autonomic dysfunction includes rectal and/or bladder anesthesia, constipation, obstipation, encopresis (i.e., fecal incontinence), enuresis (i.e., urinary incontinence), and impotence.
   - Urinary retention is the most common autonomic nervous system dysfunction associated with SCC.
   - Bowel sounds may be diminished or absent.
   - Magnetic resonance imaging (MRI) of spinal segments should be performed regardless of the level of the block. MRI can demonstrate bone metastasis without epidural components, intramedullary metastasis, and leptomeningeal tumors. MRI should image the entire spine, because 33% of patients have multiple lesions. At minimum, the symptomatic area and the thoracic and lumbar spine should be imaged, because asymptomatic cervical lesions are rare (Abdi et al., 2005; Loblaw et al., 2005).

6. CT scan provides valuable information about the vertebral columns and paravertebral structures. It is more sensitive than plain x-ray films and bone scans in distinguishing between benign and malignant lesions. Also, a CT scan is needed to plan the management of SCC.

7. A bone scan is more sensitive than plain x-ray films in detecting SCC. However, it is less sensitive than CT or MRI. A bone scan can show multiple lesions and has a diagnostic accuracy of approximately 66%.

8. Plain x-ray films image collapsed vertebral bodies in 75% of patients.

NURSING CARE AND TREATMENT

1. Administer corticosteroids to reduce edema.
2. Perform pain assessment at least q8hr.
3. Perform motor assessment (strength and movement of upper and lower extremities; deep tendon reflexes).
4. Perform sensory examination (light touch and pinprick).
5. Evaluate for bowel and bladder dysfunction.
6. Assess for ataxia.
7. Administer analgesics to reduce pain.
8. Obtain and assess: CT/MRI for location and degree of SCC.
9. Intake and output (I & O) q4-8hr.
10. Activity as tolerated.
11. Initiate a bowel regimen to prevent opioid-induced constipation.
12. Perform skin assessments if patient's mobility is decreased.
13. Initiate range-of-motion exercises if patient's mobility is decreased.

14. Anticipate the need for antiembolism stockings or sequential compression devices if the patient is on bed rest.
15. Anticipate the need for low-molecular-weight heparin therapy if the patient is on bed rest.
16. Use relaxation techniques to reduce pain and anxiety.
17. Provide a regular diet with sufficient fiber.
18. Provide a referral for rehabilitation to physical therapy and occupational therapy.
19. Provide a referral to the clinical nurse specialist for initiation and maintenance of a bladder program if neurogenic bladder occurs.

EVIDENCE-BASED PRACTICE UPDATES

1. Maintain a high index of suspicion for SCC in an oncology patient who presents with back pain. The most common error in the management of SCC is failure to diagnose this oncologic emergency! It is imperative to diagnose SCC as soon as symptoms occur to prevent permanent neurologic damage.
2. Management of SCC is based on several interrelated factors, including the patient's primary tumor, the level of the SCC, the rapidity of the onset of symptoms, the degree and duration of the blockage, and the patient's general condition.
3. Corticosteroids (e.g., dexamethasone) are used to inhibit the production of prostaglandins, which results in a decrease in edema (Loblaw et al., 2005; Schiff, 2003; Abrahm, 2004; Gabriel & Schiff, 2004; Prasad & Schiff, 2005).
   • The optimal dosing of dexamethasone is not known. A common protocol is a bolus dose of 96 mg or 100 mg administered intravenously, followed by 24 mg given orally QID for 3 days, followed by 48 mg, 32 mg, 16 mg, 4 mg, and 2 mg, each given for 2 days.
4. RT usually is directed at the painful sites and includes ports one or two vertebral bodies above and below the site of SCC. Most treatments are 2500 to 3600 cGy in 10 to 15 fractions. An alternative approach is to administer 800 cGy in 2 fractions 1 week apart (Loblaw et al., 2005; Prasad & Schiff, 2005; Abrahm, 2004; Gabriel & Schiff, 2004; Schiff, 2003). For metastatic SCC in patients with non-small cell lung cancer, administration of 800 cGy for 1 day has been effective (Rades et al., 2006).
5. Laminectomy historically has been used as the initial approach to the treatment of SCC. In recent years, corticosteroids and RT have become the standard treatment for SCC because laminectomy alone or with RT did not show any benefit (Klimo & Schmidt, 2004; Maranzano et al., 2003). Recently, a randomized clinical trial compared the effects of surgery followed by RT to RT alone for the management of SCC. Significantly more patients in the group that had surgery followed by RT were able to walk after treatment (84%) than in the group that had RT alone (57%) (Patchell et al., 2005).
6. A current animal study has shown that a prostaglandin E2 receptor subtype agonist increases blood flow to the nerve roots in cauda equina compression (Sekiguchi et al., 2006), possibly indicating a new treatment for SCC in humans.

TEACHING AND EDUCATION

Pain: *Rationale*: Report any changes in the intensity or location of your pain. The pain will decrease in intensity after administration of steroids and the start of RT. Ask for pain medication.

Weakness: *Rationale*: Report any changes in the strength or mobility of your arms or legs to the nurse immediately.

Constipation/fecal incontinence: *Rationale*: It is important to tell the nurse if you notice any changes in your ability to have a bowel movement.

Urinary retention/incontinence: *Rationale*: It is important to tell the nurse if you cannot urinate or become incontinent.

Tests and procedures: *Rationale*: You may need x-ray films or CT or MRI scans of you back to determine where the tumor is pressing on your spinal cord.

Treatments: *Rationale*: You will be treated with steroids to reduce the swelling in your spinal cord. In addition, you will receive RT to shrink the tumor.

Maintenance of mobility and rehabilitation: *Rationale*: If weakness develops, it will be important for you to maintain your mobility. You will need to do routine exercises to maintain the strength in your upper and lower extremities. After your treatment, you will be referred to physical therapy and occupational therapy as needed.

NURSING DIAGNOSES

1. **Chronic pain** related to SCC
2. **Impaired physical mobility** related to SCC
3. **Disturbed sensory perception** related to SCC
4. **Constipation** related to decreased mobility, opioid analgesics, and/or SCC
5. **Impaired urinary elimination** related to SCC

EVALUATION AND DESIRED OUTCOMES

1. SCC will be diagnosed and treated within 24 hours.
2. The patient will know the signs and symptoms of SCC and present for an assessment as soon as symptoms occur.
3. Baseline neurologic functioning will be maintained or restored after treatment.
4. The patient's pain will be well controlled with analgesics and other treatments (i.e., the worst pain will be less than 4 on a 0 to 10 scale).
5. The patient will report regular bowel movements and good bowel motility with or without the use of a routine bowel regimen.
6. A bladder program will be established immediately in patients with a neurogenic bladder and the patient will be free of the problems of distention, overflow, or incontinence.
7. The patient will be free of pressure ulcers.

DISCHARGE PLANNING AND FOLLOW-UP CARE

- Prescribe a pain medication regimen.
- If the patient has residual neurologic deficits, the following resources may be needed:
  - Physical and occupational therapy referrals to evaluate the home for modifications and safety.
  - Wheelchair, cushion, transfer board, and instructions for family on transfer techniques.
  - Hospital bed.
  - Bladder management program and equipment.
  - Bowel management program and equipment.
  - Skin care regimen and equipment.

- Instruct patient to call the health care provider immediately about any changes in pain or mobility.
- Follow-up appointment at physician's office 1 to 2 weeks after discharge.
- Home health nursing visits for assessment of neurologic status and pain, as well as effectiveness of bowel, bladder, and skin care protocols.
- Consider the need for referral to hospice care, depending on the patient's prognosis.

REVIEW QUESTIONS

QUESTIONS

1. The most common site of spinal cord compression is:
   1. Thoracic area
   2. Lumbosacral area
   3. Cervical area
   4. It occurs equally in all three areas.

2. The most common error clinicians make with regard to SCC is:
   1. Use of the incorrect diagnostic test.
   2. Failure to diagnose SCC.
   3. Prescription of incorrect treatment.
   4. Lack of follow-up care.

3. The most frequent initial symptom of SCC is:
   1. Constipation
   2. Weakness
   3. Pain
   4. Shortness of breath

4. SCC that impinges on the corticospinal tracts would cause all of the following symptoms *except*:
   1. Spasticity
   2. Hyperreflexia
   3. Positive Babinski's sign
   4. Atrophy

5. The posterior columns of the spinal cord transmit which sensation:
   1. Pain
   2. Temperature
   3. Light touch
   4. Proprioception

6. The test that provides the *least* information to assist the clinician in making a diagnosis of SCC is:
   1. Plain radiograph
   2. Bone scan
   3. CT scan
   4. MRI

7. Mrs. Smith, who is 65 years old, has a history of metastatic breast cancer.

She comes to the office for a routine follow-up visit. She tells you that for the past 2 weeks she has had pain in the middle of her back that is increasing in intensity everyday. Based on this report, you would:
   1. Schedule a follow-up visit in 1 week.
   2. Perform a physical examination and prescribe an MRI.
   3. Prescribe an analgesic medication.
   4. Tell her that her symptoms are most likely the result of overactivity.

8. Mrs. Smith is diagnosed with SCC in the fifth and sixth thoracic vertebrae. Her treatment plan will include all of the following *except*:
   1. Corticosteroids
   2. Radiation therapy
   3. Analgesic medications
   4. Systemic chemotherapy

9. The estimated incidence of SCC caused by cancer is:
   1. Less than 1%
   2. 5%
   3. 15%
   4. 25%

10. Which signs and symptoms of SCC are most indicative of advanced compression:
   1. Severe pain
   2. Numbness and tingling
   3. Weakness
   4. Bowel and bladder dysfunction

ANSWERS

1. *Answer: 1*
   Rationale: In about 70% of patients, SCC occurs in the thoracic area; in 20% it occurs in the lumbosacral area; and in 10% it occurs in the cervical area.

2. *Answer: 2*
Rationale: The most common error in the management of SCC is failure to diagnose this oncologic emergency.

3. *Answer: 3*
Rationale: Pain is the initial symptom of SCC in 83% to 95% of patients.

4. *Answer: 4*
Rationale: The corticospinal tracts conduct impulses from the brain to the motor neurons in the ventral grey matter of the spinal cord. Damage to these tracts results in a loss of control over voluntary movements.

5. *Answer: 4*
Rationale: The posterior columns are involved in the transmission of the sensation of our body in space (i.e., proprioception).

6. *Answer: 1*
Rationale: Plain radiographs are falsely negative in 17% of patients with SCC. More than 50% of the bone needs to be destroyed before a plain radiograph detects the changes indicative of SCC.

7. *Answer: 2*
Rationale: Pain occurs as the initial symptom of SCC in 83% to 95% of patients. Because undiagnosed SCC can result in severe neurologic deficits, the patient needs a complete physical examination, with emphasis on the neurologic examination, and an appropriate diagnostic workup.

8. *Answer: 4*
Rationale: In most cases, the treatment of SCC focuses on the management of the SCC, not on the underlying tumor.

9. *Answer: 2*
Rationale: The estimated incidence of SCC related to cancer is 2.5% to 5%.

10. *Answer: 4*
Rationale: Bowel and bladder dysfunction are late signs of SCC and indicate that the autonomic nervous system is impaired.

REFERENCES

Abdi, S., Adams, C. I., & Foweraker, K. L., et al. (2005). Metastatic spinal cord syndromes: Imaging appearances and treatment planning. *Clinical Radiology, 60*(6):637-647.

Abrahm, J. L. (2004). Assessment and treatment of patients with malignant spinal cord compression. *Journal of Supportive Oncology, 2*(5):377-388, 391; discussion, 391–373, 398, 401.

Chang, C. Y., Hung, G. Y., & Hsu, W. M., et al. (2006). Retinoblastoma with spinal recurrence presenting as spinal cord compression. *Journal of the Formosan Medical Association, 105*(6):497-502.

Gabriel, K., & Schiff, D. (2004). Metastatic spinal cord compression by solid tumors. *Seminars in Neurology, 24*(4):375-383.

Klimo, P., Jr., & Schmidt, M. H. (2004). Surgical management of spinal metastases. *Oncologist, 9*(2):188-196.

Loblaw, D. A., Perry, J., & Chambers, A., et al. (2005). Systematic review of the diagnosis and management of malignant extradural spinal cord compression: The Cancer Care Ontario Practice Guidelines Initiative's Neuro-Oncology Disease Site Group. *Journal of Clinical Oncology, 23*(9):2028-2037.

Maranzano, E., Trippa, F., & Chirico, L., et al. (2003). Management of metastatic spinal cord compression. *Tumori, 89*(5):469-475.

Miele, V. J., Price, K. O., & Bloomfield, S., et al. (2006). A review of intrathecal morphine therapy related granulomas (review). *European Journal of Pain, 10*(3):251-261.

Patchell, R. A., Tibbs, P. A., & Regine, W. F., et al. (2005). Direct decompressive surgical resection in the treatment of spinal cord compression caused by metastatic cancer: A randomised trial. *Lancet, 366*(9486):643-648.

Prasad, D., & Schiff, D. (2005). Malignant spinal cord compression. *Lancet Oncology, 6*(1):15-24.

Rades, D., Staplers, L. J., & Schulte, R., et al. (2006). Defining the appropriate radiotherapy regimen for metastatic spinal cord compression in non-small cell lung cancer patients. *European Journal of Cancer, 42*(8):1052-1056.

Schiff, D. (2003). Spinal cord compression. *Neurologic Clinics, 21*(1):67-86, viii.

Sekiguchi, M., Konno, S., & Kikuchi, S. (2006). Effects on improvement of blood flow in the chronically compressed cauda equina: Comparison between a selective prostaglandin E receptor (EP4) agonist and a prostaglandin E1 derivate. *Spine, 31*(8):869-872.

Spiritual Distress in People with Cancer

MARTHA MERAVIGLIA • CAROL D. GASKAMP • REBECCA R. SUTTER

DEFINITIONS AND CHARACTERISTICS

From the earliest associations of nursing with religious orders to the emerging field of parish nursing, nurses, especially oncology nurses, have recognized the importance of spirituality in health and healing. Assessment of spirituality beyond knowing the patient's denominational affiliation is now considered an expected aspect of care in health care facilities accredited by The Joint Commission (TJC) (LaPierre, 2003, Staten, 2003).

Spirituality refers to the experiences and expressions of one's spirit in a unique and dynamic process that reflects faith in God or a supreme being; connectedness with oneself, others, nature, or God; and integration of the dimensions of mind, body, and spirit (Meraviglia, 1999 & 2004). The definitions and classifications established by the North American Nursing Diagnosis Association (NANDA) include three diagnoses related to spirituality: *spiritual distress* was introduced in 1978; *readiness for enhanced spiritual well-being* was accepted in 1994; and *risk for spiritual distress* was included in 1998.

An adult diagnosed with a terminal or life-threatening illness, such as cancer, is at risk for spiritual distress. NANDA defines spiritual distress as "the impaired ability to experience and integrate meaning and purpose in life through... connectedness with self, others, art, music, literature, nature, or a power greater than oneself" (NANDA, 2005). Spiritual distress is also referred to in the literature as *spiritual pain, spiritual suffering,* and *spiritual disequilibrium.* A recent analysis of the concept identifies negative consequences of spiritual distress as a false sense of hope, increased somatic complaints and symptom distress, harm to oneself, and suicide (Ackley & Ladwig, 2006; Villagomeza, 2005).

People with cancer who express feelings of impaired meaning and purpose in life, peace, or faith are experiencing spiritual distress. Additional characteristics of spiritual distress include feelings of anger, guilt, and ineffective coping with life events, such as the diagnosis and treatment of cancer (Head & Faul, 2005; NANDA, 2005; Villagomeza, 2005). O'Brien (2003) described other characteristics of spiritual distress as a deep sense of hurt from being separated from God or power greater than oneself, a sense of personal inadequacy before God and humanity; and a pervasive condition of loneliness of the spirit. The presence of these feelings in a person with cancer indicates spiritual distress and warrants a thorough assessment for evidence of negative consequences such as loneliness, social isolation, hopelessness, anxiety, and depression.

Three additional NANDA diagnoses have been added for religiosity, an important component of the care of a person with spiritual distress (NANDA, 2005). NANDA (2005) defines *religiosity* as "the reliance on beliefs and/or participation in the rituals of a particular faith tradition." The three nursing diagnoses are *readiness for enhanced religiosity, risk for impaired religiosity*, and *impaired religiosity*. The oncology nurse needs to differentiate between spiritual distress and impaired religiosity to determine the best plan of care.

RISK PROFILE

Clinical and research findings have identified the following risk factors for the development of spiritual distress in people with cancer (Head & Faul, 2005; NANDA, 2005; Villagomeza, 2005):
- Diagnosis and/or treatment of advanced or recurring cancer.
- Alterations in the usual social support network.
- Conditions that interfere with the person's ability to participate in spiritual or religious practices (e.g., institutionalization, physical impairment).
- Events that lead to the questioning of one's faith.
- Verbalization of interpersonal or emotional suffering.
- Development of cognitive impairment (e.g., confusion, dementia).
- Depression

PROFESSIONAL ASSESSMENT CRITERIA (PAC)

The following assessment criteria indicate spiritual distress and warrant a thorough spiritual assessment (Villagomeza, 2005; McClain-Jacobson et al., 2004; Murray et al., 2004):
- Inability to participate in spiritual or religious practices.
- Expression of frustration, fear, hurt, or doubt.
- Feelings of loneliness and isolation.
- Expression of lack of hope or of feeling that life is not worthwhile.
- Feelings of losing control.
- Verbalization of questions about faith or loss of faith.
- Expression of emotional suffering, such as lack of meaning, guilt, or anger.
- Evidence of anxiety and/or depression.
- Desire for hastened death.
- Suicide ideation.

A guide for assessing spiritual distress is the Brief Assessment of Spiritual Resources and Concerns (Gaskamp et al., 2004). This brief guide is an open-ended interview that helps the nurse determine whether the person is unable to practice spiritual rituals, desires spiritual rituals or support, is questioning his or her faith or experiencing a loss of faith, or expressing suffering, loss of hope, lack of meaning, or the need to find meaning in the midst of suffering (Box 44-1). The questions that make up the assessment open a conversation about spirituality between the nurse and patient and provide for further exploration of spiritual concerns and resources. If the person is cognitively impaired, information may be obtained from a family member or caregiver on the importance of spirituality and rituals, membership in a faith community, and beliefs that might affect health care decisions. Additional spirituality assessment tools are described in Box 44-2.

NURSING CARE AND TREATMENT

Providing spiritual care involves the interpersonal dimension and requires strong communication skills. Nurses need to be aware of their own spiritual histories and beliefs, because their spirituality always affects the care given to patients. Specific guidelines for ethical

| BOX 44-1 | BRIEF ASSESSMENT OF SPIRITUAL RESOURCES AND CONCERNS |

Instructions: Use the following questions as an interview guide with the person with cancer (or the caregiver if the person is unable to communicate).
- Does your religion/spirituality provide comfort or serve as a source of stress? (Ask the person to explain in what ways spirituality is a comfort or stressor.)
- Do you have any religious or spiritual beliefs that might conflict with health care or affect health care decisions? (Ask the person to identify any conflicts.)
- Do you belong to a supportive church, congregation, or faith community? (Ask the person how the faith community is supportive.)
- Do you have any practices or rituals that help you express your spiritual or religious beliefs? (Ask the person to identify or describe these practices.)
- Do you have any spiritual needs you would like someone to address? (Ask the person what those needs are and if referral to a spiritual professional is desired.)
- How can we (health care providers) help you with your spiritual needs or concerns?

Modified from Meyer, C. (2003). How effectively are nurse educators preparing students to provide spiritual care? *Nurse Educator, 28*(4):185-190; and Koenig, H. G. (2002). *Spirituality in patient care: Why, how, when, what?* Philadelphia: Templeton Foundation Press.

| BOX 44-2 | SPIRITUAL ASSESSMENT TOOLS |

Four Basic Content Areas for a Spiritual History (Koenig, 2002)
- Religion or spirituality as a way to cope with illness, or a source of stress.
- Member of supportive spiritual community.
- Spiritual concerns or questions.
- Spiritual beliefs that might influence health care.

Five Categories for Assessing Spiritual Needs (LaPierre, 2003)
- Capacity to love and be loved.
- Search for meaning, purpose, truth, and balance.
- Performing spiritual practices or rituals.
- Experience of transcendence, awe, or fear.
- Evil as the experience of the opposite of how spirituality is usually defined.

(Meyer, 2003)
- Religion/spirituality as comfort or cause of stress.
- Beliefs that might conflict with medical care or affect medical decisions.
- Membership in a supportive community.
- Spiritual needs someone should address.
- Practices that help express spiritual beliefs.

Spiritual Assessments Required in All Settings (Staten, 2003)
- What provides the patient with strength and hope.
- The patient's use of prayer.
- How the patient expresses spirituality.
- The patient's philosophy of life.
- Spiritual or religious support desired.
- Name of a spiritual professional.
- Meaning of suffering.
- Meaning of dying.
- Spiritual goals.
- Role of place of worship in the patient's life.
- How faith helps in coping with illness.

Continued

| BOX 44-2 | SPIRITUAL ASSESSMENT TOOLS–cont'd |

- What keeps the patient going day to day.
- What helps the patient get through the health care experience.
- How illness has affected the patient's and family's life.

Spiritual Assessment Approaches (Post et al., 2000)*
- HOPE: Sources of hope; role of organized religion; personal spirituality and practices; effects on care and decision making.
- FICA: Faith and beliefs; importance of spirituality in one's life; spiritual community support; how the person wants spirituality addressed.
- SPIRIT: Spiritual belief system; personal spirituality; integration with spiritual community; ritualized practices and restrictions; implications for care; terminal events planning.
- Single question history: "What role does spirituality or religion play in your life?"

Dimensions of Assessment (Taylor, 2002)
- Experience of God or Transcendence.
- Spirit-enhancing practices or rituals.
- Involvement in a spiritual community.
- Sense of meaning.
- Connectedness to self and others, giving and receiving love.
- Sources of hope and strength.
- Links between spirituality and health.

Topics for a Spiritual Assessment Interview (Wilkinson, 2001)
- Religious practices: What practices are important and how illness has interfered with religious practices.
- Faith: Whether faith is important and helpful; what the health care provider can do to help older adults carry out their faith.
- Referral to spiritual professional desired.
- Concept of "God" or power greater than oneself.
- Purpose and meaning in life.
- Sources of hope and strength.
- Religious practices and rituals.
- Perception of connection between health and spiritual beliefs.
- Fear of loneliness, solitude, or alienation.

*The author notes that none of these approaches has undergone rigorous psychometric testing.
  From Koenig, H. G. (2002). *Spirituality in patient care: Why, how, when, and what*. Philadelphia: Templeton Press; LaPierre, L. L. (2003). JCAHO safeguards spiritual care. *Holistic Nursing Practice, 17*(4):219; Meyer, C. L. (2003). How effectively are nurse educators preparing students to provide spiritual care? *Nurse Educator*, 28(4):185-190; Post, S. G. (2000). Physicians and patient spirituality: Professional boundaries, competency, and ethics. *Annals of Internal Medicine, 132*, 578-583. Staten, P. (2003). Spiritual assessment required in all settings. *Hospital Peer Review, 28*(4):55-57. Retrieved November 20, 2005, from www.galenet.galegroup.com; Taylor, E. J. (2002). *Spiritual care: Nursing theory, research, and practice*. Upper Saddle River, NJ: Prentice Hall; and Wilkinson, J. M. (2001). *Nursing process and critical thinking*. (3rd ed.). Upper Saddle River, NJ: Prentice Hall.

spiritual care include respecting the patient's spiritual needs and practices while maintaining the nurse's integrity. Expertise in spiritual care comes through self-awareness, education, practice, and sensitivity to others' spiritual needs.

Spiritual care is based on a whole-person perspective that views people as having integrated physical, emotional, social, and spiritual dimensions. Alterations in well-being in one dimension always affect the other dimensions. For this reason, nursing interventions directed at the spiritual dimension affect the physical, emotional, and social dimensions (Fig. 44.1). The ultimate goal in providing spiritual care is to support and enhance the patient's well-being and quality of life, which is foundational in oncology nursing

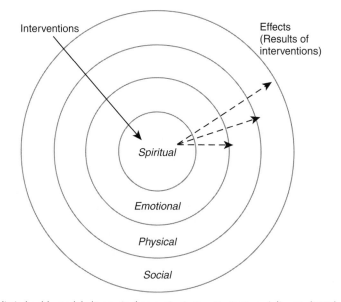

Fig. 44.1 • Holistic health model. (From Gaskamp, C., Sutter, R., & Meraviglia, M. (2004). *Promoting spirituality in the older adult: Evidence-based protocol.* Gerontological Nursing Interventions Research Center, University of Iowa College of Nursing.)

(Meraviglia et al., 2006). Spiritual care interventions for the patient with cancer focus on preventing and/or caring for spiritual distress. Nursing interventions are grouped into two broad categories, active listening and spiritual support, with specific actions directed toward feelings of loneliness, social isolation, hopelessness, anxiety, and depression.

Active Listening

1. Actively listening to the patient enables the nurse to hear, understand, interpret, and synthesize what is being said.
2. The nurse must establish a trusting relationship and provide sufficient time for the patient to interpret his or her own feelings and experiences.
3. *Presence* is an important spiritual care intervention that encompasses much more than physical presence; it includes an interpersonal relationship with sincere and genuine communication. In "being with" the patient, the nurse is fully available to hear and understand the patient's difficulties and/or suffering.
4. Being present requires knowing and being comfortable with oneself and connecting with the person through affirmation, valuing, vulnerability, empathy, serenity, and silence.
5. Caring touch, such as hand holding or touching an arm or shoulder, facilitates communication between the nurse and patient and conveys acceptance, concern, comfort, and reassurance, especially during stressful periods.
6. Nurses should listen for feelings of isolation, rejection, or abandonment by friends or family members, especially since diagnosis of the cancer. Fearfulness of becoming dependent on others or a desire to "suffer in silence" can intensify spiritual distress.
7. Allowing the patient to express his or her sense of meaning and purpose in life minimizes spiritual distress. Encouraging patients to discover the meaning of cancer is

especially beneficial. Nurses can have significant influence on reducing spiritual distress using effective interventions.

8. Oncology nurses can facilitate the search for meaning by asking probing questions, offering additional explanations and, when necessary, reframing maladaptive interpretations of life events.

9. Support groups are helpful for many people with cancer, providing them an opportunity to improve meaning by rethinking and clarifying previous experiences and identifying inner spiritual resources for living through the cancer experience.

10. Cancer support groups have positive benefits, such as successful adaptation to having cancer, reducing anxiety and depression, and improving emotional well-being and overall quality of life.

11. Maintaining strong social support can prevent feelings of social isolation and loneliness, which are known to intensify spiritual distress.

12. Interventions for patients expressing loneliness involve including family members in activities and plans, helping the patient learn new coping strategies, and referral to a mental health provider for individual psychotherapy. Feeling "connected" to other people protects against feelings of isolation and depression.

Spiritual Support

1. Spiritual support is the process of helping patients feel balance and connection with oneself, others, and God or a power greater than oneself. Spiritual support interventions include facilitating forgiveness, instilling hope, and encouraging prayer. If a patient needs more intensive assistance, the nurse can refer the person to pastoral care, a hospital chaplain, or his or her own spiritual support person.

2. Lack of forgiveness can be an overlooked aspect of spiritual distress. Oncology nurses should encourage forgiveness of others. Forgiveness promotes constructive change in a person's life and a sense of renewal, as well as reconciliation with oneself and God or a power greater than oneself.

3. Nursing actions that facilitate forgiveness include being available; listening, especially when the person expresses self-doubt or guilt; providing guidance in the forgiveness of others and self; and offering to contact another person if intensive spiritual support is indicated.

4. Patients with cancer who have spiritual distress may experience anxiety as well as depression. The anxiety and/or depression may be an underlying disorder or a result of untreated or undertreated symptoms associated with cancer, such as pain. Antianxiety and antidepressant medications may be indicated and can take days to weeks to become effective.

5. Effective nonpharmacologic interventions for anxiety and depression include neurosensory stimulation through music, massage therapy, and aromatherapy; referral to a mental health provider; and/or psychotherapy.

6. Feelings of hopelessness can be relieved by nursing actions directed at fostering and/or redefining hope during the cancer experience.

7. Initially the nurse needs to assess the person's source of hope, such as faith in God or a power greater than oneself, a sense of a positive future, or the availability of personal choices.

8. Nurses can explore past experiences and systems of meaning with the patient to understand the person's personal values and to reinforce successful coping strategies.

9. Nurses can also assist patients with spiritual distress to redefine their source of hope and learn new coping strategies for dealing with personal losses, such as loss of health and/or independence.

10. Supporting patients' prayer beliefs and practices can relieve feelings of spiritual distress. Nurses who participate in prayer with patients enhance the patient's trust, self-worth, hope, and well-being.
11. Nursing actions for prayer include offering to pray, meditate, or read spiritual texts, arranging for another spiritual care provider to do so, and respecting a person's time for quietness and prayer.

EVIDENCE-BASED PRACTICE UPDATES

1. People with cancer and their family members want their spiritual needs to be addressed by oncology care providers (Balboni et al., 2007; Taylor & Mamier, 2005).
2. People with cancer feel that their spiritual needs are not supported by religious community or oncology nurses and/or physicians (Balboni et al., 2007).
3. Oncology nurses view spiritual issues as important but report lack of confidence and time constraints as barriers to providing spiritual care to people with cancer (Highfield, 2000; Kristeller et al., 1999).
4. A sense of spiritual well-being has a positive impact on emotional well-being and adjustment to cancer (McClain-Jacobson et al., 2004; McClain et al., 2003).
5. Spiritual distress is associated with poorer health outcomes, including emotional despair, depression, suicidal thoughts, and substance abuse (NCI, 2006b; Hills et al., 2005; Larson & Larson, 2003; Pargament et al., 2001).
6. Having a sense of one's meaning in life has been found to be positively related to emotional well-being and negatively related to the physical symptoms of cancer (Meraviglia, 2004 & 2006).
7. More prayer activities and experiences have been reported to be positively related to emotional well-being in people with lung and breast cancer (Meraviglia, 2004 & 2006).
8. Many cancer survivors report positive psychospiritual outcomes from their experience with having cancer, such as re-evaluating life priorities, greater appreciation of relationships, improved spiritual well-being, and greater life satisfaction (Zebrack & Chesler, 2002; Cordova et al., 2001).

NURSING DIAGNOSES

1. **Spiritual distress** related to feelings of anxiety, hopelessness, loneliness/social isolation, and/or chronic or life-threatening illness
2. **Risk for spiritual distress** related to diagnosis of life-threatening cancer secondary to history of substance abuse, depression, minimal social support, and/or absence of spiritual health
3. **Anxiety** related to situational crisis and spiritual conflict secondary to diagnosis of cancer
4. **Hopelessness** related to feelings of spiritual distress, loss of belief in God or power greater than oneself, negative life review, and/or advanced stage of cancer
5. **Risk for loneliness** related to minimal social support, feelings of abandonment, spiritual suffering, and/or loss of independence

EVALUATION AND DESIRED OUTCOMES

1. Feelings of spiritual distress will be reduced, as evidenced by verbalization of feelings of connectedness with self, others, and/or God or a power greater than oneself.

2. Spiritual well-being will be present, as evidenced by verbalization of meaning and purpose in life, acceptance of health status, expression of forgiveness and/or spiritual wholeness.
3. The patient will express reduced feelings of anxiety and a greater sense of peace and serenity.
4. A sense of hopefulness and concern for others will replace the patient's previous expressions of isolation, a limited future, and diminished personal energy.
5. The patient will experience social and spiritual connectedness to family, friends, health care providers, and/or God or will feel that a power greater than oneself is present.

DISCHARGE PLANNING AND FOLLOW-UP CARE

- Caregiver to assist spiritually with active listening and spiritual support.
- Referral to a spiritual professional, such as a pastor, priest, or rabbi, for ongoing spiritual assessment and support.
- Recommend that patient and caregivers read online information (Cancer Source, 2006; National Cancer Institute, 2006).
- Contact health care provider or spiritual professional if feelings of spiritual distress return.

REVIEW QUESTIONS

QUESTIONS

1. **Spirituality includes which of the following:**
   1. Emotional well-being
   2. Physical health
   3. Connection with oneself
   4. Faith in the environment

2. **Spiritual distress is also known as:**
   1. Spiritual unhappiness
   2. Spiritual pain
   3. Spiritual equilibrium
   4. Spiritual well-being

3. **The impaired ability to experience connectedness with others, nature, God, or oneself is called:**
   1. Spiritual distress
   2. Spiritual unhappiness
   3. Spiritual well-being
   4. Spiritual equilibrium

4. **Negative consequences of experiencing spiritual distress during cancer treatment include all of the following *except:***
   1. Hopeless feelings
   2. Physical complaints
   3. Decreased pain
   4. Depression

5. **People with cancer are at risk for developing spiritual distress because:**
   1. They have to take chemotherapy, which makes them feel very sick.
   2. They have to face their own mortality.
   3. They question the existence of God.
   4. They have to be hospitalized for extended periods.

6. **The recommended tool for assessing the presence of spiritual distress is:**
   1. Brief Assessment of Spiritual Resources and Concerns
   2. Hope Index
   3. The single question, "What role does spirituality or religion play in your life?"
   4. Spiritual Distress Scale

7. **Nursing interventions for spiritual distress are classified into which categories:**
   1. Active listening and presence
   2. Presence and cancer support groups
   3. Social support and forgiveness
   4. Spiritual support and active listening

8. **Oncology nurses who want to provide spiritual care must have:**
   1. Spiritual well-being
   2. Effective communication skills
   3. Patience
   4. Strong faith in God or a power greater than oneself

9. **Spiritual care of the person experiencing spiritual distress should focus on:**
   1. Relief of only the person's physical pain.
   2. Listening and hearing only the person's emotional pain.
   3. Encouraging expression of the meaning in life.
   4. Financial management of illness as it relates only to suicide.

10. **Oncology nurses primarily mention which of the following as being a barrier to providing spiritual care to their patients:**
    1. They are uncomfortable talking about spiritual problems.
    2. They are unaware of spiritual issues.
    3. They lack confidence.
    4. They are not interested.

ANSWERS

1. *Answer: 3*
   Rationale: Connection with oneself, others, nature, or God or a power greater than oneself is central to the concept of spirituality.

2. *Answer: 2*
   Rationale: Spiritual distress is also called spiritual pain, spiritual suffering, and spiritual disequilibrium in the current literature.

3. *Answer: 1*
   Rationale: NANDA defines spiritual distress as the "impaired ability to experience and integrate meaning and purpose in life through... connectedness with self, others, art, music, literature, nature, or a power greater than oneself."

4. *Answer: 3*
   Rationale: Spiritual distress during cancer has many negative consequences,

including a false sense of hope, physical complaints, symptom distress, anxiety, depression, loneliness, social isolation, hopelessness, thoughts of harming oneself, and suicide. Decreased physical pain is not one of the negative consequences.

5. *Answer: 2*
   Rationale: Research has shown that being diagnosed with a life-threatening disease such as cancer leads people to face their own mortality and reprioritize their life, which can negatively affect their spiritual condition for a period of time.

6. *Answer: 1*
   Rationale: The Brief Assessment of Spiritual Resources and Concerns guide can inform the nurse if the person is unable to practice spiritual rituals, desires spiritual support, is questioning his or her faith, or experiencing lack of meaning or hope.

7. *Answer: 4*
   Rationale: Actively listening to what the patient is saying and providing spiritual support are the main categories of spiritual care.

8. *Answer: 2*
   Rationale: Providing spiritual care involves the interpersonal dimension, therefore effective communication skills and the ability to establish a trusting relationship are extremely important.

9. *Answer: 3*
   Rationale: Spiritual care is "whole person" care, therefore all dimensions of the person have to be considered in relieving spiritual distress. Nursing interventions directed at the physical can affect the spiritual dimension, and spiritual care interventions can affect the emotional and/or social dimensions.

10. *Answer: 3*
    Rationale: Several research studies have reported the most common reasons oncology nurses give for not providing spiritual care are lack of confidence and time constraints.

REFERENCES

Ackley, B., & Ladwig, G. (2006). *Nursing diagnosis handbook: A guide to planning care.* (7th ed.). St. Louis: Mosby.

Balboni, T., Vanderwerker, L., & Block, S., et al. (2007). Religiousness and spiritual support among advanced cancer patients and associations with end-of-life treatment preferences and quality of life. *Journal of Clinical Oncology, 25*(5):555-560.

Cancer Source. (2006). Coping spirituality and prayer. Retrieved July 20, 2006. from http://www.cancer-source.com/Search/34,23396-1.

Cordova, J. J., Cunningham, L. L., & Carlson, C. R., et al. (2001). Posttraumatic growth following breast cancer: A controlled comparison study. *Health Psychology, 20*:176-185.

Gaskamp, C., Sutter, R., & Meraviglia, M. (2004). *Promoting spirituality in the older adult: Evidence-based protocol.* Gerontological Nursing Interventions Research Center, University of Iowa College of Nursing.

Head, B., & Faul, A. (2005). Terminal restlessness as perceived by hospice professionals. *American Journal of Hospice and Palliative Care, 22*:277-282.

Highfield, M. E. (2000). Providing spiritual care to patients with cancer. *Clinical Journal of Oncology Nursing, 4*(3):115-120.

Hills, J., Paice, J. A., & Cameron, J. R., et al. (2005). Spirituality and distress in palliative care consultation. *Journal of Palliative Medicine, 8*(4):782-788.

Koenig, H. G. (2002). *Spirituality in patient care: Why, how, when, and what.* Philadelphia: Templeton Press.

Kristeller, J. L., Zumbrun, C. S., & Schilling, R. F. (1999). "I would if I could": How oncologists and oncology nurses address spiritual distress in cancer patients. *Psycho-Oncology, 8*:451-548.

LaPierre, L. L. (2003). JCAHO safeguards spiritual care. *Holistic Nursing Practice, 17*(4):219.

Larson, D. B., & Larson, S. S. (2003). Spirituality's potential relevance to physical and emotional health: A brief review of quantitative research. *Journal of Psychology and Theology, 31*(1):37-51.

McClain, C. S., Rosenfeld, B., & Breitbart, W. (2003). Effect of spiritual well-being on end-of-life despair in terminally ill cancer patients. *Lancet, 361*:1603-1607.

McClain-Jacobson, C., Rosenfeld, B., & Kosinski, A., et al. (2004). Belief in an afterlife, spiritual well-being and end-of-life despair in patients with advanced cancer. *General Hospital Psychiatry, 26*:484-486.

Meraviglia, M. (1999). Critical analysis of spirituality and its empirical indicators: Prayer and meaning in life. *Journal of Holistic Nursing, 17*:18-33.

Meraviglia, M. (2004). The effects of spirituality on well-being in people with lung cancer. *Oncology Nursing Forum, 31*(1):89-94.

Meraviglia, M. (2006). Effects of spirituality for breast cancer survivors. *Oncology Nursing Forum, 33*(1):E1-E7.

Meraviglia, M., Sutter, R., & Gaskamp, C. (2006). *Providing spiritual care to the terminally ill older adult: Evidence-based protocol.* Gerontological Nursing Interventions Research Center, University of Iowa College of Nursing (in review).

Meyer, C. L. (2003). How effectively are nurse educators preparing students to provide spiritual care? *Nurse Educator, 28*(4):185-190.

Murray, S. A., Kendall, M., & Boyd, K. (2004). Exploring the spiritual needs of people dying of lung cancer or heart failure: A prospective qualitative interview study of patients and their caregivers. *Palliative Medicine, 18*(1):39-45.

National Cancer Institute. (2006). *Spirituality in cancer care (PDQ).* (Health professional version). Retrieved July 20, 2006 from http://www.cancer.gov/cancertopics/pdq/supportivecare/spirituality/HealthProfessional/page1.

North American Nursing Diagnosis Association (NANDA) International. (2005). *Nursing diagnoses: Definitions and classifications 2005-2006.* Philadelphia: NANDA.

O'Brien, M. E (2003). *Spirituality in nursing: Standing on holy ground.* (2nd ed.). Boston: Jones & Bartlett.

Pargament, K. I., Koenig, H. G., & Tarakeshwar, N., et al. (2001). Religious struggle as a predictor of mortality among medically ill elderly patients: A two-year longitudinal study. *Archives of Internal Medicine, 161*:1881-1885.

Post, S. G., Puchalski, G. M., & Larson, D. B. (2000). Physicians and patient spirituality: Professional boundaries, competency, and ethics. *Annals of Internal Medicine, 132,* 578-583.

Staten, P. (2003). Spiritual assessment required in all settings. *Hospital Peer Review, 28*(4):55-57. Retrieved November 20, 2005, from www.galenet.galegroup.com.

Taylor, E. J (2002). *Spiritual care: Nursing theory, research, and practice*. Upper Saddle River, NJ: Prentice Hall.

Taylor, E. J, & Mamier, I. (2005). Spiritual care nursing: What cancer patients and family caregivers want. *Journal of Advanced Nursing, 49*(3):260-267.

Villagomeza, L. R. (2005). Spiritual distress in adult cancer patients: Toward conceptual clarity. *Holistic Nursing Practice, 19*:285-294.

Wilkinson, J. M (2001). *Nursing process and critical thinking*. (3rd ed.). Upper Saddle River, NJ: Prentice Hall.

Zebrack, B. J., & Chesler, M. A. (2002). Quality of life in childhood cancer survivors. *Psycho-Oncology, 11*:132-141.

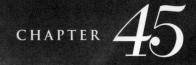

CHAPTER 45

SUICIDAL IDEATION

KATHLEEN MURPHY-ENDE

PATHOPHYSIOLOGICAL MECHANISMS

Suicide is the act of killing oneself on purpose. The term *suicide* stems from the Latin words *sui*, meaning "self," and *caedere*, meaning "to kill." Suicidal ideation is the thought of harming or killing oneself. Suicidal behavior includes acts of intentional attempts to inflict self-death.

Most people have causal fleeting thoughts of suicide at times of frustration, grief, and disappointment. Suicidal ideation and behavior in the general population have multiple causes, such as proximal stressors or triggers and predisposition. No single pathophysiologic mechanism causes suicidal ideation or behavioral attempts; the personal life history and physical, psychological, spiritual, and social factors collectively influence an individual's beliefs about self-destruction.

Psychiatric illness is a major contributing factor in most suicides in the general population. The mood disorders, including major depression and bipolar illness, are most associated with suicide (Bertolote et al., 2003). Psychological autopsy studies, performed to discover the state of mind of the person before death, suggest that 90% of completed suicides had one or more mental illness, such as major depression or alcoholism (Luoma, 2003). Other contributing factors included the availability of lethal means, alcohol and drug abuse, lack of access to psychiatric treatment, attitude toward suicide, lack of help-seeking behavior, physical illness, marital status, age, and gender (Mann, 2002).

The desire of patients with advanced cancer for a hastened death is related to psychological distress, such as depression and anxiety (Mystakidou et al., 2005). Specific concerns also are related to thoughts of suicide, including unrelieved pain, poorly managed symptoms, depression, a sense of loss of control, a feeling of being a burden to others, being dependent for personal care, and loss of dignity (Eisenberg, 1992).

Depression rates in patients with cancer are high; nearly half of these patients show symptoms during screening (Carroll et al., 1993), and the prevalence is 25% in the palliative care setting (Martin & Jackson, 2000). Unfortunately, a high percentage of those who received a psychiatric diagnosis experienced a significant amount of cancer-related pain (Derogatis et al., 1998); however, the symptoms of depression may be a consequence of uncontrolled pain.

Another factor that influences suicidal ideation is a perceived loss of control. Patients with cancer who were accepting and adaptable were less likely to commit suicide than those who exhibited a need to be in control (Farberow et al., 1971). Suicidal ideation stems from stressful life events and/or mood or psychiatric disorders, and the factors involved in suicidal behavior seem to be related to impulsivity, hopelessness and/or pessimism, access to lethal means, and imitation.

Adolescents with cancer deal with a realm of psychosocial issues related to their developmental phase and individual characteristics. Suicidal ideation and attempts in this population are rare. Often the adolescent believes that his or her disease and life are more determined by fate, luck, or God than by the adolescent's control. These young patients' belief that the disease is outside their control and the lack of cognitive maturity needed to plan and implement a lethal attempt may account for the low incidence of suicide in the pediatric oncology population. Refusal of cancer treatment by adolescents is not a means of attempting suicide (NCI, 2006).

Patients' preference for limiting life-sustaining treatment is a different concept from suicidal ideation and should be honored. Euthanasia and physician-assisted suicide (PAS) are distinctly different from suicidal ideation. However, the research exploring patients' desire or request for PAS has provided insight into the reasoning of those who want to end their life. Euthanasia, the intentional bringing about of a patient's death for his or her own sake, either by killing (active) the patient or allowing the patient to die (passive), can be classified as voluntary, nonvoluntary, or involuntary. Physician-assisted suicide refers to a physician acting to aid a patient's request to end his or her life; it is legal only in the state of Oregon. Unfortunately, medically ill patients' requests for PAS are not rare (Stoudemire, 1996).

EPIDEMIOLOGY AND ETIOLOGY

The exact number of people who contemplate suicide is unknown. However, suicide rates in the general population may provide some insight into the scope of the problem. A review of the literature shows that more than 90% of those who commit suicide had a psychiatric illness. Approximately 50% of suicides are associated with a major depressive episode (Lagomasino & Stern 1998).

Approximately 10% to 15% of bipolar patients commit suicide (Hirschfeld et al., 2003). Because suicide is highly associated with depression, it is noteworthy that 15% to 25% of patients with cancer experience depression (Lloyd-Williams & Freidman, 2001; Henriksson et al., 1995).

The prevalence of suicidal ideation in the cancer population is difficult to determine because it is not always assessed or recorded in patients. However, the rate as determined from nurse reports in hospitalized patients with cancer was 11% (Pasacreta & Massie, 1990); in ambulatory and hospitalized patients with cancer pain, it was 16% (Breitbart et al., 1992). In the palliative care unit, Brown and colleagues (1986) found a suicidal ideation rate of 20%.

The prevalence of suicidal ideation or attempts in childhood cancer is unknown. Research exploring the prevalence of suicidal ideation is limited, because the clinical impression may not accurately reflect the patient's suicidal thoughts, and patients may not feel comfortable sharing suicidal thoughts with the researcher.

Suicide rates are also difficult to obtain accurately, because it often goes unrecognized and underreported. Intentional overdoses by the terminally ill may not be recognized or cited as the cause of death. Suicide in cancer patients occurs most frequently in the advanced stage (Fox et al., 1982). Considering all medical conditions, cancer and AIDS are associated with the highest rates of suicide and requests for hastened death (Louhiviour & Hakama, 1997; Kizer et al., 1988; Marzuk et al., 1988; Fox et al., 1982). The number of patients with cancer who actually commit suicide is small, but the relative risk of suicide in these patients is twice that of the general population (Breitbart, 1993).

The etiology of suicidal ideation in patients with cancer may be highly variable. It includes psychological distress, the patient's coping ability, the individual's medical condition and physical well-being, and social and spiritual factors (Box 45-1). A sense of hopelessness correlated more with suicidal ideation in terminally ill cancer patients than did depression (Chochinov et al., 1998). Patients with advanced cancer who express suicidal ideation are likely to be experiencing underrecognized and undertreated physical

BOX 45-1	FACTORS THAT MAY INFLUENCE THE DESIRE TO HASTEN DEATH IN PATIENTS WITH CANCER

Psychological Factors
- Mood
- Depression
- History of mental illness
- Family history of suicide
- Previous suicidal attempts
- Anxiety
- Loss of autonomy
- Loss of sense of control
- Hopelessness
- Loss of independence
- Fear of being a burden
- Loss of dignity
- Delirium
- Personality disorder
- Inability to participate in pleasurable activities

Physical Factors
- Terminal stage
- Poor prognosis
- Advanced disease
- Pain
- Dyspnea
- Fatigue
- Insomnia
- Nausea
- Inability to eat or swallow
- Poor physical functioning
- Immobility
- Paralysis
- Loss of bowel or bladder control
- Amputation
- Loss of eyesight or hearing
- Older age
- Substance abuse

Spiritual Factors
- Decreased spiritual well-being
- Existential distress
- Guilt
- Lack of spiritual resources

Social Factors
- Lack of social support
- Isolation
- Altered communication
- Inability to participate in social activities
- Recent death of a friend or spouse

symptoms or psychiatric disturbances. Suicidal ideation is relatively infrequent in cancer and is limited to those who have advanced disease, are hospitalized, in palliative care settings, or have pain or depression (Breitbart, 1993). Refusal of cancer treatment, noncompliance, and requests for allowing a natural death should not be equated with suicidal ideation, and the reason for these decisions should be explored further, misconceptions corrected, and decisions respected.

RISK PROFILE

- Terminal stage of cancer (Breitbart et al., 2004).
- Advanced illness (Blound, 1985).
- Pre-existing psychopathology.
- Personality disorder (Breitbart, 1987 & 1990).
- Pain (Breitbart, 1990).
- Unrelenting physical symptoms (Foley, 1991).
- Terminal phase of a progressive chronic illness (Valente & Trainor, 1998).
- Hopelessness (Chochinov et al., 1998).
- Pancreatic, head and neck, and gastrointestinal cancers (Holland, 2002).
- Cancer associated with heavy and prolonged tobacco and alcohol use, impaired function, and facial disfigurement (Farberow et al., 1971).
- Loss of autonomy (Oregon Department of Human Services, 2003).
- Loss of sense of control (Farberow et al., 1971).
- Poor physical functioning (Akechi et al., 2001).
- Decreased ability to participate in enjoyable activities (Oregon Department of Human Services, 2003).

- Loss of dignity (Oregon Department of Human Services, 2003).
- Depression (Massie et al., 1994).
- Delirium (Breitbart, 1990).
- Fatigue (Breitbart, 1987).
- Previously conveyed suicidal thoughts or plans (Blound, 1985).
- Fear of being a burden on others (Block, 2000; Eisenbergh, 1992).
- Poor social support (Pearlman et al., 2000).
- History of previous suicide attempts.
- Older age (sixth and seventh decades) (Louhivouri & Hakama, 1997).

PROGNOSIS

The goal of identifying suicidal ideation in patients with cancer is to prevent suicide. Most causes of suicidal ideation, such as pain and depression, are treatable. Morbidity is higher in cancer patients with depression or uncontrolled symptoms than in those without symptoms. Nursing care should be aimed at reducing morbidity by identifying patients at high risk and providing aggressive symptom management and psychosocial support.

PROFESSIONAL ASSESSMENT CRITERIA (PAC)

1. Identify cancer patients at risk (see Risk Profile section), so that prevention and psychosocial interventions can be initiated.
2. If a patient has made direct statements about suicidal intent, further assessment must be done immediately (Box 45-2).
3. All patients with cancer should be screened for depression and suicidal ideation. Many patients with advanced terminal disease experience a spectrum of suicidal thoughts, ranging from fleeting thoughts of death to hastening death or suicidal intention; it is important to assess the level of deliberate self-harm. The discussion and questions should start with general and unthreatening questions (Box 45-2).
4. Assessment tools for depression include the Hospital Depression Assessment Scale and the Geriatric Depression Scale.
5. An assessment tool for hopelessness is the Beck Hopelessness Scale.
6. Obtain a psychiatric history, including a history of depression, mental illness, substance abuse, previous suicidal attempts, or a family history of suicide.
7. Assess pain and other physical symptoms; evaluate the level of distress the symptoms are causing the patient.
8. Review the patient's current medications and consider discontinuing medications that may cause depression.

NURSING CARE AND TREATMENT

1. For suicidal patients, document the psychiatric consultation request, patient behavior (statement that captures thoughts or plans), suicide precautions (actions taken to protect the patient), and interventions used to promote safety (type of restraint and rationale).
2. For suicidal patients, initiate one-to-one observation status or admit or transfer the patient to the inpatient psychiatric unit. Explain the purpose of suicide precautions and the goal of keeping the patient safe. Remove all potentially dangerous items from the room. Follow the institution's policy for suicide precautions.

| BOX 45-2 | ASSESSING SUICIDAL IDEATION AND RISK IN CANCER PATIENTS |

Approach

Evaluation of a patient's suicidal thoughts should include sensitive exploration of the topic of self-inflicted death.

- Clarify what the patient is saying about thoughts of ending his or her life.
- Support the patient's need to express emotions and validate the person's feelings. Identify specific factors that may be contributing to the patient's suffering and demonstrate your commitment to providing care that will enhance his or her quality of life.
- Evaluate the patient's mental status and decision-making capacity.
- Treat the factors contributing to the patient's suffering.
- Refer the patient to the appropriate health care team members (psychiatrist or psychiatric nurse practitioner, pain clinical nurse specialist, pastoral care, or social worker).

Questions to Help Assess Suicidal Intent

1. It sounds as if you have been through a lot of changes and issues related to your illness and treatment. Tell me how it has been for you.
2. Do you ever feel hopeless?
3. Do you ever wish you could go to sleep and never wake up?
4. Have you ever had thoughts of harming yourself?
   If yes: What would you do to harm yourself?
5. Do you have a person you could call if you felt tempted to harm yourself?
   If no: What stops you from harming yourself?
6. Have you ever thought of suicide?
   If yes: How likely are you to act on your thoughts? Do you have a plan/means to carry this out? What specifically would you do to end your life? Do you have a person you could call if you were thinking about suicide?
7. Have you ever acted on your plans?
   If no: What has stopped you from taking your life?

3. Assess and document the current level of suicide intent on a consistent analog scale (e.g., 0 to 10, with 0 meaning no thoughts of suicide and 10 meaning constant thoughts of suicide). Use the comparison to help the patient understand the factors may or may underlie his or her thoughts about suicide or depression (Captian, 2006).
4. Establish a trusting and safe relationship with the patient and family. Include the family in the plan of care.
5. Assist with physical impairments or deficits induced by cancer or its treatment (e.g., mobility, bowel and bladder function, hygiene).
6. Minimize confusion and sedation from medications or sleep deprivation.
7. Ensure pain and symptom management.
8. Encourage support from family and friends to prevent feelings of isolation or abandonment.
9. Administer medications (antidepressants and anxiolytics); monitor for side effects and evaluate the drugs' effectiveness.
10. For outpatients, refer patients who have expressed or are suspected of suicidal ideation, or who have made a suicide attempt, to a psychiatrist, psychiatric nurse practitioner, or psychologist for diagnostic evaluation and recommendations.

EVIDENCE-BASED PRACTICE UPDATES

1. The increased desire to hasten death was associated with higher levels of depression, more hours required for caregiving, and greater marital satisfaction in males with

advanced cancer (Ransom et al., 2006). Nurses should consider the aspects of the marital and caregiving relationships that may cause a patient distress at the thought of dying and leaving them.

2. Of patients with cancer, 25% (Martin & Jackson, 2000) to nearly 50% (Carroll et al., 1993) experience depression.

3. A history of depression increases the risk for recurrent depression (Pignone et al., 2002).

4. Nurses tend to underestimate the level of depressive symptoms in patients with cancer who are depressed (Martin & Jackson 2000; McDonald et al., 1999).

5. Patients with cancer rarely commit suicide without some degree of premorbid psycho-pathology that places them at increased risk.

6. In a Swedish study, half of all cancer suicides had previously expressed suicidal thoughts or plans to their relatives (Blound, 1976).

7. A 2-year review (2000-2002) of 1000 studies on the relationship between religion and mental health found that religious people are less suicidal (Wallis, 2005).

8. It is a myth that asking patients with cancer about suicidal thoughts causes them to consider suicide (Rosenfeld et al., 2002).

9. Appropriate psychiatric interventions help alleviate or diminish suicidal ideation (Breitbart, 1987).

10. Hospice workers, working with a patient who requests a hastened death, experience an ethical dilemma and feel conflicted about honoring the patient's autonomy versus promoting a death (Harvath et al., 2006).

11. Listening to patients' expressed desire for a hastened death helps nurses understand what the patients are requesting. In a phenomenologic inquiry involving terminally ill patients who expressed a desire for a hastened death, a number of themes were communicated: a manifestation of the will to live, a dying process that was so difficult that early death was preferred, an intolerable immediate situation, a way of drawing attention to the patient as a unique individual, a gesture of altruism, an attempt to manipulate the family to avoid abandonment, and a cry depicting the misery of the situation (Coyle, 2004).

TEACHING AND EDUCATION

1. Depression is treatable. Symptoms to look for include feeling sad, empty, or numb; sleeping a lot or having trouble sleeping; feeling hopeless, helpless, worthless, or guilty; feeling angry or moody or crying easily; chronic worrying and panic attacks; avoiding friends; feeling alone even when with others; loss of interest in previously enjoyed activities; difficulty concentrating or making decisions; a change in eating habits not related to health; recurring headaches, backaches, or stomach aches without a medical cause; alcohol or drug abuse; thinking about suicide.

2. Warning signs of suicide include talking or writing about suicide; previous suicidal thoughts or attempts at suicide; admitting to feeling worthless or helpless; self-destructive behavior; and giving away personal items.

3. Sometimes family and friends withdraw prematurely from a patient with cancer who has advanced disease or symptoms, causing the patient to feel isolated or abandoned. A social support system may act as a buffer against isolation.

4. Resources are available as a source of help:
   - American Suicide Foundation, 1045 Park Avenue, Suite 3C, New York, NY 10028. Phone: 212-410-0352. This organization supports research, education, and treatment programs with the goal of preventing suicide. A newsletter is available for those concerned about suicide and those who have lost a loved one to suicide. On request,

the foundation will provide informational material, including a list of local support groups for survivors of suicide.

- Choice in Dying, 200 Varick Street, 10th floor, New York, NY 10014-4810. Phone: 800-989-WILL (9455). This organization provides information on end of life issues other than assisted suicide, from living wills to choosing whether to die in a hospital or at home. It provides a range of services, from free counseling about end of life issues to public education, through a national network of volunteer speakers. Informational materials are provided on request.

5. **Web sites for information:**
   - American Association of Suicidology: http://www.suicidology.org
   - American Foundation for Suicide Prevention: http://www.afsp.org
   - Helping Others Prevent & Educate about Suicide (HOPES): www.hopes-wi.org
   - National Center for Health Statistics: http://www.cdc.gov/nchs/fastats/suidice.htm
   - National Institute of Mental Health: http://www.ninh.nih.gov/suicideprevetnion/suifact.cfm
   - North Carolina Wesleyan College Faculty, psychological autopsy: http://faculty.ncwc.edu/toconnor/psy/psylect04.htm.

NURSING DIAGNOSES

1. **Risk for self-directed violence** related to suicidal ideation
2. **Ineffective coping** related to stressors associated with advanced cancer
3. **Self-care deficit** related to physical immobility and symptoms
4. **Grieving** related to cumulative losses
5. **Spiritual distress** related to terminal condition and fear of dying

EVALUATION AND DESIRED OUTCOMES

1. Suicidal ideation, gestures, or attempts will be identified, and safety precautions and evaluation and treatment will be initiated immediately.
2. Depression and anxiety will be identified and treated.
3. Pain and physical symptoms will be controlled, and the patient will report relief of symptoms.
4. The patient will be protected from self-harm.
5. The nurse will remain objective in caring for patients who express a desire to die, with a continual assessment of suicide risk.
6. The patient and family will verbalize an understanding of suicidal ideation and resources to assist in coping with these feelings.

DISCHARGE PLANNING AND FOLLOW-UP CARE

- Contact names and numbers of people and resources for psychological crisis.
- Follow-up appointment with psychiatrist or psychiatric nurse practitioner.
- Follow-up appointment for oncology care with physician or nurse practitioner.
- Home will be safeguarded from weapons and lethal substances.
- Home care nursing services will be notified of patient's risk factors for suicide.
- Plan of care for symptom management will be shared with all health care providers.
- Patient will be sent home or to another care facility with a list of medications, the rationales for their use, and their side effects.

REVIEW QUESTIONS

QUESTIONS

1. **A major risk factor for suicide in patients with cancer is:**
   1. New diagnosis of cancer
   2. Currently being treated for depression
   3. Uncontrolled pain
   4. Breast cancer

2. **The most appropriate response to a patient's expression of suicidal thoughts is:**
   1. "Euthanasia is something that you should talk to your health care provider about because it is legal is some states."
   2. "Requests for physician-assisted suicide are legal only in the state of Oregon."
   3. "It is not unusual for people experiencing cancer to have fleeting thoughts of self-harm or ending their life. Let me ask you a few more questions about how you are feeling."
   4. "I see from your chart that you are Jewish; does your religion condone suicide?"

3. **Risk factors for suicide in the general population include:**
   1. History of childhood abuse
   2. Depression
   3. Socioeconomic status
   4. Race

4. **Risk factors for suicide in those with cancer include:**
   1. Younger age
   2. Early stage of the disease (new diagnosis)
   3. Unemployed status
   4. Hopelessness

5. **Assessing suicidal ideation and risk in patients with advanced cancer should include:**
   1. Screening for depression
   2. Assessing the patient's level of hopelessness

   3. Assessing the patient's level of pain
   4. All of the above

6. **Which of the following statements is** *true:*
   1. Asking patients about thoughts of suicide should be discouraged because it may give them ideas to inflict self-harm.
   2. Asking patients about suicide should be discouraged because it implies that they are in a bad situation for which suicide is the only solution.
   3. All patients being screened for cancer should be asked about suicidal ideation at the time of screening.
   4. Obtaining a history of depression, mental illness, substance abuse, and suicidal ideation is appropriate in patients suffering with symptoms or in advanced disease states.

7. **What other information should initially be obtained from patients who appear depressed:**
   1. List of all medications
   2. List of allergies
   3. Family history of thyroid disease
   4. Insurance coverage for counseling

8. **Priority nursing care for patients who have expressed suicidal ideation is aimed at:**
   1. Telling the family or significant other what the patient has expressed and including them in on the plan of care.
   2. Immediately applying restraints to keep the patient from committing suicide.
   3. Administering antidepressants and medications for anxiety as ordered.
   4. Further assessing the patient's suicidal intention and referring the patient to a psychiatrist or psychiatric nurse practitioner.

9. **The best way to prevent suicide is:**
   1. Give all cancer patients the suicide hot line number.
   2. Warns families of patients with advanced disease to frequently check the patient while at home.
   3. Identify those at risk and make certain they get proper treatment.
   4. There is no way to prevent suicide, and it is a person's legal right to take their own life.

10. **The role of the certified psychiatric mental health nurse practitioner in the oncology population includes:**
   1. Assessing patients' psychiatric status.
   2. Prescribing antidepressants.
   3. Providing counseling services to patients and families with cancer.
   4. All of the above

ANSWERS

1. *Answer: 3*
   Rationale: Uncontrolled cancer pain has been noted in numerous studies to be associated with suicidal ideation.

2. *Answer: 3*
   Rationale: Reassuring the patient that these thoughts are normal and immediately assessing for suicide risk is the most appropriate response. Euthanasia is illegal in the United States. Although PAS may be legal in Oregon, stating this does not gather information about the patient's feelings or intentions. Assessing spirituality is important and should be incorporated into the assessment, after risk has been evaluated.

3. *Answer: 2*
   Rationale: Depression is a risk factor for suicide in the general population.

4. *Answer: 4*
   Rationale: Hopelessness is associated with suicidal ideation in cancer patients. Advanced age (sixth and seventh decades) and advanced disease are associated risk factors. Employment status has not been studied.

5. *Answer: 4*
   Rationale: All of the factors listed should be assessed when working with patients with advanced disease.

6. *Answer: 4*
   Rationale: Answer choice 4 is a true statement. No evidence indicates that asking patients about suicide gives them ideas of self-harm.
   Although cancerscreening may be stressful, it is not noted to be a time of high risk for suicide. Patients with symptoms and advanced disease are at highest risk

7. *Answer: 1*
   Rationale: Numerous medications can cause depression, and the health care provider should consider eliminating suspected agents if possible. Insurance information is useful but is not the first priority.

8. *Answer: 4*
   Rationale: It is not unusual for patients with advanced cancer to have fleeting thoughts of self-harm or hastening death. The registered nurse should further explore the patient's intention of harm and then make the appropriate referrals as needed.

9. *Answer: 3*
   Rationale: It is important to help those who are at risk by providing psychological support and symptom management so that quality of life improves. Answer choices 1 and 2 are not practical or realistic and are likely to give the wrong message to those undergoing cancer treatment. Suicide is not legal, and research documents that most suicidal ideation or attempts are associated with distressing symptoms that usually can be controlled.

10. *Answer: 4*
   Rationale: The psychiatric nurse practitioner is an excellent resource for patients, families, and staff to help evaluate and treat psychiatric conditions.

REFERENCES

Akechi, T., Hitoshi, O., & Yamawaki, S., et al. (2001). Why do some cancer patients with depression desire an early death and others do not? *Psychosomatics, 42*(2):141-145.

Bertolote, J. M., Fleischmann, A., & DeLeo, D., et al. (2003). Suicide and mental disorders: Do we know enough? *British Journal of Psychiatry, 183:*382-383.

Block, S. D. (2000). Assessing and managing depression in the terminally ill patient. ACP-ASIM End-of-Life Care Consensus Panel. *Annals of Internal Medicine, 132:*209-218.

Blound, C. (1976). Suicide and cancer. II. Medical and care factors in suicide by cancer patients in Sweden. *Journal of Psychosocial Oncology, 3:*17-30.

Blound, C. (1985). Medical and care factors in suicides caused by cancer patients in Sweden. *Journal of Psychosocial Oncology, 3:*31-52.

Breitbart, W. (1987). Suicide in the cancer patient. *Oncology, 1:*49-54.

Breitbart, W. (1990). Cancer pain and suicide. In K. Foley (Ed.), *Advances in pain research and therapy,* (pp. 399-412). Vol 16. New York: Raven Press.

Breitbart, W. (1993). Suicide risk and pain in cancer and AIDS patient. In C.R. Chapman & K. Foley (Eds.), *Current and emerging issues in cancer pain: Research and practice.* New York: Lippincott Raven.

Breitbart, W., Chochinov, H. M., & Passik, S. (2004). Psychiatric symptoms in palliative medicine. In D. Doyle G. Hanks & N. Cherny, et al. (Eds.), *Oxford textbook of palliative medicine.* (p. 755) (3rd ed.). Oxford: University Press.

Breitbart, W., Passik, S. D., & Eller, K., et al. (1992). Suicidal ideation in AIDS: The roles of pain and mood (abstract). *145th Annual Meeting of the American Psychiatric Association.* May 20, 1992. Washington, D. C.

Brown, J. H., Henteleff, P., & Barakat, S., et al. (1986). Is it normal for terminally ill patient to desire death? *American Journal of Psychiatry, 143:*208-211.

Captian, C. (2006). Is your patient a suicide risk? *Nursing 2006, 36*(8):43-47.

Carroll, B. T., Kathol, R. G., & Noyes, R., Jr., et al. (1993). Screening for depression and anxiety in cancer patients using the hospital anxiety and depression scale. *General Hospital Psychiatry, 15:*69-74.

Chochinov, H. M., Wilson, K. G., & Enns, M., et al. (1998). Depression, hopelessness and suicidal ideation in the terminally ill. *Psychosomatics, 39:*366-370.

Coyle, N. (2004). Expressed desire for hastened death in seven patients living with advanced cancer: A phenomenologic inquiry. *Oncology Nursing Forum, 31*(4):699-706.

Derogatis, L. R., Morrow, G. R., & Fetting, J., et al. (1998). The prevalence of psychiatric disorders among cancer patients. *Journal of the American Medical Association, 249:*751-757.

Eisenberg, L. (1992). Treating depression and anxiety in primary care: Closing the gap between knowledge and practice. *New England Journal of Medicine, 326:*180-184.

Farberow, N. L. et al. (1971). An 8-year survey of hospital suicides. Suicide and Life-threatening Behavior, 1:20.

Foley, K. M. (1991). The relationship of pain and symptom management to patient requests for physician-assisted suicide. *Journal of Pain and Symptom Management, 6:*289-297.

Fox, B. H., et al. (1982). Suicide rate among cancer patients in Connecticut. *Journal of Chronic Diseases, 35:*85-100.

Harvath, T., Miller, L., & Smith, K., et al. (2006). Dilemmas encountered by hospice workers when patients wish to hasten death. *Journal of Hospice and Palliative Nursing, 8*(4):200-209.

Henriksson, M. M., Isometsa, E. T., & Heitanen, P. S., et al. (1995). Mental disorders in cancer suicides. *Journal of Affective Disorders, 36:*11-20.

Hirschfeld, R. M., Lewis, L., & Vornik, L. A. (2003). Perceptions and impact of bipolar disorder: How far have we really come? Results of the Not Depressive and Manic Depressive Association 2000 Survey of Individuals with Bipolar Disease. *Journal of Clinical Psychology, 64:*425-432.

Holland, J. C. (2003). Psychological aspects of cancer. In J. F. Holland & E. Frei (Eds.), *Cancer medicine* (pp. 1039-1054). (6th ed.). Philadelphia: Lea & Febiger.

Kizer, K. W., Green, M., & Perkins, C. I., et al. (1988). AIDS and suicide in California. *Journal of the American Medical Association, 260:*1981.

Lagomasino, I. T., & Stern, T. A. (1998). Approach to the suicidal patient. In T.A. Stern J.B. Herman & P.L. Slavin (Eds.), *MGH guide to psychiatry in primary care.* New York: McGraw-Hill.

Lloyd-Williams, M., & Friedman, T. (2001). Depression in palliative care patients: A prospective study. *European Journal Cancer Care (England), 10*(4):270-274.

Louhivouri, K. A., & Hakama, J. (1997). Risk of suicide among cancer patients. *American Journal of Epidemiology, 109*:59-65.

Luoma, J. B. (2003). Contact with mental health and primary care providers prior to suicide: A review of the evidence. *American Journal of Psychiatry, 160*(5):1012-1013.

Mann, J. (2002). A current perspective of suicide and attempted suicide. *Annals of Internal Medicine, 136*:302-311.

Martin, A. C., & Jackson, K. C. (2000). Depression in palliative care patients. *Journal of Pharmaceutical Care in Pain and Symptom Control, 7*:71-89.

Marzuk, P. M., Teirney, H., & Tardiff, K., et al. (1988). Increased risk of suicide in persons with AIDS. *Journal of the American Medical Association, 259*:1333-1337.

Massie, M. J., Gagnon, M. D., & Holland, J. C. (1994). Depression and suicide in patients with cancer. *Journal of Pain and Symptom Management, 9*(5):325-339.

McDonald, M., Passik, S. D., & Dugan, W., et al. (1999). RN recognition of depression in patients with cancer. *Oncology Nursing Forum, 21*:493-499.

Mystakidou, K., Rosenfeld, B., & Katsouda, E., et al. (2005). Desire for death near the end of life: The role of depression, anxiety and pain. *General Hospital Psychiatry, 27, 4.*

National Cancer Institute (NCI). (2006). Pediatric considerations for suicidality. Depression (PDQ). (Health professional version). Retrieved April 20, 2007, from www.cancer.gov.

Oregon Department of Human Services. (2003). Death with dignity annual report, 2003. Retrieved July 1, 2006, from http://www.dhs.state.or.us/publichealth/chs/pas/ar-index.cfm.

Pasacreta, J. V., & Massie, M. J. (1990). Nurses reports of psychiatric complications in patients with cancer. *Oncology Nursing Forum, 17*:347-353.

Pearlman, R. A., Cain, K. C., & Starks, H., et al. (2000). Preferences for life-sustaining treatments in advanced planning and surrogate decision making. *Journal of Palliative Medicine, 3*:37-48.

Pignone, M., Gaynes, B. N., & Rushton, J. L., et al. (2002). Screening for depression: Systematic evidence review no. 6 (prepared by the Research Triangle Institute, University of North Carolina Evidence-Based Practice under contract no. 290-97-0011). AHPQ Publication No. 02-S002. Rockville, MD: Agency for Healthcare Research and Quality.

Ransom, S., et al. (2006). The desire of terminally ill patients to hasten dying. *Annals of Behavioral Medicine, 31*(1):63-69.

Rosenfeld, B., et al. (2002). Suicide, assisted suicide and euthanasia in the terminally ill. In H. M. C. Chochinov & W. Breitbart (Eds.), *Handbook of psychiatry in palliative medicine* (pp. 51-62). New York: Oxford University Press.

Stoudemire, A. (1996). Epidemiology and psychopharmacology of anxiety in medical patients. *Journal of Clinical Psychiatry, 57*(Suppl. 7):977-989.

Valente, S. M., & Trainor, D. (1998). Rational suicide among patients who are terminally ill. *AORN Journal, 68*:252-264.

Wallis, C. (2005). The new science of happiness. *Time, 165*:25-28.

Superior Vena Cava Syndrome

MOLLY LONEY • NANCY KELLY

PATHOPHYSIOLOGICAL MECHANISMS

Superior vena cava syndrome (SVCS) is a partial or complete obstruction of the blood flow returning to the heart from the head, neck, upper thorax, and upper extremities. Because the superior vena cava (SVC) is located within the narrow space of the mediastinum, any intraluminal or extraluminal compression impairs venous drainage and results in venous congestion, with engorgement of the supplying veins.

As the congestion increases, so does venous pressure behind the compression, and blood may be shunted to adjacent collateral pathways to maintain blood return to the right atrium (Moore, 2005; Haapoja & Blendowski, 1999). The collateral circulation usually bypasses the obstructed SVC through the azygos, internal mammary, thoracic, vertebral, and subcutaneous veins. If any of these vessels are not patent or if the level of compression is below the azygos vein, compensation is challenged, and more acute symptoms result as blood is shunted through the inferior vena cava (Flounders, 2003; Yahalom, 2001; Haapoja & Blendowski, 1999).

Rising venous pressure and venous stasis in the head and upper torso result in third spacing of fluid into adjacent tissue. Fluid accumulation only adds to the vena caval compression and may compress other vital structures in the mediastinum, resulting in pleural or pericardial effusions. If the obstruction of venous blood flow is severe and the collateral circulation pathways are inadequate, cardiac filling and output decline, leading to impaired cerebral perfusion. These sequelae often are accompanied by thrombosis and both laryngeal and cerebral edema, which further place the patient at risk for acute respiratory, cardiovascular, and neurologic distress (Moore, 2005; Flounders, 2003; Myers, 2001; Haapoja & Blendowski, 1999).

EPIDEMIOLOGY AND ETIOLOGY

As an oncologic emergency, SVCS is relatively rare, affecting only 3% to 4% of cancer patients. Three basic types of occlusion can result in SVCS: (1) extraluminal compression caused by a mass, metastases, fibrosis, or one or more enlarged lymph nodes; (2) intraluminal obstruction caused by a mass invading the vessel wall or thrombosis; and (3) intraluminal response to infection or inflammation (Miaskowski, 1999; Hogan & Rosenthal, 1998; Joyce & Cunningham, 1998).

Approximately 15% to 22% of all cases of SVCS are associated with benign conditions, primarily infection or thrombosis; cancer accounts for 78% to 85% of SVCS cases (Drews, 2006). Lung cancer and lymphoma, especially with right-side perihilar adenopathy, account for most cancer-related cases of SVCS. Small cell and squamous cell lung cancers are the most common histological types, because they tend to develop centrally in the pulmonary bed (Drews, 2006; Hogan & Rosenthal, 1998). Because of the right lung's proximity to the SVC, right-side lung cancer is four times more likely to be associated with SVCS than left-side lung cancer. Other cancers that may be associated with SVCS include Kaposi's sarcoma, thymoma, germ cell tumors, and cancers in which nodal mediastinal metastasis is a potential risk (Drews, 2006; Tyson, 2004; Flounders, 2003; Joyce & Cunningham, 1998).

RISK PROFILE

- Age and gender (Haapoja & Blendowski, 1999):
  - Average age is 40 to 70 years.
  - SVCS is three times more to likely to occur in men.
- Benign conditions associated with SVCS (Drews, 2006; Krimsky et al., 2002; Miaskowski, 1999):
  - Aortic aneurysm
  - Infections
    - Involving the structures in the mediastinum (i.e., mediastinitis, tuberculosis, actinomycosis, aspergillosis, and blastomycosis).
    - Resulting from contagious spread from a lung, pleural, or skin infection (i.e., nocardiosis).
  - Thyroid disorders (i.e., goiter).
  - Sclerosing cholangitis.
  - Sarcoidosis
  - Vascular fibrosis after thoracic radiation.
  - Central venous catheters or tunneled venous ports in patients with the following conditions (Rice et al., 2006; Moore, 2005; Tyson, 2004; Flounders, 2003; Haapoja & Blendowski, 1999):
    - Hypercoagulable state.
    - Damage to the intima of the SVC by the venous catheter.
    - Pacemaker
    - Venous stasis from extraluminal compression of the SVC.
    - Inadequate flushing of the venous catheter or port.
- Malignant causes of SVCS (Drews, 2006; Flounders, 2003; Lonardi et al., 2002; Yahalom, 2001; Haapoja & Blendowski, 1999):
  - Most common in men age 50 to 70 years with primary or metastatic tumors involving the mediastinum.
  - Lung cancer:
    - Small cell lung cancer (SCLC) is more common than non-small cell lung cancer (NSCLC).
    - Non-small cell lung cancer of squamous cell histology
  - Non-Hodgkin's lymphoma:
    - Diffuse large cell type (i.e., primarily large cell lymphoma with sclerosing).
    - Lymphoblastic type.
  - Metastases to the mediastinum from primary cancers (Joyce & Cunningham, 1998):
    - Breast cancer
    - Esophageal cancer
    - Colon cancer
    - Testicular cancer
    - Kaposi's sarcoma
    - Thymoma
    - Germ cell cancer

PROGNOSIS

Although SVCS can be accompanied by distressing symptoms, it rarely presents as a life-threatening emergency (Tyson, 2004). Most patients usually respond to treatment for SVCS, with relief of symptoms or tumor regression if cancer is present. Death from venous obstruction alone has not been described in the medical literature. Mortality comes from concurrent or advanced stages of disease, such as cancer in the mediastinum (Bierdrager, et al., 2005; Myers, 2001; Haapoja & Blendowski, 1999).

The prognosis depends on how rapidly the obstruction develops the degree of vena caval blockage, and compensation by collateral circulation. If venous return can be maintained and hypoxia prevented, heart failure and organ damage can be prevented even with acute onset. The overall prognosis also depends on the underlying disease and its histology, if malignant. Benign causes can be easily treated, and these patients have a favorable prognosis; likewise for patients with lymphoma and small-cell lung cancer. Patients with mediastinal metastases have limited long-term response. Although early diagnosis and treatment of SVCS may not bring long-term survival, quality of life can be improved with palliation (Drews, 2006; Moore, 2005; Lonardi et al., 2002; Myers, 2001; Yahalom, 2001).

PROFESSIONAL ASSESSMENT CRITERIA (PAC)

The range and severity of symptoms in SVCS depend on how rapidly the obstruction develops, its underlying cause, its location and whether it extends into the mediastinum, the presence of laryngeal edema, the availability of collateral circulation, and the amount of venous hypertension (Drews, 2006; Moore, 2005; Flounders, 2003; Yahalom, 2001; Haapoja & Blendowski, 1999).

Symptoms can arise suddenly or gradually. Because the course of SVCS can vary greatly from one patient to another, identifying a baseline assessment for each individual is important. Early recognition prompts early treatment and can often prevent symptoms from progressing to life-threatening airway obstruction, congestive heart failure, and cerebral hypoxia (Flounders, 2003; Haapoja & Blendowski, 1999).

Although debate persists about which symptoms present early in SVCS, the cluster of hallmark symptoms include dyspnea, facial edema or head fullness, cough, upper extremity edema, and upper torso vein engorgement. Most signs and symptoms worsen when the patient bends over or is in the supine position. Some patients may experience symptoms of SVCS only in the morning after rising (Drews, 2006; Moore, 2005; Flounders, 2003: Myers, 2001; Haapoja & Blendowski, 1999). Table 46-1 presents a more detailed list of some of the clinical signs and symptoms, and Table 46-2 lists the diagnostic and differential tests for SVCS.

NURSING CARE AND TREATMENT

SVCS has many potential causes, therefore identification of its underlying etiology is important in directing treatment, especially because the syndrome may be the first sign of disease (Wudel & Nesbitt, 2001; Yahalom, 2001).

1. Vital signs: Assess for hypertension, tachycardia, tachypnea, and/or fever. Monitor every 15 minutes if the patient is in acute distress.
2. Elevate the head of the bed to high Fowler's position so that gravity can help reduce pulmonary congestion.

Table 46-1	POSSIBLE SIGNS AND SYMPTOMS OF SVCS	
System	**Subjective Assessment**	**Objective Assessment**
General	C/O hoarseness, chest pain, pain at site of goiter or thrombosis	Enlarged, nontender lymph nodes
Skin	C/O ruddy complexion	Plethora (facial erythema) or skin tone change in upper torso, reddish palms and mucous membranes, "looks healthier" with fewer visible age lines and wrinkles
HEENT	C/O headache, visual changes, mood changes, difficulty swallowing, nasal stuffiness	Mood or behavior changes, enlarged lymph nodes in the neck, periorbital edema, edema of the conjunctivae
Respiratory	C/O dyspnea, "catching" breath, nonproductive cough, breathing hard or fast, fatigue, throat spasms	Acute dyspnea, SOB, stridor, crackles on auscultation, tachypnea, decreased lung expansion, dyspnea on exertion, decreased pulse oximetry level, cyanosis (nail bed first), paroxysmal nocturnal dyspnea (increased dyspnea when lying down), laryngospasms and sternal retractions on inspiration, right-side pleural effusion
Cardiovascular	C/O palpitations, dizziness, Stoke's sign (tight collar, unable to button shirt at neck), neck and/or head fullness, rings on hands feel tight, ear fullness, chest or breast edema, orthopnea	Acute tachycardia; bounding pulse; initial hypertension then hypotension; possibly orthostatic blood pressures; BP may be higher in upper extremities than in lower extremities; increased jugular venous distension/pressure; edema in the face, neck, chest, and/or arms; early morning periorbital edema; decreased neck flexibility; epistaxis; difficulty with peripheral venipuncture; hand veins do not collapse when the hands are raised over the head; frequent IV infiltrations on right side
GI	C/O dysphagia, poor appetite, nausea, heartburn	Weight gain over 1 to 2 weeks
GU	C/O "not voiding much"	Urine output <30 mL/hr
Musculoskeletal	C/O upper body aches, stiffness, weakness, fatigue	Decreased range of motion in upper extremities, decreased ability to perform ADLs
Neurologic	Family reports intermittent confusion, C/O decreased ability to concentrate, headache, lethargy, visual changes	Mood swings, delirium, altered cognition, altered level of consciousness (can progress to stupor and coma), altered vision, Horner's syndrome (unilateral ptosis with constricted pupil), seizures, death
Psychosocial	C/O restlessness, apprehension, anxiety, premonition of doom, irritability	Visibly restless, anxious

Data from Haapoja, I., & Blendowski, C. (1999). Superior vena cava syndrome. *Seminars in Oncology Nursing*, 15(3):183-189; Hemann, R. (2001). Superior vena cava syndrome. *Clinical Excellence for Nurse Practitioners*, 5(2):85-87; Merrill, P. (2000). Oncologic emergencies. *Primary Care Practice*, 4(4):400-409; Moore, S. (2005). Superior vena cava syndrome. In C. Henke Yarbro, M. Hansen, & M. Goodman, et al. (Ed.), *Cancer nursing: Principles and practice* (pp. 925-939). Sudbury, MA: Jones & Bartlett; and Tyson, L. (2004). Oncologic urgencies and emergencies. In N. Houlihan, (Ed.), *Lung cancer* (pp. 45-55). Pittsburgh: Oncology Nursing Society.

Table 46-2 DIAGNOSTIC AND DIFFERENTIAL TESTS FOR SUPERIOR VENA CAVA SYNDROME

Test	Risk	Findings
CBC with diff	Minimal	Monitor for anemia or infection. WBC count may be elevated. Hgb and Hct may be low.
PT/PTT/INR	Minimal	Monitor for clotting times, pulmonary embolism, hypercoagulable state, DIC. Results may be elevated. Obtain baseline data for possible thrombolytic therapy.
Fibrin split products	Minimal	Assess for s/s of DVT, DIC, PE. May be positive test. Obtain baseline data.
Fibrinogen	Minimal	Monitor for DVT, DIC, PE. Obtain baseline data.
Chemistries	Minimal	Monitor for hypovolemia. BUN/creatinine may be elevated. Obtain baseline values for renal function. Monitor for hyponatremia, hypokalemia, hypo magnesia, hypokalemia. Obtain baseline data.
ABGs	Minimal	Monitor for degree of respiratory compromise. May indicate poor perfusion. Obtain baseline data.
Biopsy	Moderate to high risk, depending on degree of respiratory compromise and risk of bleeding	Obtain and assess biopsy results if a mass is present; may indicate cancer diagnosis.
ECG	Minimal	Monitor rhythms for tachycardia and atrial fibrillation or myocardial injury/ischemia. Obtain baseline data.
CT scan	Minimal	Differentiates internal or external compression; identifies mass and surrounding structures; localizes tumor area for biopsy.
CXR	Minimal	Identifies presence of mediastinal mass, if SVC is caused by a tumor or lymphadenopathy. Normal CXR may indicate cause is thrombus or radiation fibrosis.
CT-guided biopsy	Moderate to high risk, depending on degree of respiratory compromise and risk of bleeding	Obtain to evaluate the cancer diagnosis (histologic diagnosis).
MRI	Minimal	Multidimensional image of the vena cava and source of obstruction; noninvasive tool to identify vascular pathways and mediastinal structures.
Contrast venography	Moderate, depending on the risk of bleeding	Detects compromise in the circulation and collateral venous development.

Data from Chernecky, C., & Berger, B. (2004). *Laboratory and diagnostic procedures*. Philadelphia: W. B. Saunders; and Moore, S. (2005). Superior vena cava syndrome. In C. Henke Yarbro, M. Hansen, & M. Goodman, et al. (Ed.). *Cancer nursing: Principles and practice* (pp. 925-939). Sudbury, MA: Jones & Bartlett.

3. Obtain and interpret O_2 saturation (signs of hypoxia include restlessness, dyspnea, anxiety, and cyanosis) and ABGs (hypoxia, acidosis).
4. Measure dyspnea on a 0 to 10 scale (0 = no dyspnea and 10 = severe dyspnea) at least every shift unless the patient is in acute distress.
5. Administer oxygen to treat hypoxia. Suction as needed for difficulty handling secretions. Have airway at bedside.
6. Assess for any laryngeal or tracheal edema, hoarseness, difficulty swallowing, stridor, headache, visual changes, changes in mood or orientation, delirium, palpitations, dizziness, epistaxis, nonproductive cough, crackles, adventitious breath sounds, decreased chest expansion, neck and chest vein engorgement, and edema (face, neck, upper torso, upper extremities).
7. Anticipate STAT radiation therapy or stent placement for acute distress from increased intracranial pressure, laryngeal edema, or airway obstruction (Moore, 2005).
8. Avoid any venous constriction. Take BP in nonaffected upper extremity or in lower extremity. Keep legs flat or below heart level.
9. Obtain and maintain venous access in nonaffected upper extremity via 18-gauge peripheral IV in an adult or via a venous access device (VAD).
10. Obtain and monitor laboratory test results: CBC, diff, chemistries, BUN/creat, PT/PTT/INR, fibrin split, fibrinogen, thyroid studies. NOTE: Blood for PT determinations should be drawn 5 hours after IV administration of heparin and 24 hours after subcutaneous administration of heparin, or the PT will be lengthened. Many Chinese herbals prolong bleeding, and coffee or herbal coffee can falsely decrease the INR. The INR increases with the use of feverfew, garlic, gingko biloba, ginseng, or ginger (Chernecky & Berger, 2004).
11. Obtain and/or assess: Chest x-ray film, CT/MRI of the chest for venous congestion, pleural or pericardial effusion, cardiomegaly, mediastinal widening, mediastinal mass, lymphadenopathy, and/or tracheal compression. If a mass is suspected, obtain a biopsy.
12. Anticipate possible administration of (Myers, 2001; Wudel & Nesbitt, 2001):
    • Corticosteroids for inflammation.
    • Antiarrhythmic medication, depending on the rhythm of ECG changes and heart strain.
    • Broad-spectrum antibiotics IVPB for signs of infection or fever.
    • Itraconazole IVPB for histoplasmosis from fibrosing mediastinitis.
    • Diuretics with dietary sodium and fluid restriction. Note that overhydration can exacerbate symptoms (Haapoja & Blendowski, 1999).
    • Radiation therapy, once a cancer diagnosis has been confirmed, with high-dose fractions for 2 to 3 days, followed daily by standard fractions for the total prescribed dose (Donato et al., 2001).
      • Chemotherapy may be used in combination with radiation therapy for treating underlying cancer
      • Heparin by continuous IV infusion until the INR is 2 to 3 (Moore, 2005); also rt-PA (tissue plasminogen) IVP for risk of thrombosis or occlusion. Contraindicated if patient has brain or spinal cord metastases, past CVA, or history of bleeding (Haapoja & Blendowski, 1999).
      • Warfarin 1 mg PO daily starting with heparin to help maintain INR. NOTE: In patients receiving heparin, concurrent therapy with warfarin or fluoxetine can increase PT slightly (Chernecky & Berger, 2004).
      • Warfarin 1 mg PO daily with monthly urokinase IVP may be used for prophylaxis in patients at risk for SVCS (Drews, 2006).
      • With IV heparin, monitor for ecchymosis and inflammation, which may indicate extravasation. If present, stop the infusion and apply ice or a cold pack to the site.

- Monitor fibrinogen, PTT, and INR every 6 hours during therapy (Moore, 2005). Note the influence of some medications and herbals on lab test results (Chernecky & Berger, 2004).

13. Monitor for side effects of radiation therapy (esophagitis, cough, nausea, skin reaction, and fatigue) and/or chemotherapy (myelosuppression, nausea and vomiting, stomatitis, esophagitis, and alopecia) (Spira & Ettinger, 2004; Tyson, 2004; Myers, 2001).

14. Monitor for any medication side effects (e.g., mood swings, involuntary muscle activity, glycosuria, insomnia, dehydration or pulmonary edema, thrombosis with risk of pulmonary embolus, venous congestion, and bleeding).

15. Intake and output every hour initially (until patient is stabilized), then every 2 hours.

16. Anticipate possible placement of an intraluminal stent for acute symptoms, refractory disease, recurrence after radiation therapy, or risk of intolerance of other therapy (Drews, 2006; Greillier et al., 2004). A stent is contraindicated if the tumor has invaded the SVC (Moore, 2005).
    - A stent may be used in combination with radiation therapy or chemotherapy.
    - IV heparin may be used during stent placement, but warfarin is often used for 3 to 6 months after placement (Moore, 2005).
    - Balloon angioplasty may be done to completely reopen the occluded SVC.
    - Monitor for:
        - Postoperative hematoma, infection, deep vein thrombosis, transient renal insufficiency, or pleuritic chest and/or shoulder pain. Administer analgesics PRN (Moore, 2005; Myers, 2001). Monitor for possible respiratory depression.
        - Rare complications, including pulmonary edema, stent migration, stent fracture, or cardiac and respiratory distress from cardiac tamponade (stent penetration through vena caval wall into the pericardial sac) (Dinkel et al., 2003; Myers, 2001).

17. Offer calm and supportive environment to reduce the patient's anxiety.
    - Use relaxation techniques (e.g., imagery, music therapy).
    - Administer antianxiety agents (i.e., Ativan PO or IV) PRN as prescribed.

18. Assess and offer support to the patient and family in meeting spiritual needs.

19. Refer the patient to the clinical nurse specialist, social worker, dietician, pastoral care professional, home health nurse, and/or hospice as indicated.

EVIDENCE-BASED PRACTICE UPDATES

1. Intravascular devices are the most common benign etiology of SVCS, followed by fibrosing mediastinitis (Rice et al., 2006).

2. Stenting as a first-line therapy in patients with non-small cell lung cancer achieves quick resolution of SVCS without immediate or delayed complications (Greillier et al., 2004; Urruticoechea, Mesia, Domiguez, et.al., 2004)).

3. Unilateral stent placement in the treatment of malignant SVCS achieved greater patency and fewer complications than bilateral stent therapy (Dinkel et al., 2003).

4. Palliative stenting can be useful as a first-line therapeutic measure before antitumor therapy for quick symptom response without serious complications; the results are better than those obtained with radiation therapy or chemotherapy alone (Bierdrager et al., 2005).

5. Treatment with short-course, large fraction radiation therapy in patients over 70 years old who had solid malignancy–related SVCS achieved symptomatic relief of SVCS with mild systemic effects (i.e., chest pain, fever). These patients also had greater tolerance of treatment and minimal side effects (Lonardi et al., 2002).

TEACHING AND EDUCATION

Dyspnea: *Rationale:* We may need to give you oxygen to help you feel less short of breath and to help your heart pump more easily. Keeping the tube or mask on gives you extra oxygen while we reduce your swelling. Minimize your activity when you feel short of breath.

Anxiety: *Rationale:* When you are short of breath, you may sometimes feel anxious and restless. These feelings can make you breathe faster, making you more uncomfortable. To break this cycle, try slow, deep-breathing exercises, guided imagery, watching TV, listening to music, or taking antianxiety medication prescribed by your health care provider. Let your nurse and physician know how you are feeling.

Nutrition and fluids: *Rationale:* Eat small meals high in calories and protein. Your health care team wants you to limit liquids and salt to help reduce your swelling.

Tests: *Rationale:* You may need x-ray films, CT scans, or an MRI scan of your chest, as well as an ECG or heart monitor to watch your heart rhythm. Also, blood samples may need to be drawn from a vein in your nonswollen arm, from the PortaCath, or from your wrist.

Procedures: *Rationale:* A biopsy of your lungs or chest lymph nodes may be required to help your physician identify the reason your blood is backing up and causing the swelling. A specially trained physician will give you a numbing medication and then insert a tube into your airway (or a needle into your chest) to collect a tissue sample. The sample can be studied under a microscope to determine the disease that is causing your symptoms.

Signs to report: *Rationale:* High pressure can occur in your superior vena cava from blood backing up. Because the superior vena cava is a major vein that returns blood from your upper extremities to your heart, high pressure can cause swelling in your face, neck, head, chest, arms, and/or hands. It is important to tell your nurse or physician if you have:
- Swelling, changes in your vision, changes in your mood or thinking, a persistent cough, periods of confusion, difficulty passing urine, or seizures.
- Shortness of breath, difficulty swallowing or talking, a very rapid heart rate, dizziness, chest pain, or extreme weakness.

Safety precautions: *Rationale:* Let your nurse or family know right away if you feel dizzy or have any changes in your thinking or vision. Call for help in getting out of bed or going to the bathroom to prevent falls. Avoid coughing, sneezing, bending over, or straining when trying to have a bowel movement. Any of these normal activities can increase the pressure in your head and chest, making you more uncomfortable.

Reducing swelling: *Rationale:* Keeping the head of your bed elevated will help make it easier for you to breathe. Avoid tight clothing and rings, because these can cause more blood to back up. Keep your legs flat and below your heart to help your blood circulate better. Your physician or nurse may prescribe steroids and a diuretic to help reduce the swelling (Walton, 2005).

Radiation therapy: *Rationale:* Your physician has decided that the best way to ease your symptoms is to use concentrated x-ray beams, or radiation therapy, to shrink the mass pressing on your superior vena cava. Radiation therapy usually helps you feel better in 2 to 3 days (Myers, 2001). (Review the potential side effects with the patient and family.)

Chemotherapy: *Rationale:* Your physician has decided that the best way to ease your symptoms is to use a strong medication to shrink the mass pressing on your superior vena cava. Chemotherapy usually can help you feel better in 7 to 10 days (Walton, 2005). (Review the potential side effects of specific agents with the patient and family.)

Anticoagulant and thrombolytic therapy: *Rationale:* Your physician has decided that your symptoms may be caused by blockage from a blood clot, which is preventing some of your blood from circulating, and that the best way to treat this is with medication. This medicine will help break down the clot and prevent clotting in the future. Call your nurse or physician if you feel dizzy, have bruising, or have blood in your urine, stool, or phlegm (spit).

Stent placement: *Rationale:* To open up your blocked superior vena cava, a specially trained physician will give you numbing medication and insert a small catheter with a balloon into the vessel through the skin in your chest. This is done under fluoroscopy in the x-ray department. The balloon may be inflated to help open the blockage. Stent placement usually helps you feel better in 1 to 3 days (Bierdrager et al., 2005). Let your nurse know right away if you have any chest or shoulder pain so that you can be given pain-relieving medication.

Recurrence: *Rationale:* Watch for any signs that may indicate that superior vena cava syndrome is recurring. These signs include difficulty breathing, shortness of breath, swelling in your face, neck, chest, arms, or fingers, and cough. Call your physician right away if you notice these signs.

Web sites for information:
- American Cancer Society: www.cancer.org
- American Lung Association: www.lungusa.org
- National Cancer Institute: www.cancer.gov
- Cleveland Clinic Foundation: www.chemocare.com

NURSING DIAGNOSES

1. **Decreased cardiac output** related to decreased venous return
2. **Ineffective tissue perfusion** related to cardiovascular dysfunction and/or cerebral tissue perfusion related to venous congestion
3. **Ineffective breathing pattern** related to decreased tissue perfusion and/or airway compression
4. **Anxiety** related to hypoxia
5. **Deficient knowledge** related to signs and symptoms to report for intervention (Hunter, 2005; Carpenito-Moyet, 2005)

EVALUATION AND DESIRED OUTCOMES

1. The patient will rate dyspnea, cough, fatigue, hoarseness, and anxiety each as less than 3 on a 0 to 10 scale. (Assess for improvement and offer supportive care if symptoms persist.)
2. O_2 saturation will be greater than 92%, ABGs will be within patient's baseline, and respiratory function will be maintained.
3. The patient will have no edema (head, neck, upper torso, or upper extremities), head or neck erythema, chest pain, distended jugular or chest veins, headache, visual

changes, mood changes, enlarged lymph nodes in the neck, throat spasm, dysphagia, or ptosis.

4. CBC, platelets, differential, electrolytes, liver enzymes, PT/PTT/INR, fibrin split product, fibrinogen, BUN, creatinine, and thyroid studies will be done to monitor values.
5. INR will be within the range of 2 to 3 (Moore, 2005).
6. CXR/CT/MRI findings will be within normal limits.
7. The patient and family will deny changes in ADLs and cognitive functioning.

DISCHARGE PLANNING AND FOLLOW-UP CARE

- Home oxygen via tube or mask as prescribed for advanced malignancy.
- Scheduled radiation therapy or chemotherapy as indicated.
- Weekly home health nursing visits for at least 1 to 2 months for assessment of pulmonary and cardiac symptom relief or progression, anticoagulation therapy, antianxiety interventions, and evaluation of medications prescribed and herbals taken.
- Family or caregiver assistance with meal preparation, ADLs, safety precautions, and household maintenance if needed.
- Follow-up visit to physician's office within 1 week of discharge. Discuss hospice referral as an option for advanced cancer or SVCS that is not responding to treatment.
- Follow-up:
  - CBC, platelets, PT/PTT/INR within 1 week of discharge.
  - CXR, CT scan, PT/PTT/INR, CBC, platelets, and/or electrolytes if symptoms recur.
- Monitor for late side effects of mediastinal radiation therapy: pneumonitis, pulmonary fibrosis, ulceration or stenosis of the esophagus, spinal cord myelopathy, brachial plexopathy, cardiac changes (Moore, 2005; Flounders, 2003; Miaskowski, 1999).

REVIEW QUESTIONS

QUESTIONS

1. **Superior vena cava syndrome (SVCS) is primarily a disorder involving:**
   1. Venous congestion
   2. Hypovolemia
   3. Pulmonary edema
   4. Dysrhythmias

2. **A mechanism that can cause compression of the SVC is:**
   1. Congestive heart failure
   2. Extrinsic or invasive tumor
   3. Hepatomegaly
   4. Cerebral edema

3. **A patient with severe onset of respiratory symptoms may be experiencing difficulty compensating with SVCS because:**
   1. Anxiety increases hypoxia.
   2. Venous pressure is low.
   3. Cardiac output has not increased.
   4. Collateral circulation has not developed.

4. **Risk factors for developing SVCS include:**
   1. Sarcoidosis and recent myocardial infarction
   2. Mediastinitis and lymphoma
   3. Tuberculosis and malnutrition
   4. Coronary artery disease and goiter

5. **Hallmark signs of SVCS include:**
   1. Shortness of breath, hypotension, and facial edema
   2. Dyspnea, facial edema, and neck vein engorgement
   3. Tachypnea, cough, and headache
   4. Upper extremity edema, anxiety, and lymphadenopathy

6. **The overall prognosis for patients with SVCS depends on whether:**
   1. The SVCS is caused by cancer involving the mediastinum.
   2. The SVCS is caused by thrombosis.

3. The peripheral circulation is adequate.
4. The diagnostic workup includes invasive tests.

7. **Diagnostic tests for SVCS include:**
   1. CBC, diff, and cardiac enzymes
   2. CT scan, chest x-ray film, and pulmonary function tests
   3. PTT/INR, chest x-ray film, and biopsy
   4. ECG, head CT scan, and chemistries

8. **The top priority nursing intervention for acute onset SVCS is:**
   1. Maintaining venous return from the lower extremities
   2. Maintaining a patent airway
   3. Preventing overhydration
   4. Correcting electrolyte imbalances

9. **Possible treatments for SVCS may include:**
   1. Radiation therapy, chemotherapy, and bypass surgery
   2. Anticoagulants, thrombolytics, and IV fluid bolus
   3. Stent placement, steroids, and a diuretic
   4. Radiation therapy, antibiotics, and vein stripping

10. **Important precautions to highlight in teaching the patient with SVCS include:**
    1. Elevate your head and feet to prevent swelling.
    2. Avoid getting out of bed in the morning.
    3. Refuse any invasive diagnostic tests.
    4. Avoid straining or bending.

ANSWERS

1. *Answer: 1*
   Rationale: SVCS results from blockage and congestion of venous blood flow returning from the body to the heart through the SVC.

2. *Answer: 2*
   Rationale: Causative mechanisms of SVCS include compression by an extrinsic or invasive tumor, infection, inflammation, central venous catheter or pacemaker thrombosis, and thrombosis in the SVC.

3. *Answer: 4*
   Rationale: Acute onset SVCS causes severe respiratory symptoms because collateral circulation around the compressed or obstructed SVC has not had time to develop.

4. *Answer: 2*
   Rationale: Risk factors for SVCS include sarcoidosis, mediastinitis, lymphoma, tuberculosis, and goiter. Recent MI, malnutrition, and coronary artery disease may exacerbate SVCS but are not causes of the syndrome.

5. *Answer: 2*
   Rationale: Hallmark signs of SVCS include dyspnea, facial edema or head fullness, cough, upper extremity edema, and neck vein engorgement.

6. *Answer: 1*
   Rationale: The overall prognosis for patients with SVCS depends on the underlying cause (the prognosis is worse if mediastinal cancer is the cause), the patient's age and gender, the speed of onset, the degree of vena caval blockage, the adequacy of collateral circulation around the SVC, and whether a tissue sample can be obtained for diagnosis.

7. *Answer: 3*
   Rationale: Diagnostic tests for SVCS include CBC, diff, CT scan of the chest, chest x-ray film, PTT/INR, biopsy (if tumor is suspected), ECG, and chemistries.

8. *Answer: 2*
   Rationale: Because of the high risk of airway obstruction and hypoxia with acute onset SVCS, maintaining a patent airway is the top nursing priority.

9. *Answer: 3*
   Rationale: Possible treatments for SVCS may include radiation therapy, chemotherapy, anticoagulant and thrombolytic therapy, stent placement, steroids, diuretics, and antibiotics. IV fluid bolus is contraindicated to prevent overhydration, which can exacerbate symptoms.

10. *Answer: 4*

Rationale: Important precautions to highlight in teaching the patient ways to prevent complications of SVCS include elevating the head to maintain the airway and prevent venous congestion in head and neck; asking for help when getting out of bed if dizzy; and avoiding straining or bending, which could increase intracranial pressure. Elevating the feet only reduces venous return.

REFERENCES

Bierdrager, E., Lampmann, L., & Lohle, P., et al. (2005). Endovascular stenting in neoplastic superior vena cava syndrome prior to chemotherapy or radiotherapy. *Journal of Medicine, 63*(1):20-23.

Carpenito-Moyet, L. (2005). *Handbook of nursing diagnosis.* Philadelphia: Lippincott Williams & Wilkins.

Chernecky, C., & Berger, B. (2004). *Laboratory and diagnostic procedures.* Philadelphia: W. B. Saunders.

Dinkel, H., Mettke, B., & Schmid, F., et al. (2003). Endovascular treatment of malignant superior vena cava syndrome: Is bilateral wall stent placement superior to unilateral placement? *Journal of Endovascular Therapy, 10*(4):788-797.

Donato, V., Bonfili, P., & Bulzonetti, N., et al. (2001). Radiation therapy for oncological emergencies. *Anticancer Research, 21*(3C):2219-2224.

Drews, R. (2006). Superior vena cava syndrome. UpToDate. Retrieved April 24, 2006, from http://www.up-todateonline.com/utd/content/topic.do?topicKey=genl_onc/8555&view.

Flounders, J. (2003). Oncology emergency modules: Superior vena cava syndrome. *Oncology Nursing Forum, 30*(4):1-11.

Greillier, L., Barlesi, F., & Doddoli, C., et al. (2004). Vascular stenting for palliation of superior vena cava obstruction in non-small cell lung cancer patients: A future "standard" procedure? *Respiration, 71*(2):178-183.

Haapoja, I., & Blendowski, C. (1999). Superior vena cava syndrome. *Seminars in Oncology Nursing, 15*(3):183-189.

Hemann, R. (2001). Superior vena cava syndrome. *Clinical Excellence for Nurse Practitioners, 5*(2):85-87.

Hogan, D., & Rosenthal, L. (1998). Oncologic emergencies in the patient with lymphoma. *Seminars in Oncology Nursing, 14*:312-320.

Hunter, J. (2005). Structural emergencies. In J. Itano & K. Takoa (Eds.), *Core curriculum in oncology nursing* (pp. 340-356). St. Louis: Mosby.

Joyce, M., & Cunningham, R. (1998). Metastases that interfere with circulation. *Seminars in Oncology Nursing, 14*:230-239.

Krimsky, W., Behrens, R., & Kervliet, G. (2002). Oncologic emergencies for the internist. *Cleveland Clinic Journal of Medicine, 69*(3):209-222.

Lonardi, F., Gioga, G., & Agus, G., et al. (2002). Double-flash, large-fraction radiation therapy as palliative treatment of malignant superior vena cava syndrome in the elderly. *Support Care Cancer, 10*:156-160.

Merrill, P. (2000). Oncologic emergencies. *Primary Care Practice, 4*(4):400-409.

Myers, J. (2001). Oncologic complications. In S. Otto (Ed.), *Oncology nursing* (pp. 521-527). St. Louis: Mosby.

Miaskowski, C. (1999). Oncologic emergencies. In C. Miaskowski & P. Buchsel (Eds.), *Oncology nursing assessment and clinical care* (pp. 221-243). St. Louis: Mosby.

Moore, S. (2005). Superior vena cava syndrome. In C. Henke Yarbro M. Hansen & M. Goodman M., et al. (Eds.), *Cancer nursing: Principles and practice* (pp. 925-939). Sudbury, MA: Jones & Bartlett.

Rice, T., Rodriguez, R., & Light, R. (2006). The superior vena cava syndrome: Clinical characteristics and evolving etiology. *Medicine, 85*(1):37-42.

Spira, A., & Ettinger, D. (2004). Multidisciplinary management of lung cancer. *New England Journal of Medicine, 350*:379-392.

Tyson, L. (2004). Oncologic urgencies and emergencies. In N. Houlihan (Ed.), *Lung cancer* (pp. 45-55). Pittsburgh: Oncology Nursing Society.

Urruticoechea, A., Mesia, R., & Domiguez, J., et al. (2004). Treatment of malignant superior vena cava syndrome by endovascular stent insertion: Experience of 52 patients with lung cancer. *Lung Cancer, 43*(2):209-214.

Walton, A. (2005). Superior vena cava syndrome: An education sheet for patients. *Clinical Journal of Oncology Nursing, 9*(4):479-480.

Wudel, L., & Nesbitt, J. (2001). Superior vena cava syndrome. *Current Treatment Options in Oncology, 2*(1):77-91.

Yahalom, J. (2001). Oncologic emergencies: Superior vena cava syndrome. In V. DeVita S. Hellman & S. Rosenberg (Eds.), *Cancer: Principles and practice of oncology* (pp. 2609-2616). Philadelphia: Lippincott Williams & Wilkins.

Syndrome of Inappropriate Antidiuretic Hormone (SIADH)

JEANNE HELD-WARMKESSEL

PATHOPHYSIOLOGICAL MECHANISMS

The human body is approximately 60% water, which is contained within two major compartments, the extracellular fluid and the intracellular fluid (Guyton & Hall, 2000). The fluid inside the cells is called *intracellular fluid;* the *extracellular fluid* is found outside the cells, in the plasma and the interstitial fluid. Most of the body's fluids are intracellular fluids.

Dissolved as ions or solutes in the water are electrolytes, which are separated by a cell membrane; this helps keep the ions in their appropriate compartment. Intracellular ions consist mostly of potassium and phosphate ions, with lesser amounts of magnesium and sulfate ions; these ions are found to a lesser extent in the extracellular fluid. The chief ions of the extracellular fluid are sodium and chloride (Guyton & Hall, 2000). The number of solutes dissolved in water is termed *osmoles*, and the osmolarity of a solution is based on the number of solutes in the solution.

The body has a variety of homeostatic mechanisms to maintain a balance between the cellular compartments. Thirst is a major mechanism of fluid intake. Fluids and electrolytes are lost through the skin, lungs, renal system, and gastrointestinal tract. The cells regulate water passage across the cell membrane to maintain isotonicity between the intracellular and extracellular fluids (Guyton & Hall, 2000). *Osmosis* is the process by which water moves. If one compartment has too much or too little of an ion concentration, water moves between compartments to restore balance.

The kidneys regulate the amount of water and solutes in the body. When the body has too little water, the posterior pituitary gland secretes and releases antidiuretic hormone (ADH), which allows the kidneys to reabsorb water; when the body has too much water, ADH release stops, and the kidneys excrete the excess water. Water and sodium ions have a close alliance, therefore if the amount of water is reduced, the sodium concentration increases; ADH is released and causes more water to be reabsorbed by the kidneys and less water to be excreted (Guyton & Hall, 2000).

In SIADH, the body secretes ADH (also known as vasopressin) inappropriately from the hypothalamus, resulting in water reabsorption by the kidneys and increased body water with increased intracellular and extracellular water (Flounders, 2003). The excess water dilutes the sodium in the extracellular compartment, causing hyposmolarity and movement of water into the intracellular compartment. As a result, the patient has a fluid volume excess intracellularly and a low solute (sodium) concentration extracellularly (Flounders, 2003).

In summary, ADH secretion results in increased water absorption by the kidneys, causing hypervolemia and dilutional hyponatremia. Therefore some signs of hypervolemia are seen, including weight gain, normal or elevated blood pressure, and changes in mental status (Trimarchi, 2006). However, heart failure, edema, and ascites are not normally seen (Flounders, 2003), because most of the water is intracellular.

EPIDEMIOLOGY AND ETIOLOGY

Although frequently a paraneoplastic syndrome, SIADH has both malignant and nonmalignant causes. The most common malignant causes are small cell lung cancer (SCLC), followed by GI and GU cancers. Approximately 3% to 15% of patients with SCLC develop SIADH (Lokich, 1982). SCLC cells produce ectopic ADH, resulting in SIADH (Gandhi & Johnson, 2006). Two alkylating agents, ifosfamide and cyclophosphamide, are associated with SIADH, as are carboplatin (Yokoyama et al., 2005; Chu & DeVita, 2004), cisplatin (Yamamoto et al., 2005; Chu & DeVita, 2004), and the monoclonal antibody alemtuzumab (Kunz & Bannerji, 2005). SIADH has numerous causes and risk factors (Box 47-1). Antidepressants, especially the selective serotonin reuptake inhibitors (SSRIs), and anticonvulsants are also known causes (Table 47-1).

BOX 47-1	PARTIAL RISK PROFILE FOR SIADH

Malignant Conditions
- Lung cancers
  - Small cell
  - Non-small cell
- Gastrointestinal cancers
  - Duodenal
  - Pancreas
  - Colon
  - Carcinoid
  - Esophageal
- Genitourinary cancers
  - Ovarian
  - Bladder
  - Ureter
  - Prostate
- Other cancers
  - Brain, brain metastases, carcinomatous meningitis, neuroblastoma
  - Breast
  - Sarcomas
  - Lymphomas and leukemias
  - Other small cell tumors
  - Mesothelioma
  - Thymoma
  - Head and neck

Nonmalignant Conditions
- Central nervous system
  - Head trauma
  - Infection
  - Meningitis
  - Encephalitis
  - Intracranial bleeding

Continued

BOX 47-1	**PARTIAL RISK PROFILE FOR SIADH—cont'd**

- Abscess
- CVA
- Polydipsia
- Pulmonary
  - Pneumonia
  - Abscess
  - Tuberculosis
  - Asthma
  - Infections
  - Pneumothorax
  - Respiratory failure
- Peripheral neuropathy
- Infections
  - AIDS
- Hypotension, dehydration
- Severe pain
- Pain from abdominal or chest surgery
  - Pituitary surgery
- Smoking
- Emotional stress
- Hemorrhage
- Medications
  - Antineoplastics:
  - Ifosfamide
  - Cyclophosphamide
  - Vincristine
  - Vinblastine
  - Cisplatin
  - Carboplatin
  - Melphalan
  - Monoclonal antibody:
  - Alemtuzumab
  - Narcotics and acetaminophen
  - Non-steroidal anti-inflammatory agents
  - Anesthetic agents
  - Anticonvulsants (Table 47-1)
  - Antidepressants
  - Barbiturates
  - Selective serotonin reuptake inhibitors (Table 47-1)
  - Antipsychotics
  - Diuretics
  - Oral hypoglycemics
- Chemotherapy-induced nausea
- Exogenous hormones
- Nicotine, cigarette smoking

Data from Kraft, M. D., Btaiche, I. F., & Sacks, G. S., et al. (2005). Treatment of electrolyte disorders in adult patients in the intensive care unit. *American Journal of Health-System Pharmacy, 62*:1663-1682; Robertson, G. L. (2005). Disorders of the neurohypophysis. In D. L. Kasper, E. Braunwald, & A. S. Fauci, et al. (Eds.), *Harrison's principles of internal medicine* (pp. 2097-2104). (16th ed). New York: McGraw-Hill; Poe, C. M., & Taylor, L. M. (1989). Syndrome of inappropriate antidiuretic hormone: Assessment and nursing implications. *Oncology Nursing Forum, 16*:373-381; Keenan, A. M. M. (1999). Syndrome of inappropriate antidiuretic hormone in malignancy. *Seminars in Oncology Nursing, 15*:160-167; Richerson, M. T. (2004). Electrolyte imbalances. In C. H. Yarbro, M. H. Frogge, & M. Goodman (Eds.), *Cancer symptom management* (pp.440-453). (3rd ed.). Sudbury, MA: Jones & Bartlett; Flounders, J. A. (2003). Syndrome of inappropriate antidiuretic hormone. *Oncology Nursing Forum, 30*(3):E63-E68. Retrieved May 25, 2006, from http://www.ons.org/publications/journals/ONF/Volume30/Issue3/pdf/381.pdf; and Rose, B. D. (2006). Causes of the SIADH. UpToDate. Retrieved May 24, 2006, from http://www.uptodateonline.com.

Table 47-1	SSRI ANTIDEPRESSANT AND ANTICONVULSANT MEDICATIONS KNOWN TO CAUSE SIADH		
Generic Name	**Trade Name**	**Medication Category**	**Reference**
Carbamazepine	Tegretol	Anticonvulsant	Llinares-Tello et al., 2005
Levetiracetam	Keppra	Anticonvulsant	Nasrallah & Silver, 2005
Amitriptyline	Apo-amitriptyline	SSRI	Miehle et al., 2005
Citalopram hydrochloride	Celexa	SSRI	Miehle et al., 2005
Duloxetine	Cymbalta	SSRI	Maramattom, 2006
Escitalopram oxalate	Lexapro	SSRI	Miehle et al., 2005
Fluoxetine hydrochloride	Prozac	SSRI	Maramattom, 2006
Paroxetine mesylate	Paxil	SSRI	Alvarez Perez et al., 2004

RISK PROFILE

- **Age:** Older adults and children are more prone to developing symptoms (Berl & Verbalis, 2004). The prevalence of hyponatremia in elderly individuals living in long-term care facilities in Taipei was reported as 31.3% (Chen et al., 2006), and abnormal sodium levels are commonly found in elderly patients (Tareen et al., 2005; Kugler & Hustead, 2000).
- **Female gender:** Menstruating patients have a greater risk of SIADH-related neurotoxicity (Ayus et al., 1992).
- **Chemotherapy:** Treatment with ifosfamide, cyclophosphamide, carboplatin, or cisplatin.
- **Monoclonal antibody:** Alemtuzumab (Campath) can induce SIADH (Kunz & Bannerji, 2005).
- **Bone marrow transplantation:** The prevalence of SIADH in post stem cell transplant (SCT) patients is 11.4%. SIADH is a common complication, especially in children under 4 years of age and after SCT from an HLA-mismatched donor (Kobayashi et al., 2004). SIADH precedes varicella-zoster virus reactivation months after autologous stem cell transplantation for leukemia (Vinzio et al., 2005).
- Rate and severity of reduced extracellular osmolality (Berl & Verbalis, 2004):
  - The faster the onset of low osmolality, the greater the risk of neurologic symptoms (Berl & Verbalis, 2004).
  - The lower the serum osmolality, the greater the risk of neurologic symptoms (Berl & Verbalis, 2004).
- **Medications:** Use of Ecstasy, treatment with SSRIs or anticonvulsants.
- Cytomegalovirus (CMV) associated with acute pandysautonomia has been reported (Sato et al., 2004).

PROGNOSIS

For patients with cancer and SIADH, the mortality rate ranges from 5% to 55% (Berl, 1990; Sterns, 1987; Arieff et al., 1976). SIADH is a poor prognostic factor and is associated with advanced disease (Berl & Verbalis, 2004).

PROFESSIONAL ASSESSMENT CRITERIA (PAC)

SIADH is frequently detected through diagnostic studies in patients with few symptoms. A high degree of suspicion is required by the health care provider.

1. Laboratory values (Gobel, 2005; Richerson, 2004; Flounders, 2003;): The serum sodium level cannot be used as the sole test to diagnose SIADH; hyposmolality must also be present (Flounders, 2003). Lab values should be assessed daily.
   - Low serum sodium level (less than 130 to 134 mEq/L).
   - Serum hyposmolality (less than 275 to 280 mOsm/kg).
   - Urine hyperosmolality (greater than 300 to 330 mOsm/kg).
   - High urine sodium level (greater than 20 to 25 mEq/L).
   - Urine specific gravity greater than 1.015.
   - Decreased serum values for BUN, creatinine, uric acid, and electrolytes.
   - Normal thyroid, adrenal, cardiac, liver, and kidney function.
   - Normal blood glucose (Robertson, 2005).
2. Clinical manifestations (signs and symptoms) and patient assessment of signs and symptoms (Table 47-2). The development of clinical signs and symptoms is related to how quickly the serum sodium falls and how low it falls in relation to the reduced osmolality of the extracellular fluid (Berl & Verbalis, 2004; Keenan, 1999). Most clinical manifestations are related to the brain; neurologic function is affected by the excess amount of water in the brain cells, which causes these cells to swell (intracellular

Table 47-2 CLINICAL SIGNS AND SYMPTOMS OF SIADH

	Severity		
	Mild	**Moderate**	**Severe**
Serum sodium level (mEq/L)	125-134	115-124	< 115
Clinical manifestations	No symptoms (possible) Dysgeusia (unpleasant sweet taste)	Dysgeusia (unpleasant sweet taste)	Dysgeusia (unpleasant sweet taste)
Neurologic	Headache Mild changes in mental status, such as confusion, trouble concentrating, disorientation, sleepiness	Worsening mental status Confusion Lethargy Loss of deep tendon reflexes Changes in personality Irritability	Coma Seizures Death (rare)
Gastrointestinal	Anorexia Nausea Weight gain	Thirst Impaired taste Nausea Vomiting Diarrhea Abdominal cramps	
Constitutional	Weakness Fatigue Muscle cramps		
Genitourinary		Oliguria Incontinence	

Data from Keenan, A. M. M. (1999). Syndrome of inappropriate antidiuretic hormone in malignancy. *Seminars in Oncology Nursing, 15:*160-167; Poe, C. M., & Taylor, L. M. (1989). Syndrome of inappropriate antidiuretic hormone: Assessment and nursing implications. *Oncology Nursing Forum, 16:*373-381; Richerson, M. T. (2004). Electrolyte imbalances. In C. H. Yarbro, M. H. Frogge, & M. Goodman (Eds.), *Cancer symptom management* (pp. 440-453). (3rd ed.). Sudbury, MA: Jones & Bartlett; Flombaum, C. D. (2000). Metabolic emergencies in the cancer patient. *Seminars in Oncology, 27:*322-334; Panayiotou, H., Small, S. C., & Hunter, J. H., et al. (1995). Sweet taste (dysgeusia): The first symptom of hyponatremia in small cell carcinoma of the lung. *Archives in Internal Medicine, 155*(12):1325-1328; Nakazato, Y., Imai, K., & Abe, T., et al. (2006). Unpleasant sweet taste: A symptom of SIADH caused by lung cancer. *Journal of Neurology, Neurosurgery and Psychiatry, 77*(3):405-406.

fluid expansion). Extracellular fluid excess typically is not seen, therefore patients do not usually develop peripheral edema or heart failure from fluid overload (Flounders, 2003).

3. History or current diagnosis of one or more of the know SIADH etiologies (see Box 47-1).
4. Vital signs may reflect fluid volume excess (increased blood pressure may be present).
5. Weight is increased.
6. Review and evaluation for medications known to cause SIADH (see Table 47-1).

NURSING CARE AND TREATMENT

Treatment decisions are made based on the patient's symptoms, the severity and duration of the hyponatremia, and the risk of neurologic complications (Berl & Verbalis, 2004).

1. Baseline patient assessment, including hydration level (check skin turgor and mucous membrane moisture), weight, medical history, medication review and laboratory study evaluation (Langfeldt & Cooley, 2003).
2. Prone-to-fall precautions; safety assessment, monitoring, and precautions. Patients are at increased risk of falling even with mild hyponatremia (Decaux, 2006). Seizure precautions when the serum sodium level is less than 125 mEq/L. Measures to reduce hazards of immobility (Poe & Taylor, 1989).
3. Assessment of signs and symptoms, paying particular attention to neurologic functioning, every 4 to 8 hours. Neurologic assessments may be needed more frequently in patients with low serum sodium levels. Assess breath sounds for fluid overload (Poe & Taylor, 1989). Other systems requiring ongoing assessment and monitoring include cardiac, gastrointestinal, renal, and muscular systems (Flounders, 2003).
4. Chemotherapy for treatment of underlying or causative malignancy, with radiation for brain metastases per medical oncology (Arnold et al., 2005). Radiation therapy, surgery, or other treatment for malignancy.
5. Daily weights. I & O every 4 to 8 hours. Vital signs every 4 hours. Monitor for fluid volume excess. Monitor lab work results.
6. Discontinue causative medications, if possible. If not possible, monitor fluid and electrolyte balance and weight every 8 or 12 hours and initiate precautions for seizure management and patient safety (Poe & Taylor, 1989).
7. Fluid restriction of 500 to 1000 mL/day (Berl & Verbalis, 2004; Poe & Taylor, 1989; Lokich, 1982) should correct serum sodium in 3 to 10 days. Institute when the serum sodium level is 125 to 134 mEq/L. Calculate the amount of fluid by subtracting 500 mL from the 24-hour urine output; the result is the amount of the fluid restriction (Robertson, 2005). More severe fluid restriction is needed for lower serum sodium levels; the goal is a negative fluid balance (Keenan, 1999).
8. If fluid restriction is unsuccessful, demeclocycline 600-1200 mg/day PO in divided doses reduces the effect of ADH on the renal tubules; this treatment usually is effective in 3 to 7 days or longer (Arnold et. al., 2005; Robertson, 2005; Berl & Verbalis, 2004; Flounders, 2003). The dose is reduced for renal and liver impairment (this drug is known to cause hepatotoxicity). Other side effects include nausea, vomiting, diarrhea, photosensitivity, and infections (Micromedex, 2006). It also may cause renal toxicity, especially at higher doses, therefore renal function needs to be monitored (Micromedex, 2006; Keenan, 1999). If the medication is effective, it is continued and fluid restriction may be stopped. In some patients, the fluid restriction may be stopped when demeclocycline is started.
9. For life-threatening hyponatremia, intravenous hypertonic saline (3%) with intravenous furosemide may be given. Care must be taken to avoid too rapid correction of the serum

sodium level (when hyponatremia has been present for 1 to 2 days) and the hyposmolality to prevent central pontine myelinolysis, which occurs with too rapid shrinking of the brain cells (Sterns & Silver, 2006). This treatment is done in intensive care. The rate of continuous intravenous infusion of 3% saline is equal to or less than 0.05 mL/kg body weight/minute and is monitored every 2 hours by STAT assessments of the serum sodium level (Robertson, 2005) and other electrolytes. The infusion is stopped when the serum sodium level increases by 12 mmol/L; or when the serum sodium level rises to 130 mmol/L (Robertson, 2005). Monitor strict I & O and watch for diuresis, which increases with the rise in the serum sodium level. This is also an indication to stop the 3% saline infusion. Monitor the patient for changes in neurologic status.

10. Other treatments that have been used include oral urea (30-60 g in 100 mL of water daily), furosemide (40 mg/day) with salt tablets (200 mEq/day) (Berl & Verbalis, 2004), and oral urea (30% to 50% solution) for use in children (Huang et al., 2006). 11. Clinical trials are investigating the use of vasopressin agents (lixivaptan, conivaptan, tolvaptan) to treat low sodium levels (Palm et al., 2006). Conivaptan helps promote the excretion of water while sparing electrolytes (Raftopoulos, 2007). The dose is 20 mg IV over 30 minutes. This is followed by a continuous infusion of 20 mg over 24 hours administered for 1-3 more days. The maximum dose is 40 mg per day for a maximum of 4 days (Micromedex, 2007).

EVIDENCE-BASED PRACTICE UPDATES

1. Morbidity and mortality may result from too rapid correction of hyponatremia (Nguyen & Kurtz, 2005).
2. No guidelines or consensus statements are available regarding the best treatment for SIADH (Adrogué & Madias, 2000).

TEACHING AND EDUCATION

1. Etiology of SIADH: Signs and symptoms to report to the health care provider, including alterations in mental status, increased weight, decreased urine output, thirst, and any other signs and symptoms (Langfeldt & Cooley, 2003; Poe et al., 1989).
2. Safety and seizure precautions and seizure management (Landfeldt & Cooley, 2003). Pressure reduction and hazards of immobility (Poe & Taylor, 1989).
3. Purpose of fluid restriction; how to space fluids throughout the day; and oral care measures (e.g., oral rinses, use of sugar-free gum and candy) to manage thirst sensations. The patient should avoid water and consume fluids containing electrolytes and nutrients. The patient should avoid smoking and using tobacco products because they may dry the mouth (Langfeldt & Cooley, 2003). The patient also needs to know how to measure urine output and the importance of this measurement (Poe & Taylor, 1989)
4. Medications used to manage SIADH (i.e., dose, frequency, side effects, and side effect management).
   - Demeclocycline should be taken on an empty stomach with enough fluid to reduce irritation of the esophagus. Dairy products and calcium-containing products, antacids, and products or medications that contain iron should be avoided. The drug should be taken 1 hour before or 2 hours after food (Micromedex, 2006).
5. **Web sites for information:**
   - UCLA Endocrinology: http://www.endocrinology.med.ucla.edu/siadh.htm
   - National Library of Medicine: http://www.nlm.nih.gov/medlineplus/ency/article/
   - emedicine: http://www.emedicine.com/emerg/topic784.htm
   - University of Chicago: http://home.uchicago.edu/~adam cifu/

NURSING DIAGNOSES

1. **Excess fluid volume** related to excess ADH
2. **Risk for injury** related to risk of seizures
3. **Risk for injury** related to altered neurological status
4. **Altered comfort** related to dry mouth
5. **Altered coping** related to potentially life-threatening paraneoplastic syndrome

EVALUATION AND DESIRED OUTCOMES

1. Abnormal laboratory values will return to normal. (Monitor for normalization of serum sodium and urine osmolality.)
2. The patient's weight will be reduced.
3. The patient will be protected against harm, as evidenced by absence of seizures, falls, and hazards of immobility.
4. The patient and family will verbalize how to manage fluid restriction and medications and the signs and symptoms to report to the health care provider.

DISCHARGE PLANNING AND FOLLOW-UP CARE

- Prescriptions for medications (Is the patient able to obtain and afford the medications?)
- Equipment for measuring urine output.
- Prescriptions for blood work and urine osmolality.
- Dates and times to return for next cycle of chemotherapy or when to return for radiation therapy. (Is transportation required?)
- Education related to notifying the health care provider about signs and symptoms of returning or worsening SIADH (e.g., weight gain, reduced urine output), or side effects related to medications, chemotherapy, or radiation therapy.

REVIEW QUESTIONS

QUESTIONS

1. **An early sign or symptom of SIADH might be:**
    1. Inability to remember one's home address
    2. Oliguria
    3. Thirst
    4. Diarrhea

2. **SIADH is a paraneoplastic syndrome *most* commonly associated with which of the following malignancies:**
    1. Lung
    2. Pancreas
    3. Prostate
    4. Head and neck

3. **Which of the following antineoplastics are** commonly associated with SIADH:
    1. Vincristine and vinorelbine
    2. Ifosfamide and cyclophosphamide
    3. Melphalan and Alkeran
    4. 5-Floururacil and mitomycin

4. **Which of the following patients is *most* at risk of developing SIADH:**
    1. A 56-year-old male with newly diagnosed stage I colon cancer.
    2. A 46-year-old female with newly diagnosed stage II breast cancer.
    3. An 86-year-old female with relapsed/recurrent small cell lung cancer.
    4. A 77-year-old male with stage IV non-small cell lung cancer.

5. **Which of the following laboratory values indicates a diagnosis of SIADH:**
   1. Serum sodium, 121 mEq/L; serum osmolality, 300 mOsm/kg; urine osmolality, 275 mOsm/kg; urine sodium, 5 mEq/L.
   2. Serum sodium, 139 mEq/L; serum osmolality, 270 mOsm/kg; urine osmolality, 275 mOsm/kg; urine sodium 10mEq/L.
   3. Serum sodium 134 mEq/L; serum osmolality 281 mOsm/kg; urine osmolality 299 mOsm/kg; urine sodium, 19 mEq/L.
   4. Serum sodium, 121 mEq/L; serum osmolality, 245 mOsm/kg; urine osmolality, 400 mOsm/kg; urine sodium, 40 mEq/L.

6. **An important nursing intervention for the patient with SIADH is:**
   1. Safety and seizure precautions
   2. A low-sodium diet
   3. Force fluids
   4. Bed rest

7. **Which medication may be prescribed for patients with SIADH:**
   1. Demeclocycline (Declomycin)
   2. Tetracycline (Sumycin)
   3. Ifosfamide (Ifex)
   4. Vinblastine (Velban)

8. **A common complaint from patients on fluid restriction is:**
   1. Frequent urination
   2. Diarrhea
   3. Dry mouth
   4. Itching

9. **At the time of discharge, the patient should be able to verbalize:**
   1. How to drive home.
   2. Signs and symptoms to report to the health care provider.
   3. How to check the urine specific gravity.
   4. The amount of sodium commonly found in foods.

10. **Which finding may present in the patient with SIADH:**
    1. Edema
    2. Weight gain
    3. Rales
    4. Pleural effusions

ANSWERS

1. *Answer: 1*
   Rationale: Inability to remember where you live indicates impaired neurologic function, one of the first signs of SIADH. The other symptoms occur later, with more moderate SIADH.

2. *Answer: 1*
   Rationale: Small cell lung cancer is the most common malignancy associated with SIADH. Although the other cancers listed are possible causes, they are not the most common.

3. *Answer: 2*
   Rationale: Ifosfamide and cyclophosphamide are known causes of SIADH.

4. *Answer: 3*
   Rationale: The elderly, females, and patients with small cell lung cancer are at the greatest risk. The elderly patient with non-small cell lung cancer is at risk, but the risk is lower than for patient #3. The other patients are at lower risk.

5. *Answer: 4*
   Rationale: Answer choice 4 is the only that includes all the criteria for the diagnosis of SIADH. In all the other answer choices, at least one of the lab values does not fit the criteria.

6. *Answer: 1*
   Rationale: Patients with SIADH are at risk of falling and for seizures, depending on the severity of the hyponatremia. The other responses are incorrect. Fluids are restricted in patients with SIADH. A low-sodium diet would not be appropriate, nor would bed rest, because the patient is at risk for the hazards of immobility.

7. *Answer: 1*
   Rationale: Tetracycline is not used in the treatment of SIADH, and both ifosfamide and vinblastine are known causes of SIADH.

8. *Answer: 3*
   Rationale: Reduced oral intake causes the mouth and mucous membranes to feel dry and the patient to feel thirsty. Diarrhea is a symptom of SIADH. The other responses are incorrect.

9. *Answer: 2*
Rationale: The patient needs to know what to report to the health care provider with regard to side effects of medications and signs and symptoms of recurrent/relapsed SIADH. The other responses are incorrect. The patient should not be driving home from the hospital. The urine specific gravity is not checked in the home, and the amount of sodium found in foods is not important in the care of the patient.

10. *Answer: 2*
Rationale: Patients with SIADH do not usually have peripheral edema, signs of heart failure, or third spacing of fluids.

REFERENCES

Adrogué, H. J., & Madias, N. (2000). Hyponatremia. *New England Journal of Medicine, 342*(21):1581-1589.

Alvarez Perez, P., Rubio Nazabal, E., & Lopez, M. E., et al. (2004). Inappropriate secretion of antidiuretic hormone secondary to paroxetine (Spanish). *Anales de Medicina Interna 21*(10):519.

Arieff, A. I., Llach, F., & Massry, S. G. (1976). Neurological manifestations and morbidity of hyponatremia: Correlation of brain water and electrolytes. *Medicine, 55*(2):121-129.

Arnold, S. M., Lieberman, F. S., & Foon, K. A. (2005). Paraneoplastic syndromes. In V. T. DeVita, S. Hellman, & S. A. Rosenberg (Eds.), *Cancer: Principles and practice of oncology* (pp. 2189-2211). (7th ed.). Philadelphia: Lippincott Williams & Wilkins.

Ayus, J. C., Wheeler, J., & Arieff, A. I. (1992). Post-operative hyponatremic encephalopathy in menstruant women. *Annals of Internal Medicine, 117*:891-897.

Berl, T. (1990). Treating hyponatremia: What is all the controversy about? *Annals of Internal Medicine, 113*:417-419.

Berl, T., & Verbalis, J. (2004). Pathophysiology of water metabolism. In B. M. Brenner (Ed.), *Brenner and Rectors the kidney* (pp. 857-919). Philadelphia: W. B: Saunders.

Chen, L. K., Lin, M. H., & Hwang, S. J., et al. (2006). Hyponatremia among institutionalized elderly in two long-term care facilities in Taipei. *Journal of the Chinese Medical Association, 69*(3):115-119.

Chu, E., & DeVita, V. T (2004). *Cancer chemotherapy drug manual 2004.* Sudbury, MA: Jones & Bartlett.

Decaux, G. (2006). Is asymptomatic hyponatremia really asymptomatic? *American Journal of Medicine, 119*:S79-S82.

Flounders, J. A. (2003). Syndrome of inappropriate antidiuretic hormone. *Oncology Nursing Forum 30*(3):E63-E68. Retrieved May 25, 2006, from http://www.ons.org/publications/journals/ONF/Volume30/Issue3/pdf/381.pdf.

Gandhi, L., & Johnson, B. E. (2006). Paraneoplastic syndromes associated with small cell lung cancer. *Journal of the National Comprehensive Cancer Network, 4*(6):631-638.

Gobel, B. H. (2005). Metabolic emergencies. In J. K. Itano & K. N. Taoka (Eds.), *Core curriculum for oncology nursing* (pp. 383-421). (4th ed.). St. Louis: Mosby.

Guyton, A. C., & Hall, J. E. (2000). *Textbook of medical physiology.* (10th ed.). Philadelphia: W. B. Saunders.

Huang, E. A., Feldman, B. J., & Schwartz, I.D., et al. (2006). Oral urea for the treatment of chronic syndrome of inappropriate antidiuresis in children. *Journal of Pediatrics, 148*(1):128-131.

Keenan, A. M. M. (1999). Syndrome of inappropriate antidiuretic hormone in malignancy. *Seminars in Oncology Nursing, 15*:160-167.

Kobayashi, R., Iguchi, A., & Nakajima, M., et al. (2004). Hyponatremia and syndrome of inappropriate antidiuretic hormone secretion complicating stem cell transplantation. *Bone Marrow Transplantation, 34*(11):975-979.

Kugler, J. P., & Hustead, T. (2000). Hyponatremia and hypernatremia in the elderly. *American Family Physician, 61*(12):3623-3630.

Kunz, J. S., & Bannerji, R. (2005). Alemtuzumab-induced syndrome of inappropriate antidiuretic hormone. *Leukemia and Lymphoma, 46*(4):635-637.

Langfeldt, L. A., & Cooley, M. E. (2003). Syndrome of inappropriate antidiuretic hormone secretion in malignancy: Review and implications for nursing management. *Clinical Journal of Oncology Nursing, 7*:425-430.

Llinares-Tello, F., Hernandez-Prats, C., & Cervera-Juan, A., et al. (2005). Syndrome of inappropriate antidiuretic hormone secretion secondary to carbamazepine (Spanish). *Revista de Neurologia, 40*(12):768.

Lokich, J. J. (1982). The frequency of clinical biology of ectopic hormone syndromes of small cell carcinoma. *Cancer, 50:*2111-2114.

Maramattom, B. V. (2006). Duloxetine-induced syndrome of inappropriate antidiuretic hormone secretion and seizures. *Neurology, 66*(5):773-774.

Micromedex. (2006). Demeclocycline. Retrieved July 24, 2006, from http://www.thomsonhc.com/hcs/librarian/ ND_PR/Main/SBK/2/PFPUI/FZ3yvGr1qcXnll/ND_PG/PRIH/CS/CD696F/ND_T/HCS/ND_P/Main/ DUPLICATIONSHIELDSYNC/D39E1D/ND_B/HCS/PFActionId/hcs.common.RetrieveDocumentCommon/ DocId/163685/ContentSetId/42/SearchTerm/DEMECLOCYCLINE/SearchOption/BeginWith.

Micromedex. (2007). Conivaptan. Retrieved December 6, 2007 from http://www.thomsonhc.com/hcs/ librarian/ND_PR/Main/SBK/2/PFPUI/Yn129H22bnTDmI/ND_PG/PRIH/CS/877F9D/ND_T/HCS/ ND_P/Main/DUPLICATIONSHIELDSYNC/7841D3/ND_B/HCS/PFActionId/ hcs.common.RetrieveDocumentCommon/DocId/2449/ContentSetId/31#secN66027

Miehle, K., Paschke, R., & Koch, C. A. (2005). Citalopram therapy as a risk factor for symptomatic hyponatremia caused by the syndrome of inappropriate secretion of antidiuretic hormone (SIADH): A case report. *Pharmacopsychiatry, 38*(4):181-182.

Nasrallah, K., & Silver, B. (2005). Hyponatremia associated with repeated use of levetiracetam. *Epilepsia, 46*(6):972-973.

Nguyen, M. K., & Kurtz, I. (2005). An analysis of current quantitative approaches to the treatment of severe symptomatic SIADH with intravenous saline therapy. *Clinical and Experimental Nephrology, 9:*1-4.

Palm, C., Pistrosch, F., & Herbrig, K., et al. (2006). Vasopressin antagonists as aquaretic agents for the treatment of hyponatremia. *American Journal of Medicine, 119:*S87-S92.

Panayiotou, H., Small, S. C., & Hunter, J. H., et al. (1995). Sweet taste (dysgeusia): The first symptom of hyponatremia in small cell carcinoma of the lung. *Archives of Internal Medicine, 155*(12):1325-1328.

Poe, C. M., & Taylor, L. M. (1989). Syndrome of inappropriate antidiuretic hormone: Assessment and nursing implications. *Oncology Nursing Forum, 16:*373-381.

Raftopoulos, H. (2007). Diagnosis and management of hyponatremia in cancer patients. *Supportive Care Cancer, 15:*1341-1347.

Richerson, M. T. (2004). Electrolyte imbalances. In C. H. Yarbro, M. H. Frogge, & M. Goodman (Eds.), *Cancer symptom management* (pp. 440-453). (3rd ed.). Sudbury, MA: Jones & Bartlett.

Robertson, G. L. (2005). Disorders of the neurohypophysis. In D. L. Kasper, E. Braunwald, & A. S. Fauci et al. (Eds.), *Harrison's principles of internal medicine* (pp. 2097-2104). (16th ed.). New York: McGraw-Hill.

Sato, H., Kamoi, K., & Saeki, T., et al. (2004). Syndrome of inappropriate secretion of antidiuretic hormone and thrombocytopenia caused by cytomegalovirus infection in a young immunocompetent woman. *Internal Medicine, 43*(12):1177-1182.

Sterns, R. H. (1987). Severe symptomatic hyponatremia: Treatment and outcomes. *Annals of Internal Medicine, 107:*656-664.

Sterns, R. H., & Silver, S. M. (2006). Brain volume regulation in response to hypo-osmolality and its correction. *American Journal of Medicine, 119:*512-516.

Tareen, N., Martins, D., & Nagami, G., et al. (2005). Sodium disorders in the elderly. *Journal of the National Medical Association, 97*(2):217-224.

Trimarchi, T. (2006). Endocrine problems in critically ill children: An overview. *AACN Clinical Issues: Advanced Practice in Acute and Critical Care, 17*(1):66-78.

Vinzio, S., Lioure, B., & Enescu, I., et al. (2005). Severe abdominal pain and inappropriate antidiuretic hormone secretion preceding varicella-zoster virus reactivation 10 months after autologous stem cell transplantation for acute myeloid leukemia. *Bone Marrow Transplantation, 35*(5):525-527.

Yamamoto, Y., Kokubo, A., & Yonekawa, M., et al. (2005). Syndrome of inappropriate secretion of antidiuretic hormone suddenly occurring in a case following chemotherapy (Japanese). *Gan To Kagaku Ryoho* [Japanese Journal of Cancer and Chemotherapy] 32(1):107-109.

Yokoyama, Y., Shigeto, T., & Futagami, M., et al. (2005). Syndrome of inappropriate secretion of antidiuretic hormone following carboplatin-paclitaxel administration in a patient with recurrent ovarian cancer. *European Journal of Gynaecological Oncology, 26*(5):531-532.

Tumor Lysis Syndrome

BRENDA K. SHELTON

PATHOPHYSIOLOGICAL MECHANISMS

The term *tumor lysis syndrome* (TLS) is used to describe the clinical consequences of serum accumulation of excessive cell lysis products. When cells die, the internal components are released into the serum circulation; these include potassium, phosphates, and nucleic acids. Normally the kidneys efficiently clear these byproducts so that no serum elevation occurs. However, when cell lysis exceeds the kidneys' capacity or when the patient has pre-existing renal dysfunction, the cell byproducts cause clinical electrolyte disorders, with or without renal dysfunction (Davidson et al., 2004). According to Fernandez and colleagues (2006), clinical TLS is defined by specific laboratory evidence plus one or more of the following criteria: a serum creatinine greater than 1.5 times the upper limit of normal, cardiac dys-rhythmia or sudden death, and seizure. These criteria are outlined in the Cairo-Bishop grading system (Table 48-1).

Tumor lysis syndrome can be seen as early as 6 hours after initiation of antineoplastic therapy, although the peak incidence occurs within the first 24 to 48 hours (Secola, 2006; Davidson et al., 2004). In unusual cases, signs and symptoms may persist for 5 to 7days. The onset and duration of symptoms vary, depending on the tumor burden and its respon-siveness to therapy. Rapidly responding tumors create a larger number of lysis products in a shorter time, which increases the risk of clinical effects.

EPIDEMIOLOGY AND ETIOLOGY

The patients most likely to develop TLS are those who have rapidly proliferating tumors, those who are highly sensitive and responsive to the antineoplastic therapy, and those with renal compromise. Hematologic malignancies are the most common reported risk factors, although TLS has been reported in a variety of other malignancies as well. The incidence perceptually decreased as a result of greater recognition of risk factors and implementation of preventive strategies. However, some believe that more effective antineoplastic therapies actually may have caused a higher incidence of TLS, although in a milder form (Reedy, 2006). Survival also has improved, increasing from 5% to 8% in the 1980s to the current 20% to 30%. This may be related to early pheresis management of high white blood cell counts in acute leukemia and newer renal replacement therapies (Cairo, 2006; Mato et al., 2006).

RISK PROFILE

- Individuals with rapidly proliferating white blood cells, such as the blasts (immature cells) associated with acute leukemia or Burkitt's lymphoma, are at risk (Secola, 2006).

Table 48-1	**CAIRO-BISHOP GRADING CRITERIA FOR TLS**			
Grade	**Laboratory Evidence**	**Creatinine Level**	**Cardiac Dysrhythmias**	**Seizures**
0	−	< 1.5× the upper limit of normal	None	None
1	+	1.5 × the upper limit of normal	Intervention not indicated	None
2	+	> 1.5-3 × the upper limit of normal	Nonurgent medical intervention indicated.	One brief generalized seizure (or seizures) well controlled, or infrequent focal motor seizures that do not interfere with ADLs.
3	+	> 3-6 × the upper limit of normal	Symptomatic and incompletely controlled medically or controlled with a device.	Seizure in which consciousness is altered; poorly controlled seizure disorder; breakthrough generalized seizures despite medical intervention.
4	+	> 6 × the upper limit of normal	Life-threatening	Seizures of any kind that are prolonged, repetitive, or difficult to control.
5	+	Death	Death	Death

Data from Cairo, S. E., & Bishop, M. (2004). Tumor lysis syndrome: New therapeutic strategies and classification. *British Journal of Haematology, 127*:3-11.

In some of these individuals, high cell turnover exists even before treatment, which means that a degree of tumor lysis is seen at diagnosis. This usually worsens after definitive treatment causes more rapid lysis (Fernandez et al., 2006).

- Other tumors with high growth fractions (e.g., small cell lung cancer, testicular cancer, medulloblastoma, neuroblastoma) may also cause tumor lysis as a result of the rapid cell turnover rate (Rampello et al., 2006; Reedy, 2006).
- A large tumor mass, as indicated by high serum LDH levels, represents a greater risk of the development of TLS. LDH levels greater than 1500 mg/dL represent a greater risk for TLS (Cairo, 2006; Jeha, 2006; Rampello et al., 2006).
- Tumors that are highly responsive to antineoplastic therapy may also cause TLS. Tumor types that have been reported in the literature to induce TLS include breast carcinoma, Hodgkin's and Non-Hodgkin's lymphoma, medulloblastoma, melanoma, ovarian carcinoma, renal cell carcinoma, rhabdomyosarcoma, sarcoma, seminoma, small cell lung cancer, and thymoma (Cairo, 2006; Rampello et al., 2006; Yahata et al., 2006).
- Several monoclonal antibodies that target cell surface markers on tumor cells have been reported to cause acute tumor lysis. These include rituximab, campath, and bortezomib (Kenealy et al., 2006).
- Hypovolemia and dehydration lead to higher concentrations of cell lysis products, which can exacerbate the tendency for tumor lysis.
- Renal dysfunction predisposes individuals to tumor lysis as a result of a reduced glomerular filtration rate and decreased clearance of metabolic products.

8. Steroid-sensitive tumors have been reported to produce tumor lysis even after hormonal replacement or premedication-dose dexamethasone (Chanimov et al., 2006).

PROGNOSIS

Although TLS has been associated with poor long-term outcomes, this often is due to its association with severe and advanced malignant disease rather than inadequate treatment of the complication. Only 30% of patients with TLS have severe symptoms such as dysrhythmias or renal failure, and only 5% to 8% of all patients with TLS die of the syndrome (Reedy, 2006). TLS complications reportedly are more severe in elder adults and children (Reedy, 2006).

The Cairo-Bishop grading system, mentioned previously, defines the severity of TLS based on the key clinical findings (see Table 48-1). Laboratory findings, renal dysfunction, cardiac dysrhythmias, and neuromuscular abnormalities are used to determine the severity score (Cairo & Bishop, 2004).

PROFESSIONAL ASSESSMENT CRITERIA (PAC)

A complete physical examination and evaluation of common diagnostic findings before antineoplastic therapy is started help differentiate the clinical findings associated with TLS. Initial and ongoing assessment of the following clinical criteria are important (Table 48-2).

1. Intake and output measurement. Large quantities of fluid are administered to enhance renal clearance of lysis products; intake greater than output is a high risk.
2. Urine output is an extremely important specific aspect of the intake and output totals. Elevated uric acid and calcium-phosphate precipitants may both cause oliguria, therefore a reduction in urine output could be a significant sign of renal impairment.
3. The pulse rate and regularity are important indicators of dysrhythmias, which can occur as a result of hypocalcemia and hypokalemia.
   - If pulse irregularities occur, continuous cardiac monitoring is recommended to provide consistent feedback about the presence of dangerous rhythm disturbances, such as ventricular tachycardia or heart block, which can occur with TLS.
4. Blood pressure assessment helps verify complications such as hypervolemia (hypertension) or dysrhythmias (hypotension).
5. Edema may reflect fluid volume overload.
6. Respiratory assessment for rate and quality can reflect the workload of breathing. Oxygen saturation monitoring can reveal hypoxemia. Tachypnea and dyspnea provide information about compensation for pH imbalance or fluid overload.
7. When possible, the central venous pressure is monitored to assess for fluid volume overload and to adjust the rate of fluid administration. A normal central venous pressure is 0 to 6 mm Hg or 5 to 10 cm H_2O. Patients with TLS usually require central venous pressures that are slightly higher to ensure continuous urine flow.
8. Muscle tone may vary, depending on the predominant electrolyte manifestation. Muscle cramping and tetany can occur as a result of hypocalcemia, and weakness or hypotonia is present with hyperkalemia.
9. The abdomen should be assessed for large tumor masses, hepatomegaly, or splenomegaly; these are indicative of a large tumor burden, which increases the risk for TLS (Secola, 2006).

Table 48-2   CLINICAL MANIFESTATIONS OF TUMOR LYSIS SYNDROME

Abnormal Laboratory Finding	Clinical Manifestations	Management
Potassium >5.5 mEq/L or >25% increase from baseline	• Increased bowel sounds • Abdominal cramping and diarrhea • Nausea • Muscle weakness, flaccidity • Fatigue • Paresthesias • Progressive ECG changes: First stage—peaked T waves, shortened PR interval, ST depression Second phase—widened QRS, prolonged PR interval, decreased amplitude of P wave; Third phase—flattened QRS into ventricular fibrillationz • Palpitations • Tachycardia (atrial, supraventricular, or ventricular) • Increased premature beats (atrial, junctional, or ventricular)	• Kayexylate given orally or by enema to bind with K+ ions and remove them via loose stool. • Sodium bicarbonate (1 mEq/kg) to cause potassium ions to move into the cells. • Calcium gluconate 1 amp (4.5 mEq) given intravenously (this is not the preferred choice if symptoms are mild or the only ECG change is peaked T waves). • Dextrose 50% and regular insulin 10 units given intravenously. • Force sodium-based fluids to enhance electrolyte excretion. • Loop diuretics (e.g. furosemide). • Dialysis.
Phosphate >8 mg/dL or 25% increase from baseline	• Renal dysfunction • Muscle weakness • Joint pain • Limited joint movement • Pruritus • Red eye or conjunctivitis • Mental status changes ranging from mild confusion to obtundation or seizures • Cataracts • Paresthesias • Prolonged QT segment on ECG • Leukopenia • Thrombocytopenia • Hypocalcemia	• Force sodium-based fluids to enhance electrolyte excretion. • Phosphate binding agents (e.g., aluminum hydroxide). • Dialysis. • Bone marrow growth factors.

Uric acid >8 mg/dL or increase from baseline	• Renal dysfunction, as evidenced by elevated creatinine • Oliguria, anuria • Hematuria • Enlarged, tender kidney with possible tubular obstruction	• Allopurinol • Rasburicase (Elitek) • Force fluids • Diuretics • Dialysis
Calcium <8 mg/dL or 25% decrease from baseline	• Muscle contraction/tetany • Painful twitching/fasciculation of small muscles • Increased deep tendon reflexes • Abdominal cramping, diarrhea, increased bowel sounds • Irritable heart rhythms (tachycardia, atrial fibrillation/flutter, premature beats) • Nausea	• Calcium replacement only after phosphorus has been reduced, • Phosphorus reduction.
Arterial pH <7.25	• Bradycardia, junctional rhythm, heart block • Hypotension • Cyanosis • Smooth muscle contraction (abdominal, uterine cramping)	• Increase blood volume with fluids, blood products, and colloids. • Maximize oxygenation of tissues with oxygen supplements if levels are deficient. • Support blood pressure with vasopressors (e.g., dopamine, norepinephrine). • Sodium bicarbonate 1 mEq/kg given intravenously.

Data from Fitzpatrick, L. A. (2002). Hypocalcemia: Diagnosis and treatment. Retrieved November 28, 2006, from www.Endotext.com; Garth, D. (2006). Hyperkalemia. Retrieved January 8, 2007, from www.emedicine.com/EMERG/topic261.htm; Kaplow, R. (2002a). Pathophysiology, signs, and symptoms of acute tumor lysis syndrome. *Seminars in Oncology Nursing, 18*(3):6-11; Lederer, E., & Ouseph, R. (2004). Hyperphosphatemia. Retrieved January 8, 2007, from www.emedicine.com/med/topic1097.htm; Patterson, L. A., & DeBlieux, P. M. C. (2006). Hyperphosphatemia. Retrieved January 9, 2007, from www.emedicine.com/emerg/topic266.htm; and Rampello, E., Fricia, T., & Malaguarnera, M. (2006). The management of tumor lysis syndrome. *Nature Clinical Practice in Oncology, 3*(8):438-447.

10. Gastrointestinal distress, represented by anorexia, nausea, vomiting, and diarrhea, is a common symptom of TLS. These signs are due to the multitude of metabolic imbalances rather than one specific abnormality.

11. The serum chemistry should be monitored once to three times daily, depending on the degree of risk for TLS. Monitoring is more intense during the peak periods of occurrence (between 24 and 48 hours). Common electrolyte abnormalities include hyperkalemia, hyperphosphatemia, and hypocalcemia. More severe hyperphosphatemia is common in patients with therapy-induced TLS (Fernandez et al., 2006).

12. High phosphate levels are common with TLS. Close monitoring for a decline in phosphate levels, which indicates the end of TLS, allows for discontinuation of phosphate-binding therapies before a rebound hypophosphatemia is induced by overtreatment. The severity of hyperphosphatemia predicts the degree of hypocalcemia because of the inverse relationship of calcium and phosphate. High phosphate levels cause bone resorption or urinary excretion of calcium.

13. A method of calculating the risk of calcium-phosphate salt precipitants is calculation of the calcium-phosphorous solubility product. The formula is:

$$\text{Serum calcium} \times \text{Serum phosphorus}$$

If the product is greater than 60, the risk of precipitation is high (Secola, 2006).

14. Uric acid is monitored daily. It reflects the end product of nucleic acid conversion to xanthine oxidase after release from destroyed tumor cells, and it increases the risk of renal failure. Uric acid levels that remain less than 9.8 mg/dL connote a better prognosis (Cairo, 2006). Higher uric acid levels occur in spontaneous TLS that develops before initiation of antineoplastic therapy (Fernandez et al., 2006). Specific therapies directed at preventing hyperuricemia or reducing uric acid levels are administered and should be discontinued when the TLS has resolved.

15. Serum blood urea nitrogen and creatinine levels are monitored at least daily during the high-risk period for tumor lysis. Renal failure is an infrequent but possible complication, and these laboratory values are the most accurate indicators of early renal insufficiency.

16. Arterial blood gases may be evaluated to assess pH balance and the degree of compensation by the respiratory system. Severe metabolic acidosis may occur with high uric acid levels, renal insufficiency, and fluid imbalances. If metabolic acidosis is severe, the respiratory workload to attempt to clear the acid may produce hypoxemia. To avoid frequent arterial blood punctures, the venous pH may be used for intermittent monitoring to validate the stability of the pH level.

17. LDH levels are indicative of the amount of tumor, and these levels are monitored daily during the period of high risk for TLS to assess tumor reduction (Secola, 2006).

18. In the past, the urine pH level has been used to titrate bicarbonate infusions. However, with decreased use of preventive bicarbonate infusions, this laboratory monitoring practice is not often performed.

19. If renal insufficiency occurs, a renal ultrasound examination is performed to rule out an obstructive process. Although unusual, uric acid crystallization and calcium-phosphate precipitation may cause kidney stones. The treatment for obstruction caused by stones is significantly different from that used for acute renal failure caused by tubular necrosis.

NURSING CARE AND TREATMENT

As a result of advanced risk profiling and vigilant diagnostic surveillance, TLS is rarely an unexpected crisis. High-risk patients are managed aggressively, as if they have TLS. Early recognition of clinical and laboratory changes permits adjustment of fluids, electrolyte management, and administration of xanthine oxidase inhibitors, as well as initiation of early renal replacement therapy (Kaplow, 2002b).

1. TLS can be prevented with careful monitoring of electrolytes and fluid administration. Recognition and direct management of the risk factors for TLS can also reduce the risk. Patients with acute leukemia and a high white blood cell count may receive leukapheresis to remove some of the excess malignant white blood cells and to reduce the number of cells to lyse (Secola, 2006; Doane, 2002).

2. High-volume fluid administration during the high-risk period for TLS aids renal clearance of cell lysis byproducts. The infusion rate is titrated to achieve a urine output greater than 100 to 200 mL/hr and a stable central venous pressure of 6 to 12 mm Hg (Koduri, 2005; Gobel, 2002). Normal saline is most often used; however, with high infusion rates and in patients with hyperphosphatemia, half normal saline (0.45%) may be more appropriate to maximize dilute urine and minimize sodium wasting (Koduri, 2005).

3. As long as renal function is preserved, loop diuretics are administered to enhance urinary flow. Loop diuretics may also be helpful in controlling hyperkalemia, but they may worsen hypocalcemia.

4. Because the primary clinical crisis associated with TLS is renal failure, therapies targeted at preventing renal toxins (e.g., uric acid) are started before antineoplastic therapy. Table 48-3 presents a comparison of allopurinol and rasburicase, two agents used to manage elevated uric acid levels.

Table 48-3	COMPARISON OF ALLOPURINOL AND RASBURICASE	
Parameter	**Allopurinol**	**Rasburicase**
Mechanism of action	Blocks xanthine oxidase and prevents the production of uric acid but does not reduce uric acid already present.	Promotes excretion of uric acid in the urine via a nonactive metabolite.
Administration	Loading dose of 300-800 mg by mouth or 200-400 mg IV for first 1-2 days, then 300-600 mg daily until TLS is complete or 3-5 days after the end of treatment.	Intravenous: 0.15-0.2 mg/kg daily for 5 days; efficacy of a single dose has been documented.
Onset, peak, and duration of effect	Onset of action 1-4 days, reduces uric acid 50% at 5 days; peak effect is 2-3 days; duration of effect is 1-3 weeks.	Onset of action approximately 4 hours, with peak occurring within 24 hours. Duration is approximately 5 days.
Adverse effects	Bone marrow suppression, skin rash, vasculitis, gastrointestinal distress, hepatic centrolobar necrosis	Hypersensitivity, gastrointestinal distress, rash, hemolytic anemia myoclonus, increased spasticity
Drug interactions	Decreases metabolism (higher blood levels): azathioprine, mercaptopurine Increases half-life: warfarin, theophylline Increases serum level: cyclosporine Increases rash: amoxicillin, ampicillin	None known

Data from Brant, J. M. (2002). Rasburicase: An innovative new treatment for hyperuricemia associated with tumor lysis syndrome. *Clinical Journal of Oncology Nursing, 6*(1):12-16; Jeha, S. (2006). Current and emerging treatment options for patients with tumor lysis syndrome. *Johns Hopkins Advanced Studies in Nursing, 4*(3):49-57; Kaplow, R. (2002a). Intravenous allopurinol. *Clinical Journal of Oncology Nursing, 6*(2):110-112; Pui, C. H. (2001). Urate oxidase in the prophylaxis or treatment of hyperuricemia: The United States experience. *Seminars in Hematology, 38*(4 Suppl. 10):13-21; Smalley, R. V., Guaspari, A., & Haase-Statz, S., et al. (2000). Allopurinol: Intravenous use for prevention and treatment of hyperuricemia. *Journal of Clinical Oncology, 18*(8):1758-1763; and Del Toro, G., Morris, E., & Cairo, M. S. (2005). Tumor lysis syndrome: Pathophysiology, definition, and alternative treatment approaches. *Clinical Advances in Hematology and Oncology, 3*(1):54-61.

- The conversion of nucleic acids to xanthine oxidase can be prevented by administration of allopurinol. However, this drug does not convert existing uric acid and therefore is not the best treatment choice once the uric acid level exceeds 9 mg/dL. In patients who are unable to take oral medications, intravenous allopurinol is now available (Kaplow, 2002a).
- Rasburicase is a miscellaneous intravenous drug that enhances the breakdown of uric acid via an enzymatic pathway, mimicking normal mechanisms. It is useful when the uric acid level is already elevated (Shonkwiler, 2006; Brant, 2002).

5. High phosphate levels usually are balanced in the body by a reduction in calcium. A rapid rise in phosphate may result in calcium-phosphate precipitants that cause renal failure. Oral phosphate-binding agents (e.g., aluminum hydroxide) are used to lower the excess phosphate levels. Calcium-phosphate precipitants are a common complication if hypocalcemia is clinically symptomatic and calcium is replenished before the phosphate level is lowered. Phosphate-binding agents are discontinued a few days after tumor lysis resolves.

6. Hyperkalemia can be treated by various therapies that enhance excretion or temporarily shift potassium into the cells.
   - Definitive excretion of excess potassium via the stool is accomplished by administration of oral or enema resin kayexalate.
   - Loop diuretics may also aid urinary excretion of excess potassium.
   - The most effective means of temporarily shifting potassium into the cells is calcium replenishment. Calcium gluconate 4.5 mEq (1 ampule) is administered by a short intravenous infusion. This must be undertaken cautiously if hyperphosphatemia is present.
   - Administration of sodium bicarbonate 1 mEq/kg is effective at immediately shifting potassium into the cells, but its duration of action is only hours, therefore it cannot be the only therapy used.
   - For immediate short-term shifting of potassium into the cells, glucose is administered, in the form of dextrose 50% 50 mL followed by regular insulin 10 units given subcutaneously. This therapy is effective only for 1 to 4 hours and must be followed by definitive removal of potassium.

7. Cautious red blood cell replacement may be implemented. Unless the patient has symptomatic anemia, blood cell transfusions are held until the electrolyte abnormalities and renal failure have resolved, because banked blood contains lysed red blood cells that are releasing potassium, as well as citrate preservative, which further reduces calcium.

8. Cautious calcium replacement therapy may be instituted after normalization of the phosphate level. Calcium gluconate 1 ampule (4.5 mEq) given intravenously over 1 hour is the preferred method of replacement. It is gentler and less dramatic in effect than calcium chloride (14.5 mEq), which should be reserved for a life-threatening situation. As the TLS resolves, phosphate becomes corrected, and electrolyte shifting therapies wear off, the calcium levels may vary. Unless the patient is symptomatic, active calcium replacement may not be the preferred option of therapy.

9. The definitive treatment for removing lysis byproducts is renal replacement therapy. Hemodialysis is the most efficient means of removing creatinine, fluid, and uric acid. However, the continuous removal of electrolytes and solutes achieved by continuous renal replacement therapy (CRRT) may be advantageous in TLS when the pathophysiology involves constant release of electrolytes (Briglia, 2005). Patients receiving CRRT usually are managed by the bedside critical care nurse rather than dialysis nurses. Special care for these patients includes:
   - Maintenance of a large-bore central venous catheter to ensure the integrity of the tubing; prevention of accidental disconnection; and strict infection control.

- Troubleshooting alarms that signal pressure changes in the lines or filter.
- Conscientious assessment of the vital signs and fluid balance to prevent excess fluid removal.
- Daily weighing of the patient.
- Strict measurement of intake and output, totaled at least three or four times a day.
- Monitoring of electrolytes, pH, and glucose levels, which may become abnormal during the dialysis process.
- Implementation of body warming procedures if heat loss through the circuit becomes a clinical problem. (The nurse must be aware of how hypothermia or its treatment may mask or provide false-positive temperature readings.)

EVIDENCE-BASED PRACTICE UPDATES

1. Both tumor characteristics and therapy characteristics contribute to the predictability of TLS. Historically, the literature has focused on the host- and tumor-based risk factors. However, as more targeted antineoplastic therapies, which cause cell-specific apoptosis, are licensed for use, a higher incidence of TLS in a wider variety of patient populations is likely to be seen.
2. The traditional standard of care has been to administer a large volume of fluids and bicarbonate to treat the acidosis that accompanies high uric acid levels. However, we now better understand the complex interactions in TLS, and we know that pH correction with sodium bicarbonate may counteract nucleic acid–related acidosis, but at the same time, it increases the calcium-phosphate product and deposition of calcium-phosphate precipitants (Secola, 2006).
3. Until recently, the available medications only permitted treatment that blocked further breakdown of xanthine oxidase into uric acid. A newer medication, rasburicase, directly blocks xanthine oxidase conversion, thereby more rapidly and effectively reducing uric acid levels. Use of rasburicase is indicated only when the uric acid is already high (greater than 9 mg/dL) (Brant, 2002).
4. Continuous renal replacement therapy for treatment of ongoing electrolyte disturbances during TLS provides continuous removal of metabolic byproducts, an advancement that has become universally available only during the past decade (Briglia, 2005).

TEACHING AND EDUCATION

Water intake: *Rationale:* You must drink a large amount of water every day, approximately 1 gallon. This will increase the glomerular filtration rate and improve the clearance of electrolytes that accumulate from tumor lysis. Water is the best replacement therapy, because many other flavored drinks and soda contain undesirable electrolytes.

Dietary restrictions: *Rationale:* Avoid foods that are high in phosphate or potassium (Table 48-4).

Medications: *Rationale:* While you are at risk for TLS, be sure to take only the medications prescribed for you. Over-the-counter medications, vitamins, and herbal supplements may exacerbate the electrolyte disorders associated with TLS.

Outpatients: *Rationale:* Because you are at risk for TLS, you may need to return for follow-up blood tests to your assess electrolyte levels and renal function for 2 days after therapy. If the test results are normal, you may not need to see your health care provider until your next cycle. However, evidence of TLS may necessitate additional follow-up.

Table 48-4	CONDITIONS, MEDICATIONS, AND DIETARY FACTORS TO AVOID IN PATIENTS AT RISK FOR TUMOR LYSIS SYNDROME	
Rationale	**Conditions/Medications/Foods**	
Causes or exacerbates hyperkalemia	• ACE inhibitors • Aminocaproic acid (Amicar) • Amphetamines • Antifungals • Beta blockers • Blood products • Cyclosporine • Fludarabine • Heparin • Indomethacin • Interferon • Ketorolac • Lithium • Mannitol • Neuromuscular blocking agents • Nifedipine • Penicillin G • Pentamidine • Propofol • Rituximab • Spironolactone • Tacrolimus • Thalidomide • Trimethoprim	• Bran, bran wheat, bran flakes • Green leafy vegetables • Fruits: apricots, citrus, currants, bananas, figs, kiwi, raisins, strawberries • Iron • Nuts • Salt substitutes • Tomatoes • Veal
Causes or exacerbates hyperphosphatemia	• Etidronate • Fludarabine • Foscarnet • Interferon alpha • Leuprolide • Minocycline • Rituximab • Sodium phenylbutyrate	• Baking powder • Beans • Beer • Bran: rice, wheat • Brewer's yeast • Carbonated beverages (cola or pepper type) • Cheese (American, cheddar, cream, mozzarella) • Chinese cabbage • Chocolate, cocoa • Corn • Fish (especially cod) • Milk • Mollusks • Mushrooms • Organ meats • Peas, fresh • Sardines • Seaweed • Squash • Vitamin D supplements • Watercress • Zucchini
Causes or exacerbates hyperuricemia	• Alcohol, especially beer • Aspirin • Corticosteroids	• Fruits • Milk • Niacin

Table 48-4	CONDITIONS, MEDICATIONS, AND DIETARY FACTORS TO AVOID IN PATIENTS AT RISK FOR TUMOR LYSIS SYNDROME—cont'd	
Rationale	**Conditions/Medications/Foods**	
	• Cyclosporine • Diuretics, thiazide • Hypertension • Hypothyroidism • Lead exposure • Leukemia • Lymphoma • Obesity • Psoriasis • Renal insufficiency	• Vegetables
Causes or exacerbates hypocalcemia	• Aminoglycosides • Amphotericin B • Amyloidosis • Bisphosphonates (etidronate, pamidronate, zoledronate) • Cyclosporine • Dark carbonated drinks • Diuretics • Estrogen replacement therapy • Gadolinium for MRI • Hepatitis • Human immunodeficiency virus (HIV) infection • Hypoparathyroidism • Insulin-dependent diabetes • Magnesium depletion • Neck irradiation • Pancreatitis • Pentamidine • Phenobarbital • Plasmapheresis • Phenytoin • Radiographic contrast dyes • Sarcoidosis • Transfusion of a large amount of blood	• Vitamin D deficiency

Data from Fernandez, P. C., Larson, R. A., & Agus, Z. S. (2006). Tumor lysis syndrome, 2006. UpToDate. Retrieved November 1, 2006, from www.utd.com; Fitzpatrick, L. A. (2002). Hypocalcemia: Diagnosis and treatment. Retrieved November 28, 2006, from www.Endotext.com; Koduri, P. R. (2005). Hyperphosphatemia and tumor lysis syndrome. *Annals of Hematology, 84*:696-698; Lederer, E., & Ouseph, R. (2004). Hyperphosphatemia. Retrieved January 8, 2007, from www.emedicine.com/med/topic1097.htm; Nutrition Data. (2006). Foods high in phosphorus. Retrieved January 9, 2007, from www.nutritiondata.com; Weight Loss for All. (2005). Foods high in potassium. Retrieved January 9, 2007, from www.weightlossforall.com; and U. S. D. A. Agricultural Service. (2005). USDA national database for standard reference;/retrieved August 27, 2007 from www.nal.usda.gov/fnic/foodcomp/search.

NURSING DIAGNOSES

1. **Readiness for enhanced fluid balance** related to altered fluid and electrolyte balance, more than required
2. **Impaired urinary elimination** related to reduced renal clearance
3. **Decreased cardiac output** related to potential for decreased cardiac output related to dysrhythmias that occur with electrolyte or aid-base disturbances

4. **Ineffective breathing pattern**, tachypnea and dyspnea, related to fluid overload and acidosis
5. **Acute confusion** related to potential for altered mental status resulting from metabolic imbalance

EVALUATION AND DESIRED OUTCOMES

1. Electrolytes (potassium, phosphate, and calcium) and uric acid will normalize (this is the best indicator of resolution of TLS).
2. Normal blood urea nitrogen and creatinine levels will be maintained (this indicates prevention or resolution of renal insufficiency).
3. Stabilization of LDH levels will parallel the normalization of electrolytes (lower LDH indicates removal of tumor cells).

DISCHARGE PLANNING AND FOLLOW-UP CARE.

- TLS is most common in the first cycle of therapy, although if the tumor relapses, repetitive TLS can occur. Patients may demonstrate TLS with one therapy, yet not with another. For example, a patient's first chemotherapy regimen may not produce TLS if it does not effectively reduce the tumor burden. The second therapy, if more effective, may induce TLS. Patients in established remission are unlikely to have TLS and clinicians may not elect to institute monitoring measures.
- Follow-up monitoring of the return to normal renal function may be necessary. Renal dosing of other medications may be required until the BUN and creatinine are normal.

REVIEW QUESTIONS

QUESTIONS

1. **The nurse should closely monitor which of the following patients for TLS:**
   1. A 24-year-old with Hodgkin's lymphoma receiving Adriamycin, bleomycin, vincristine, and dexamethasone (ABVD) chemotherapy.
   2. A 32-year-old man with stage IV testicular cancer receiving high-dose chemotherapy.
   3. A 56-year-old woman with non-small cell lung cancer receiving chemotherapy and radiation therapy.
   4. A 78-year-old man with colorectal cancer with lung and liver metastases receiving chemotherapy and biotherapy.

2. **The clinical finding *most* likely to enhance the risk of TLS in a patient being treated for active cancer is:**
   1. Older age
   2. Anemia

   3. Hyperglycemia
   4. Hypovolemia

3. **TLS is *most* likely to occur within what period after initiation of highly active antineoplastic therapy:**
   1. 2 to 4 hours
   2. 6 to 12 hours
   3. 24 to 48 hours
   4. 72 to 96 hours

4. **The *most* sensitive indicator of early onset TLS is:**
   1. Acidosis
   2. Hyperkalemia
   3. Elevated creatinine
   4. Elevated LDH

5. **An assessment finding indicative of the electrolyte disturbances associated with TLS is:**
   1. Irregular pulse
   2. Absent bowel sounds
   3. Disorientation
   4. Constipation

6. **The *most* effective intervention to prevent TLS or reduce the risk of it developing is:**
   1. Oxygen therapy
   2. Preventive intravenous bicarbonate infusion
   3. Forced fluids
   4. Diuretics

7. **An important adverse effect of allopurinol that nurses must be able to recognize in patients receiving anticancer therapy is:**
   1. Rash
   2. Bone marrow suppression
   3. Dystonia
   4. Oral mucositis

8. **High-volume intravenous fluids are administered and titrated according to:**
   1. Weight
   2. The goal of even intake and output
   3. Osmolarity
   4. Brisk urine output

9. **A common electrolyte abnormality with TLS is:**
   1. Hypokalemia
   2. Hyponatremia
   3. Hypocalcemia
   4. Hypophosphatemia

10. **Which of the following conditions or diseases and their treatments can exacerbate hypocalcemia in a patient with TLS:**
    1. Obesity
    2. Epilepsy
    3. Migraine headache
    4. Acute depression

ANSWERS

1. *Answer: 2*
   Rationale: Patients with a high tumor burden, rapid proliferation, or high growth fractions are most likely to develop tumor lysis. Patient 2 has all of these risk factors, which are independent of the patient's age, type of therapy, or stage of the disease trajectory.

2. *Answer: 4*
   Rationale: Specific variables enhance the risk of tumor lysis or increase the severity of the syndrome. These variables usually involve the rate of production or clearance of toxic metabolites or their dilution in the bloodstream. Hypovolemia depletes the vascular fluid, causing hemoconcentration of electrolytes and metabolic toxins that are already excessive.

3. *Answer: 3*
   Rationale: The usual time frame for therapy-responsive tumors to begin lysing and to accumulate if not cleared by the kidneys is 24 to 48 hours.

4. *Answer: 2*
   Rationale: Hyperkalemia is an immediate and direct reflection of cell lysis. High LDH increases the risk of TLS, but its presence is not an indicator of the disorder. Acidosis and elevated creatinine are secondary clinical effects that occur only when the metabolic byproducts are not cleared.

5. *Answer: 1*
   Rationale: The most symptomatic clinical findings in electrolyte disturbances manifest as neuromuscular dysfunction. Changes in neuromuscular activity most often affect muscle strength, gastrointestinal peristalsis, and rhythmogenicity of the heart. The precise electrolyte disturbances of TLS—hyperkalemia, hypocalcemia, and hyperphosphatemia—produce increased muscular contractility and irritability and increased peristalsis. This means that the most common clinical finding would be an irregular pulse.

6. *Answer: 3*
   Rationale: The primary clinical problems associated with TLS are excess electrolytes in the circulating bloodstream. In the past, bicarbonate was viewed as an important preventive measure to reduce uric acid crystallization in the kidneys. However, the latest research demonstrates that this measure may increase calcium-phosphorus calcification deposits. Increased fluid intake is the most effective measure to enhance renal excretion of excess electrolytes without further loss of normal electrolytes. Diuretics may cause unnatural loss of calcium that is already low.

7. Answer: 2

Rationale: Patients receiving allopurinol to reduce the serum uric acid level may experience a variety of nonspecific adverse effects that also are common with antineoplastic therapy. The most significant side effects are gastrointestinal distress, interstitial nephritis, and bone marrow suppression; these effects may have implications for discontinuing allopurinol or other medications because of drug toxicity.

8. Answer: 4

Rationale: Although the administration of IV fluids may influence multiple clinical parameters, the objective of increased renal filtration and excretion of uric acid and electrolytes is best assessed through the volume of urine output. Weight and intake-output records reflect total fluid volume but not necessarily perfusing blood volume. Laboratory test results such as the creatinine level and osmolarity become abnormal only with significant renal impairment.

9. Answer: 3

Rationale: The electrolyte abnormalities present with TLS reflect the shift of electrolytes from lysed cells into the circulating serum. Because cells contain large amounts of potassium and phosphorus, these levels become elevated as tumor cells lyse. The calcium level declines as the body either excretes calcium or returns it to bone in an effort to maintain the normal inverse relationship of calcium and phosphorous. Sodium normally is an extracellular ion that is not significantly altered in TLS.

10. Answer: 2

Rationale: Phenobarbital and phenytoin, which are often used to treat epilepsy, are two common causes of exacerbation of hypocalcemia in patients with TLS.

REFERENCES

Brant, J. M. (2002). Rasburicase: An innovative new treatment for hyperuricemia associated with tumor lysis syndrome. *Clinical Journal of Oncology Nursing, 6*(1):12-16.

Briglia, A. E. (2005). The current state of nonuremic applications for extracorporeal blood purification. *Seminars in Dialysis, 18*(5):380-390.

Cairo, S. E. (2006). Preventing and managing tumor lysis syndrome: A case review. Retrieved September 25, 2007rom www.CMEZone.com.

Cairo, M. S., & Bishop, M. (2004). Tumor lysis syndrome: New therapeutic strategies and classification. *British Journal of Haematology, 127*:3-11.

Chanimov, M., Koren-Michowitz, M., & Cohen, M. L., et al. (2006). Tumor lysis syndrome induced by dexamethasone. *Anesthesiology, 105*(3):633-634.

Davidson, M. B., Thakkar, S., & Hix, J. K., et al. (2004). Pathophysiology, clinical consequences, and treatment of tumor lysis syndrome. *American Journal of Medicine, 116*:546-554.

Doane, L. (2002). Overview of tumor lysis syndrome. *Seminars in Oncology Nursing, 18*(3):2-5.

Fernandez, P. C., Larson, R. A., & Agus, Z. S. (2006). Tumor lysis syndrome 2006. UpToDate. Retrieved November 1, 2006, from www.utd.com.

Gobel, B. H. (2002). Management of tumor lysis syndrome: Prevention and treatment. *Seminars in Oncology Nursing, 18*(3):12-16.

Jeha, S. (2006). Current and emerging treatment options for patients with tumor lysis syndrome. *Johns Hopkins Advanced Studies in Nursing, 4*(3):49-57.

Kaplow, R. (2002a). Intravenous allopurinol, *Clinical Journal of Oncology Nursing, 6*(2):110-112.

Kaplow, R. (2002b). Pathophysiology, signs, and symptoms of acute tumor lysis syndrome. *Seminars in Oncology Nursing, 18*(3):6-11.

Kenealy, M. K., Prince, H. M., & Honemann, D. (2006). Tumor lysis syndrome after treatment with bortezomib for multiple myeloma. *Pharmacotherapy, 26*(8):1205-1206.

Koduri, P. R. (2005). Hyperphosphatemia and tumor lysis syndrome. *Annals of Hematology, 84*:696-698.

Mato, A. R., Riccio, B. E., & Qin, L., et al. (2006). A predictive model for the detection of tumor lysis syndrome during AML induction therapy. *Leukemia and Lymphoma, 47*(5):877-883.

Rampello, E., Fricia, T., & Malaguarnera, M. (2006). The management of tumor lysis syndrome. *Nature Clinical Practice: Oncology, 3*(8):438-447.

Reedy, A. M. (2006). Targeting tumor lysis syndrome: new therapeutic options. *Advanced Studies in Nursing, 4*(3):38-40, 61-62.

Secola, R. (2006). Tumor lysis syndrome: nursing management and new therapeutic options. *Advanced Studies in Nursing, 4*(3):41-48, 616-2.

Shonkwiler, E. (2006). Targeting tumor lysis syndrome. *ONS News, 21*(8 Suppl.):49-50.

Yahata, T., Nishikawa, N., & Aoki, Y., et al. (2006). Tumor lysis syndrome associated with weekly paclitaxel treatment in a case with ovarian cancer. *Gynecology and Oncology, 103*(2):752-754.

TYPHLITIS IN PEDIATRICS

KACI L. OSENGA

PATHOPHYSIOLOGICAL MECHANISMS

The term *typhlitis* (from the Greek word *typhlon*, for cecum) was first used by Wagner and colleagues (1970) to describe a necrotizing inflammation of the cecum that was diagnosed in leukemic children undergoing chemotherapy who were in the terminal stages of the disease (Abramson et al., 1983). Also known as *neutropenic enterocolitis* and *ileocecal syndrome*, typhlitis is a potentially life-threatening necrotizing inflammation of the cecum, terminal ileum, or colon. It initially was recognized at autopsy as a complication of childhood leukemia, but it now is known to occur in both adults and children with a variety of hematologic and solid tumor malignancies, in individuals with acquired immunodeficiency syndromes, and as a complication of bone marrow transplantation (McCarville et al., 2005). The appendix usually is only secondarily involved in the inflammatory process (Abramson et al., 1983).

The exact pathogenesis of typhlitis remains unclear and is likely multifactorial. It is believed to begin with mucosal damage, followed by inflammation and edema of the bowel wall, which progresses to ulceration, necrosis, and perforation (Paulino et al., 1994). The cecum is the portion of the lower gastrointestinal tract most vulnerable to developing neutropenic enterocolitis because it is the least vascularized and most distensible region of the colon (Wang & Fadare, 2004). The cecum normally is an area of relative stasis, and chemotherapeutic agents themselves have direct toxic effects on the bowel that may cause vascular changes and ileus (Ikard, 1981; Slavin et al., 1978).

Because most cases of typhlitis have occurred in patients with leukemia who received chemotherapy, one hypothesis of the pathologic etiology of this process is that cytotoxic chemotherapeutic agents are a significant factor in its development. Chemotherapy medications may predispose the cecum to breaks in the mucosal layers of the bowel wall. These interruptions in the cecal wall integrity may serve as portals of entry into the bowel wall for bacteria and fungi (Wang & Fadare, 2004). Chemotherapeutic agents such as cytosine arabinoside, topotecan, atovaquone, PEG-asparaginase, idarubicin, daunorubicin, methotrexate, vincristine, paclitaxel, doxorubicin, and steroids have been implicated in the development of typhlitis (McCarville et al., 2005; Wang & Fadare, 2004).

In addition to mucosal damage, chemotherapeutic drugs induce profound neutropenia. Together, ileal stasis and the resultant distention lead to relative mucosal ischemia which, in the presence of chemotherapeutically induced mucosal damage and agranulocytopenia, allow bacterial, fungal, or viral overgrowth (Abramson et al., 1983). Bacterial or fungal invasion of the cecal mucosa may progress from inflammation to full-thickness infarction and perforation. *Pseudomonas* species, *Escherichia coli*, and other gram-negative bacteria, *Staphylococcus aureus*, alpha-hemolytic streptococci, and *Clostridium* species are common bacterial pathogens. Necrosis of the mucosal surface of the ileocecal region provides a favorable environment for the spores of *Clostridium* species to germinate and may be the portal of entry into the bloodstream (Wang & Fadare, 2004). *Candida* and *Aspergillus* species are the major fungal pathogens, and *Cytomegalovirus* organisms may also be present in large numbers (Pizzo & Poplack, 2002; Newbold et al., 1987; Abramson et al., 1983).

In a systematic review of adults with neutropenic enterocolitis, Cardona and colleagues (2005) found that most blood cultures from these patients were negative; 31% grew gram-negative organisms, 9% grew gram-positive organisms, 7.2% grew anaerobes, and 0.9% grew *Candida* organisms. Of reported stool cultures, 59.6% were negative, 18.8% showed gram-negative organisms, 11.7% showed anaerobes, 7.4% showed *Candida* organisms, and 3.2.% showed gram-positive organisms (Cardona et al., 2005). McCarville and coworkers (2005) reported that blood cultures obtained from 89 episodes of typhlitis in pediatric patients were positive only 8% of the time; isolated organisms included *E. coli*, *Klebsiella* and *Enterococcus* species, staphylococci, and streptococci. Of 92 stool cultures done, 20% were positive for *Clostridium difficile*.

EPIDEMIOLOGY AND ETIOLOGY

Although typhlitis has been reported in adults, it is more commonly reported in children (Varki et al., 1979; Exelby et al., 1975; Wagner et al., 1970; Bierman, 1960). It is difficult to determine accurate prevalence rates for typhlitis and necrotizing enterocolitis. This uncertainty stems from the nonspecific features of the illness and similarities to other acute abdominal syndromes in immunocompromised patients. Also, because few accurate clinical tests are available, pathologic confirmation of the diagnosis may be lacking (Urbach & Rotstein, 1999).

When Wagner and colleagues first described typhlitis in the 1970s, it was considered a terminal disease. This group reported on clinical and autopsy material from 191 cases (children with leukemia) from Texas Children's Hospital from 1958 to 1970. During that time, there were 19 cases of advanced typhlitis, representing approximately 10% of the studied sample (Wagner et al., 1970).

In 1962 Amromin and Solomon reported the frequency of typhlitis in patients with ALL to be 22% (Amromin & Solomon, 1962). Moir and Bale (1976) reported an autopsy-based descriptive series that suggested an incidence of neutropenic enterocolitis of up to 32% among treated leukemia patients.

Sloas and colleagues (1993) diagnosed typhlitis in 24 of 6911 children treated for cancer between 1962 and 1992, with an overall incidence of 0.35%. The incidence was significantly higher (2.1%) among children treated for acute leukemia (Sloas et al., 1993). Sloas and coworkers also noted an increase in the incidence of typhlitis during the final years of the study; this corresponded to a period when patients with AML were treated with high doses of cytarabine and etoposide.

Cartoni and colleagues (2001) reported a 6% incidence of neutropenic enterocolitis between 1995 and 1998 among 1450 patients, most of whom were adults with acute leukemia or chronic myeloid leukemia in blast crisis, and all of whom were treated with aggressive chemotherapy.

In 2000 Jain and colleagues reported on a series of 180 children treated for ALL between 1990 and 1995. The incidence of typhlitis in this group was 6.1%. The median age at which typhlitis developed was 6 years, with a range of 4 to 12 years. Four of the 11 children with typhlitis were over age 10. Seventy-three percent of the children with typhlitis suffered from severe neutropenia, defined as an absolute neutrophil count (ANC) less than $10^8/L$ (Jain et al., 2000).

Similar to the work of Sloas and colleagues, McCarville and coworkers reviewed the records of patients treated for cancer at St. Jude Children's Research Hospital. This retrospective review of 3171 children showed that 83 (2.6%) had developed typhlitis (McCarville et al., 2005). In this study, the only demographic variable associated with the development of typhlitis was age. On average, patients with leukemia or lymphoma who developed typhlitis were older than those who did not, whereas in the group of children with solid tumors, younger patients were more likely to develop typhlitis. Overall, patients older than 16 years of age were at significantly greater risk than younger patients. Similarly, McCarville and colleagues (2005) found that the duration of typhlitis significantly increased with increasing age (P = 0.04); this suggests that not only are older children at greater risk of developing typhlitis, but also that they may not respond as well as younger children to management.

It generally is believed that the incidence of typhlitis is related to the intensity of chemotherapy and the degree of immunosuppression (Baerg et al., 1999). With this in mind, Otaibi and colleagues (2002) reviewed a 7-year experience with typhlitis in the bone marrow transplantation program at the Alberta Children's Hospital in Calgary, Alberta. From 1993 to 2000, 142 transplantations were performed at this institution. Of these, 97 patients had abdominal pain, and five patients had radiographically proven typhlitis. In this study, abdominal pain was very common after bone marrow transplantation, and typhlitis was relatively rare (3.5%) (Otaibi et al., 2002).

The exact pathogenesis of typhlitis remains unclear. Cytotoxic chemotherapy may cause intestinal ulcerations which, in the presence of neutropenia, retard healing. Simultaneously, bacterial and fungal invasion may occur, leading to varying degrees of intestinal inflammation. If the inflammation is only mild, it may remain limited to the mucosa. However, it may progress to transmural inflammation, necrosis, and perforation, especially if the neutropenia is severe (ANC less than 10^8/L) and prolonged (longer than 7 days) (Jain et al., 2000).

RISK PROFILE

- **Immunosuppression:** Malignant diseases warranting aggressive chemotherapy, including bone marrow transplantation; HIV; transplant recipients on immunosuppressive therapy; and aplastic anemia.
- **Neutropenia:** Severe neutropenia is defined as an ANC less than 10^8/L.
- **Duration of neutropenia:** The risk of typhlitis is higher with neutropenia that lasts longer than 7 days (McCarville et al., 2005; Jain et al., 2000).
- **Age:** On average, patients with leukemia or lymphoma who developed typhlitis were older than those who did not; in the solid tumor group, younger patients were more likely to develop typhlitis (McCarville et al., 2005).
- **Bowel wall thickness:** Based on ultrasound imaging, a bowel wall thickness equal to or greater than 0.3 cm, along with clinical signs and symptoms of typhlitis (fever, abdominal pain, diarrhea, nausea, and vomiting), correlates with the duration of typhlitis (McCarville et al., 2005).
- **Medications/chemotherapeutic drugs:** See Box 49-1 (Cardona et al., 2005; McCarville et al., 2005).

PROGNOSIS

Historically typhlitis was considered a terminal event. Although this is no longer the case, the outcome for these patients remains variable. Moir and Bale (1976) reported mortality rates ranging from 50% to 100%. Wade and colleagues (1992) reported a mortality rate of 63% in their series of 22 patients, and Jain and coworkers (2000) reported a rate of 45% in

BOX 49-1	DRUGS ASSOCIATED WITH DEVELOPMENT OF TYPHLITIS

- Atovaquone
- Carboplatin
- Cyclophosphamide
- Cytosine arabinoside
- Daunomycin
- Docetaxel
- Doxorubicin
- G-CSF
- Hydrocortisone
- Idarubicin
- Methotrexate
- Paclitaxel
- PEG-asparaginase
- Topotecan
- Vincristine

their small series of 11 patients. However, McCarville and colleagues (2005) found a mortality rate of only 2% in their series of 92 patients.

PROFESSIONAL ASSESSMENT CRITERIA (PAC)

1. Classic symptoms are abdominal pain, fever, abdominal tenderness (especially in the right lower quadrant), watery or bloody diarrhea, nausea, vomiting, and neutropenia (McCarville et al., 2005).
2. Neutropenia (ANC less than $10^8/L$) (Jain et al., 2000; Pizzo & Poplack, 2002; Urbach & Rotstein, 1999).
3. Current treatment with chemotherapy or an immunosuppressed state.
4. Bowel wall thickness equal to or greater than 0.3 cm on either CT or ultrasound imaging is suggestive of typhlitis (McCarville et al., 2005). CT scans may demonstrate a diffusely thickened cecum and ascending colon. The colonic wall may be homogeneously thickened, or it may contain areas of decreased attenuation, reflecting edema or necrosis. CT scans may also demonstrate intramural or intraluminal hemorrhages, mucosal ulcerations, free air, or abscesses (Wang & Fadare, 2004). Characteristic findings on ultrasound are a thickened, echogenic cecum and redundant mucosa in parts of the terminal ileum (Jain et al., 2000).
5. Evidence of sepsis (i.e., fever, hypotension, tachycardia).
6. Palpable mass (inflamed cecum) in the right lower quadrant (Urbach & Rotstein, 1999).
7. Pneumatosis intestinalis (air in the bowel wall) in the area of the cecum has been observed (Urbach & Rotstein, 1999).

NURSING CARE AND TREATMENT

1. Vital signs: Assess for hypotension, tachycardia, tachypnea, and fever (evidence of sepsis).
2. Hold chemotherapy.
3. Obtain and assess blood counts (evaluate for evidence of infection and neutropenia) and coag studies (evidence of DIC).

4. Assess for abdominal pain on a 5-point Faces Scale.
5. Assess for abdominal tenderness.
6. Obtain and assess: Abdominal x-ray film, abdominal ultrasound, abdominal CT scans (evaluate for dilated loops of bowel; bowel wall thickening, especially cecal thickening; and pneumatosis intestinalis).
7. Administer broad-spectrum antibiotics to cover for gram-negative, gram-positive, and *Clostridia* organisms (e.g., vancomycin, tobramycin, ceftazidime, and meropenem) (McCarville et al., 2005; Meyerovitz & Fellows, 1984).
8. Add antifungal coverage to initial regimen if the patient remains febrile after 72 hours (McCullough, 2003).
9. Diet: NPO and total parenteral nutrition.
10. Assess for need for surgical intervention based on gastrointestinal bleeding despite granulocyte recovery; thrombocytopenia and coagulopathy; free intraperitoneal air (which suggests bowel perforation); and clinical deterioration during medical therapy (Shamberger et al., 1986).
11. Maintain venous access via peripheral IV or central venous catheter (if already in place).
12. Administer IV fluids.
13. Intake and output every 2 to 8 hours.
14. Assess the need for gastric decompression with an NG tube.

EVIDENCE-BASED PRACTICE UPDATES

1. Ultrasound imaging is superior to CT scans for evaluation of pediatric patients with suspected typhlitis (McCarville et al., 2005).
2. Bowel wall thickness, as measured by ultrasound imaging, has correlated with the duration of typhlitis (McCarville et al., 2005).
3. Lower threshold of bowel wall thickness (equal to or greater than 0.3 cm) is suspect for typhlitis (McCarville et al., 2005; Teefey et al., 1987).
4. Combination antibiotics are used to cover gram-negative, gram-positive, and anaerobic organisms; antifungals can be added to cover fungi (Cardona et al., 2005; McCarville et al., 2005).
5. No difference in outcomes is seen with or without the use of growth factors (Cardona et al., 2005; McCarville et al., 2005).

TEACHING AND EDUCATION

Discontinuation of chemotherapy: *Rationale:* Chemotherapy can cause further damage to the mucosa and exacerbate the inflammation of the bowel wall.

IV fluid administration: *Rationale:* When a person does not eat or drink, has a fever, or has vomiting or diarrhea, fluid and other substances, such as salt, potassium, and bicarbonate, need to be replaced.

Nutrition: *Rationale:* Bowel rest, including gastric decompression with parenteral nutrition in the interim. Patients with typhlitis are not likely to tolerate feeding and often have significant gastrointestinal symptoms.

Tests and procedures: *Rationale:* Your child probably will need abdominal x-ray films, ultrasound scans, or CT scans. These imaging studies will be used to evaluate for inflammation and the integrity of the bowel wall. These studies are not painful and can help the medical team determine the appropriate treatment for you.

Medicines: *Rationale:* Your child will be taking a number of different antibiotics. Typhlitis is thought to be caused by bacteria in the bowel wall. Because a variety of organisms are responsible for typhlitis, several different antibiotics are used to ensure adequate coverage.

Nasogastric tube (NG)/NPO status: *Rationale:* Because the bowel walls are inflamed, it is important to minimize any pressure that could cause a tear or rupture, which could lead to infection. The NG tube is used to remove the bowel fluid that naturally accumulates even when one is not eating or drinking.

Pain monitoring and treatment: *Rationale:* It is important to watch for changes in your child's level of pain so that medication can be given to keep your child comfortable.

Surgical consult: *Rationale:* The goal of care is to help the bowel heal without an operation; however, sometimes surgery is needed. The surgeon visits frequently to help evaluate whether the condition is worsening to the point where surgery is needed.

Frequent physical exams and radiographic tests: *Rationale:* The purpose of frequent monitoring and tests is to look for increased pressure in the bowel, to evaluate the effectiveness of the treatment, and to determine whether the current medications and treatment plan need to be changed or whether surgery is needed.

NURSING DIAGNOSES

1. **Acute Pain** related to inflammation and edema of the bowel wall
2. **Risk for infection** related to inflammation, edema, ulceration, necrosis and/or perforation of the intestinal wall
3. **Acute pain** related to intestinal perforation resulting from ulceration and/or necrosis of the intestinal wall
4. **Imbalanced nutrition: less than body requirements** related to inflammation, edema, ulceration, necrosis and/or perforation of the intestinal wall, and/or need for gastric decompression
5. **Deficient knowledge** related to diagnosis, treatment, and therapies for leukemia in adults or children

EVALUATION AND DESIRED OUTCOMES

1. The patient will have acceptable pain scores (i.e., 2 or lower on a 5-point pain scale).
2. The patient will remain afebrile; vital signs will be stable and the patient will be afebrile for 24 hours before discharge.
3. The patient will have no abdominal pain; the abdomen will remain soft and nontender to palpation with no evidence of guarding or rebound. Bowel sounds will be present.
4. The serum electrolyte panel values will return to normal within 48 hours of IV fluid replacement.
5. The patient will tolerate oral intake with no evidence of nausea or vomiting. If the patient receives hyperalimentation, his or her weight will remain stable.
6. The patient and/or family will verbalize understanding of radiographic evaluations, diagnosis of typhlitis, therapies, and potential complications.

DISCHARGE PLANNING AND FOLLOW-UP CARE

- Follow-up with physician 1 to 2 weeks after discharge.
- Call health care provider immediately if patient develops a fever higher than 38° Celsius, abdominal pain, nausea, vomiting, or diarrhea.
- Parenteral nutritional support if patient is unable to take adequate oral nutrition.

REVIEW QUESTIONS

QUESTIONS

1. Which of the following is *not* another term for typhlitis:
   1. Neutropenic enterocolitis
   2. Necrotizing enterocolitis
   3. Ileocecal syndrome
   4. Terminal colitis

2. Typhlitis has been shown to occur in which of the following clinical scenarios:
   1. A 12-year-old with sickle cell anemia
   2. A 35-year-old with a brain tumor
   3. A 5-year-old with leukemia
   4. A 1-month-old with meningitis

3. Which part of the intestinal tract is most susceptible to developing typhlitis:
   1. Stomach
   2. Cecum
   3. Rectum
   4. Duodenum

4. Several hypotheses attempt to explain the pathophysiology of typhlitis. Which of the following is *not* correct:
   1. Blunt trauma to the abdomen causes damage to the cecum, thus causing inflammation in the surrounding tissues.
   2. Chemotherapy may predispose the cecum to breaks in the mucosa, which serve as portals of entry for bacteria and fungi.
   3. Mucosal damage occurs to the gut wall, followed by inflammation and edema of the bowel wall, which can progress to ulceration, necrosis, and perforation.
   4. Chemotherapy may cause an ileus and vascular changes to the cecum. This, along with distention of the cecum and neutropenia, allow for invasion of bacteria and fungi.

5. Which of the following bacterial organisms have *not* been identified as pathogens associated with typhlitis:
   1. *E. coli*
   2. *Stenotrophomonas*
   3. *Pseudomonas*
   4. *Clostridia*

6. Jane, a 5-year-old female, was recently diagnosed with acute lymphoblastic leukemia. She will receive several different chemotherapeutic drugs in an attempt to cure her disease. Which of the following drugs places her at risk of developing typhlitis:
   1. Mercaptopurine
   2. Allopurinol
   3. Cytosine arabinoside
   4. CCNU

7. You are caring for a child in the intensive phase of chemotherapy who was admitted for fever and neutropenia. The boy recently completed a course of high-dose methotrexate and has been neutropenic for approximately 9 days. As you assess the patient, he complains of abdominal tenderness and nausea. Which of the following is the *most* appropriate next step in caring for this patient:
   1. Recommend a lumbar puncture
   2. Recommend a colonoscopy
   3. Recommend abdominal imaging with ultrasound or CT scan
   4. Recommend a stronger dose of opioids

8. The *most* appropriate imaging technique for confirming a diagnosis of typhlitis is:
   1. Plain film
   2. PET scan
   3. Gallium scan
   4. Ultrasound

9. Which of the following findings is *not* universally seen on the CT scans of patients with typhlitis:
   1. Thickened bowel wall
   2. Mucosal ulceration
   3. Bowel wall edema
   4. Pneumatosis intestinalis

10. You are caring for a 13-year-old male with acute lymphoblastic leukemia who was admitted for abdominal pain and fever. You are very suspicious that he has typhlitis. He and his parents are very concerned and anxious about him not getting his chemotherapy and about the chances of his leukemia returning. The *most* appropriate thing to tell this anxious family about the hold on the patient's chemotherapy is:
   1. "I will talk to the team and advocate for the continuation of chemotherapy, since we certainly don't want your leukemia to come back."
   2. "That is a very good question. I can see how the return of the leukemia would be frightening. Right now, chemotherapy could make the process in his abdomen much worse."
   3. "That's a very good question. Why don't you discuss it with your doctors?"
   4. "The chemotherapy may interfere with your antibiotics, which may reduce the effectiveness of the chemotherapeutic drugs."

ANSWERS

1. *Answer: 4*
   Rationale: Other acceptable terms for typhlitis include *neutropenic enterocolitis, necrotizing enterocolitis,* and *ileocecal syndrome.*

2. *Answer: 3*
   Rationale: Typhlitis has been known to occur in both adults and children with a variety of hematologic and solid malignancies and acquired immunodeficiency syndromes, and as a complication of bone marrow transplantation.

3. *Answer: 2*
   Rationale: The cecum is the portion of the lower intestinal tract that is most vulnerable to the development of typhlitis.

4. *Answer: 1*
   Rationale: Blunt trauma to the abdomen is not a mechanism associated with the development of typhlitis.

5. *Answer: 2*
   Rationale: Pseudomonas, E. coli, and other gram-negative bacteria; S. aureus; alpha-hemolytic streptococci; and Clostridium species are common bacterial pathogens associated with typhlitis.

6. *Answer: 3*
   Rationale: See Box 49-1 for a list of drugs often associated with the development of typhlitis.

7. *Answer: 3*
   Rationale: In this scenario, this child is demonstrating classic symptoms of typhlitis: fever, neutropenia, abdominal tenderness, and nausea. The index of suspicion should be high for typhlitis, and the most appropriate next step is to image the abdomen.

8. *Answer: 4*
   Rationale: The most appropriate imaging technique to confirm a diagnosis of typhlitis is ultrasound.

9. *Answer: 4*
   Rationale: Pneumatosis intestinalis is not universally seen on the CT scans of patients with typhlitis.

10. *Answer: 2*
    Rationale: Chemotherapy is held with suspicion of typhlitis because of the concern of worsening mucosal damage to the bowel and prolonged neutropenia.

REFERENCES

Abramson, S. J., Berdon, W. E., & Baker, D. H. (1983). Childhood typhlitis: Its increasing association with acute myelogenous leukemia: Report of five cases. *Radiology, 146*(1):61-64.

Amromin, G. D., & Solomon, R. D. (1962). Necrotizing enteropathy: A complication of treated leukemia or lymphoma patients. *Journal of the American Medical Association, 182:*23-29.

Baerg, J., Murphy, J. J., & Anderson, R. (1999). Neutropenic enteropathy: A 10-year review. *Journal of Pediatric Surgery, 34*(7):1068-1071.

Bierman, H. R. (1960). The ileocecal syndrome in the leukopathic condition. *Clinical Research, 13:*134.

Cardona, A. F., Ramos, P. L., & Casasbuenas, A. (2005). From case reports to systematic reviews in neutropenic enterocolitis. *European Journal of Haematology, 75*(5):445-446.

Cartoni, C., et al. (2001). Neutropenic enterocolitis in patients with acute leukemia: Prognostic significance of bowel wall thickening detected by ultrasonography. *Journal of Clinical Oncology, 19*(3):756-761.

Exelby, P. R., et al. (1975). Management of the acute abdomen in children with leukemia. *Cancer, 35*(3):826-829.

Ikard, R. W. (1981). Neutropenic typhlitis in adults. *Archives of Surgery, 116*(7):943-945.

Jain, Y., Arya, L. S., & Kataria, R. (2000). Neutropenic enterocolitis in children with acute lymphoblastic leukemia. *Pediatric Hematology and Oncology, 17*(1):99-103.

McCarville, M. B., et al. (2005). Typhlitis in childhood cancer. *Cancer, 104*(2):380-387.

McCullough, K. D., (2003). Neutropenic enterocolitis. *Current Treatment Options in Infectious Diseases, 5*(5):367-375.

Meyerovitz, M. F., & Fellows, K. E. (1984). Typhlitis: A cause of gastrointestinal hemorrhage in children. *American Journal of Roentgenology, 143*(4):833-835.

Moir, D. H., & Bale, P. M. (1976). Necropsy findings in childhood leukaemia, emphasizing neutropenic enterocolitis and cerebral calcification. *Pathology, 8*(3):247-258.

Newbold, K. M., Lord, M. G., & Baglin, T. P. (1987). Role of clostridial organisms in neutropenic enterocolitis. *Journal of Clinical Pathology, 40*(4):471.

Otaibi, A. A., et al. (2002). Neutropenic enterocolitis (typhlitis) after pediatric bone marrow transplant. *Journal of Pediatric Surgery, 37*(5):770-772.

Paulino, A. F., et al. (1994). Typhlitis in a patient with acute lymphoblastic leukemia prior to the administration of chemotherapy. *American Journal of Pediatric Hematology and Oncology, 16*(4):348-351.

Pizzo, P. A., & Poplack, D. G. (2002). *Principles and practice of pediatric oncology.* (4th ed.). Philadelphia: Lippincott Williams & Wilkins.

Shamberger, R. C., et al. (1986). The medical and surgical management of typhlitis in children with acute nonlymphocytic (myelogenous) leukemia. *Cancer, 57*(3):603-609.

Slavin, R. E., Dias, M. A., & Saral, R. (1978). Cytosine arabinoside induced gastrointestinal toxic alterations in sequential chemotherapeutic protocols: A clinical-pathologic study of 33 patients. *Cancer, 42*(4):1747-1759.

Sloas, M. M., et al. (1993). Typhlitis in children with cancer: A 30-year experience. *Clinical Infectious Diseases, 17*(3):484-490.

Teefey, S. A., et al. (1987). Sonographic diagnosis of neutropenic typhlitis. *American Journal of Roentgenology, 149*(4):731-733.

Urbach, D. R., & Rotstein, O. D. (1999). Typhlitis. *Canadian Journal of Surgery, 42*(6):415-419.

Varki, A. P., Armitage, J. O., & Feagler, J. R. (1979). Typhlitis in acute leukemia: Successful treatment by early surgical intervention. *Cancer, 43*(2):695-697.

Wade, D. S., Nava, H. R., & Douglass, H. O., Jr. (1992). Neutropenic enterocolitis: Clinical diagnosis and treatment. *Cancer, 69*(1):17-23.

Wagner, M. L., et al. (1970). Typhlitis: A complication of leukemia in childhood. *American Journal of Roentgenology, Radium Therapy, and Nuclear Medicine, 109*(2):341-350.

Wang, S., & Fadare, O. (2004). Pathologic quiz case: An 11-year-old boy with acute-onset right lower abdominal pain—typhlitis (neutropenic enterocolitis). *Archives of Pathology and Laboratory Medicine, 128*(2):239-240.

A

Academy of Neurology, guidelines for anticonvulsant use, 461
Acidosis, 553. *See also* Lactic acidosis, Type B
Active listening, 503-504
Activity, with congestive heart failure (CHF), 245
Acute graft versus host disease. *See* Graft versus host disease (GVHD)
Acute lung injury (ALI), 15
Acute pancreatitis
  chemotherapy/biotherapy causes of, 5
  complications of, 2t
  discharge plan/follow-up care, 10
  drugs associated with, 3b
  epidemiology/etiology, 3
  evaluation/desired outcomes, 9-10
  evidence-based practice updates, 8
  Glasgow (IMRIE) criteria for severity of, 6b
  laboratory values with, 7t
  nursing care and treatment, 7-8
  nursing diagnoses, 9
  pathophysiologic mechanisms, 1, 3
  professional assessment criteria (PAC), 5-6
  prognosis, 4-5
  risk profile, 4
  teaching/education of patients, 9
Acute respiratory distress syndrome (ARDS)
  clinical disorders associated with, 14t
  discharge plan/follow-up care, 22
  epidemiology/etiology, 15-16

Acute respiratory distress syndrome (ARDS) *(Continued)*
  evaluation/desired outcomes, 21
  evidence-based practice updates, 21
  nursing assessment, 20-21
  nursing care and treatment, 18-21
  nursing diagnoses, 21
  other names for, 15
  pathophysiological mechanisms, 13-15
  professional assessment criteria (PAC), 17-18
  prognosis, 17
  risk profile, 16-17
  signs/symptoms of, 18
  teaching/education of patients, 21
ADH (antidiuretic hormone), 99, 315
Adolescents. *See* Pediatric patients
Adrenal metastases, hyperkalemia and, 299
Advance directives, 150, 175
Age factors. *See also* Pediatric patients
  carotid artery rupture (CAR) risk, 60
  cognitive function in elderly patients, 74-75
  depression in elderly patients, 84
  hypernatremia in elderly patients, 318
  for sepsis, 471
  in superior vena cava syndrome (SVCS), 522
  for syndrome of inappropriate antidiuretic hormone (SIADH), 537
  typhlitis in pediatric patients, 562
Agency for Health Care Policy and Research (AHCPR), 87
Agitation, management of, 153-154

Note: Page numbers followed by f indicates figures; t, tables; b, boxes.